EMERGENCY DERMATOLOGY

MANY PHYSICIANS and patients do not believe that dermatology involves life-threatening situations. However, there are many emergencies that the dermatologist needs to address and many cutaneous diseases in the emergency room that require rapid dermatologic consultation. The dermatologist is frequently the first physician to examine such patients before a hospital admission and also the first to identify a critical situation, stabilize the patient, and choose urgent and appropriate intervention. The first chapters of this book are directed toward those dermatologists who care for hospitalized patients with severe and dangerous skin diseases. Later chapters are intended for all physicians, including dermatologists, who wish to hone their diagnostic skills, expand their knowledge and understanding of pathological events, and learn treatment options available for acute life-threatening skin diseases. This book brings together top dermatologists from around the world to address the complicated and multifaceted field of dermatologic emergencies for the practicing dermatologist and emergency physician.

Ronni Wolf, MD, is Associate Clinical Professor and Head of the Dermatology Unit at Kaplan Medical Center, Rechovot, Israel, and the Hebrew University–Hadassah Medical School, Jerusalem, Israel.

Batya B. Davidovici, MD, is Physician in the Dermatology Unit at Kaplan Medical Center, Rechovot, Israel.

Jennifer L. Parish, MD, is Assistant Clinical Professor of Dermatology and Cutaneous Biology at Jefferson Medical College of Thomas Jefferson University, Philadelphia, Pennsylvania, and Assistant Professor of Dermatology, Tulane University School of Medicine, New Orleans, Louisiana.

Lawrence Charles Parish, MD, MD(hon), is Clinical Professor of Dermatology and Cutaneous Biology and Director of the Jefferson Center for International Dermatology at Jefferson Medical College of Thomas Jefferson University, Philadelphia, Pennsylvania. Dr. Parish is also Visiting Professor of Dermatology at Tulane University School of Medicine, New Orleans, Louisiana.

EMERGENCY
DERMATOLOGY

Edited by

Ronni Wolf

Kaplan Medical Center

Batya B. Davidovici

Kaplan Medical Center

Jennifer L. Parish

Jefferson Medical College of Thomas Jefferson University
and Tulane University School of Medicine

Lawrence Charles Parish

Jefferson Medical College of Thomas Jefferson University
and Tulane University School of Medicine

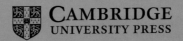

CAMBRIDGE UNIVERSITY PRESS
Cambridge, New York, Melbourne, Madrid, Cape Town, Singapore,
São Paulo, Delhi, Dubai, Tokyo, Mexico City

Cambridge University Press
32 Avenue of the Americas, New York, NY 10013-2473, USA

www.cambridge.org
Information on this title: www.cambridge.org/9780521717335

First published 2010

Printed in China by Everbest

A catalog record for this publication is available from the British Library.

Library of Congress Cataloging in Publication data

Emergency dermatology / edited by Ronni Wolf ... [et al.].
p.   ;   cm.
Includes bibliographical references and index.
ISBN 978-0-521-71733-5 (hardback)
1. Dermatology.   2. Medical emergencies.   I. Wolf, Ronni.
[DNLM: 1. Skin Diseases – therapy.   2. Emergencies.   3. Emergency Treatment.   WR 140 E53 2009]
RL72.E443   2009
616.5'025 – dc22   2009007871

ISBN 978-0-521-71733-5 Hardback

Contents

Contributors

Samuel H. Allen, FRCP
Department of Infectious Diseases
Ayrshire & Arran
Scotland, United Kingdom

Sapna Amin, MD
Department of Dermatology
Baylor College of Medicine
Houston, Texas

Lucio Andreassi, MD
Department of Dermatology
University of Siena
Siena, Italy

Adone Baroni, MD, PhD
Department of Dermatology
Second University of Naples
Naples, Italy

Kazal R. Bhowmik, MBBS
Paddington Testing Company, Inc.
Philadelphia, Pennsylvania

Kristen Biggers, MD
West Virginia University School of Medicine
Morgantown, West Virginia

Roberta Bilenchi, MD
Department of Dermatology
University of Siena
Siena, Italy

Georgeta Bocheva, MD, PhD
Department of Pharmacology
Medical University–Sofia
Sofia, Bulgaria

Elisabetta Buommino, PhD
Department of Experimental Medicine
  Microbiology and Clinical Microbiology
  Section
Second University of Naples
Naples, Italy

Sueli Coelho Carneiro, MD, PhD
Sector of Dermatology
Federal University of Rio de Janeiro
Hospital Universitario Clementino Fraga Filho
School of Medicine
Rio de Janeiro State University
Rio de Janeiro, Brazil

Brandon Christianson, MD
Department of Otolaryngology/Head and Neck Surgery
University of Texas Southwestern Medical Center
Dallas, Texas

Richard B. Cindrich, MD
Department of Medicine
Bronx Lebanon Hospital Center
Albert Einstein College of Medicine
Bronx, New York

Gwynn Coatney, DO
Department of Family Medicine
University of Medicine and Dentistry of New Jersey
Stratford, New Jersey

Carlos Gustavo Costanza, MD
Sector of Dermatology
Federal University of Rio de Janeiro
Hospital Universitario Clementino Fraga Filho
School of Medicine
Rio de Janeiro, Brazil

Batya B. Davidovici, MD
Dermatology Unit
Kaplan Medical Center
Rechovot, Israel

Giovanna Donnarumma, PhD
Department of Experimental Medicine
  Microbiology and Clinical Microbiology Section
Second University of Naples
Naples, Italy

Dirk M. Elston, MD
Department of Dermatology
Geisinger Medical Center
Danville, Pennsylvania

Aron J. Gewirtzman, MD
Division of Dermatology
Albert Einstein College of Medicine
Bronx, New York

Ryan Hawley, DO
Samaritan Medical Center
Watertown, New York

Serge A. Jabbour, MD
Department of Medicine
Division of Endocrinolgy
Jefferson Medical College of Thomas Jefferson University
Philadelphia, Pennsylvania

Pierre-Henri Jarreau, MD, PhD
Department of Neonatal Medicine
Port-Royal Hospital
Paris, France

Jana Kazandjieva, MD, PhD
Department of Dermatology
Medical University–Sofia
Sofia, Bulgaria

Sadiye Keskin, MD
Department of Dermatology
Cerrahpasa Medical Faculty
Istanbul University
Istanbul, Turkey

Kishore Kumar, MBBS, FCPS
Assistant Registrar
Burn and Plastic Surgery Unit
Dhaka Medical College Hospital
Dhaka, Bangladesh

Marina Landau, MD
The Dermatology Unit
Wolfson Medical Center
Holon, Israel

Jasna Lipozenčić, MD, PhD
University Hospital Center Zagreb and
University Department of Dermatology and Venereology
School of Medicine
University of Zagreb
Zagreb, Croatia

Maryann Mikhail, MD
Department of Dermatology
St. Luke's–Roosevelt Hospital Center
Beth Israel Medical Center
New York, New York

Larry E. Millikan, MD
Department of Dermatology
Tulane University School of Medicine
New Orleans, Louisiana

Robert A. Norman, DO, MPH
Department of Dermatology
College of Osteopathic Medicine
Nova Southeastern University
Fort Lauderdale, Florida

Daniel H. Parish, MD, JD
Department of Dermatology and Cutaneous Biology
Jefferson Medical College of Thomas Jefferson University
Philadelphia, Pennsylvania
Formerly, Assistant United States Attorney
Northern District of Illinois
Chicago, Illinois

Jennifer L. Parish, MD
Department of Dermatology and Cutaneous Biology
Jefferson Medical College of Thomas Jefferson University
Philadelphia, Pennsylvania
Department of Dermatology
Tulane University School of Medicine
New Orleans, Louisiana

Lawrence Charles Parish, MD, MD(hon)
Department of Dermatology and Cutaneous Biology
Jefferson Medical College of Thomas Jefferson University
Philadelphia, Pennsylvania
Department of Dermatology
Tulane University School of Medicine
New Orleans, Louisiana

Geeta Patel, DO
Montgomery Regional Hospital
Blacksburg, Virginia

Brenda L. Pellicane, MD
Department of Dermatology
Wayne State University School of Medicine
Dearborn, Michigan

Lion Poles, MD
Deputy Director General
Kaplan Medical Center, Rechovot and the
    Ministry of Health, Israel

Kyrill Pramatarov, MD, PhD
Department of Dermatology
Medical University–Sofia
University Hospital Lozenetz
Sofia, Bulgaria

Marcia Ramos-e-Silva, MD, PhD
Sector of Dermatology
Federal University of Rio de Janeiro
Hospital Universitario Clementino Fraga Filho
School of Medicine
Rio de Janeiro, Brazil

Arie Roth, MD
Division of Cardiology
Tel Aviv Sourasky Medical Center
Sackler Faculty of Medicine
Tel Aviv University
Tel Aviv, Israel

Hirak B. Routh, MBBS
Paddington Testing Company, Inc.
Philadelphia, Pennsylvania

Donald Rudikoff, MD
Division of Dermatology
Bronx Lebanon Hospital Center
Albert Einstein College of Medicine
Bronx, New York

Eleonora Ruocco, MD, PhD
Department of Dermatology
Second University of Naples
Naples, Italy

Vincenzo Ruocco, MD
Department of Dermatology
Second University of Naples
Naples, Italy

Margaret T. Ryan, MD
Department of Medicine
Division of Endocrinology
Riddle Memorial Hospital
Media, Pennsylvania

Sonia Sangiuliano, MD
Department of Dermatology
Second University of Naples
Naples, Italy

Vincent Savarese, MD
Division of Endocrinology
Department of Medicine
Jefferson Medical College of Thomas Jefferson
    University
Philadelphia, Pennsylvania

Noah Scheinfeld, MD, JD
Department of Dermatology
Columbia University College of Physicians and Surgeons
New York, New York

Virenda N. Sehgal, MD, FNASc, FAMS, FRAS (Lond.)
Skin Institute and School of Dermatology
Greater Kailash
New Delhi, India

Haim Shmilovich, MD
Division of Cardiology
Tel Aviv Sourasky Medical Center
Sackler Faculty of Medicine
Tel Aviv University
Tel Aviv, Israel

Govind Srivastava, MD, MNAMS
Skin Institute and School of Dermatology
Greater Kailash
New Delhi, India

Anne Marie Tremaine, MD
Department of Dermatology
University of California–Irvine School of Medicine
Irvine, California

Nikolai Tsankov, MD, PhD, DrSci
Department of Dermatology
Tokuda Hospital–Sofia
Sofia, Bulgaria

Maria Antoinetta Tufano, MD
Department of Experimental Medicine
    Microbiology and Clinical Microbiology
    Section
Second University of Naples
Naples, Italy

Yalçin Tüzün, MD
Department of Dermatology
Cerrahpasa Medical Faculty
Istanbul University
Istanbul, Turkey

Stephen Tyring, MD, PhD
Center for Clinical Studies
Departments of Dermatology, Microbiology and
    Molecular Genetics, and Internal Medicine
University of Texas Health Science Center
Houston, Texas

Snejina Vassileva, MD, PhD
Department of Dermatology
Medical University–Sofia
Alexandrovska University Hospital
Sofia, Bulgaria

Daniel Wallach, MD
Department of Dermatology
Tarnier Hospital
Paris, France

Michael Waugh, MB, FRCP, FRCPI, FAChSHM, Dip Ven DHMSA
Genito-Urinary Medicine
Nuffield Hospital
Leeds, United Kingdom

Jeffrey M. Weinberg, MD
Department of Dermatology
Columbia University College of Physicians and Surgeons
Department of Dermatology
St. Luke's–Roosevelt Hospital Center
Beth Israel Medical Center
New York, New York

Ronni Wolf, MD
Head, Dermatology Unit
Kaplan Medical Center
Rechovot, Israel
Hebrew University–Hadassah Medical School
Jerusalem, Israel

Preface

"Dermatology is the best specialty. The patient never dies – and never gets well." (anonymous)

Many physicians and patients believe that dermatology does not involve life-threatening situations and that it is, like beauty, only skin deep (e.g., it is mainly an aesthetic specialty). Although the horrors of the syphilitics and the lepers of medieval times no longer exist, there are contemporary emergencies with which the dermatologist needs to contend, as well as cutaneous diseases that require rapid management.

Although the dermatologist is not likely to be the primary care physician responsible for the severely ill patients in the hospital setting, the skin disease specialist is still frequently the first clinician to examine these patients before hospital admission. The specialist may be responsible for making the initial diagnosis; for differentiating mundane skin ailments from more serious, life-threatening conditions; and also for being the first to identify a critical situation, to stabilize the patient, and to choose urgent and appropriate interventions.

Dermatologic emergencies and life-threatening skin diseases should be spared the "atrophy" that threatens knowledge that is not applied in everyday practice and fails to be refreshed from time to time. Dermatologists have no choice but to continue to be on the front line of diagnosing and treating all skin diseases, especially the more severe and acute ones.

This book brings together the top "players" in the lively, complicated, and multifaceted field of dermatologic emergencies and life-threatening skin diseases with the purpose of assisting the practicing physician in coping with dermatologic conditions that require urgent intervention. Although this book is intended primarily for dermatologists, it should also be of help to family practitioners, internists, and all those who practice in emergency rooms, intensive care units, and burn units in differentiating between skin diagnoses. Treating a severely ill dermatologic patient is always multidisciplinary teamwork. Although the trained eyes of the dermatologists and their extensive knowledge about diseases of the skin are indispensable for rapid and correct diagnosis and management of a dermatological emergency, fundamental knowledge of internal medicine, including cardiology, nephrology, and rheumatology, is also essential in this setting. This volume is intended to update and refresh what dermatologists and nondermatologists need to know for dealing with critically ill dermatologic patients. *Emergency Dermatology* should provide the link to the experience, expertise, and skills of various disciplines with the aim of guiding the medical caretakers of patients who are in true dermatological crises.

There are plenty of available dermatology textbooks. Some encompass widespread fields of dermatology (e.g., *Fitzpatrick's Dermatology in General Medicine*) whereas others are devoted to special issues, such as dermatopathology, contact dermatitis, dermatologic surgery, photodermatology, and many others. There is currently no publication that covers all aspects of critically ill dermatologic patients. In *Emergency Dermatology*, we have attempted to retrieve and organize the relevant information and available knowledge on this specific niche of medicine and to fill the gap in available reference material to guide the medical caretakers of patients who are in true dermatological crises. Although we have strived for completeness, we recognize that certain entities have not been addressed as completely as some readers may wish; however, it is not our intention to provide an encyclopedic textbook, but rather a more usable volume.

We are indebted to all the distinguished international specialists who have consented to give of their valuable time and vast experience to cover this complex and vital issue in a systematic and practical manner and who have produced such a comprehensive, state-of-the-art reference source of which we believe we can all be proud. If this book helps practicing physicians, both dermatologists and nondermatologists alike, to cope with dermatologic emergencies by knowing what to do whenever they encounter severely ill patients with complicated skin diseases and reach the correct decisions in urgent and critical situations, it will all have been worth the effort.

CHAPTER 1

Cell Injury and Cell Death

Adone Baroni

Eleonora Ruocco

Maria Antonietta Tufano

Elisabetta Buommino

WHEN CELLS are damaged, as often occurs during trauma and metabolic stress, the organism has to choose whether to repair the damage by promoting cell survival or remove irreparably injured cells. Cell injury occurs when an adverse stimulus reversibly disrupts the normal, complex homeostatic balance of the cellular metabolism. In this case, after injury the cells attempt to seal breaks in their membranes, chaperone the removal or refolding of altered proteins, and repair damaged DNA. On the contrary, when cell injury is too extensive to permit reparative responses, the cell reaches a "point of no return" and the irreversible injury culminates in programmed cell death (PCD). Specific properties or features of cells make them more or less vulnerable to external stimuli, thus determining the kind of cellular response. In addition, the characteristic of the injury (type of injury, exposure time, or severity) will also affect the extent of the damage.

We present a short overview of the best-known PCD pathways. We emphasize the apoptotic pathway, considered for years the hallmark of PCD, and the different stimuli that produce cell injury.

CELL INJURY

The survival of multicellular organisms depends on the function of a diverse set of differentiated cell types. After development is complete, the viability of the organism depends on the maintenance and renewal of these diverse lineages. Within each lineage homeostasis is maintained through a delicate balance between cell proliferation and cell death.[1] Disorders of either process have pathological consequences and can lead to disturbed embryogenesis, neurodegenerative diseases, or the development of cancer.[2] Therefore, the equilibrium between life and death is tightly controlled, and faulty elements can effectively be eliminated by PCD, a term that well defines the planned sequence of physiological cellular autodestruction, which requires both energy expenditure and a specific enzymatic network. Cell death is an essential strategy for the control of the dynamic balance of the living system, and it is the ultimate result of most physiological as well as pathological processes. Skulachev aptly described the concept of cell death using the metaphor of the "Samurai law of biology" (i.e., it is better to die than to be wrong), showing that the suicide program is a way to purify cells of damaged organelles and tissues of unwanted cells that use up valuable substrates and nutrients.[3,4] Likewise, cell death also has value for the species, as it provides a mechanism for eliminating terminally injured individuals who consume necessary society resources or harbor toxic pathogens.[3,5] Death, therefore, appears as the unique solution to eliminate what is unwanted or dangerous to the "community."

In past decades, PCD was mainly associated with apoptosis, a death process characterized by morphological changes such as shrinkage of the cell, condensation of chromatin, and disintegration of the cell into small fragments (so-called "apoptotic bodies") that are removed by phagocytosis. On the contrary, necrosis was considered as an alternative passive cell death occurring in an accidental, violent, or chaotic way.[6] Necrosis, however, has been recently recognized as a specific form of cell death with distinct morphological features.[7,8] It is now known that cell death cannot readily be classified as "apoptosis" or "necrosis," and alternative types of PCD have been described.[9–11] Different PCD pathways exist, either mediated by caspases (a specific family of cysteine proteases, as in apoptosis) or caspase-independent (such as autophagic cell death [ACD], paraptosis, and programmed necrosis).[1] Death patterns may overlap or integrate, reflecting the high flexibility in cell responses to various circumstances and stimuli (Figure 1.1).

Cell injury occurs as a result of physical, chemical, or biological insults or as a result of vital substrate deficiency. The cellular response to injury can be adaptive when it is designed to restore homeostasis and protect the cell from further injury. In this context, the gene transcriptional activity is modified in favor of vital genes.[5] If the genetic and metabolic adaptive responses are inadequate

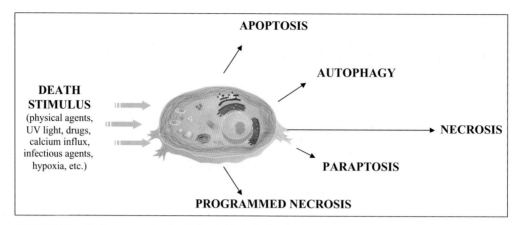

FIGURE 1.1: *Various models of cell death (© Quill Graphics, www.cellsalive.com).*

for a given injury, or if injury accumulation reaches a critical level, the damaged cells commit suicide.[3] Cell injury can, therefore, be reversible (sublethal) or irreversible (lethal). Cells may be reversibly injured, but if severely injured, they may be unable to recover and cell death will occur. The death stimuli are diverse and include normal physiological signals, such as hormones that trigger deletion of cells during differentiation or involution of tissues and organs, maturation of organ systems as, for example, in the immune system, and removal of cells that have sustained some form of damage.[2] Alternatively, cells already may be primed to undergo cell death, with the withdrawal of important extracellular components, such as serum or growth factors, providing the signal.[12] Other death stimuli also are important from a biomedical perspective. These include physical agents (ultraviolet [UV] light causing damage to the skin, hyperthermia, cold, and trauma), cytotoxic drugs, calcium influx, glucocorticoids, infectious agents (bacteria, virus, yeast), and hypoxia. The stimuli that initiate the death pathways vary widely with the affected cells.[13] In particular, various stimuli (e.g., cytokines, heat, irradiation, pathogens) can cause both apoptosis and necrosis in the same cell population (Figure 1.1). Apoptosis can be induced by a lower concentration or level of almost all the stimuli that cause necrosis.[14] This means that the mechanism of self-destruction can be activated by a relatively mild stimulus. Whereas mild hypoxia produced symptoms of apoptosis, severe hypoxia produced infarction and necrosis;[15] similarly, exposure to temperatures between 37°C and 43°C induced apoptosis in lymphocytes, and exposure to higher temperatures induced necrosis.[16] Therefore, the character of the injury will determine the pattern of cell death evoked. This aspect is important to highlight. The three main features of injury are type of injury, exposure time, and severity.

Type of Injury

The injury can be, for example, physical, chemical, or toxic, but the response will be different for different cell types.

In fact, some cells will be more susceptible than others to agents (heart muscle cells are more susceptible than connective tissue cells to oxygen depletion).

Exposure Time

The length of exposure to a particular stimulus will affect the chances of cell survival. Relatively resistant cells will be damaged if the duration of exposure is prolonged.

Severity

The ability of a cell to survive an injury also will depend on its severity; if the withdrawal of growth factor is partial, the cell is still able to survive for a long period (depending on cellular resistance), but if it is complete, cell death occurs in a very short time with modalities that vary from cell to cell.

We now describe some models of cellular death, taking into consideration that a clear-cut definition cannot be given because of the overlapping of the different programs of cell death.

Apoptosis. Cells have different ways of committing suicide and may select the fastest and most effective of the options available. Apoptosis has been considered for years as the PCD paradigm and is still considered one of the main pathways activated during stressful conditions, although alternative pathways were recently identified.[1] The term "apoptosis" derives from the ancient Greek word used to describe the "falling off" or "dropping off" of petals from flowers or leaves from trees, to emphasize the normal physiological nature of the process.[17] In 1972 this kind of cell death was first described[17] and noted that it was truly distinct from necrosis, underscoring the importance of apoptosis in human medicine. As part of the immune response, apoptosis allows the elimination of virally infected and cancer cells or the deletion of unnecessary or potentially dangerous lymphocytes.[18] Defects of apoptotic cell death may promote tumor or autoimmune disease development. The apoptotic process has been shown to proceed

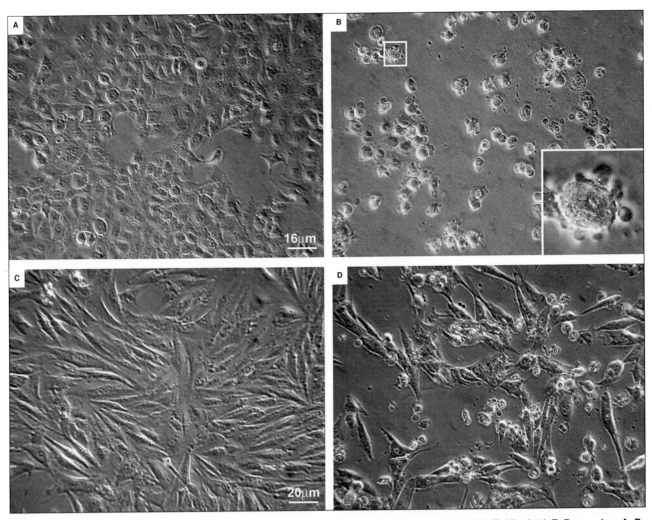

FIGURE 1.2: *Morphological changes occurring in A549 (human carcinoma lung cell line) (panel B) (R. Nicoletti, E. Buommino, A. De Filippis, M. P. Lopez-Gresa, et al. World J Microbio and Biotechnol. 2008; 24: 189–95) and NCI (human mesothelioma cell line) (panel D) cells (E. Buommino, I. Paoletti, A. De Filippis, R. Nicoletti, et al. Cell Prolif. forthcoming 2010), treated with proapoptotic metabolites, with a particular of membrane budding shown in panel B; panel A and C show the morphology of A549 and NCI untreated cells, respectively. Magnification: 20X.*

via a number of discrete steps. Cells undergoing apoptosis are characterized morphologically by cell shrinkage, chromatin condensation, loss of contact with neighboring cells and the extracellular matrix (Figure 1.2), [19] actin cleavage,[20] and biochemically by DNA laddering (Figure 1.3).[19] The last is a peculiarity of most apoptotic pathways. The double-stranded linker deoxyribonucleic acid (DNA) between nucleosomes is cleaved at regularly spaced internucleosomal sites, giving rise to DNA fragments representing the length of nucleosomes (180–200 base pairs).[13] Molecular characterization of this process identifies a specific DNase (caspase-activated DNase) that cleaves chromosomal DNA in a caspase-dependent manner.[21] Other features of apoptosis are early depolymerization of cytoskeletal proteins, loss of phospholipid symmetry in plasma membrane with the outer layer exposure of phosphatidylserine (PS) residues, and the appearance of a smooth-surfaced protuberance of the plasma membrane

with its preserved integrity. The fragmentation of both nucleus and whole cell then produces membrane-bound bodies in which the organelles are intact to form apoptotic bodies (Figure 1.2 [inset]).[22] This is also called the "budding phenomenon" and should not be confused with blebs, fluid-filled structures typically devoid of organelles.[6] The apoptotic bodies are cleared from tissues by professional phagocytes, such as macrophages, but also epithelial cells and even fibroblasts have been shown to clear apoptotic bodies.[23,24] Phagocytosis is initiated by the exposure of the PS receptor located on the membrane of the phagocytes and vitronectin receptors, resulting in a cell-signaling response.[22] The apoptotic pathway and the engulfment process are part of a continuum that helps ensure the noninflammatory nature of this death paradigm. Studies in mammals have highlighted the importance of proper disposal of apoptotic bodies by phagocytic cells.[24] The suppression of proinflammatory factors is necessary during apoptotic

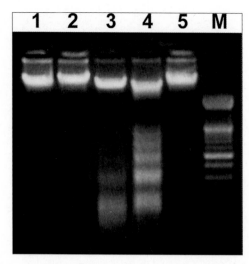

FIGURE 1.3: DNA feature of HeLa cells treated or not with 3-O-methylfunicone. DNA fragmentation induced in OMF treated cells after 48 and 72 h (lane 3 and 4, respectively). Lane 1, untreated cells; lane 2, cells treated for 24 h; lane 5, negative control (absolute ethanol). M, 100 bp ladder (Roche Diagnostics) used as MW-marker. (E. Buommino, R. Nicoletti, G. M. Gaeta, M. Orlando et al. Cell Proliferation. 2004; 37:413–26)

body clearance. This suppression is accomplished at least in part by a release of antiinflammatory factors including transforming growth factor β and IL-10 by macrophages engaged in corpse engulfment. Furthermore, regulatory mechanisms help ensure that, when phagocytosing dendritic cells present peptides from apoptotic bodies to T cells, no immune reaction against self-peptides is initiated. Defects in the clearance of corpses are predicted to create a proinflammatory milieu that may predispose to autoimmune disorders.

A cascade of genes is activated as a consequence of the induction of a defined genetic program in which caspases have a prominent role. Caspases are cysteine proteases (preexisting as inactive zymogen precursors in the cell) that cleave substrates at critical aspartic acid residues.[18] Activation of caspases is the central event in apoptosis, leading to the cleavage of numerous proteins involved in the cell structure, cell-cycle control, and DNA synthesis and repair. The initiator caspases (caspase-2, -8, -9, and -10) are activated by interaction with caspase adapters, whereas the effector caspases (caspase-3, -6, and -7) are downstream of the activator caspases and act to cleave various cellular targets and substrates and induce cell death.[18] The enzyme poly(adenosine diphosphate [ADP]-ribose) polymerase, or PARP, was one of the first proteins identified as a substrate for caspases. PARP is involved in the repair of DNA damage. It functions by catalyzing the synthesis of PARP and by binding to the DNA strand breaks and modifying nuclear proteins.[25] The ability of PARP to repair DNA damage is prevented following cleavage of PARP by caspase-3. The inflammatory caspases are involved in cytokine activation and are represented by caspases-1, -4, -5, -11, -12, -13, and -14.

Caspases can be activated through three main pathways: an "extrinsic" death receptor (DR)–mediated process and two "intrinsic pathways," a mitochondria-mediated– and an endoplasmic reticulum (ER)–mediated pathway (Figure 1.4).[1,18]

The extrinsic pathway involves the surface DRs, a subfamily of the tumor necrosis factor receptor (TNF-R) superfamily activated in response to specific extracellular signals.[26] To date, eight DRs have been identified, namely, Fas (CD95, Apo-1), TNF-related apoptosis-inducing ligand (TRAIL)-receptors 1 (TRAIL-R1) (DR4) and 2 (DR5, Apo-2), TNF-R1, TRAMP (WSL-1, Apo-3), EDAR, p75 neurotrophin receptor (p75NTR), and DR6.[26] Despite their name, not all of these receptors induce apoptosis, but they may trigger specific signaling pathways that result in a variety of cellular outcomes. The DRs comprise three domains: an extracellular cysteine-rich domain for ligand binding, a transmembrane domain, and an intracellular death domain (DD), which is required for apoptotic signal transduction.[26] The DR TNF ligand (TNF-L), Fas ligand (FasL), and TRAIL induce apoptosis by binding to their cell membrane receptors. Following ligand binding, a conformational change in the intracellular domains of the receptors reveals the presence of a "death domain," which allows the recruitment of various apoptotic proteins to the receptor. This protein complex is known as the death-inducing signaling complex (DISC). The final step in this process is the recruitment of one of the caspases, typically caspase-8, to the DISC. This recruitment results in the activation of caspase-8 and the initiation of apoptosis.

Interestingly, there are also decoy receptors (DcRs) that compete to bind ligands to DRs, allowing the cell to escape death ligand–induced killing. DcR1 and DcR2 compete with DR4 or DR5 to bind to TRAIL. DcR3 competes with Fas to bind to the FasL.

The intrinsic cell death pathway involves the mitochondria and ER. The mitochondria-mediated pathway is induced by lethal intracellular signals such as oncogenic transformation and DNA damage. Mitochondria contain many proapoptotic proteins such as apoptosis-inducing factor (AIF), cytochrome c, and Smac/DIABLO.[27] The last is a protein that directly neutralizes inhibitors of apoptotic proteins (IAPs), such as survivin, originally described as an inhibitor of apoptosis proteins with a cell-cycle–specific function.[28] AIF, cytochrome c, and Smac/DIABLO are released from the mitochondria following the formation of a pore in the mitochondrial membrane called the permeability transition (PT) pore. These pores are thought to form through the action of the proapoptotic members of the bcl-2 family of proteins, which in turn are activated by apoptotic signals such as cell stress, free radical damage, or growth factor deprivation.[29] In particular, AIF and Smac/DIABLO were also reported to be involved in the mitochondrial death pathway related not to apoptosis but to the apoptosis-like death pathway.[30] The release of cytochrome c from the mitochondria is a

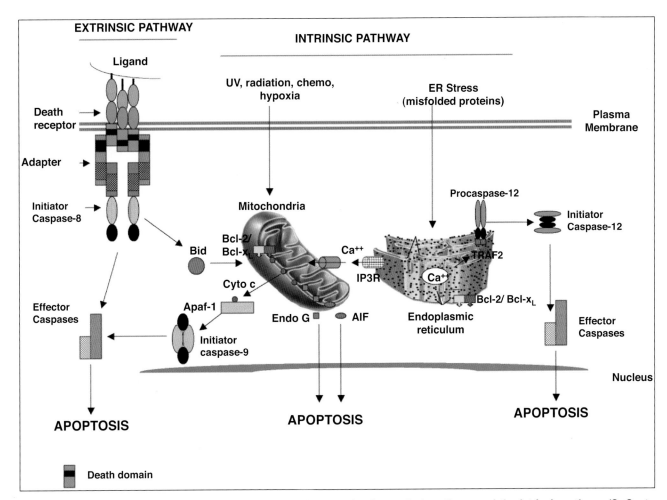

FIGURE 1.4: *The two main pathways for the initiation of apoptosis: the extrinsic pathway and the intrinsic pathway (S. Gupta, A. Agrawal, S. Agrawal, H. Su et al. Immunity & Ageing 2006; 3:5 doi:10.1186/1742-4933-3-5).*

particularly important event in the induction of apoptosis. When cytochrome *c* has been released into the cytosol it interacts with a protein called Apaf-1. This interaction leads to the recruitment of procaspase-9 into a multiprotein complex with cytochrome *c* and Apaf-1 called the apoptosome. Specifically, adenosine triphosphate (ATP) is required for the formation of the apoptosome, necessary for the activation of caspase-9 and the induction of apoptosis. If damage to the mitochondria is such that the ATP levels are insufficient to complete the apoptotic process, the mode of death may be directed toward necrosis.

The bcl-2 proteins are a family of proteins involved in the response to apoptosis. Some of these proteins (such as bcl-2 and bcl-X_L) are antiapoptotic, whereas others (such as Bad, Bax, or Bid) are proapoptotic. The sensitivity of cells to apoptotic stimuli can depend on the balance of pro- and antiapoptotic bcl-2 proteins. When there is an excess of proapoptotic proteins, the cells are more sensitive to apoptosis, but when there is an excess of antiapoptotic proteins, the cells will tend to be more resistant. An excess of

proapoptotic bcl-2 proteins at the surface of the mitochondria is thought to be important in the formation of the PT pore.[29] The proapoptotic bcl-2 proteins are often found in the cytosol, where they act as sensors of cellular damage or stress. Following cellular stress they relocate to the surface of the mitochondria, where the antiapoptotic proteins are located. This interaction between proapoptotic and antiapoptotic proteins disrupts the normal function of the antiapoptotic bcl-2 proteins and can lead to the formation of pores in the mitochondria and the release of cytochrome *c* and other proapoptotic molecules from the intermembrane space. This in turn leads to the formation of the apoptosome and the activation of the caspase cascade. The *bcl-2* gene has been shown to be transcriptionally repressed by *p53*.[31] The *p53* tumor suppressor gene codes for the p53 protein and plays an important role in the control of the cell cycle, apoptosis, senescence, differentiation, and accelerated DNA repair.[32] DNA damage caused by exposure to ionizing radiation, UV light, or some exogenous or endogenous chemical mutagens, which results in DNA strand breakage, can trigger an accumulation of *p53*. This

TABLE 1.1: Different Characteristics of the Cell Death Pathways

Types, characteristics	Apoptosis	Autophagic cell death	Paraptosis	Programmed necrosis	Necrosis
Triggers	Death receptors, trophic factor withdrawal, DNA damage, viral infections, etc.	Serum amino acid starvation, protein aggregates	Trophotoxicity	Ischemia, excitotoxicity	Excessive damage by physical or chemical injury, high intensities of pathological insult
Plasma membrane	Membrane-bound apoptotic bodies, blebbing	Elongation and invagination, blebbing	Shrinkage	Rapid loss of plasma membrane integrity	Rapid disintegration
Nucleus	Chromatin condensation, internucleosomal DNA cleavage (ladder)	Pyknosis in some cases, but neither prevalent nor striking, no DNA laddering	Late disintegration	No chromatin condensation, in some cases chromatin clustering to loosen speckles	Karyolysis
Cytoplasm	Condensation and shrinkage, cytoskeleton collapse	Vacuolization, autophagosome and autolysosome formation	Vacuolization	Swelling, extensive vacuolization	Condensation, loss of structure, fragmentation, swelling
Organelles	Preservation	Enwrapped by membrane sac. Autodigestion	Swelling	Swelling	Condensation and final disintegration

gene can activate transcription of growth regulatory genes such as *p21 WAF1/Cip1*, *GADD-45*, and *cyclin G*, resulting in G_1 growth arrest, presumably to allow for repair of damaged DNA. If irreparable DNA damage exists, the cell becomes committed to the apoptosis pathway and is deleted by the system. For this reason, p53 is known as the "guardian of the genome." Mutant p53 proteins may allow an escape from this surveillance mechanism and generation of a malignant phenotype.

The ER is another important sensor of cellular stress that can withhold protein synthesis and metabolism to restore cellular homeostasis. Misfolded proteins are constantly produced; these proteins trigger a protective stress response, known as the unfolded protein response. Although this response may put off a cellular catastrophe for a short time, if the damage to ER is too extensive, the damage can initiate PCD via the unfolded protein response or via release of calcium into the cytoplasm.[33] Thus caspase-12 is activated, which then engages caspase-9 and leads to the effector cascade recruitment.[34] In addition, an intracellular calcium influx caused by ER stress induces the activation of a family of cytosolic proteases, the calpains (calcium-activated neutral proteases), which normally reside in the cytosol as inactive zymogenes.[35,36] Calpains, kept in control by their natural inhibitor calpastatin, have been shown to act downstream of caspase. In fact, it has been demonstrated that vitamin D compounds trigger cell death in MCF-7 cells via calpains and independent of caspase activation, thus indicating a role of ER in certain types of caspase-independent cell death.[37] Disorders such as Alzheimer disease, Parkinson disease, Huntington disease, amyotrophic lateral sclerosis, and prion protein disease all share the common features of accumulation and aggregation of misfolded proteins.[38]

OTHER FORMS OF PCD

Compared to apoptosis, relatively little is known about autophagic PCD and paraptosis, and even less is known about other nonapoptotic forms of PCD. Most of what is known is based on morphological descriptions. The exact phenotype of a dying cell is certainly dependent on many different factors that include the cell type, the cellular context, and the specific death stimulus.[30] Characteristic changes that differ in the various forms also include modifications of the cell shape and architecture, such as alterations of the cytoskeleton (Table 1.1). Any questions about the other forms of cell death remain unanswered: How important is the activation of the different PCD for the organism, and are all the mediators that trigger one type of death or another known? To these and other questions we will try to give an answer.

ACD

ACD is a long-known nonapoptotic cell death modality, also called type II cell death (to distinguish it from apoptosis or type I cell death).[39] Phagocytosis and autophagy are two well-known processes involved, respectively, in the removal of extracellular organisms and the destruction of organisms in the cytosol. Autophagy, for either metabolic regulation or defense, involves the formation of a double membrane called the autophagosome, which then fuses with lysosomes to degrade the contents, a process that has similarities to phagosome maturation. Autophagy is, in fact, normally activated during starvation by nutrient sensors to allow the recycling of substrates and organelles and to ensure the metabolic precursor.[40] Autophagy is also a means to eliminate dysfunctional organelles and allow a turnover of long-living proteins, thus preventing their pathological accumulation in the cells. Consequently, the cell "cannibalizes itself" from the inside (autophagy = "self-eating" in Greek). When this self-eating reaches excessive levels it may progress toward ACD, occurring in response to prolonged deprivation or stress, during embryogenesis, in adult tissue remodeling, in human diseases, or during cytotoxic drug treatment.[39] Autophagy is often observed when massive cell elimination is needed or when phagocytes do not have easy access to the dying cells. ACD is differentiated from apoptosis by certain peculiarities, including autophagosome and/or autolysosome formation, a vast autodigestion of organelles, a preserved nucleus until late stages (with the absence of DNA laddering), and cytoskeleton preservation until the final stages. In contrast to apoptosis, ACD occurs in a caspase-independent pathway. Interestingly, autophagy can be a factor in both the promotion and prevention of cancer, and its role may be altered during tumor progression.[41] The first autophagy gene identified in humans was *Beclin 1*. The heterogeneous disruption of this gene leads to increased tumorigenesis in mice.[42] Beclin 1 is inhibited by its interaction with Bcl-2, which thus not only functions as an apoptotic suppressor, but also as an antiautophagic factor.[43] Another aspect to be considered is that some malignant cell types respond to anticancer agents by triggering autophagy, indicating the potential utility of ACD induction in cancer therapy. Cancer cells may need autophagy to survive nutrient-limiting and low-oxygen conditions, and autophagy may protect cancer cells against ionizing radiation by removing damaged elements. The precise role of this cell death is, therefore, not yet fully understood, but it is important to underline that autophagy and apoptosis can be observed simultaneously in the same tissue, and, in some cases, autophagy may precede and later trigger apoptosis when the autophagic capacity is overwhelmed.[39] In other settings, autophagy has been observed to delay or antagonize apoptosis, and there are also examples in which the two processes can be mutually exclusive.[39]

PARAPTOSIS

Recently, a novel nonapoptotic PCD process designated paraptosis was described by Sperandio and colleagues.[10]

The features of paraptosis differ from those of apoptosis and involve cytoplasmic vacuolation, mitochondrial swelling, the absence of caspase activation, and typical nuclear changes including pyknosis and DNA fragmentation.[10] There is increasing evidence that this alternative, nonapoptotic PCD exists in parallel with apoptosis. The neuropeptide substance P and its receptor, neurokinin-1, mediate a nonapoptotic form of PCD resembling paraptosis in some cases.[44] Activated microglia trigger neuronal cell death with ultrastructural characteristics of marked vacuolation and slightly condensed chromatin following the blockage of the caspase cascade.[45] In addition, ceramide induces nonapoptotic PCD with necrosis-like morphology in human glioma cells in the presence of pan-caspase inhibitors or during overexpression of bcl-X_L.[46] These examples support the theory that cells have other intrinsic programs for death that are distinct from apoptosis. This death program can be mediated by mitogen-activated protein kinases and can be triggered by the TNF-R family member *TAJ/TROY*, capable of inducing apoptosis independent of DNA fragmentation and caspase activation, and the insulin-like growth factor I receptor.[1,47] The idea that PCD might be induced by hyperactivation of a trophic factor receptor (trophotoxicity) is compatible with an earlier observation that some trophic factors may increase neuronal cell death, for example, that induced by excitotoxicity.[48] Such an effect might be protective against neoplasia in that it may eliminate cells that would otherwise undergo autocrine loop–stimulated oncogenesis. The resulting program would necessarily be nonapoptotic because trophic factors inactivate apoptotic signaling.

NECROSIS AND PROGRAMMED NECROSIS

For a long time necrosis was considered as an alternative to apoptosis.[7,8] Recently, necrosis, once thought of as simply a passive, unorganized way to die, has emerged as an alternative form of PCD, the activation of which might have important biological consequences, including the induction of an inflammatory response.[49] The term necrosis has, therefore, been wrongly used for years to define an alternative mode of cell death. It is now evident that we cannot refer to necrosis to mean a particular program of death and that this term should be used to describe what happens after a cell is dead. It is, therefore, more correct to use the term "programmed necrosis" or "necrosis-like PCD" when we describe certain kinds of cell death governed by a specific genetic program and quite different from classical apoptosis or not falling within the cell death pathways described earlier in this chapter.[6] There are many examples of programmed necrosis being a normal physiological and regulated (programmed) event. Signaling pathways (e.g., DRs, kinase cascades, and mitochondria) participate in both processes, and, by modulating these pathways, it is possible to switch between apoptosis and programmed necrosis. Moreover, antiapoptotic mechanisms (e.g., bcl-2/bcl-x proteins, heat shock proteins) are equally effective in protecting against apoptosis and programmed necrosis. There are several examples of necrosis during embryogenesis, normal tissue renewal, and the immune response.[7] The core events of programmed necrosis are bioenergetic failure and rapid loss of plasma membrane integrity. These events can result from specific molecular events that occur in the dying cell, including increased mitochondrial reactive oxygen species production, channel-mediated calcium uptake, activation of nonapoptotic proteases, and/or enzymatic destruction of cofactors required for ATP production. Karyolysis of the nucleus occurs as a consequence of the complete dissolution of the chromatin due to the activity of specific DNase. In addition, these necrotic mediators are often induced in the dying cell simultaneously and enhance each other's ability to initiate the demise of the cell.[50] Calpain and lysosomal cathepsin activation have been shown to contribute to necrotic cell death. Due to the immunogenic potential of the necrotic cell debris removal, the target induction of programmed necrosis is gaining attention among immunologists and oncologists in cancer immunotherapy.[51] At this point, it is important to note that, to complicate the intricate net of terminologies used to define the area of apoptosis versus necrosis, the term "oncosis" (from the Greek word for swelling), a form of cell death activated by ischemia, has also been used through the years to define all the situations in which marked cellular swelling occurred. Extensive literature on the morphological criteria for oncosis exists, but the biochemical pathway(s) of oncosis has not yet been described. Oncosis is thought to be mediated by a failure of plasma membrane ionic pumps. One potential mediator of oncosis is a calpain-family protease (possibly a mitochondrial calpain), which suggests that oncosis may turn out to be related to, or synonymous with, a calcium-activated programmed necrosis cell death. Majno and Joris proposed this term for designating any programmed cellular suicide characterized by a marked swelling, whereas the term "necrosis" refers to the features that appear after the cell has died.[6] Necrosis may be either oncotic or apoptotic in origin. In this context, oncosis comprises the prelethal changes leading to ischemic or coagulation necrosis, whereas necrosis describes a morphology but not a process, thus underscoring the final feature of a dead cell.

APOPTOSIS AND HUMAN DISEASES

Nonregulated apoptosis involves different pathophysiological situations such as malignant and premalignant conditions, neurological disorders (e.g., Alzheimer disease, prion-associated disorders), heart disease (ischemic cardiac damage, chemotherapy-induced myocardial suppression), immune system disorders (e.g., acquired immune deficiency syndrome [AIDS], type I diabetes, systemic lupus erythematosus [SLE], Sjögren syndrome), intestinal disorders, and kidney disease.[2] In particular, diseases characterized by the accumulation of cells include cancer, autoimmune diseases, and certain viral illnesses. Cell accumulation can result from either increased proliferation or the failure of cells to undergo apoptosis in response to appropriate stimuli.

Cell Death in Cancer

Tumor growth occurs when the cellular birth rate exceeds the death rate. Control of cell growth is important in the process of normal development and tissue homeostasis, and in pathological conditions such as neoplasia. Growth arrest and cell death are also important in normal and neoplastic growth.

Inactivation of apoptosis is a hallmark of cancer, an obligate ritual in the malignant transformation of normal cells. By inactivating apoptosis, cancer cells enhance their chances of survival and increase their resistance to chemotherapeutic agents. Because apoptosis is a gene-controlled process, it is susceptible to genetic manipulation for therapeutic purposes, such as in cancer treatment. The acquisition of resistance to apoptosis is important in the transition from normal melanocyte to melanoma. Apoptosis is, in fact, critical for epidermal homeostasis, representing a key protective mechanism removing premalignant cells that have acquired mutations.[52]

Melanoma is the most aggressive form of skin cancer, notoriously resistant to current modalities of cancer therapy and known to be a tumor with an elevated metastatic ability.[53] Although today melanoma is more often diagnosed in an early stage of disease and therefore shows a better overall survival, when tumor cells are detected in the regional lymph node, the patient has a poorer prognosis. One of the earliest events in melanoma progression involves the unregulated proliferation of melanocytes. In this stage of melanoma progression, the cells lose their ability to maintain the cell-cycle controls that function in normal unstimulated melanocytes. This loss of cell-cycle control can lead to sustained proliferation, decreased apoptosis, or both. It also has been reported that melanocytes displayed a broad expression of apoptotic inhibitors to maintain their longevity, at the cost of the nonelimination of damaged cells, thus resulting in a high probability of developing melanoma.[52] In contrast, keratinocytes are more prone to undergoing apoptosis to ensure a rapid turnover and efficiently remove damaged cells and meet their functional needs in the skin. Melanoma cells are resistant to a wide range of antineoplastic treatments because of their ability to evade the cytotoxic action of different insults such as DNA damage, microtubule destabilization, or topoisomerase inhibition,[53] showing, in contrast, strong resilience. In fact, melanoma cells in vivo demonstrate low levels of spontaneous apoptosis compared with other tumor cell types, and resistance to apoptosis is associated with increased resistance to chemotherapeutic agents.[54] The knowledge acquired about the altered apoptotic mechanism in melanoma has focused the attention of researchers on molecules able to compensate for or bypass the cell death defects and on the development of new chemotherapeutic strategies that facilitate the death of cancer cells.

Cell Death and Autoimmune Disorders

Physiological regulation of cell death is essential for the removal of potentially autoreactive lymphocytes during development and for the removal of excess cells after the completion of an immune response. Failure to remove autoimmune cells that arise during development or that develop as a result of somatic mutation during an immune response can result in autoimmune disease.[55] Upregulated levels of soluble Fas, which might competitively inhibit FasL–Fas interactions, have been documented in many autoimmune disorders such as rheumatoid arthritis, SLE, and pemphigus vulgaris (PV).[56] PV is a chronic autoimmune cutaneous disease characterized by circulating autoantibodies that cause blisters and erosions on the skin and mucous membranes.[57] Circulating autoantibodies bind with the epidermal cell membrane and cause cell–cell detachment (acantholysis), leading to epidermal tissue damage. In recent years, the idea that apoptosis might play a central role in the induction of acantholysis has gained momentum. In support of this supposition, a study by Weiske and colleagues demonstrated the proteolytic cleavage of desmoglein 3 (PV antigen) by caspase-3 during apoptosis, thereby causing desmosome disruption only after the induction of apoptosis.[58]

In a past study, we showed the ability of pemphigus serum and captopril to induce apoptosis in human keratinocytes.[59] In particular, the authors demonstrated that a drug (captopril) or antibodies (PV serum) acting, respectively, by a biochemical or immunological mechanism induced acantholysis through the same genetic program leading to PCD. Of interest is a contribution published by Arredondo and colleagues demonstrating the therapeutic action of intravenous immunoglobulin (IVIg) in PV.[60] In the plethora of biological effects exerted by IVIg administration (acceleration of the clearance of autoantibodies, modulation of serum levels of proinflammatory cytokines, induction of immunocompetent cell death), an array of antiapoptotic effects should also be mentioned. IVIg inactivates FasL, protects target cells from apoptosis by upregulating Bcl-2 expression, interferes with TNF-α and interferon-γ signaling pathways, and increases sensitivity to corticosteroid action, thus strengthening the idea that apoptosis may play an important role in the onset of the disease.

CONCLUSIONS

Even in diseases in which the affected cells have been shown to die with "apoptotic morphology," one cannot exclude the possibility that a caspase-independent cell death program occurs in concert with a caspase-dependent program.[61] The knowledge of the genetic program underlying the onset of the disease might help the researcher to use the appropriate genetic therapy by inhibiting one pathway or another. In such cases, it is important to understand whether a program of death is controlled by caspase activation. The inhibition of the caspase cascade to control apoptosis induction in some degenerative diseases can delay (but not prevent) the progression of the disease if some other caspase-independent program of death is operating. The occurrence of one or another of the different programs of cell death is an important aspect to take into account. In fact, one of the cancer therapy approaches is to kill cancer cells by apoptosis. It is also known that cancer cells are selected for their acquired resistance to apoptosis. It is, therefore, important to be able to exploit other genetic programs to complement or integrate apoptosis and perhaps open new frontiers for tumor therapy.

Despite the numerous models proposed to categorize PCD, it is difficult to give one single definition, and probably also incorrect, due to the overlap and shared signaling pathways of the different death programs. It has, therefore, been postulated that the dominant cell death phenotype triggered by cytotoxic agents is determined by the most readily available death program.[62] Besides caspases, a broad spectrum of proteases can carry out PCD, with the participation of different cellular organelles, including mitochondria, lysosomes, or ER, which can act independently or actively collaborate with each other. The multicellular organism can take advantage of the existence of multiple death pathways because they offer protection, for example, against the development of malignant diseases. Many difficulties and obstacles have to be overcome before a cell becomes a tumor cell, and this in part explains the rarity of cancer, considering the number of cell divisions and mutations that occur during human life. The control of PCD may ultimately offer a new perspective in cancer immunotherapy, but also in the treatment of autoimmune diseases and neurodegenerative disorders.

REFERENCES

1. Broker LE, Kruyt FAE, Giaccone G. Cell death independent of caspases: a review. Clin Cancer Res. 2005;11:3155–62.
2. Barr PJ, Tomei LD. Apoptosis and its role in human disease. Biotechnology. 1994;12:487–93.
3. Skulachev VP. The programmed death phenomena, aging, and the Samurai law of biology. Exp Gerontol. 2001;36:996–1024.
4. Skulachev VP. Programmed death phenomena: from organelle to organism. Ann NY Acad Sci. 2002;959:214–37.

5. Cobb JP, Hotchkiss RS, Karl IE, Buchman TG. Mechanism of cell injury and death. Br J Anaesth. 1996;77:3–10.

6. Majno G, Joris I. Apoptosis, oncosis, and necrosis. An overview of cell death. Am J Pathol. 1995;146:3–15.

7. Proskuryakov SY, Konoplyannikov AG, Gabai VL. Necrosis: a specific form of programmed cell death? Exp Cell Res. 2003;283:1–16.

8. Fietta P. Many ways to die: passive and active cell death styles. Riv Biol. 2006;99:69–83.

9. Blagosklonny MV. Cell death beyond apoptosis. Leukemia. 2000;14:1502–8.

10. Sperandio S, de Belle I, Bredesen DE. An alternative, non apoptotic form of programmed cell death. Proc Natl Acad Sci USA. 2000;97:14376–81.

11. King KL, Cidlowski JA. Cell cycle and apoptosis: common pathways to life and death. J Cell Biochem. 1995;58:175–80.

12. Raff MC. Social controls on cell survival and cell death. Nature. 1993;356:397–400.

13. Sen S. Programmed cell death: concept, mechanism and control. Biol Rev. 1992;67:287–319.

14. Lennon SV, Martin SJ, Cotter TG. Dose-dependent induction of apoptosis in human tumor cell lines by widely diverging stimuli. Cell Prolif. 1991;24:203–14.

15. Kerr JFR. Shrinkage necrosis: a distinct mode of cellular death. J Pathol. 1971;105:13–20.

16. Shrek R, Chandra S, Molnar Z, Stefani SS. Two types of interphase death of lymphocytes exposed to temperatures of 37–45°C. Radiat Res. 1980;82:162–70.

17. Kerr JFR, Willie AH, Currie AR. Apoptosis: a basic biological phenomenon with wide-ranging implications in tissue kinetics. Br J Cancer. 1972;26:239–57.

18. Chang HY, Yang X. Proteases for cell suicide: functions and regulation of caspases. Microbiol Mol Biol Rev. 2000;64:821–46.

19. Barrett JC, Annab LA, Alcorta D, et al. Cellular senescence and cancer. Cold Spring Harbor Symposia on Quantitative Biology Vol LIX. 1994.

20. Guenal I, Risler Y, Mignotte B. Down-regulation of actin genes precedes microfilament network disruption and actin cleavage during p53-mediated apoptosis. Br J Cell Sci. 1997;110:489–95.

21. Nagata S. Apoptotic DNA fragmentation. Exp Cell Res. 2000;256:12–8.

22. Van Cruchten S, Van Den Broeck W. Morphological and biochemical aspects of apoptosis, oncosis, and necrosis. Anat Histol Embryol. 2002;31:214–23.

23. Platt N, da Silva RP, Gordon S. Recognizing death: the phagocytosis of apoptotic cells. Trends Cell Biol. 1998;8:365–72.

24. Savill J, Fadok V. Corpse clearance defines the meaning of cell death. Nature. 2000;407:784–8.

25. West JD, Ji C, Marnett LJ. Modulation of DNA fragmentation factor 40 nuclease activity by poly(ADP-ribose) polymerase-1. J Biol Chem. 2005;280:15141–7.

26. Contassot E, Gaide O, French LE. Death receptors and apoptosis. Dermatol Clin. 2007;25:487–501.

27. Susin SA, Zamzami N, Castedo M, et al. The central executioner of apoptosis: multiple connections between protease activation and mitochondria in Fas(Apo-1(CD95- and ceramide-induced apoptosis. J Exp Med. 1997;186:25–37.

28. Temme A, Rieger M, Reber F, et al. Localization, dynamics and function of survivin revealed by expression of functional survivinDsRed fusion proteins in the living cell. Mol Biol Cell. 2003;14:78–92.

29. Nouraini S, Six E, Matsuyama S, et al. The putative pore-forming domain of Bax regulates mitochondrial localization and interaction with Bcl-X$_L$. Mol Cell Biol. 2000;20:1604–15.

30. Leist M, Jäättelä M. Four deaths and a funeral: from caspases to alternative mechanisms. Nat Rev Mol Cell Biol. 2001;2:589–98.

31. Sabbatini P, Chiou SK, Rao L, White E. Modulation of p53-mediated transcriptional repression and apoptosis by the adenovirus E1B 19k protein. Mol Cell Biol. 1995;15:1060–70.

32. Oren M. Decision making by p53: life, death and cancer. Cell Death Differ. 2003;10:431–42.

33. Breckenridge DG, Germain M, Mathai JP, et al. Regulation of apoptosis by endoplasmic reticulum pathways. Oncogene. 2003;22:8608–18.

34. Rao RV, Poksay KS, Castro-Obregon S, et al. Molecular components of a cell death pathway activated by endoplasmic reticulum stress. J Biol Chem. 2004;279:177–87.

35. Guroff G. A neutral, calcium-activated proteinase from the soluble fraction of the brain. J Biol Chem. 1964;239:149–55.

36. Wang KK. Calpain and caspase: can you tell the difference? Trends Neurosci. 2000;23:20–6.

37. Mathiasen IS, Lademann U, Jäättelä M. Apoptosis induced by vitamin D compounds in breast cells is inhibited by bcl-2 but does not involve known caspases or p53. Cancer Res. 1999;59:4848–56.

38. Taylor JP, Hardy J, Fischbeck KH. Toxic proteins in neurodegenerative disease. Science. 2002;296:1991–5.

39. Gozuacik D, Kimchi A. Autophagy as a cell death and tumor suppressor mechanism. Oncogene. 2004;23:2891–906.

40. Danial NN, Korsmeyer SJ. Cell death: critical control points. Cell. 2004;116:205–19.

41. Shintani T, Klionsky DJ. Autophagy in health disease: a double-edged sword. Science. 2004;306:990–6.

42. Yue Z, Jin S, Yang C, et al. Beclin 1, an autophagy gene essential for early embryonic development, is a haplo-insufficient tumor suppressor. Proc Natl Acad Sci USA. 2003;100:15077–82.

43. Pattingre S, Tassa A, Qu X, et al. Bcl-2 antiapoptotic proteins inhibit Beclin 1-dependent autophagy. Cell. 2005;122:927–39.

44. Castro-Obregon S, Del Rio G, Chen SF, et al. A ligand-receptor pair that triggers a non-apoptotic form of programmed cell death. Cell Death Differ. 2002;9:807–17.

45. Tanabe K, Nakanishi H, Maeda H, et al. A predominant apoptotic death pathway of neuronal PC12 cells induced by activated microglia is displaced by a non-apoptotic death pathway following blockage of caspase-3-dependent cascade. J Biol Chem. 1999;274:15725–31.

46. Mochizuki T, Asai A, Saito N, et al. Akt protein kinase inhibits non-apoptotic programmed cell death induced by ceramide. J Biol Chem. 2002;277:2790–7.

47. Eby MT, Jasmin A, Kumar A, et al. A novel member of the tumor necrosis factor receptor family, activates the c-Jun N-terminal kinase pathway and mediates caspase-independent cell death. J Biol Chem. 2000;275:15336–42.

48. Koh JY, Gwang BJ, Lobner D, Choi DW. Potential necrosis of cultured cortical neurons by neurotrophins. Science. 1995;268:573–5.

49. Edinger AL, Thompson CB. Death by design: apoptosis, necrosis and autophagy. Curr Opin Cell Biol. 2004;16:663–9.

50. Zong WX, Thompson CB. Necrotic death as a cell fate. Genes Dev. 2006;20:1–15.

51. Sauter B, Albert ML, Francisco L, et al. Consequences of cell death: exposure to necrotic tumor cells, but not primary tissue cells or apoptotic cells, induces the maturation of immunostimulatory dendritic cells. J Exp Med. 2000;191:423–34.

52. Bowen AR, Hanks AN, Allen SM, et al. Apoptosis regulators and responses in human melanocytic and keratinocytic cells. J Invest Dermatol. 2003;120:48–55.

53. Soengas MS, Lowe SW. Apoptosis and melanoma chemoresistance. Oncogene. 2003;22:3138–51.

54. Johnstone RW, Ruefli AA, Lowe SW. Apoptosis: a link between cancer genetics and chemotherapy. Cell. 2002;108:153–64.

55. Thompson CB. Apoptosis in the pathogenesis and treatment of disease. Science. 1995;267:1456–62.

56. Puviani M, Marconi A, Cozzani E, Pincelli C. Fas ligand in pemphigus sera induces keratinocyte apoptosis through the activation of caspase-8. J Invest Dermatol. 2003;120:164–7.

57. Korman N. Pemphigus. J Am Acad Dermatol. 1988;18:1219–38.

58. Weiske J, Schoneberg T, Shroder W, et al. The fate of desmosomal proteins in apoptotic cells. J Biol Chem. 2001;276:41175–81.

59. Baroni A, Buommino E, Paoletti I, et al. Pemphigus serum and captopril induce hsp 70 and inducible nitric oxide synthase overexpression, triggering apoptosis in human keratinocytes. Br J Dermatol. 2004;150:1070–80.

60. Arredondo J, Cheryavsky AI, Karaouni A, Grando SA. Novel mechanism of target cell death and survival and of therapeutic action of IVIg in pemphigus. Am J Pathol. 2005;167:1531–44.

61. Kitanaka C, Kuchino Y. Caspase-independent programmed cell death with necrotic morphology. Cell Death Differ. 1999;6:508–15.

62. Bursch W. The autophagosomal-lysosomal compartment in cell death. Cell Death Differ. 2001;8:569–81.

CHAPTER 2

Clean and Aseptic Technique at the Bedside

Sapna Amin

Aron J. Gewirtzman

Stephen Tyring

CUTANEOUS SURGICAL INTERVENTIONS are becoming more and more popular as this area of dermatology continues to rapidly expand. Dermatologists are performing progressively more surgical procedures in their private offices.[1] A survey performed by the American Society of Dermatologic Surgery (ASDS) in 2003 revealed that 3.9 million procedures were performed that year by participating ASDS members.[2] These outpatient procedures allow the dermatologist to provide more comprehensive care to the patient and present the patient with a more affordable option, because outpatient procedures under local anesthesia are less expensive than in the hospital setting.[1,3]

With the upsurge in the number of cutaneous surgeries, an important goal remains to keep patients free of nosocomial and surgical site infections (SSIs). Traditionally, dermatologic procedures and surgeries have benefited from relatively low infection rates,[2,4] despite varying infection-control practices.[1] Strict adherence to aseptic technique is required to maintain this low rate of infectious complications. In addition to the principles of asepsis, the surgeon must also minimize patient and environmental risk factors, achieve adequate preoperative preparation, decide if antibiotic prophylaxis is necessary, as well as maintain proper surgical suite protocol and surgical technique.

SURGICAL SITE INFECTIONS

Postoperative infections after dermatologic procedures are rare. These surgeries are largely considered either "clean" or "clean-contaminated," with infection rates of less than 5%[5] and 5%–10%, respectively.[2] Studies examining the rate of infectious complications following dermatologic procedures have indicated an even lower incidence in this field. Two studies reported infectious complication rates of 2% following outpatient dermatologic procedures,[6,7] and another study describing the complications following Mohs Micrographic Surgery showed an infection rate of 1.6%.[8]

Complication rates have been shown to be higher in dermatology inpatients. A recent study examining the complication rate of diagnostic skin biopsies performed on inpatients found that 29% of patients developed postoperative complications, with 93% of these complications being wound infections.[9] This increased rate may be attributable to differences in the patient population. Dermatology inpatients are more likely to be widely colonized with *Staphylococcus aureus*, to have extensive skin disease, and/or to be systemically unwell.[9,10]

Clinically, SSIs are recognized by the extrusion of pus from a wound that may also exhibit some of the cardinal signs of inflammation in the surrounding skin: redness, heat or warmth, swelling, and pain. Patients may also display systemic signs of infection, such as fever or chills. Laboratory confirmation is also necessary to make the diagnosis. Bacterial cultures taken from the site should demonstrate a concentration of at least 100,000 colony-forming units per square centimeter. Treatment of infected wounds requires effectively reducing the bacterial concentration, and debridement is the most important method of achieving this. Other techniques include the use of topical antibacterials, frequent dressing changes, and biologic dressings.

The most common cause of wound infections is the patient's endogenous skin flora,[11,12] with the absolute most common pathogen being *S. aureus*.[11,13] These microorganisms tend to colonize the uppermost layers of the skin and hair follicles; approximately 10%–20% of bacteria penetrate deeper into the hair follicles, however, where they can escape routine disinfection methods. Despite sterilization and disinfection procedures, the skin remains contaminated because these elusive organisms are a viable source of recolonization after the removal of superficial bacteria.[14]

Researchers have suggested that the rate of SSIs might be decreased further by decreasing the number of skin flora.[11]

PATIENT RISK FACTORS

Many factors contribute to the likelihood of a patient contracting a surgical wound infection. Patient-specific characteristics often cannot be eliminated or modified and must be dealt with on an individual basis. The most common patient-specific risk factors encountered are specific medical conditions that decrease the immune status of the individual.[15-17] Diabetes mellitus, for example, has been shown to increase the risk of infection and to have a negative effect on wound healing. Smoking also has been shown to have similar harmful effects, perhaps from the nicotine-induced vasoconstriction, reducing blood flow to the skin. In a study examining risk factors for SSIs, diabetes, obesity, and smoking all were found to be independent risk factors. Patients should be encouraged to abstain from smoking in the perioperative period as this will decrease the risk of SSI and tissue necrosis.[13,18,19] Other risk factors include an immunocompromised state secondary to a variety of causes (e.g., human immunodeficiency virus/acquired immune deficiency syndrome [HIV/AIDS], corticosteroids, malignancy, advanced age) and concomitant infections, such as urinary tract infections, which must be treated before the surgical procedure is performed. Patients with concurrent infections have a markedly increased risk for developing SSIs, even if the infection is distantly located from the wound.[15-17] Location of surgery also contributes to the risk of SSI development. Due to vascular factors, the lower extremities pose the highest risk[18,20] whereas the well-vascularized face presents the lowest risk of infection.[18]

ENVIRONMENTAL RISK FACTORS

Factors extrinsic to the patient also contribute to the development of SSIs. These environmental risk factors can often be modified and/or eliminated to decrease the patient's risk of acquiring infection.

DECONTAMINATION OF SURGICAL EQUIPMENT

Surgical procedures involve the use of instruments that may come into contact with patient skin, mucous membranes, and/or sterile body cavities. Viable microorganisms and spores must be removed from reusable surgical equipment after each use to decrease the risk of infection and prevent cross-contamination between patients. Microbial decontamination may be achieved by cleaning, disinfection, and/or sterilization.[21-23]

Cleaning

Cleaning removes viable microorganisms and the organic matter in which they survive from the surfaces of medical equipment. Although cleaning does not kill these bacteria, spores, or viruses, it remains an essential part of the decontamination process as the removal of these surface organisms facilitates disinfection and sterilization of equipment. Organic matter may interfere with adequate decontamination by inactivating disinfectants and sterilants and preventing direct contact with microbial cells. Cleaning is most effective when performed as soon as possible after equipment use. Cleaning should only be performed as the sole method of decontamination on noncritical items – that is, items that come into contact only with normal and intact patient skin. In general, automated cleaning methods, such as washer disinfectors and ultrasonic cleaners, are superior and preferable to manual methods (paper towels, wet wipes, etc.) as these methods produce standardized results.[21-24]

Disinfection

Disinfection refers to the chemical destruction of the majority of viable microorganisms residing on a given surface. Although some spores may also be targeted, disinfection alone does not reliably kill or inactivate all spores and viruses. In situations where sterilization by steam under pressure (autoclaving) is inappropriate or could damage medical equipment, the disinfection process may be utilized to decontaminate semicritical and critical items that have been exposed to nonintact patient skin, mucous membranes, or sterile body cavities. Disinfectants may be compromised by some organic matter, highlighting the importance of proper cleaning prior to disinfection. Disinfection may be achieved by either chemical or physical processes, with the latter being preferred as they are more amenable to monitoring and standardization.[21-24]

Sterilization

Sterilization refers to the complete destruction or elimination of all transmissible organisms from a surface, including bacteria, spores, viruses, and fungi. Given its thoroughness, this process is appropriate for critical equipment and instruments. Many different types of sterilization exist; the most commonly used methods for surgical equipment include autoclaving, dry heat, ethylene oxide, and irradiation.[21,22,24]

PREOPERATIVE SKIN ANTISEPSIS

Alcohol

Alcohol is one of the oldest and most effective antiseptics available. It is abundant, rapid acting, and inexpensive. It is appropriate for use in minor, clean procedures, and has germicidal properties against most bacteria, fungi, and viruses. Some bacterial spores may show resistance. Its use is often limited, however, by its flammability and potential for skin irritation.[16,17]

Iodinated Preparations

Betadine and other iodophors have broad-spectrum antimicrobial activity. These compounds are rapid acting and are bactericidal within minutes; however, iodinated compounds are effective only when dry, and they lose their bactericidal effect when removed from the skin. They also leave a yellowish discoloration on the skin, are irritating, and are inactivated by contact with blood and other serum proteins. Although iodophors are relatively safe, when used chronically in pregnant women, associated hypothyroidism has been reported in neonates.[16,17,25]

Chlorhexidine

Chlorhexidine gluconate (CHG) is active against a wide range of gram-positive and -negative bacteria, viruses, and yeast. It is rapid acting, does not stain the skin, and is not inactivated by contact with blood or other serum proteins. An additional benefit of CHG is that it demonstrates prolonged antimicrobial activity by binding to the stratum corneum of the skin, allowing for efficacy even after removal. In comparison with the iodophors, CHG has been shown to lead to a greater reduction in bacterial counts and demonstrates a cumulative effect after repeated exposure. Cases of keratitis and ototoxity have been reported after prolonged, direct contact with patients' eyes and tympanic membranes. The majority of these instances occurred in patients exposed to CHG while under general anesthesia, who were unable to respond to the antiseptic-induced irritation.[16,17,26–28]

Preparation of the Skin

Before prepping the skin with antiseptic, all visible dirt and organic matter should first be removed. Antiseptic should then be applied to the area where the skin incision will be made, extending outward in concentric circles. A large enough area should be prepped so that the incision can be extended or new incisions/drain sites can be made if necessary.[16,17]

Hair Removal. Hair that may contaminate the operative site should be removed with scissors or by clipping prior to the procedure. Shaving of the area should not be performed within 24 hours of the surgical procedure as open skin, cuts, and scratches increase the risk of infection. If shaving is necessary to remove the hair, the skin should first be scrubbed with an antiseptic and then shaved immediately prior to the procedure. Adhesive tape can then be used to remove excess pieces of hair.[16,17]

Hand Washing. The majority of hospital-acquired infections are thought to be transmitted via the hands of health care workers. As many as 10,000 colony-forming units can be transmitted by brief hand contact alone![29] Studies

have found hand washing to be the most effective method of reducing hospital-acquired infections.[30] These results assume satisfactory hand-washing methods are undertaken; past studies have shown that adequate washing is hardly achieved and that approximately 89% of staff do not cleanse the entire hand surface.[15,31] Hands should be washed before and after each patient contact.[32] Three varieties of hand-washing agents are currently available.

Plain Soaps

Plain soaps derive their cleaning activity from their detergent bases. Soap and water are most effective in removing dirt, soil, and some organic substances. Although soaps have no inherent antimicrobial activity and cannot remove resident microorganisms, they can eliminate transient microorganisms from the hands;[21,32,33] however, hand washing with soap can also cause an increase in the total number of bacteria on the hands.[15,34] This paradoxical increase has been explained by enhanced release of bacterial particles from the skin after hand washing. Soaps may also contaminate the hands if the source has become extrinsically contaminated. Several cases of extrinsic contamination of nonmedicated liquid soaps with *Serratia marcescens* have been previously documented.[35,36]

Antiseptic Detergents. Antiseptic detergents, like plain soap and water, are also effective at removing dirt and soil. These agents do have antimicrobial activity and are more effective in removing both transient and resident microorganisms from the hands.[15,21,34]

Alcohol-Based Hand Rubs. Alcohol-based hand rubs are the most effective at removing microorganisms from the hands and reducing hand flora. These solutions have germicidal activity against a broad range of gram-positive and -negative bacteria, including some multidrug-resistant pathogens. Alcohols are also active against certain viruses when tested in vitro. To be most effective, these hand rubs should contain 60%–95% alcohol.[17] Additionally, these agents are simple and quick to use and require less effort than traditional soaps, which may lead to increased compliance with hand washing. Alcoholic hand rubs should not be used on visibly soiled hands as these agents are not effective at removing dirt or other physical contaminants. In this case, hands should first be washed with soap and water before applying the alcohol-based hand rub.[16,21,34]

Scrubbing. "Scrubbing" refers to the process by which members of the surgical team who will be in contact with the sterile field or instruments significantly decrease the bacterial counts on the hands and forearms. Although the majority of dermatologic surgeries are performed on an outpatient basis, some procedures require the dermatologist to perform the traditional surgical scrub.

Three types of antiseptics exist for scrubbing: aqueous scrubs, alcohol rubs, and alcohol rubs with additional active ingredients. Aqueous scrubs are water-based preparations with active ingredients such as CHG and povidone–iodine. Alcohol rubs, described earlier in this chapter, are also approved for the purpose of scrubbing. The third class of antiseptic is a modification of the alcohol rub with the addition of active ingredients (usually CHG or povidone–iodine) to impart greater antimicrobial activity.[28] CHG and povidone–iodine are the recommended antiseptics for scrubbing in the United States.[17]

The quality and effectiveness of scrubbing is also affected by factors other than the choice of antiseptic. The condition of the skin on the hands, the scrubbing technique and duration, and the gowning and gloving technique must all be considered. Although studies have not yet shown an optimum duration of scrubbing, it has been shown that scrubbing for 2 minutes is as effective as for 10 minutes. The first scrub of the day should always be the most thorough, and it is at this time that surgical team members should thoroughly clean under their fingernails. The hands and forearms should then be vigorously cleaned with a brush up to the elbows and rinsed. Hands and arms should be held up with the elbows flexed, avoiding contamination, until dried with sterile towels immediately before dressing in a sterile gown and gloves.[17]

WOUND CLASSIFICATION

Antibiotic selection to prevent wound infection first requires a discussion of wound types. Clean wounds (class I) refer to surgical sites without contamination that do not involve entry into the gastrointestinal, respiratory, or urinary tracts. No inflammation is present at the wound. Risk of infection is less than 5%. Most dermatologic surgeries fall into this category. Clean-contaminated wounds (class II) involve controlled entry into the gastrointestinal, respiratory, or urinary tracts without spillage or gross contamination. The risk of infection of dermatologic surgery into a class II wound is approximately 10%. Contaminated wounds (class III) occur by various means: breaks in sterile technique, spillage of gastrointestinal or urinary tract contents, or traumatic accidents. This category also includes wounds with nonpurulent discharge. The infection rate from dermatologic surgery in a class III wound is 20–30%. Finally, dirty wounds (class IV) include wounds with purulent discharge, fecal contamination, foreign bodies, or necrotic tissue or entry into a perforated viscus. Risk of infection is 40%.[16,37]

ANTIMICROBIAL SELECTION

Whether to use antibiotic prophylaxis in dermatological surgery is a frequent topic of debate. As discussed earlier in this chapter, most dermatological procedures are performed on class I or class II wounds and carry an inherent risk of postoperative infection of no greater than 10%. Although it is clear that antibiotic prophylaxis can reduce this already low infection rate, antimicrobials themselves may cause problems. Use of antimicrobials can add to the number of adverse drug events and allergic reactions, promote drug-resistant organisms, and interact with concomitant medications, in addition to adding cost.[5,16,38] Antimicrobial prophylaxis should not be used routinely for dermatological procedures, but rather in a select group of patients at high risk for SSI or other infectious complications.

Class I wounds do not require antimicrobial prophylaxis, nor do most cases of class II wounds. Antimicrobials may be beneficial for class II wounds in which oronasal or anogenital mucosae are breached or for large axillary or inguinal wounds.[16] In class III and IV wounds, antimicrobials serve a therapeutic rather than prophylactic purpose, and should be used routinely.

Besides reducing SSIs, another reason dermatologists often use antimicrobial prophylaxis is for the prevention of infection at a distant site such as a heart valve or prosthetic joint.[16,39] Endocarditis or seeding of a prosthetic joint theoretically can be caused by bacteremia induced during skin surgery. The incidence of bacteremia during skin surgery has been found to be only 0.7%,[40] which compares favorably to the 0%–2.1% incidence of bacteremia in random blood cultures of healthy volunteers.[41] The routine use of antimicrobial prophylaxis during dermatological procedures in otherwise healthy individuals for prevention of endocarditis or joint infection seems unwarranted. In fact, no randomized clinical trial to date has established that antimicrobial prophylaxis prevents endocarditis.[42]

Should the decision to use antimicrobials be made, the next most important step is to use them optimally. Effective prophylaxis provides a high blood and tissue level of antimicrobial at the time of anticipated bacteremia.[39] Antimicrobials given at the conclusion of a procedure are not as effective in preventing infection, and after the wound is closed there is generally no longer any risk of contamination.[16] A large loading dose of the appropriate antimicrobial should be given approximately 1 hour before surgery.

The route of antimicrobial prophylaxis is generally thought of as either oral or intravenous. Intraincisional antimicrobial prophylaxis injected along with buffered lidocaine and epinephrine has also shown to reduce wound infection. Benefits of intraincisional antimicrobial prophylaxis include immediate delivery to the site where it is needed, ease of use (in the same syringe as anesthetic), enhanced compliance, and relatively low cost.[43] Additionally, because the dose of intraincisional antimicrobials is low compared with the amount necessary in oral or intravenous prophylaxis and is applied locally, the risk of systemic side effects and bacterial resistance is theoretically lower. Intraincisional antimicrobials are not widely used currently, but their potential benefits warrant further investigation. In the future, they may become more common as an alternative to traditional prophylaxis.

For class III and IV wounds, in which antimicrobial use is recommended routinely, the choice of antimicrobials should be based on the presumed organism causing the infection. If a wound culture with sensitivities is available prior to a procedure, this should obviously be taken into account prior to antimicrobial selection. In absence of wound culture results, first-generation cephalosporins are a good choice because of their excellent coverage of staphylococcal organisms (the most common cause of wound infection) as well as common gram-negatives such as *Escherichia coli* and some *Proteus* species.[5] Penicillins, especially beta-lactamase–resistant variants are also good choices. Many patients have penicillin sensitivity, and due to cross-reactivity with cephalosporins, both of these first-line choices would be inappropriate for these patients. In these cases, macrolides (e.g., erythromycin) or quinolones (e.g., ciprofloxacin) can be used. Current American Heart Association guidelines recommend amoxicillin as the first choice for standard prophylaxis (or ampicillin for patients unable to take oral medications), with clindamycin as an alternative for patients with penicillin allergy.[42]

CONCLUSIONS

With the number of dermatological procedures being performed increasing each year, ensuring a minimal amount of nosocomial and SSIs is important, while understanding the inherent risk factors of a procedure and that using proper aseptic technique can help prevent such complications. Surgical equipment decontamination, preoperative skin asepsis, and proper hand washing are all techniques that can keep infections to a minimum. Antimicrobial prophylaxis is generally unnecessary for dermatological procedures, as the risk of adverse events due to the antimicrobials often outweighs the benefit of further reducing an already low incidence of infection.

REFERENCES

1. Rogues AM, Lasheras A, Amici JM, et al. Infection control practices and infectious complications in dermatological surgery. J Hosp Infect. 2007;65:258–63.
2. Aasi SZ, Leffell DJ. Complications in dermatologic surgery: how safe is safe? Arch Dermatol. 2003;139:213–14.
3. Salopek TG, Slade JM, Marghoob AA, et al. Management of cutaneous malignant melanoma by dermatologists of the American Academy of Dermatology. II. Definitive surgery for malignant melanoma. J Am Acad Dermatol. 1995;33:451–61.
4. Haas AF, Grekin RC. Practical thoughts on antibiotic prophylaxis. Arch Dermatol. 1998;134:872–3.
5. Babcock MD, Grekin RC. Antibiotic use in dermatologic surgery. Dermatol Clin. 2003;21:337–48.
6. Amici JM, Rogues AM, Lasheras A, et al. A prospective study of the incidence of complications associated with dermatological surgery. Br J Dermatol. 2005;153:967–71.
7. Futoryan T, Grande D. Postoperative wound infection rates in dermatologic surgery. Dermatol Surg. 1995;21:509–14.
8. Cook JL, Perone JB. A prospective evaluation of the incidence of complications associated with Mohs micrographic surgery. Arch Dermatol. 2003;139:143–52.
9. Wahie S, Lawrence CM. Wound complications following diagnostic skin biopsies in dermatology inpatients. Arch Dermatol. 2007;143:1267–71.
10. Helbling I, Muston HL, Ferguson JE, McKenna M. Audit of admissions to dermatology beds in Greater Manchester. Clin Exp Dermatol. 2002;27:519–22.
11. Cantlon CA, Stemper ME, Schwan WR, Hoffman MA, Qutaishat SS. Significant pathogens isolated from surgical site infections at a community hospital in the Midwest. Am J Infect Control. 2006;34:526–9.
12. Finn L, Crook S. Minor surgery in general practice–setting the standards. J Public Health Med. 1998;20:169–74.
13. Maragh SL, Otley CC, Roenigk RK, Phillips PK. Antibiotic prophylaxis in dermatologic surgery: updated guidelines. Dermatol Surg. 2005;31:83–91.
14. Davis CP. Normal flora. In: Baron S, editor. Medical microbiology. 4th ed. Galveston, TX: The University of Texas Medical Branch at Galveston; 1996.
15. Aseptic technique. In: Dougherty L, Lister S, editors. The Royal Marsden Hospital manual of clinical nursing procedures. 6th ed. Oxford: Blackwell. 2004. 50–63.
16. Hurst EA, Grekin RC, Yu SS, Neuhaus IM. Infectious complications and antibiotic use in dermatologic surgery. Semin Cutan Med Surg. 2007;26:47–53.
17. Mangram AJ, Horan TC, Pearson ML, et al., The Healthcare Infection Control Practices Advisory Committee. Guidelines for prevention of surgical site infection, 1999. Atlanta, GA: Centers for Disease Control and Prevention.
18. Dixon AJ, Dixon MP, Askew DA, Wilkinson D. Prospective study of wound infections in dermatologic surgery in the absence of prophylactic antimicrobials. Dermatol Surg. 2006;32:819–26; discussion 826–7.
19. Olsen MA, Lock-Buckley P, Hopkins D, et al. The risk factors for deep and superficial chest surgical-site infections after coronary artery bypass graft surgery are different. J Thorac Cardiovasc Surg. 2002;124:136–45.
20. Garland R, Frizelle FA, Dobbs BR, Singh H. A retrospective audit of long-term lower limb complications following leg vein harvesting for coronary artery bypass grafting. Eur J Cardiothorac Surg. 2003;23:950–5.
21. Hart S. Using an aseptic technique to reduce the risk of infection. Nurs Stand. 2007;21:43–8.
22. NHS Estates. Guide to decontamination of reusable surgical instruments. London: Department of Health; 2003, 39 pp.
23. Rutala WA, Weber DJ. Disinfection and sterilization in health care facilities: what clinicians need to know. Clin Infect Dis. 2004;39:702–9.
24. Spencer RC, Perry C. Decontamination of reusable surgical instruments. Hosp Med. 2001;62:662–3.

25. Danziger L, Hassan E. Antimicrobial prophylaxis of gastrointestinal surgical procedures and treatment of intraabdominal infections. Drug Intell Clin Pharm. 1987;21:406–16.

26. Perez R, Freeman S, Sohmer H, Sichel JY. Vestibular and cochlear ototoxicity of topical antiseptics assessed by evoked potentials. Laryngoscope. 2000;110:1522–7.

27. Murthy S, Hawksworth NR, Cree I. Progressive ulcerative keratitis related to the use of topical chlorhexidine gluconate (0.02%). Cornea. 2002;21:237–9.

28. Tanner J, Swarbrook S, Stuart J. Surgical hand antisepsis to reduce surgical site infection. Cochrane Database Syst Rev. 2008; CD004288.

29. Gould D, Ream E. Assessing nurses' hand decontamination performance. Nurs Times. 1993;89:47–50.

30. Gould DJ, Chudleigh J, Drey NS, Moralejo D. Measuring handwashing performance in health service audits and research studies. J Hosp Infect. 2007;66:109–15.

31. Taylor LJ. An evaluation of handwashing techniques-1. Nurs Times. 1978;74:54–5.

32. Boyce JM, Pittet D. Guideline for hand hygiene in healthcare settings. Recommendations of the Healthcare Infection Control Practices Advisory Committee and the HICPAC/SHEA/APIC/IDSA Hand Hygiene Task Force. Society for Healthcare Epidemiology of America (Association for Professionals in Infection Control/Infectious Diseases Society of America. MMWR Recomm Rep. 2002;51:1–45, quiz CE41–44.

33. Grinbaum RS, de Mendonca JS, Cardo DM. An outbreak of handscrubbing-related surgical site infections in vascular surgical procedures. Infect Control Hosp Epidemiol. 1995;16:198–202.

34. Winnefeld M, Richard MA, Drancourt M, Grob JJ. Skin tolerance and effectiveness of two hand decontamination procedures in everyday hospital use. Br J Dermatol. 2000;143:546–50.

35. Sartor C, Jacomo V, Duvivier C, et al. Nosocomial Serratia marcescens infections associated with extrinsic contamination of a liquid nonmedicated soap. Infect Control Hosp Epidemiol. 2000;21:196–9.

36. Archibald LK, Corl A, Shah B, et al. Serratia marcescens outbreak associated with extrinsic contamination of 1% chlorxylenol soap. Infect Control Hosp Epidemiol. 1997;18:704–9.

37. Bell RM. Surgical procedures, techniques, and skills. In: Lawrence PF, Beel, RM. Dayton, MT editors. Essentials of general surgery. 3rd ed. Philadelphia: Lippincott Williams & Williams: 1999. 519–62.

38. Lamberg L. Dermatologists debate sentinel node biopsy, safety of liposuction, and antibiotic prophylaxis. JAMA. 2000;283:2223–4.

39. George PM. Dermatologists and antibiotic prophylaxis: a survey. J Am Acad Dermatol. 1995;33:418–21.

40. Carmichael AJ, Flanagan PG, Holt PJ, Duerden BI. The occurrence of bacteraemia with skin surgery. Br J Dermatol. 1996;134:120–2.

41. Wilson RW, Van Scoy RE, Washington JA. Incidence of bacteremia in adults without infection. J Clin Microbiol. 1975;2:94–5.

42. Scheinfeld N, Struach S, Ross B. Antibiotic prophylaxis guideline awareness and antibiotic prophylaxis use among New York State dermatologic surgeons. Dermatol Surg. 2002;28:841–4.

43. Huether MJ, Griego RD, Brodland DG, Zitelli JA. Clindamycin for intraincisional antibiotic prophylaxis in dermatologic surgery. Arch Dermatol. 2002;138:1145–8.

CHAPTER 3

New Antimicrobials

Maryann Mikhail
Jeffrey M. Weinberg

WITH THE continuing development of clinical drug resistance among bacteria and the advent of resistance to the more recently released agents quinupristin/dalfopristin and linezolid, the need for new, effective agents to treat multidrug-resistant gram-positive infections remains important. With treatment options limited, it has become critical to identify antibiotics with novel mechanisms of activity. Several new drugs have emerged as possible therapeutic alternatives. This chapter focuses on agents newly introduced and those currently in clinical development for the treatment of skin and skin structure infections. In addition, novel antifungal agents will be reviewed, as will novel dosing of antiviral agents for herpes labialis.

NOVEL ANTIBACTERIAL AGENTS

There has been an alarming increase in the incidence of gram-positive infections, including resistant bacteria such as methicillin-resistant *Staphylococcus aureus* (MRSA) and drug-resistant pneumococci. Although vancomycin has been considered the drug of last defense against gram-positive multidrug-resistant bacteria, strains of vancomycin-resistant bacteria, including vancomycin-resistant enterococci (VRE), began to emerge by the late 1980s. More recently, strains of vancomycin-intermediate-resistant *S. aureus* (VISA) have been isolated.[1]

Gram-positive bacteria, such as *S. aureus* and *Streptococcus pyogenes*, are often the cause of both uncomplicated and complicated skin and skin structure infections. Uncomplicated infections are mild, localized to the skin, and responsive to topical or systemic antibiotics. This category includes simple abscesses, impetiginized lesions, furuncles, and cellulitis. Complicated infections are those involving deeper soft tissues and requiring surgical intervention or associated with significant systemic disease or comorbidities. Corresponding clinical entities include surgical wound infections, infected ulcers or burns, severe carbunculosis, erysipelas, and necrotizing fasciitis.

Several novel agents have emerged as possible therapeutic alternatives. These include linezolid, quinupristin/dalfopristin, daptomycin, oritavancin and dalbavancin, the quinolones (moxifloxacin and gatifloxacin), and tigecycline (Table 3.1).

LINEZOLID

Linezolid (Figure 3.1) is an oxazolidinone antibiotic shown to be effective for nosocomial and community-acquired pneumonias, vancomycin-resistant *Enterococcus faecium* (VREF) infections, and skin infections caused by certain staphylococcus or streptococcus species.[2] The oxazolidinones are a novel class of antibiotics first discovered in 1987.[3]

Mode of Action

Cellular Mechanism. Oxazolidinones, and specifically linezolid, are theorized to act by inhibiting the initiation phase of translation and thus interfering with bacterial protein synthesis.[4] It is thought that linezolid binds to the 23S portion of the 50S ribosomal subunit, preventing initiation complex formation. This early inhibition of protein synthesis is a unique mechanism and limits cross-resistance with other antimicrobial agents, because there is no preexisting resistance mechanism in nature.[4]

Pharmacokinetics. Oral bioavailability of the antibiotic in a normal host is 100%. The drug can be administered with or without meals. Food may slightly decrease the rate of absorption but has no effect on the amount of the drug absorbed. Linezolid shows a protein binding of only 31% and a half-life of 5–7 hours. At a dosing schedule of 600 mg administered orally every 12 hours, the average steady-state plasma concentrations exceed the minimum inhibitory concentration required to inhibit the growth of 90% of organisms (MIC90) for staphylococci, streptococci, and enterococci. It is primarily metabolized by oxidation of the morpholine ring, which produces two inactive metabolites. Its metabolism is unaffected by the cytochrome P450 enzyme system. Kinetics are similar in patients with mild to moderate renal or hepatic compromise. In patients older

TABLE 3.1: Novel Antibacterial Agents for Skin and Skin Structure Infections

Generic name	Brand name	Mechanism of action	Dosage	Skin infection usage
Linezolid	Zyvox®	Binds to 23S portion of the 50S ribosomal subunit and prevents initiation complex formation	400–600 mg PO/IV q12h for 10–14 d	Uncomplicated/ Complicated
Quinupristin/ Dalfopristin	Synercid®	Binds to different sites on the 50S subunit and inhibits protein synthesis	7.5 mg/kg IV q12h for at least 7 d	Complicated
Daptomycin	Cubicin®	Disrupts bacteria plasma membrane function	4 mg/kg IV q24h for 10–14 d	Complicated
Oritavancin	———	Inhibits biosynthesis of cell wall peptidoglycan	1.5–3.0 mg/kg IV qD for 3–7 d	Complicated
Dalbavancin	———	Inhibits biosynthesis of cell wall peptidoglycan	500–1000 mg IV qwk	Complicated
Moxifloxacin	Avelox®	Inhibits DNA gyrase and topoisomerase IV	400 mg PO/IV qD for 7 d	Uncomplicated
Gatifloxacin	Tequin®	Inhibits DNA gyrase and topoisomerase IV	400 mg PO/IV qD for 7–10 d	Uncomplicated
Tigecycline	Tygacil®	Inhibits protein synthesis by blocking the 30S ribosomal subunit	Initial: 100 mg, then 50 mg BID IV over 30–60 min for 5–14 d	Complicated
Retapamulin	Altabax®	Inhibits bacterial protein synthesis by interacting with the 50S ribosomal subunit	Topical application BID for 5 d	Uncomplicated (impetigo)

PO, per os (orally); IV, intravenous; DNA, deoxyribonucleic acid; BID, twice daily.

than 5 years, a dose of 10 mg/kg every 12 hours displays similar pharmacokinetic properties.[2]

In Vitro Activity. In vitro studies have shown linezolid to be effective against many antibiotic-resistant gram-positive organisms, including MRSA, penicillin-resistant *Streptococcus pneumoniae*, and VRE.[5-9] Linezolid is bacteriostatic against most susceptible organisms, but has shown bactericidal activity against *Clostridium perfringens*, *Bacteroides fragilis*, and some strains of *S. pneumoniae*.[10] In addition to its coverage of antibiotic-resistant gram-positive organisms, it has some broad-spectrum activity against gram-positive cocci, gram-negative anaerobes, and some mycobacteria. It has also shown moderate in vitro inhibitory activity against *Haemophilus influenzae* and *Moraxella catarrhalis*, although it was not effective against Enterobacteriaceae and *Pseudomonas aeruginosa*.

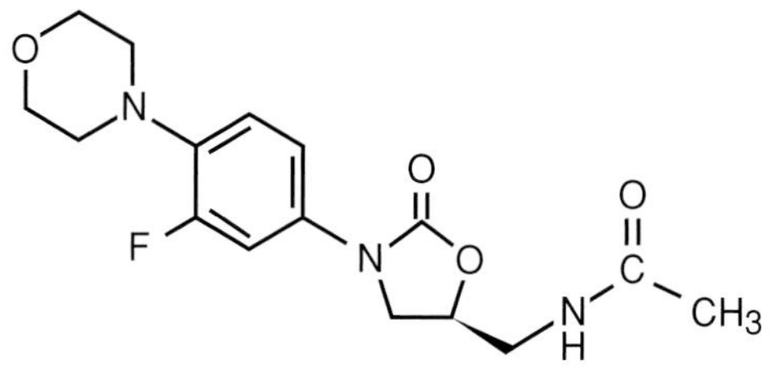

FIGURE 3.1: Linezolid.

Clinical Indications

Currently, linezolid is U.S. Food and Drug Administration (FDA) approved for the treatment of various gram-positive infections, including both hospital- and community-acquired pneumonias, complicated and uncomplicated skin and skin structure infections, and VRE infections. Studies have been conducted comparing (head to head) linezolid and standard antibiotic therapies in the treatment of skin and soft-tissue infections (SSTIs). In terms of efficacy, a double-blind, randomized study in 332 adult patients with uncomplicated skin infections (cellulitis, skin abscesses, and furuncles) secondary to staphylococcus and streptococcus compared linezolid 400 mg twice daily with clarithromycin 250 mg twice daily for a course of 7–14 days. Following treatment, 91% of the linezolid-treated patients had a clinical cure, compared with 93% in the clarithromycin group, demonstrating that linezolid is as effective as clarithromycin.[11]

Another randomized, double-blind, multicenter trial compared the efficacy and safety of linezolid, an oxazolidinone, with those of oxacillin–dicloxacillin in patients with complicated SSTIs (cSSTIs).[12] A total of 826 hospitalized adult patients were randomized to receive linezolid (600 mg intravenously [IV]) every 12 hours or oxacillin (2 grams IV) every 6 hours. Following sufficient clinical improvement, patients were switched to the respective oral agents, linezolid 600 mg orally every 12 hours or dicloxacillin 500 mg orally every 6 hours. Primary efficacy variables were clinical cure rates in both the intent-to-treat (ITT) population as well as clinically evaluable (CE) patients and microbiological success rate in microbiologically evaluable (ME) patients. Safety and tolerability were evaluated in the ITT population. Demographics and baseline characteristics were similar across treatment groups in the 819 ITT patients. In the ITT population, the clinical cure rates were 69.8% and 64.9% in the linezolid and oxacillin–dicloxacillin groups, respectively (95% confidence interval [CI], –1.58 to 11. 25; $p = .141$). In 298 CE linezolid-treated patients, the clinical cure rate was 88.6%, compared with a cure rate of 85.8% in 302 CE patients who received oxacillin–dicloxacillin. In 143 ME linezolid-treated patients, the microbiological success rate was 88.1%, compared with a success rate of 86.1% in 151 ME patients who received oxacillin–dicloxacillin. Both agents were well tolerated; most adverse events were of mild-to-moderate intensity. No serious drug-related adverse events were reported in the linezolid group.[12]

Linezolid was also found to be as effective as vancomycin in the treatment of skin and soft-tissue MRSA infections.[13,14] In VRE infections, a clinical success rate of 81% was noted, indicating that treatment with linezolid may be superior to comparator antibiotics in patients with complicated skin infections who also have comorbid conditions.[15] There have been reports of development of resistance to linezolid in some patients with *E. faecium*.[16]

Dosage Regimens

The recommended dosage of linezolid depends on the severity of the skin or soft-tissue infection. Uncomplicated infections should be treated with 400 mg every 12 hours for 10–14 days. For complicated infections, 600 mg twice daily either via IV infusion or orally is recommended. No dose adjustment is needed when switching from IV to oral therapy,[4] because the absolute bioavailability after oral dosing is nearly 100%.

Contraindications/Cautions

Linezolid is generally well tolerated, with the most common adverse effects being diarrhea (8.3%), headache (6.5%), and nausea (6.2%).[10] Because linezolid is a non-selective, reversible inhibitor of monoamine oxidase, it may interact with serotonergic or adrenergic agents.[17] Like many other antibiotics, it may cause pseudomembranous colitis, as a result of overgrowth of *Clostridium difficile*. Approximately 2% of patients develop thrombocytopenia, which appears to be dependent on duration of therapy. The effect is reversible; however, the manufacturer recommends monitoring patients with preexisting thrombocytopenia or those whose treatment will exceed 2 weeks. No deaths related to thrombocytopenia have been reported.[2]

Conclusions

Linezolid is the first of a novel class of antibiotics called oxazolidinones and is indicated for use both in uncomplicated and complicated skin and skin structure infections caused by MRSA or streptococcal species.

QUINUPRISTIN/DALFOPRISTIN

Quinupristin/dalfopristin (Figure 3.2) is a combination of two semisynthetic pristinamycin derivatives and is the first parenteral streptogramin antibacterial agent. Both quinupristin and dalfopristin have antibacterial capability individually, but demonstrate synergistic activity when used in combination. Much of the clinical experience with this antibiotic is derived from five comparative trials and an FDA-sanctioned emergency-use program for patients without alternative therapies.

Mode of Action

Cellular Mechanism. Quinupristin and dalfopristin enter bacterial cells by diffusion and bind to different sites on the 50S ribosomal subunit, resulting in an irreversible inhibition of bacterial protein synthesis.[18] Dalfopristin blocks the reaction catalyzed by the peptidyl transferase catalytic center of the 50S ribosome via inhibition of substrate attachment to the P-site and the A-site of the ribosome. Quinupristin inhibits peptide chain elongation. The synergistic effect of the combination appears to result from the fact that these compounds target early and late steps in protein synthesis.[19]

Pharmacokinetics. Quinupristin/dalfopristin is rapidly cleared from the blood and is widely distributed. It is eliminated through the bile into the feces. Its clearance may be slightly reduced in patients with severe chronic renal failure. Its pharmacokinetics are unaffected by age or gender. Quinupristin has a half-life of approximately 1 hour, and dalfopristin has a half-life of approximately 30 minutes. The postantibiotic effect of the drug is prolonged to greater than 7.4 hours against streptococci regardless of penicillin susceptibility.[20] Quinupristin/dalfopristin inhibits the biotransformation rate of cytochrome P450 substrates in vitro.

In Vitro Activity. Quinupristin/dalfopristin has inhibitory activity against a broad spectrum of gram-positive bacteria including MRSA, VREF, and drug-resistant *S. pneumoniae*. It is bactericidal against methicillin-resistant staphylococci and *S. pneumoniae* and bacteriostatic against most *E. faecium* in vitro. Quinupristin/dalfopristin also has demonstrated synergy with other antibiotics. Rifampin is synergistic with quinupristin/dalfopristin against MRSA, and doxycycline is synergistic against VREF in vitro.

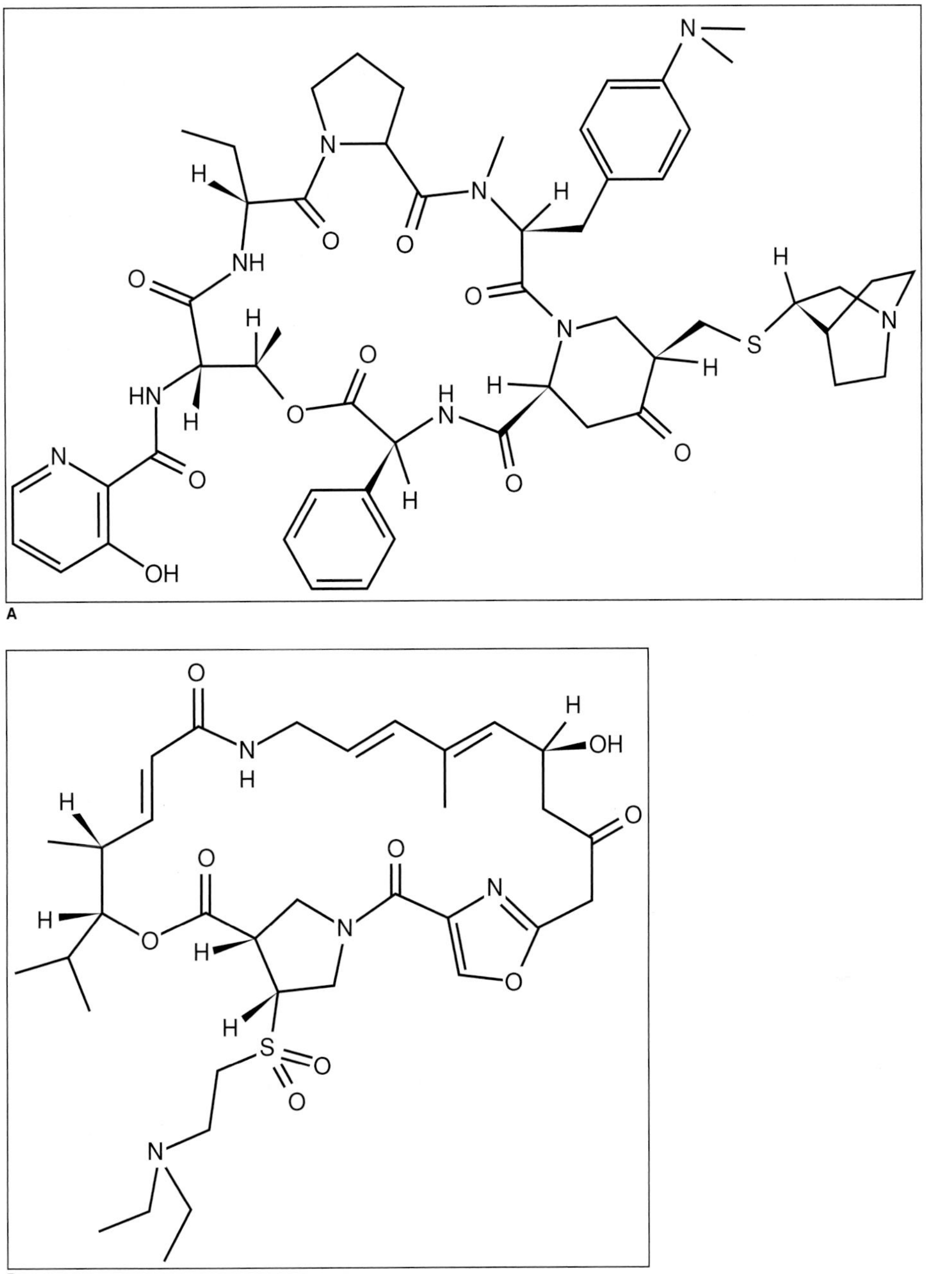

FIGURE 3.2: *Quinupristin (panel A) and dalfopristin (panel B).*

Clinical Indications

FDA indications for quinupristin/dalfopristin are serious infections associated with VREF bacteremia and complicated skin and skin structure infections caused by methicillin-sensitive *S. aureus* or *S. pyogenes*. VREF infections are difficult to treat, and few therapeutic options are currently available. These pathogens are resistant to most β-lactam and aminoglycoside antibiotics. Judicious use of vancomycin is currently being advocated to reduce the incidence of resistant organisms, but their presence continues. In 1995, quinupristin was approved for emergency use. During this emergency-use basis in the treatment of VREF infections, in which no other treatments were available, patients using quinupristin/dalfopristin had a 71% success rate[21] and a significantly lower mortality rate than did patients using other agents.[22] In another study, patients with complicated skin and skin structure infections who were given quinupristin/dalfopristin had almost identical clinical success rates (68%) when compared to those using vancomycin, oxacillin, and/or cefazolin

(71%).[23] In addition, in the treatment of patients with gram-positive nosocomial pneumonia, it was found to be as efficacious as vancomycin.[24]

Dosage Regimens

For complicated skin or skin structure infections, the recommended dose is 7.5 mg/kg IV twice daily for at least 7 days. The drug can be administered up to three times daily for bacteremic patients. Dose adjustment to 5 mg/kg is recommended for patients with hepatic insufficiency. No dose adjustment is needed for elderly or renally impaired patients.

Contraindications/Cautions

Approximately 63% of patients receiving quinupristin/dalfopristin reported at least one adverse effect. Evaluation of these adverse effects is difficult because they are often assessed in the context of severe underlying illnesses. Adverse venous events at the IV site of administration of the drug were the most common. Reports of pain and/or inflammation during its administration were reported in 34.9%–74.0% of patients.[23,25] Atrophy, edema, hemorrhage, hypersensitivity, burning, and thrombophlebitis were also reported. A statistically significant number of venous events occurred with quinupristin/dalfopristin compared with oxacillin, cefazolin, or vancomycin (66.2% vs. 28.4%).[21] Suggested but unproven management options to limit these events include administration in a larger volume of fluid or via a central line. Mild to moderate myalgias and/or arthralgias have been reported.[26] Gastrointestinal events also occurred with 4.6% of patients experiencing nausea, 2.7% experiencing vomiting and diarrhea, and 2.5% developing a rash.[27] The most common laboratory abnormalities reported were an increase in hepatic transaminases and bilirubin.[27] Use is contraindicated in patients with known hypersensitivity to streptogramins, or with any drugs metabolized by the cytochrome P450 3A4 enzyme system (some anti–human immunodeficiency virus [HIV] agents, vinca alkaloids, benzodiazepines, immunosuppressives, corticosteroids, and calcium channel blockers). In addition, particular care should be taken when using medications that prolong the QT interval (e.g., astemizole, cisapride, disopyramide, lidocaine, quinidine, and terfenadine).[27] Caution is also recommended if using cyclosporin concomitantly.[28] Resistance to quinupristin/dalfopristin has been encountered infrequently among VREF, and resistance among staphylococci is rare in the United States.[29,30]

Conclusions

Quinupristin/dalfopristin is the first parenteral streptogramin and offers a unique alternative treatment against multidrug-resistant gram-positive bacteria. Because of its potency, bactericidal activity, long postantibiotic effect, and rare resistance, it has excellent potential for treatment of serious gram-positive infections. Its efficacy should be weighed against possible adverse effects, tolerability, and interactions prior to utilizing this potent antibiotic. In seriously ill patients with unresponsive infections and minimal other potential treatment options, it should be considered the treatment of choice.

DAPTOMYCIN

Daptomycin (Figure 3.3) is a novel lipopeptide antibiotic derived from the fermentation of a strain of *Streptomyces roseosporus*. It has demonstrated potent antimicrobial activity against a wide variety of gram-positive bacteria including MRSA and VRE. Initially developed in the early 1980s,

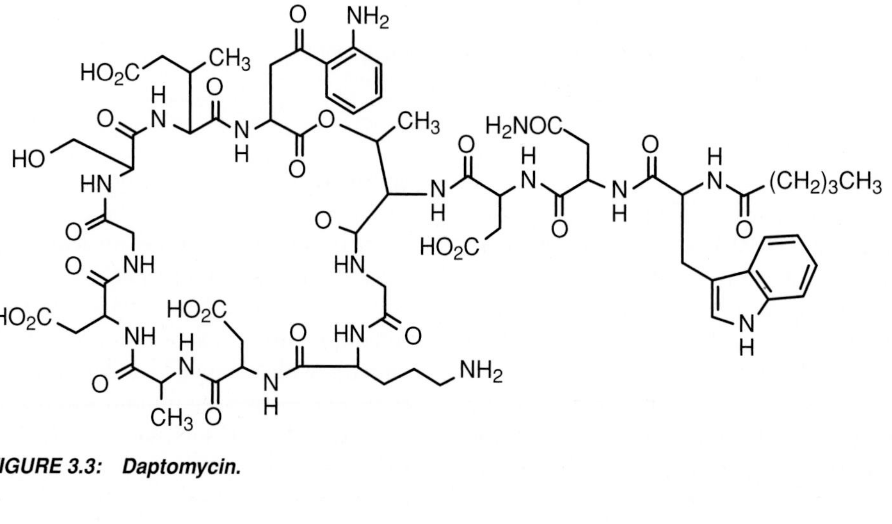

FIGURE 3.3: Daptomycin.

daptomycin was temporarily shelved due to concerns about skeletal muscle toxicity. At lower doses, this toxicity was not seen, but clinical trials using daptomycin were again halted due to treatment failures in patients with *S. aureus* endocarditis. Recently, due to the need for new agents with activity against vancomycin-resistant bacteria, this IV therapy was reevaluated and now has supportive data from phase III clinical trials.[31]

Mode of Action

Cellular Mechanism. The precise mechanism of action of daptomycin is unknown. It kills by disrupting bacteria plasma membrane function, but does not enter the cytoplasm. Proposed mechanisms include inhibition of lipoteichoic acid synthesis[32,33] and dissipation of bacterial membrane potential.[34,35]

Pharmacokinetics. Following once-daily dosing, it exhibits linear pharmacokinetics and minimal accumulation. It has a half-life of approximately 8.5 hours.[36] It is highly protein bound (94%), and its in vitro activity is altered in the presence of serum or abumin.[37,38] Daptomycin is eliminated by the kidney; therefore, dose adjustments based on creatinine clearance are required. Because hepatic metabolism of daptomycin is limited, interactions with other drugs metabolized by the liver are minimal.

In Vitro Activity. Daptomycin has rapid, concentration-dependent bactericidal activity against gram-positive organisms. Using the standard definition of a 3-log reduction in viable organisms, daptomycin (and not vancomycin) is bactericidal against both *S. aureus* and *Enterococcus faecalis*.[39] In addition, in vitro studies designed to evaluate the bactericidal activity of daptomycin (compared with vancomycin, linezolid, and quinupristin/dalfopristin) against various gram-positive organisms found that the bactericidal activity of daptomycin is improved when concentrations are ≥4 times the MIC.[40] At these levels, daptomycin and vancomycin achieved 99.9% killing of MRSA at 8 hours, which was greater than the killing seen with linezolid and quinupristin/dalfopristin. It also had greater activity against VRE at 8 hours and 24 hours when compared with linezolid and quinupristin/dalfopristin. Spontaneous acquisition of resistance is rare as long as therapeutic serum levels of daptomycin are maintained. Synergistic interactions were noted most frequently with aminoglycosides and against enterococcal organisms.

Clinical Indications

Daptomycin was recently approved for the treatment of complicated skin and skin structure infections caused by gram-positive bacteria, including those caused by MRSA and MSSA (methicillin-susceptible *S. aureus*). In early phase II trials, the clinical efficacy of daptomycin was compared with that of conventional agents such as β-lactams, semisynthetic penicillins, and vancomycin for the treatment of skin infections and bacteremia.[41] In patients with SSTIs, 2 mg/kg daily resulted in clinical cure or improvement in 29/30 patients, compared to 37/39 patients treated with conventional therapy. Two multicenter phase III trials have now been completed, involving a total of 1079 subjects with cSSTIs.[31,41] In both studies, patients were randomized for treatment with IV daptomycin (4 mg/kg, once daily) or standard treatment with a semisynthetic penicillin or vancomycin. Of all the CE patients, 89% had clinical success with daptomycin, and 88% were treated successfully with standard treatment.[31] These two groups were statistically equivalent. Of note, the group that received daptomycin required a significantly shorter course of treatment, with 63% of patients receiving daptomycin requiring only 4–7 days of treatment and 67% of patients being treated with standard therapy requiring 8 or more days of treatment.[31]

Dosage Regimens

The recommended dosage of daptomycin is 4 mg/kg IV every 24 hours for 7–14 days.[42] Because daptomycin is eliminated primarily by the kidney, a dosage modification is recommended for patients with creatinine clearance <30 mL/min, including patients receiving hemodialysis or continuous ambulatory peritoneal dialysis (CAPD). The recommended dosing regimen is 4 mg/kg once every 24 hours for patients with creatinine clearance ≥30 mL/min and 4 mg/kg once every 48 hours for patients with creatinine clearance ≥30 mL/min, including those on hemodialysis or CAPD. When possible, daptomycin should be administered following hemodialysis on hemodialysis days.[43]

Contraindications/Cautions

Daptomycin is well tolerated with an incidence and nature of serious adverse effects comparable to those seen with conventional therapy. The most frequently reported adverse events were headache and constipation in approximately 4% of patients. These events were not dose related and did not persist. Skeletal muscle has been identified as the primary target organ of daptomycin toxicity.[44] Reversible skeletal muscle toxicity occurred only at the highest dose tested (4 mg/kg every 12 hours). Transient muscle weakness and myalgia were noted, but resolved 1 week after discontinuing daptomycin. By monitoring creatine phosphokinase (CPK) levels, muscle toxicity can be prevented, as CPK elevations precede muscle toxicity. No signs of cardiac or smooth muscle toxicity were noted. In addition, once-daily dosing has been shown to minimize associated muscle toxicity.

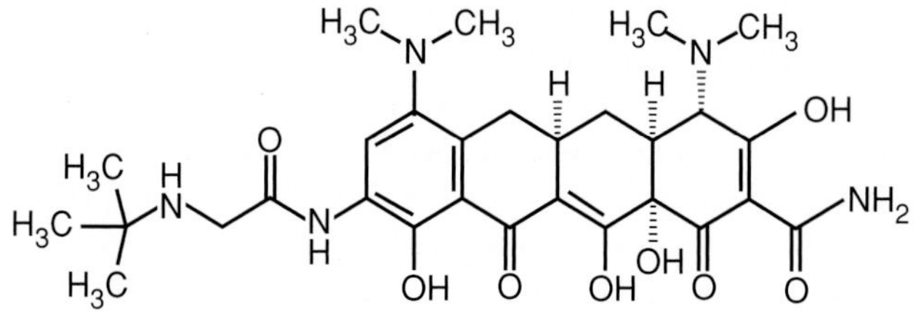

FIGURE 3.4: *Tigecycline.*

Conclusions

As resistance to conventional antibiotics increases, dapto-mycin may be a useful adjunct to our antibiotic armamen-tarium. It possesses efficacy against resistant bacteria and provides for a rapid and concentration-dependent kill time, a broad spectrum of activity, and a low frequency of resis-tance.[45]

TIGECYCLINE

Tigecycline (Figure 3.4) belongs to a novel class of antibi-otics called the glycylglycines. It was approved by the FDA in June 2005[46] for the treatment of adults 18 years old or older with complicated skin or skin structure infec-tions caused by *Escherichia coli*, *E. faecalis* (vancomycin-susceptible isolates only), *S. aureus* (methicillin-susceptible and -resistant isolates), *Streptococcus agalactiae*, *Streptococ-cus anginosus* group, *S. pyogenes*, and *B. fragilis*. It is also approved for the treatment of complicated intraabdominal infections caused by a variety of species.

Mode of Action

Cellular Mechanisms. Glycylcyclines are semisynthetic derivatives of tetracycline antibiotics in which a glycyl-amido moiety is attached at the 9 position of the D-ring of the base molecule. This modification maintains the antibacterial effect but provides stability against mecha-nisms of tetracycline resistance.[47,48] Like the tetracyclines, tigecycline is bacteriostatic and inhibits bacterial protein translation by binding to the 30S ribosomal subunit and blocking entry of amino-acyl transfer RNA molecules into the A site of the ribosome.[49]

In Vitro Activity. Tigecycline shows broad spectrum in vitro activity against gram-positive pathogens (including MRSA, methicillin-resistant *Staphylococcus epidermidis*, and VRE), gram-negative organisms (such as acinetobacter), anaerobes, and rapidly growing mycobacteria.[49] It is not active against *Pseudomonas* strains.

Pharmacokinetics. In healthy subjects given IV tigecy-cline, peak concentration is linearly proportional to doses over the range of 12.5–300 mg. Approximately 71%–89%

of tigecycline is bound to plasma proteins. Following IV administration, tigecycline serum concentrations initially decline rapidly during distribution into body tissues.[49] The mean half-life of tigecycline after a single 100-mg dose was 27.1 hours; after multiple dosing of 50 mg every 12 hours, the mean half-life was 42.4 hours.[49] Approximately 59% of the drug is eliminated by biliary and/or fecal excretion, and 33% is excreted in urine. Of the total dose, approximately 22% is excreted as unchanged tigecycline in urine.

Clinical Indications

Tigecycline is indicated for cSSTIs as well as for compli-cated intraabdominal infections. Its efficacy as monother-apy was demonstrated to be similar to combination therapy with vancomycin and aztreonam in two double-blind phase III comparison studies. Patients (total = 1116) with cSSTIs received tigecycline (100 mg, followed by 50 mg IV twice daily) or vancomycin (1 g IV twice daily) plus aztreonam (2 g IV twice daily) for up to 14 days. Clinical responses to tige-cycline and vancomycin–aztreonam at test-of-cure were similar: 79.7% (95% CI, 76.1% to 83.1%) versus 81.9% (95% CI, 78.3% to 85.1%; $p = .4183$). Adverse events were similar, with increased nausea and vomiting in the tigecy-cline group and increased rash and elevated hepatic amino-transferase levels in the vancomycin–aztreonam group.[50]

Dosage Regimens

The recommended regimen is an initial dose of 100 mg, followed by 50 mg every 12 hours. IV infusions should be administered over approximately 30–60 minutes every 12 hours. The recommended duration of treatment for cSSTIs or for complicated intraabdominal infections is 5–14 days. No dose adjustment is warranted in patients with mild-to-moderate hepatic impairment. In patients with severe liver disease, the initial dose of tigecycline should be 100 mg, followed by 25 mg every 12 hours. No dosage adjustment is necessary in patients with renal disease or in patients on hemodialysis. The safety and efficacy of tigecycline has not been tested in patients younger than 18 years.[49]

Contraindications/Cautions

In phase III clinical studies with 1415 patients, the most commonly reported adverse events were nausea (29.5%) and vomiting (19.7%). Nausea and vomiting generally occurred within the first 2 days of treatment. Only 1.3% of patients discontinued therapy due to nausea and 1.0% due to vomiting.[49]

Laboratory abnormalities reported during tigecycline treatment included increased prothrombin time and par-tial thromboplastin time, without significant bleeding episodes, increased blood urea nitrogen without con-comitant nephrotoxicity or increase in creatinine, and hyperbilirubinemia. Although in phase III clinical studies, infection-related serious adverse events were more frequently reported for subjects treated with tigecycline (6.7%) versus comparators (4.6%), the relationship of this outcome to treatment cannot be established due to differences between treatment groups at baseline.

Glycylglycines are structurally similar to tetracyclines and, therefore, may have similar adverse events such as photosensitivity, pseudotumor cerebri, and pancreatitis. Patients with a history of tetracycline hypersensitivity should be closely monitored if treated with tigecycline. Tigecycline may cause fetal harm if administered to pregnant women and may cause permanent tooth discoloration during development. It should not be administered simultaneously with amphotericin B or diltiazem. Coagulation studies should be monitored in patients on warfarin and tigecycline.[49]

Conclusions

Tigecycline monotherapy is as effective as combination therapy with vancomycin and aztreonam in the treatment of cSSTIs. This new agent thus holds promise as an alternative to the β-lactams and fluoroquinolones for the initial empiric treatment of serious dermatologic infections.[51]

RETAPAMULIN

Retapamulin (Figure 3.5) is an antibiotic ointment approved in April 2007 for the treatment of impetigo due to MSSA and *S. pyogenes*. It is a semisynthetic derivative of the compound pleuromutilin, which is isolated through fermentation from the fungus, *Clitopilus passeckerianus*.[52]

Mode of Action

Cellular Mechanisms. Retapamulin selectively inhibits bacterial protein synthesis by interacting with the ribosomal 50S subunit L3 protein to inhibit peptidyl transfer, block P-site interactions, and prevent the normal formation of active 50S ribosomal subunits.[53]

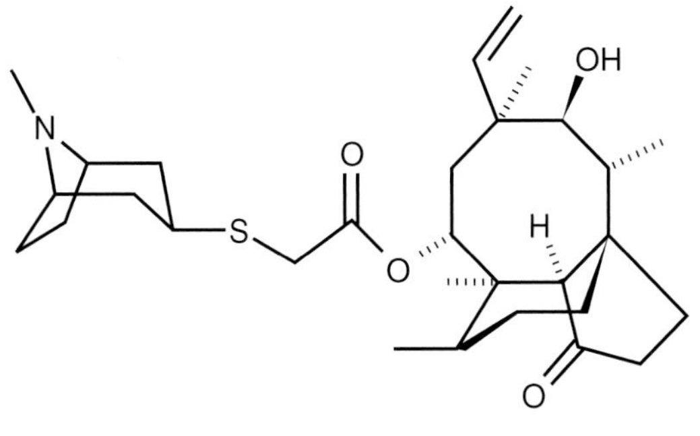

FIGURE 3.5: *Retapamulin.*

In Vitro Activity. Retapamulin is bacteriostatic against *S. aureus* and *S. pyogenes* at the retapamulin in vitro MIC for these organisms. At concentrations 1000× the in vitro MIC, retapamulin is bactericidal against these same organisms. Retapamulin demonstrates no in vitro target-specific cross-resistance with other classes of antibiotics. Two mechanisms that cause reduced susceptibility to retapamulin identified in vitro are mutations in ribosomal protein L3 or the presence of an efflux mechanism. Decreased susceptibility of *S. aureus* to retapamulin (highest retapamulin MIC was 2 mcg/mL) develops slowly in vitro via multistep mutations in L3 after serial passage in subinhibitory concentrations.[53]

Pharmacokinetics. Systemic exposure following topical application of retapamulin through intact and abraded skin was low. In a study of healthy adults, applying retapamulin ointment, 1%, once daily to intact skin (800 cm^2) and abraded skin (200 cm^2) under occlusion for up to 7 days, provided a median maximum concentration plasma value at day 7 of 3.5 ng/mL (range, 1.2–7.8 ng/mL) from intact skin and 9.0 ng/mL (range, 6.7–12.8 ng/mL) from abraded skin. Retapamulin is 94% bound to human plasma proteins regardless of concentration. Metabolism takes place mainly in the liver, and the major enzyme responsible for this is cytochrome P450 3A4. The apparent volume of distribution and retapamulin elimination in humans has not been investigated due to low systemic exposure after topical application.[54]

Clinical Indications

Retapamulin ointment is indicated for use in adults and pediatric patients 9 months old or older for the topical treatment of impetigo (up to 100 cm^2 in total area in adults or 2% total body surface area in pediatric patients 9 months old or older) due to MSSA or *S. pyogenes*.[52]

Retapamulin ointment has been studied in a multicenter, randomized, double-blind, placebo-controlled parallel-group study of adult and pediatric (9 months old or older) patients applying retapamulin ointment twice daily for 5 days for the treatment of impetigo. Of the 210 patients enrolled, 164 (78%) were younger than 13 years. Clinical success was defined as the absence of treated lesions, treated lesions that had become dry without crusts or without erythema compared with baseline, or treated lesions that improved such that no further antimicrobial treatment was required. At 2 days posttreatment, the ITT clinical population for retapamulin showed a success rate of 85.6% (119 of 139 patients) compared with the placebo group, which had a success rate of 52.1% (37 of 71 patients). A follow-up examination 9 days after treatment showed a similar trend: retapamulin with a success rate of 75.5% (105 of 139 patients) and placebo with 39.4% (28 of 71 patients).[55]

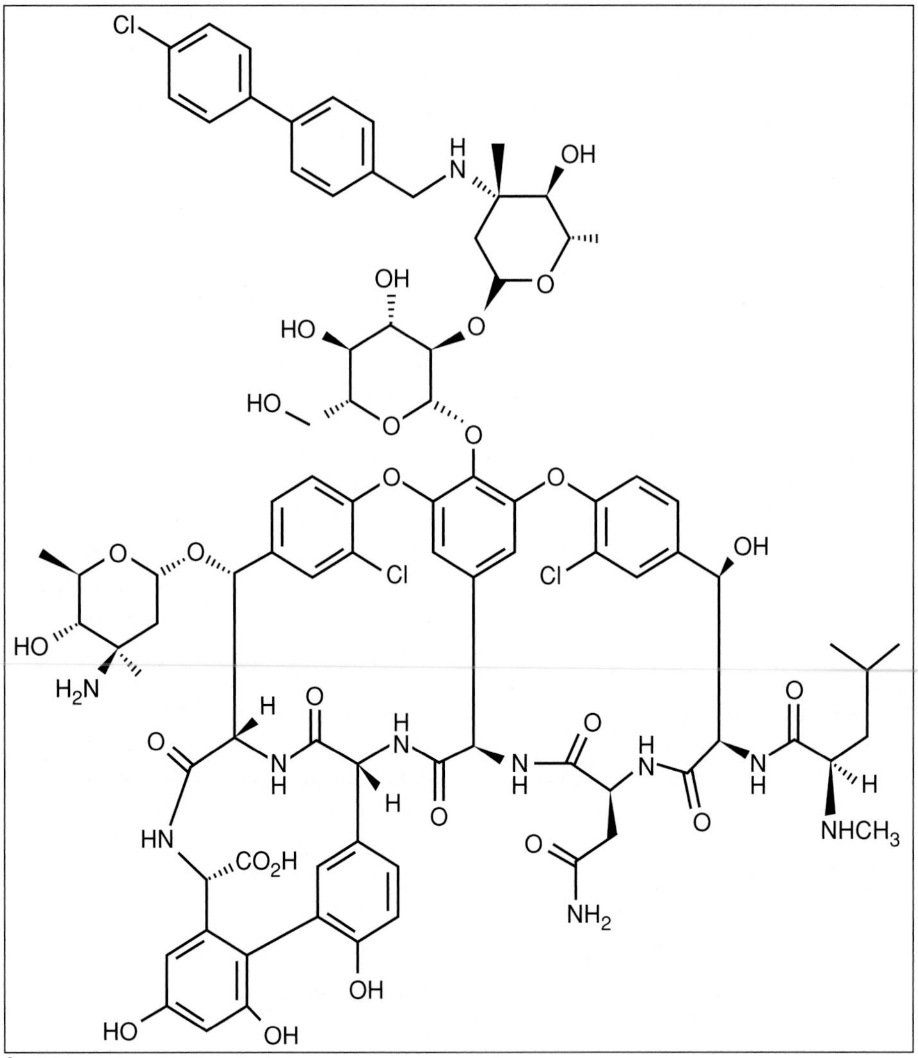

FIGURE 3.6: *Oritavancin (panel A) and dalbavancin (panel B).*

Dosage

A thin layer of retapamulin should be applied to the affected area (up to 100 cm^2 in total area in adults or 2% total body surface area in pediatric patients 9 months old or older) twice daily for 5 days. Retapamulin is dispensed as a 1% ointment in 5-, 10-, and 15-g tubes. To reduce the development of drug-resistant bacteria and maintain the efficacy of retapamulin, use should be limited to treatment or prevention of infections that are proven or strongly suspected to be caused by susceptible bacteria.[52]

Contraindications/Cautions

Retapamulin ointment is pregnancy category B; therefore, it should be used in pregnancy only when the potential benefits outweigh the risks and at the discretion of the prescribing physician.

Long-term studies in animals to evaluate carcinogenic potential have not been performed with retapamulin. It has shown no genotoxicity, and no evidence of impaired fertility has been found in either male or female rat studies.

The safety of retapamulin ointment has been assessed in a study of 2115 adult and pediatric patients who used at least one dose from a 5-day, twice-daily regimen. Adverse events rated by the investigator as drug-related occurred in 5.5% (116 of 2115) of patients treated with retapamulin ointment, the most common of which was application site irritation (1.4%). A safety profile has not been established for patients younger than 9 months.[52]

Due to low systemic exposure to retapamulin following topical application in patients, dosage adjustments for retapamulin are unnecessary when coadministered with CYP3A4 inhibitors, such as ketoconazole. From in vitro P450 inhibition studies and the low systemic

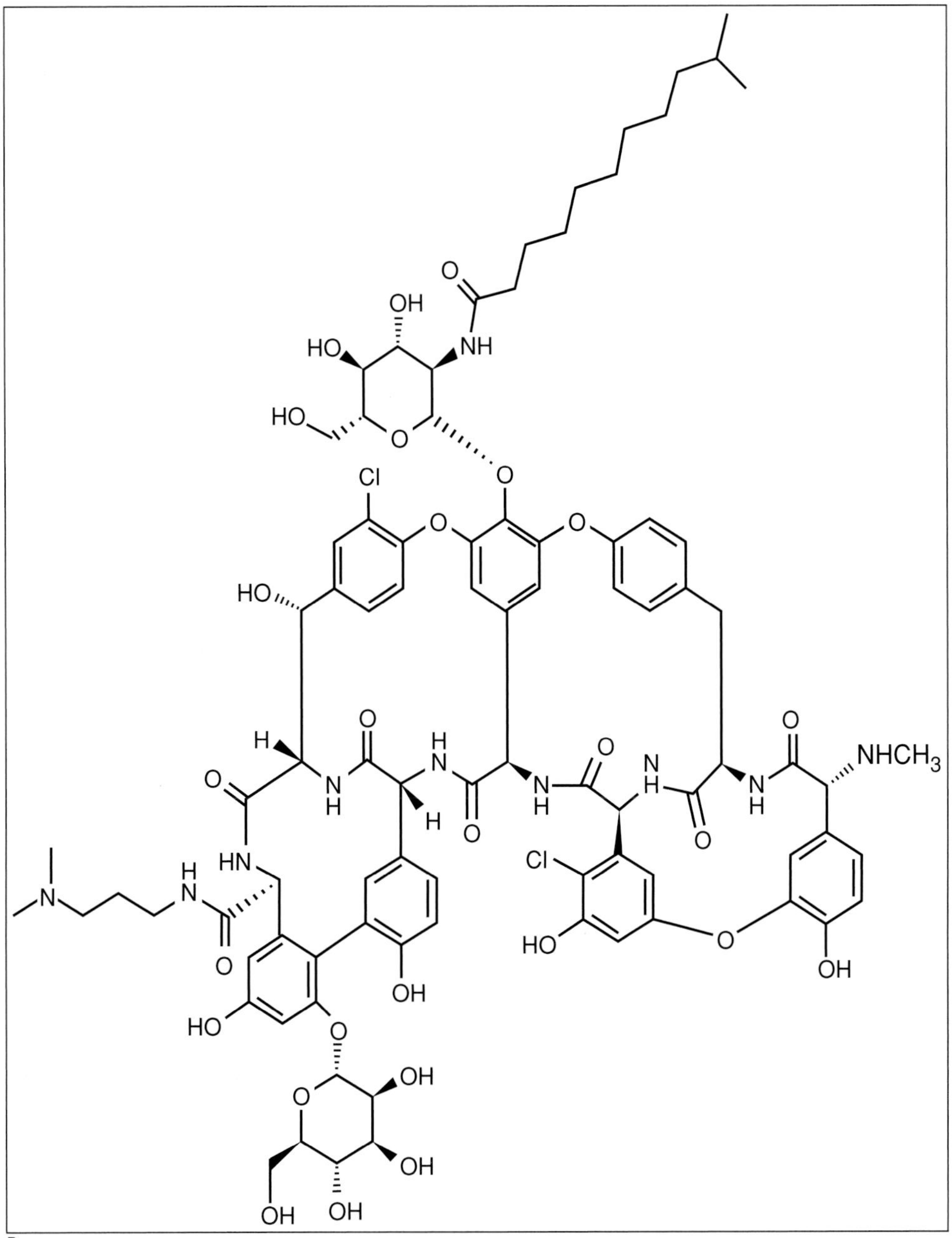

FIGURE 3.6   (continued)

exposure observed following topical application, retapamulin is unlikely to affect the metabolism of other P450 substrates. The effect of concurrent application of other topical products to the same area of skin has not been studied.[52]

ANTIBIOTICS IN DEVELOPMENT

Oritavancin (Figure 3.6A) and dalbavancin (Figure 3.6B) are two novel semisynthetic glycopeptide antibiotics, belonging to the same class as vancomycin. The antibac-

terial activity of glycopeptide antibiotics results from the inhibition of bacterial cell wall formation. More specifically, these antibiotics inhibit the biosynthesis of bacterial cell wall peptidoglycan. These two agents are currently in late stages of clinical development.

Oritavancin

Oritavancin is distinguished from vancomycin by its bactericidal activity against enterococci, *S. pneumoniae*, and staphylococci, including MRSA.[45,56,57] In animal studies

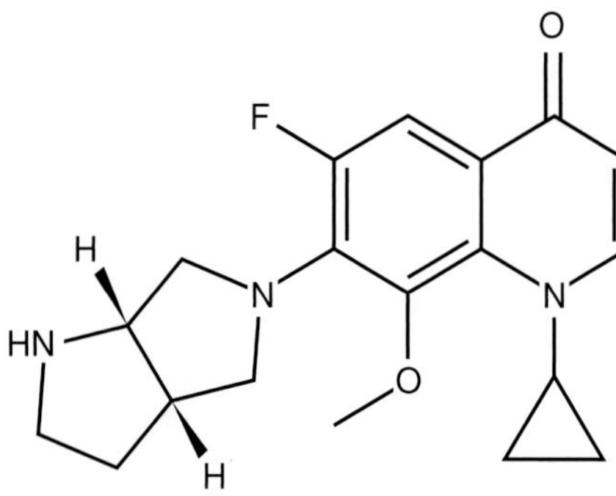

FIGURE 3.7: *Moxifloxacin.*

using rabbits as models, oritavancin was successful in the treatment of endocarditis from MRSA.[58] It also has a longer half-life (>10 days) than vancomycin, and thus can potentially offer a shorter duration of treatment.[59] In a phase III study, IV oritavancin (either 1.5 mg/kg or 3.0 mg/kg once daily) followed by placebo was compared to IV vancomycin (15 mg/kg once daily) followed by oral cephalexin in 517 patients with cSSTIs (unpublished data).[60] Efficacy was statistically equivalent in the two groups, with a 76% clinical success rate in the group that received oritavancin and 80% in patients who received vancomycin/cephalexin. Patients in the oritavancin group required an average of only 5.7 days of treatment (in those receiving the 1.5 mg/kg/d dosage) and 5.3 days of treatment (in those receiving the 3.0 mg/kg/d dosage), compared to 11.5 days in patients receiving vancomycin/cephalexin.[60]

A second phase III, double-blind, randomized trial in 1246 patients with cSSTIs corroborated that oritavancin 200 mg daily for 3–7 days IV followed by oral placebo was as effective as 10–14 days of vancomycin/cephalexin (vancomycin/cephalexin at 15 mg/kg twice daily for 3–7 days IV followed by 1000 mg twice-daily oral cephalexin). This study also demonstrated that significantly fewer patients experienced adverse events ($p < .001$) and fewer patients discontinued therapy ($p = .003$) in the oritavancin group than in the vancomycin/cephalexin group.[61]

Targanta Therapeutics submitted a new drug application to the FDA in February 2008 seeking to commercialize oritavancin in the treatment of complicated skin and skin structure infections.[62]

Dalbavancin

Dalbavancin also has been shown to be bactericidal in in vitro studies with gram-positive pathogens.[63] In animal studies, using rats as models, dalbavancin successfully treated lobar pneumonia from penicillin-resistant pneumococci.[30] In a phase I study, healthy volunteers received single IV infusions of dalbavancin in doses ranging from 70 mg to 360 mg.[63] Other subjects received dosages of 70 mg/day

for 7 days. All single and multiple dosages studied were well tolerated. Dalbavancin also was found to have a long half-life of approximately 10 days.[63] These results suggest that once-weekly dosing could be sufficient to provide trough concentrations that are bactericidal for staphylococcus.[63] In a phase II trial, 62 patients with SSTIs were treated with one of two dalbavancin-dosing regimens compared to a standard-of-care antibiotic.[64] Clinical success rates were 94.1% in patients receiving two doses of dalbavancin, given 1 week apart, 76.2% for standard-of-care treatment (dosing was daily for 7–21 days), and 64.3% for the group that received a single dose of dalbavancin (unpublished data).[64]

In a randomized, double-blind, phase III noninferiority study, two doses of dalbavancin (1000 mg given on day 1 followed by 500 mg given on day 8) were as well tolerated and as effective as linezolid given twice daily for 14 days for the treatment of patients with complicated SSTIs, including those infected with MRSA.[65]

As of December 2007, Pfizer received an approvable letter from the FDA and is in the process of providing the additional data requested.[66]

NEW INDICATIONS FOR QUINOLONES

The FDA recently added new indications for two newer generation fluoroquinolone class antibiotics. In April 2001, moxifloxacin (Figure 3.7), and in October 2002, gatifloxacin (Figure 3.8), were FDA approved for use in uncomplicated skin and skin structure infections. Several studies supported these new indications. In one multicenter trial involving 410 patients with uncomplicated SSTIs, a once-daily gatifloxacin dose of 400 mg orally had a cure rate of 91%.[67] This compared to the control group, which received a once-daily oral dose of 500 mg of levofloxacin and had a cure rate of 84%. Another study examined the efficacy of moxifloxacin versus cephalexin in patients with uncomplicated skin infections.[68] The clinical effectiveness was 90% for the group receiving oral moxifloxacin (400 mg once daily) and 91% for the group receiving oral cephalexin (500 mg three times

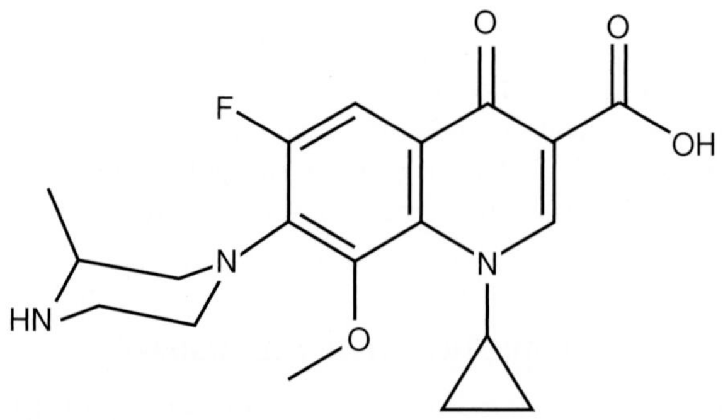

FIGURE 3.8: *Gatifloxacin.*

TABLE 3.2: Novel Antifungal Agents for Invasive Fungal Infections

Generic name	Brand name	Mechanism of action	Dosage	Indications
Voriconazole	Vfend®	Interferes with fungal cell wall synthesis by inhibiting 14α-demethylase synthesis of ergosterol	200 mg BID PO or 3–6 mg/kg BID IV for 14 d after resolution of symptoms	Candida, IFIs, drug of choice for aspergillus
Posaconazole	Noxafil®		200–400 mg BID PO	Candida, IFIs
Anidulafungin	Eraxis®	Interferes with fungal cell wall synthesis by inhibiting 1,3-β-glucan synthase synthesis of 1–3-β-glucan	50–100 mg IV q24h for 14 d after symptom resolution	Candidemia/Candidosis

BID, twice daily; PO, per os (orally); IV, intravenous; IFI, invasive fungal infection.

daily). Both groups received the antibiotics for a total of 7 days. Other studies also have supported these findings.[69]

NEW ANTIFUNGAL AGENTS

The increasing burden of invasive fungal infections (IFIs), especially among hospitalized patients with immune compromise, has created an urgent need for novel antifungal therapies (Table 3.2). The two major causes of IFI are *Candida albicans* and *Aspergillus fumigatus*, although other emerging fungi, such as non-albicans Candida (particularly *Candida glabrata*), Fusarium, and Zygomycetes, are contributing to the need to expand our armamentarium of antifungal agents.[70]

VORICONAZOLE AND POSACONAZOLE

Voriconazole (Figure 3.9) and posaconazole (Figure 3.10) are new triazole agents with broad-spectrum activity against many fungi. As with all azole antifungal agents, voriconazole and posaconazole work by interfering with synthesis of the fungal cell wall element, ergosterol, through inhibition of cytochrome P450 14α-demthylase.[71] Voriconazole was FDA approved in 2002 for primary treatment of acute invasive aspergillosis and salvage therapy for rare but serious fungal infections caused by the pathogens *Scedosporium apiospermum* and Fusarium spp. Posaconazole was approved in 2006 and is indicated for prophylaxis of invasive Aspergillus and Candida infections in patients (13 years old or older) with immune compromise as well as for the treatment of oropharyngeal candidiasis, refractory to itraconazole and/or fluconazole.[72]

Voriconazole has become the drug of choice for treatment of invasive aspergillosis. In a study comparing voriconazole with amphotericin B in 277 patients with proven or probable aspergillosis, voriconazole led to better responses and improved survival and resulted in fewer severe side effects than the standard approach of initial therapy with amphotericin B.[73] Voriconazole may be administered both orally and IV. In clinical trials, oral (200 mg twice daily) and IV (3–6 mg/kg every 12 hours) doses have produced favorable response.[74] Side effects include dose-related, transient visual disturbances, skin eruption, and elevated hepatic enzyme levels.[74]

Two randomized multicenter trials have accessed the efficacy of posaconazole (200 mg orally twice daily) in preventing IFIs compared to standard azole therapy (fluconazole or itraconazole) in high-risk patients with neutropenia or graft versus host disease (GVHD). A prospective nonblinded study in high-risk neutropenic patients with neutropenia due to either acute myelogenous leukemia or myelodysplastic syndrome randomized 602 patients to receive posaconazole (*n* = 298) or either fluconazole or itraconazole (*n* = 304) until neutrophil recovery or occurrence of an IFI for up to 84 days.[75] Proven or probable infections were diagnosed in 7 patients (2%) in the posaconazole group versus 25 (8%) in the comparator group. The majority of breakthrough infections in the fluconazole/itraconazole arm were due to aspergillosis.

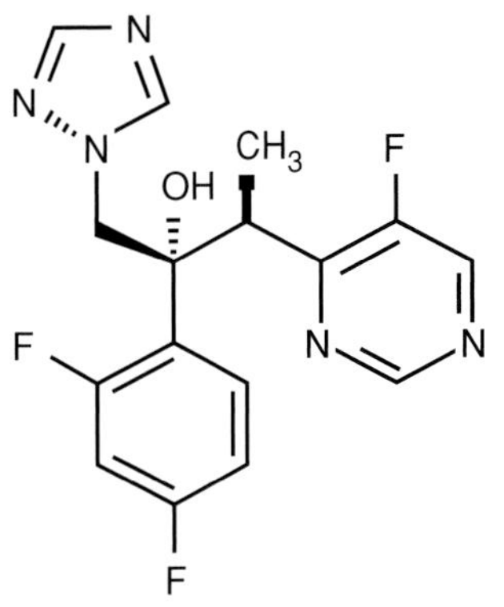

FIGURE 3.9: *Voriconazole.*

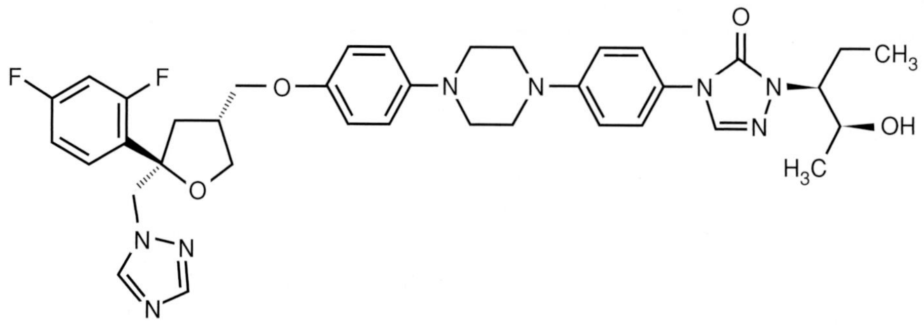

FIGURE 3.10: Posaconazole.

A double-blinded study in allogeneic hematopoietic stem cell transplant patients with GVHD compared fluconazole ($n = 299$) and posaconazole ($n = 301$) for up to 112 days or until the occurrence of an IFI. Proven or probable infections were diagnosed in 16 patients (5%) in the posaconazole group and 27 (9%) in the fluconazole group.[76]

An open-label, multicenter, case-controlled clinical trial of posaconazole as salvage therapy in patients with IFIs also has been completed for a variety of IFIs that failed primary therapy (predominantly amphotericin B regimens). Among patients with aspergillosis ($n = 107$), the global response to posaconazole therapy (800 mg/day divided doses) was 42% versus 26% response in contemporary control patients who received other licensed antifungal therapy ($p = .006$).[77]

Preliminary data also suggest that posaconazole may be an effective therapy for zygomycosis unresponsive to amphotericin B–based regimens.[78]

Posaconazole is available only as an oral suspension and requires intake with high-fat meals for absorption, limiting its utility in the critically ill patient. The major adverse effects appear to be gastrointestinal (including diarrhea, nausea, and vomiting) and rashes.[75,79]

ANIDULAFUNGIN

Anidulafungin (Figure 3.11) is a novel echinocandin approved in 2006 for the treatment of candidemia as well as for candidal esophagitis, abdominal abscesses, and peritonitis.[80] As with other echinocandins, anidulafungin blocks the synthesis of a major fungal cell wall component, 1–3-β-glucan, presumably via inhibition of 1,3-β-glucan synthase.[81]

In a multicenter, randomized, blinded trial that compared anidulafungin with fluconazole in the treatment of invasive candidosis, treatment was successful in 75.6% of patients treated with anidulafungin, as compared with 60.2% of those treated with fluconazole ($p = .01$).[82]

Another randomized, double-blind, double-dummy study compared the efficacy and safety of intravenous anidulafungin to that of oral fluconazole in 601 patients with esophageal candidiasis and found it to be statistically noninferior.[83]

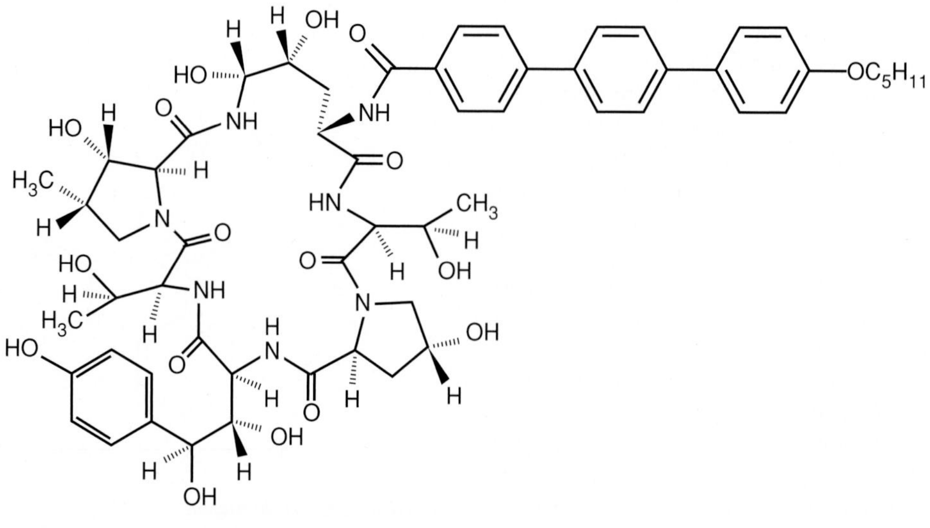

FIGURE 3.11: Anidulafungin.

TABLE 3.3: Novel Dosing of Antivirals for Herpes Labialis

Generic name	Brand name	Dosing
Famciclovir	Famvir®	1500-mg single dose
Valacyclovir	Valtrex®	2000 mg BID for 1 d

BID, twice daily.

Anidulafungin is available as an IV infusion. Dosing for esophageal candidiasis is 100 mg on day 1, then 50 mg/day. Dosing for candidemia is 200 mg on day 1, then 100 mg/day. Similar to other echinocandins, anidulafungin is well tolerated. In clinical trials, the most common side effects (<5%) are abnormal liver function tests.[83]

NEW DOSING OF ANTIVIRALS (Table 3.3)

Famciclovir

A recent study in 701 patients with herpes labialis demonstrated that famciclovir 1500-mg single-dose therapy was as efficacious as 750 mg twice daily for 1 day and reduced the time to healing of lesions by 2 days when taken within 2 hours of onset of prodromal symptoms.[84]

Valacyclovir

Two recent multicenter, randomized, double-blind, and placebo-controlled studies in 1524 and 1627 patients with herpes labialis demonstrated that high-dose therapy with valacyclovir (2000 mg twice daily for 1 day) shortened the healing time of lesions by 1 day compared with placebo and that a second day of therapy provided no additional benefit.[85]

CONCLUSIONS

SSTIs are commonly encountered in the emergency room setting. As MRSA infection becomes more prevalent and other resistant organisms continue to emerge, it is essential for physicians to be aware of newly approved antibiotics and their indications for use, dosing, and side-effect profiles. To maintain an armamentarium of useful agents, antimicrobials should be utilized only when necessary and in the context of local resistance patterns.

REFERENCES

1. Centers for Disease Control and Prevention (CDC). *Reduced susceptibility of Staphylococcus aureus to vancomycin – Japan, 1996.* MMWR Morb Mortal Wkly Rep 1997;46:624–6. Vancomycin.
2. Zyvox [package insert]. Kalamazoo, MI. Pharmacia & Upjohn Company. 2000.
3. Slee AM, Wuonola MA, McRipley RJ, et al. Oxazolidinones, a new class of synthetic antibacterial agents: in vitro and in vivo activities of DuP 105 and DuP 721. Antimicrob Agents Chemother. 1987;31:1791–7.
4. Swaney SM, Aoki H, Ganoza MC, Shinabarger DL. The oxazolidinone linezolid inhibits initiation of protein synthesis in bacteria. Antimicrob Agents Chemother. 1998;42:3251–5.
5. Eliopoulos GM, Wennersten CB, Gold HS, Moellering RC, Jr. In vitro activities in new oxazolidinone antimicrobial agents against enterococci. Antimicrob Agents Chemother. 1996;40:1745–7.
6. Ford CW, Hamel JC, Wilson DM, et al. In vivo activities of U-100592 and U-100766, novel oxazolidinone antimicrobial agents, against experimental bacterial infections. Antimicrob Agents Chemother. 1996;40:1508–13.
7. Jorgensen JH, McElmeel ML, Trippy CW. In vitro activities of the oxazolidinone antibiotics U-100592 and U-100766 against Staphylococcus aureus and coagulase-negative Staphylococcus species. Antimicrob Agents Chemother. 1997;41:465–7.
8. Mercier RC, Penzak SR, Rybak MJ. In vitro activities of an investigational quinolone, glycylcycline, glycopeptide, streptogramin, and oxazolidinone tested alone and in combinations against vancomycin-resistant Enterococcus faecium. Antimicrob Agents Chemother. 1997;41:2573–5.
9. Noskin GA, Siddiqui F, Stosor V, et al. In vitro activities of linezolid against important gram-positive bacterial pathogens including vancomycin-resistant enterococci. Antimicrob Agents Chemother. 1999;43:2059–62.
10. Clemett D, Markham A. Linezolid. Drugs. 2000;59:815–27.
11. Perry CM, Jarvis B. Linezolid: a review of its use in the management of serious gram-positive infections. Drugs. 2001;61:525–51.
12. Stevens DL, Smith LG, Bruss JB, et al. Randomized comparison of linezolid (PNU-100766) versus oxacillin-dicloxacillin for treatment of complicated skin and soft tissue infections. Antimicrob Agents Chemother. 2000;44:3408–13.
13. Stevens DL, Herr D, Lampiris H, et al. Linezolid versus vancomycin for the treatment of methicillin-resistant Staphylococcus aureus infections. Clin Infect Dis. 2002;34:1481–90.
14. Batts DH. Linezolid–a new option for treating gram-positive infections. Oncology (Williston Park). 2000;14(8 Suppl 6):23–9.
15. Wilson SE, Solomkin JS, Le V, et al. A severity score for complicated skin and soft tissue infections derived from phase III studies of linezolid. Am J Surg. 2003;185:369–75.
16. Auckland C, Teare L, Cooke F, et al. Linezolid-resistant enterococci: report of the first isolates in the United Kingdom. J Antimicrob Chemother. 2002;50:743–6.
17. Barrett JF. Linezolid Pharmacia Corp. Curr Opin Investig Drugs. 2000;1:181–7.
18. Bryson HM, Spencer CM. Quinupristin-dalfopristin. Drugs. 1996;52:406–15.
19. Cocito C, Di Giambattista M, Nyssen E, Vannuffel P. Inhibition of protein synthesis by streptogramins and related antibiotics. J Antimicrob Chemother. 1997;39 Suppl A:7–13.
20. Lamb HM, Figgitt DP, Faulds D. Quinupristin/dalfopristin: a review of its use in the management of serious gram-positive infections. Drugs. 1999;58:1061–97.

21. Landman D, Quale JM. Management of infections due to resistant enterococci: a review of therapeutic options. J Antimicrob Chemother. 1997;40:161–70.

22. Linden PK, Pasculle AW, McDevitt D, Kramer DJ. Effect of quinupristin/dalfopristin on the outcome of vancomycin-resistant Enterococcus faecium bacteraemia: comparison with a control cohort. J Antimicrob Chemother. 1997;39 Suppl A:145–51.

23. Nichols RL, Graham DR, Barriere SL, et al. Treatment of hospitalized patients with complicated gram-positive skin and skin structure infections: two randomized, multicentre studies of quinupristin/dalfopristin versus cefazolin, oxacillin or vancomycin. Synercid Skin and Skin Structure Infection Group. J Antimicrob Chemother. 1999;44:263–73.

24. Fagon J, Patrick H, Haas DW, et al. Treatment of gram-positive nosocomial pneumonia. Prospective randomized comparison of quinupristin/dalfopristin versus vancomycin. Nosocomial Pneumonia Group. Am J Respir Crit Care Med. 2000;161(3 Pt 1):753–62.

25. Moellering RC, Linden PK, Reinhardt J, et al.. The efficacy and safety of quinupristin/dalfopristin for the treatment of infections caused by vancomycin-resistant Enterococcus faecium. Synercid Emergency-Use Study Group. J Antimicrob Chemother. 1999;44:251–61.

26. Olsen KM, Rebuck JA, Rupp ME. Arthralgias and myalgias related to quinupristin-dalfopristin administration. Clin Infect Dis. 2001;32:e83–6.

27. Rubinstein E, Prokocimer P, Talbot GH. Safety and tolerability of quinupristin/dalfopristin: administration guidelines. J Antimicrob Chemother. 1999;44 Suppl A:37–46.

28. Stamatakis MK, Richards JG. Interaction between quinupristin/dalfopristin and cyclosporine. Ann Pharmacother. 1997;31:576–8.

29. Eliopoulos GM. Quinupristin-dalfopristin and linezolid: evidence and opinion. Clin Infect Dis. 2003;36:473–81.

30. Abbanat D, Macielag M, Bush K. Novel antibacterial agents for the treatment of serious gram-positive infections. Expert Opin Investig Drugs. 2003;12:379–99.

31. Wesson KM, Lerner DS, Silverberg NB, Weinberg JM. Linezolid, quinupristin/dalfopristin, and daptomycin in dermatology. Clin Dermatol. 2003;21:64–70.

32. Boaretti M, Canepari P, Lleo MM, Satta G. The activity of daptomycin on Enterococcus faecium protoplasts: indirect evidence supporting a novel mode of action on lipoteichoic acid synthesis. J Antimicrob Chemother. 1993;31:227–35.

33. Canepari P, Boaretti M, Lleo MM, Satta G. Lipoteichoic acid as a new target for activity of antibiotics: mode of action of daptomycin (LY146032). Antimicrob Agents Chemother. 1990;34:1220–6.

34. Alborn WE, Jr., Allen NE, Preston DA. Daptomycin disrupts membrane potential in growing Staphylococcus aureus. Antimicrob Agents Chemother. 1991;35:2282–7.

35. Allen NE, Alborn WE, Jr., Hobbs JN, Jr. Inhibition of membrane potential-dependent amino acid transport by daptomycin. Antimicrob Agents Chemother. 1991;35:2639–42.

36. Woodworth JR, Nyhart EH, Jr., Brier GL, et al. Single-dose pharmacokinetics and antibacterial activity of daptomycin, a new lipopeptide antibiotic, in healthy volunteers. Antimicrob Agents Chemother. 1992;36:318–25.

37. Garrison MW, Vance-Bryan K, Larson TA, et al. Assessment of effects of protein binding on daptomycin and vancomycin killing of Staphylococcus aureus by using an in vitro pharmacodynamic model. Antimicrob Agents Chemother. 1990;34:1925–31.

38. Rybak MJ, Bailey EM, Lamp KC, Kaatz GW. Pharmacokinetics and bactericidal rates of daptomycin and vancomycin in intravenous drug abusers being treated for gram-positive endocarditis and bacteremia. Antimicrob Agents Chemother. 1992;36:1109–14.

39. Tally FP, Zeckel M, Wasilewski MM, et al. Daptomycin: a novel agent for gram-positive infections. Expert Opin Investig Drugs. 1999;8:1223–38.

40. Rybak MJ, Hershberger E, Moldovan T, Grucz RG. In vitro activities of daptomycin, vancomycin, linezolid, and quinupristin-dalfopristin against Staphylococci and Enterococci, including vancomycin-intermediate and -resistant strains. Antimicrob Agents Chemother. 2000;44:1062–6.

41. Stephenson J. Researchers describe latest strategies to combat antibiotic-resistant microbes. JAMA. 2001;285:2317–8.

42. Strahilevitz J, Rubinstein E. Novel agents for resistant gram-positive infections–a review. Int J Infect Dis. 2002;6 Suppl 1:S38–46.

43. Cubicin [package insert]. Lexington, MA: Cubist Pharmaceuticals; 2003.

44. Hanberger H, Nilsson LE, Maller R, Isaksson B. Pharmacodynamics of daptomycin and vancomycin on Enterococcus faecalis and Staphylococcus aureus demonstrated by studies of initial killing and postantibiotic effect and influence of Ca2+ and albumin on these drugs. Antimicrob Agents Chemother. 1991;35:1710–16.

45. Allen NE, Nicas TI. Mechanism of action of oritavancin and related glycopeptide antibiotics. FEMS Microbiol Rev. 2003;26:511–32.

46. U.S. Food and Drug Administration Center for Drug Evaluation and Research: Priority Drug and Biologic Approvals in Calendar Year 2005. Accessed October 2, 2008. Available from: www.fda.gov/cder/rdmt/internetpriority05.htm.

47. Garrison MW, Neumiller JJ, Setter SM. Tigecycline: an investigational glycylcycline antimicrobial with activity against resistant gram-positive organisms. Clin Ther. 2005;27:12–22.

48. Bergeron J, Ammirati M, Danley D, et al. Glycylcyclines bind to the high-affinity tetracycline ribosomal binding site and evade Tet(M)- and Tet(O)-mediated ribosomal protection. Antimicrob Agents Chemother. 1996;40:2226–8.

49. Tigecycline [package insert]. Madison, NJ: Wyeth; Accessed October 2, 2008. Available from: http://www.wyeth.com/hcp/tygacil.

50. Ellis-Grosse EJ, Babinchak T, Dartois N, et al. The efficacy and safety of tigecycline in the treatment of skin and skin-structure infections: results of 2 double-blind phase 3 comparison studies with vancomycin-aztreonam. Clin Infect Dis. 2005;41 Suppl 5:S341–53.

51. Fraise AP. Tigecycline: the answer to beta-lactam and fluoroquinolone resistance? J Infect. 2006;53:293–300.

52. Altabax [package insert]. GlaxoSmithKline, Research Triangle Park, NC.

53. Jones RN, Fritsche TR, Sader HS, Ross JE. Activity of retapamulin (SB-275833), a novel pleuromutilin, against selected

resistant gram-positive cocci. Antimicrob Agents Chemother. 2006;50:2583–6.

54. Abramovits W, Gupta A, Gover M. Altabax (retapamulin ointment), 1%. Skinmed. 2007;6:239–40.

55. Oranje AP, Chosidow O, Sacchidanand S, et al. Topical retapamulin ointment, 1%, versus sodium fusidate ointment, 2%, for impetigo: a randomized, observer-blinded, noninferiority study. Dermatology. 2007;215:331–40.

56. Barrett JF. Oritavancin. Eli Lilly & Co. Curr Opin Investig Drugs. 2001;2:1039–44.

57. Mercier RC, Stumpo C, Rybak MJ. Effect of growth phase and pH on the in vitro activity of a new glycopeptide, oritavancin (LY333328), against Staphylococcus aureus and Enterococcus faecium. J Antimicrob Chemother. 2002;50:19–24.

58. Kaatz GW, Seo SM, Aeschlimann JR, et al. Efficacy of LY333328 against experimental methicillin-resistant Staphylococcus aureus endocarditis. Antimicrob Agents Chemother. 1998;42:981–3.

59. Woodford N. Novel agents for the treatment of resistant gram-positive infections. Expert Opin Investig Drugs. 2003;12:117–37.

60. Wasilewski MM, Disch D, McGill J, et al. Equivalence of shorter course therapy with oritavancin compared to vancomycin-cephalexin in complicated skin/skin structure infections. Program and abstracts of the 41st Interscience Conference on Antimicrobial Agents and Chemotherapy; 2001 Dec 16–19; Chicago, IL.

61. Giamarellou H, O'Riordan W, Haas H, et al. Phase 3 trial comparing 3–7 days of oritavancin vs. 10–14 days of vancomycin/cephalexin in the treatment of patients with complicated skin and skin structure infections (cSSSI). Abstr Intersci Conf Antimicrob Agents Chemother. Athens, Greece; 2003.

62. Targanta Therapeutics. Press release. Targanta submits oritavancin new drug application. Cambridge, MA. http://en .newspeg.com/Targanta-submits-orvita-vancin-new-drug-application-4801102.html. Accessed February 11, 2008.

63. Steiert M, Schmitz FJ. Dalbavancin (Biosearch Italia/Versicor). Curr Opin Investig Drugs. 2002;3:229–33.

64. Vesicor Inc. Press release. Vesicor announces positive phase 2 study results with dalbavancin for skin and soft tissue infections. Fremont, CA September 5, 2002.

65. Jauregui LE, Babazadeh S, Seltzer E, et al. Randomized, double-blind comparison of once-weekly dalbavancin versus twice-daily linezolid therapy for the treatment of complicated skin and skin structure infections. Clin Infect Dis. 2005;41:1407–15.

66. Pfizer Mediaroom. Pfizer receives approvable letter from FDA for Dalbavancin. New York. Available from: http://mediaroom.pfizer.com/portal/site/pfizer/index. jsp?ndmViewId=news_view&newsId=20071221005672& newsLang=en. Accessed February 2, 2008.

67. Tarshis GA, Miskin BM, Jones TM, et al. Once-daily oral gatifloxacin versus oral levofloxacin in treatment of uncomplicated skin and soft tissue infections: double-blind, multicenter, randomized study. Antimicrob Agents Chemother. 2001;45:2358–62.

68. Parish LC, Routh HB, Miskin B, et al. Moxifloxacin versus cephalexin in the treatment of uncomplicated skin infections. Int J Clin Pract. 2000;54:497–503.

69. Muijsers RB, Jarvis B. Moxifloxacin in uncomplicated skin and skin structure infections. Drugs. 2002;62:967–73.

70. Nierengarten M. Invasive fungal infections. 43rd Annual Interscience Conference on Antimicrobial Agents and Chemotherapy. September 14–17, 2003; Chicago, IL.

71. Kale P, Johnson LB. Second-generation azole antifungal agents. Drugs Today (Barc). 2005;41:91–105.

72. U.S. Food and Drug Administration. FDA approves novel medicine to prevent invasive fungal infections. September 18, 2006. [Cited February 1, 2008]. Available from: http://www. fda.gov/bbs/topics/NEWS/2006/NEW01455.html.

73. Herbrecht R, Denning DW, Patterson TF, et al. Voriconazole versus amphotericin B for primary therapy of invasive aspergillosis. N Engl J Med. 2002;347:408–15.

74. Sheehan DJ, Hitchcock CA, Sibley CM. Current and emerging azole antifungal agents. Clin Microbiol Rev. 1999;12:40–79.

75. Cornely OA, Maertens J, Winston DJ, et al. Posaconazole vs. fluconazole or –itraconazole prophylaxis in patients with neutropenia. N Engl J Med. 2007;356:348–59.

76. Ullmann AJ, Cornely OA, Burchardt A, et al. Pharmacokinetics, safety, and efficacy of posaconazole in patients with persistent febrile neutropenia or refractory invasive fungal infection. Antimicrob Agents Chemother. 2006;50:658–66.

77. Walsh TJ, Raad I, Patterson TF, et al. Treatment of invasive aspergillosis with posaconazole in patients who are refractory to or intolerant of conventional therapy: an externally controlled trial. Clin Infect Dis. 2007;44:2–12.

78. Greenberg RN, Mullane K, van Burik JA, et al. Posaconazole as salvage therapy for zygomycosis. Antimicrob Agents Chemother. 2006;50:126–33.

79. Noxafil (posaconazole) oral suspension [package insert]. Kenilworth, NJ: Schering-Plough.

80. Eraxis [package insert]. New York: Pfizer.

81. Kurtz MB, Abruzzo G, Flattery A, et al. Characterization of echinocandin-resistant mutants of Candida albicans: genetic, biochemical, and virulence studies. Infect Immun. 1996;64:3244–51.

82. Reboli AC, Rotstein C, Pappas PG, et al. Anidulafungin versus fluconazole for invasive candidiasis. N Engl J Med. 2007;356:2472–82.

83. Krause DS, Simjee AE, van Rensburg C, et al. A randomized, double-blind trial of anidulafungin versus fluconazole for the treatment of esophageal candidiasis. Clin Infect Dis. 2004;39:770–5.

84. Spruance SL, Bodsworth N, Resnick H, et al. Single-dose, patient-initiated famciclovir: a randomized, double-blind, placebo-controlled trial for episodic treatment of herpes labialis. J Am Acad Dermatol. 2006;55:47–53.

85. Spruance SL, Hill J. Clinical significance of antiviral therapy for episodic treatment of herpes labialis: exploratory analyses of the combined data from two valaciclovir trials. J Antimicrob Chemother. 2004;53:703–7.

CHAPTER 4

Immunomodulators and the "Biologics" in Cutaneous Emergencies

Batya B. Davidovici

Ronni Wolf

BIOLOGIC AGENTS are proteins or antibodies engineered to target specific molecules. They are derived from the products of living organisms. In recent years, numerous drugs of this type have been added to the therapeutic armamentarium in various disciplines of medicine. In dermatology, psoriasis is so far the only entity for which various drugs of this type are approved. Two main groups of biologic agents are used in psoriasis: The first is tumor necrosis factor (TNF) blockers, and the second group consists of inhibitors of T lymphocytes or antigen-presenting cells. Drugs from the anti-TNF group, as well as additional biological agents from other specialties, have been used off-label in numerous skin diseases – some of them are dermatologic emergencies. No doubt, the increasing development and use of these drugs will also extend the number of possible indications in numerous skin diseases. This chapter reviews the current reports on these agents and their use in various dermatologic emergencies (Table 4.1).

INFLIXIMAB

Infliximab (Remicade; Centocor, Inc., Horsham, PA) is a chimeric immunoglobulin G1 (IgG1) monoclonal antibody containing human constant regions and murine variable regions. It binds and inhibits both soluble and transmembrane TNF-α and activates lysis of cells that express transmembrane TNF-α via antibody-dependent and complement-dependent cytotoxic mechanisms.[1,2]

Indications

Indications for treating are rheumatoid arthritis (RA), psoriatic arthritis, ankylosing spondylitis, Crohn disease, ulcerative colitis, and moderate to severe plaque type psoriasis.

Dosage

Infliximab is administered as an intravenous (IV) 3–5 mg/kg (in most diseases) infusion, at initiation, week 2, and week 6 and subsequently every 8 weeks.[3]

Side Effects

Most of the side effects that have been described correspond to infusion reactions, which occur in approximately 10% of patients and tend not to be serious.[4,5]

Part of the infliximab molecule is murine in origin; hence, the development of neutralizing antibodies has been described in between 15% and 50% of cases, depending on the study.[6–9] The presence of neutralizing antibodies is associated with an increased risk of adverse effects, and a higher dose is required to control the disease.[9] The dose of infliximab is not associated with the development of antibodies, although an association has been described between low plasma levels of infliximab and the presence of antibodies.[9,10] The concomitant use of immunosuppressant drugs such as cyclosporine or methotrexate has been shown to reduce the rate of formation of neutralizing antibodies.[10,11]

Postmarketing data from infliximab-treated patients with RA, Crohn disease, or other indications for which infliximab is approved suggest a potential increased risk for events such as opportunistic infections, for example, tuberculosis, which can also present as disseminated or atypical disease,[12] lymphoma, demyelinating disease,[13–16] or congestive heart failure.[17–19] There is no evidence that TNF inhibitors increase the risk of new-onset cardiac failure in patients with RA.[20,21]

INFLIXIMAB IN DERMATOLOGIC EMERGENCIES

Blistering Diseases: Pemphigus Vulgaris

Pemphigus vulgaris (PV) is an autoimmune blistering disorder of the skin and mucous membranes that is characterized by autoantibodies directed against desmoglein (dsg) 1 and dsg 3. To date, two cases have been described of recalcitrant PV that was refractory to multiple immunosuppressant treatments and that responded rapidly to treatment with infliximab.[22,23] In both cases, the patients showed a lasting response (4 months and 104 weeks).

TABLE 4.1: Clinical Use of Immunimodulators and Biologics in Dermatologic Emergencies

	Infliximab	Etanercept	Rituximab	Intravenous immunoglobulin (IVIG)
Pemphigus vulgaris (PV)	+		++[a]	+++
Pemphigus foliaceus			+	++
Paraneoplastic pemphigus			+	
Bullous pemphigoid		+		++
Cicatrical pemphigoid	+	+		+++
Graft versus host disease	+++[b]	++	++	
SJS-TEN	++			+++[c]
Angioedema with hypereosinophilia				+

+ Weak evidence; ++ few supporting reports; +++ many supporting reports.
SJS–TEN, Stevens–Johnson syndrome and toxic epidermal necrolysis.
[a] Close surveillance for infectious complications in PV patients undergoing rituximab treatment is warranted.
[b] For patients with skin and gastrointestinal tract manifestations who have not responded to standard treatment.
[c] Because randomized, controlled, multicenter studies are lacking, treatment with IVIG cannot be considered the standard of care in these cases. Special caution is indicated in elderly patients with preexisting renal dysfunction.

Cicatricial Pemphigoid

Cicatricial pemphigoid (CP), also referred to as mucous membrane pemphigoid, is a heterogenous group of autoimmune subepithelial blistering disorders that primarily affect mucosal surfaces and, occasionally, the skin. CP was previously called benign mucousal pemphigoid; the outcome might not always be benign. Due to its scarring nature, blindness, deafness, or strictures of the pharynx, esophagus, larynx, and/or anogenital mucosa may result. Autoantibodies to β 4-integrin, α 6-integrin, bullous pemphigoid (BP) antigen (Ag) 1, BP Ag 2, and laminin 5 have been detected. Patients with ocular CP have elevated levels of serum TNF-α compared with normal controls.[24] Only one case, however, has been described of BP of the mucous membranes.[25] The process was highly aggressive and refractory to multiple immunosuppressant treatments, in which treatment with infliximab at standard dose and regimen led to remission of the disease in the oral and pharyngeal mucosa and stabilized the ocular involvement, which had led to the loss of an eye.

Acute Graft Versus Host Disease

Acute graft versus host disease (GVHD) has three different phases. TNF-α is implicated both in the first phase, in which it is released from tissues damaged by the conditioning, and the third phase, in which it is released by effector T lymphocytes from the donor, previously activated by antigen-presenting cells from the recipient and that lead to cell death via a mechanism of cytotoxicity involving TNF-α.[26]

GVHD is a serious condition in which the first-line treatment involves high doses of systemic corticosteroids followed by maintenance treatment with tacrolimus or cyclosporine. Failure to control the disease with these drugs represents a difficult therapeutic challenge.[27] Biologic agents acting against TNF-α have proven to be effective in some cases and represent a first-line option for the treatment of refractory cases. Some authors have observed greater efficacy with infliximab in cases of gastrointestinal (GI) GVHD,[28,29] suggesting that TNF-α is the main cytokine involved in the GI disease, whereas in cutaneous and hepatic GVHD, other cytokines also play an important role.[28,30]

Some case series have been published on the treatment of acute GVHD with infliximab. Most involve patients in whom severe acute disease that was refractory to traditional treatments (immunosuppressant drugs and corticosteroids) developed following bone-marrow transplant. In these case series the treatment consisted of four infusions of 10 mg/kg infliximab per week.

The most extensive series[28] included 37 patients with acute GVHD treated with infliximab, of whom 28% had corticosteroid-resistant disease. After treatment with a median of 4 weekly infusions of infliximab, 10 mg/kg, the complete response rate was 75% for skin, 81% for upper GI tract involvement, 91% for lower GI tract, and 35% for liver involvement. Twenty-two patients died during the study; in 13 of these patients, death was attributed to GVHD progression. No other adverse events were reported.

It has been reported[31] that a series of 11 patients with steroid-refractory acute GVHD, 10 of whom had grade III or IV disease were treated with infliximab. Only 2 patients had a complete response; although 5 of 9 remaining patients had a partial resolution of symptoms, all 9 eventually died. Six of these deaths were attributed to progressive GVHD and infection.

Two retrospective studies have been published in which promising results were obtained with this disease in patients refractory to corticosteroid therapy. The first was a series of 21 patients (14% grade I, 67% grade II, and 19% grade III/IV) treated with infliximab as monotherapy.[27] An overall response of 70% was obtained for cutaneous disease (67% complete response), 75% for intestinal involvement (65% complete response), and 25% for hepatic disease (25% complete response). The overall survival was 38%, but all of the patients went on to develop chronic GVHD.

The second study reported similar results in a series of 32 patients diagnosed with grade II/IV GVHD.[30] An adequate response to infliximab was obtained in 59% of the patients (19% complete responses and 40% partial responses), and all the 13 unresponsive patients died. Other series published on acute or refractory GVHD treated with infliximab encompass a total of 12 patients, of whom 10 died during follow-up, despite 8 having shown improvement with treatment.[32–34] Only two cases have been reported in which treatment of acute GVHD with infliximab (in both cases associated with adalizumab) led to a good response.[35]

A phase III study has been published comparing the efficacy of infliximab with that of standard treatment in previously untreated patients.[36] Fifty-eight patients were randomized to receive either infliximab plus methylprednisolone or methylprednisolone alone. Overall response rates were not significantly different between the two treatment arms (63% response to methylprednisolone alone compared with 66% response to a combination of methylprednisolone and infliximab). There were no differences in response by organ. This study suggests that early treatment with infliximab does not provide added benefit in patients who have not developed steroid-resistant disease.

Chronic GVHD

An initial study[28] also described 22 patients with chronic GVHD treated with a median of 4 weekly 10 mg/kg infusions of infliximab in addition to prednisone and other immunosuppressive therapy. Researchers observed a response rate of 57% for skin disease and 92% for GI tract disease in these patients. Eleven patients died, with GVHD identified as the cause of death in 7 patients. Another study, which describes 10 patients with steroid-dependent chronic GVHD treated with etanercept, reported more than 50% alleviation of symptoms in 5 of 8 patients who were able to be evaluated and a steroid dose reduction in 6 patients.[37] Finally, Reidi and colleagues[38] reported a series of 13 patients, including 8 patients with chronic GVHD, who received infliximab salvage therapy. Patients received a median of 4 weekly 10 mg/kg infusions, and responses were observed in 7 of 8 patients with skin disease who could be evaluated, 6 of 7 patients with GI tract disease, and 0 of 4 patients with liver disease.

Infliximab was well tolerated in most cases. It is not easy to reach a conclusion regarding whether it increases the risk of infection, because patients with refractory GVHD are immunocompromised and it is difficult to determine the extent to which infliximab is involved. A retrospective cohort study concluded that infliximab was associated with an increased risk of invasive fungal infections; this result suggests that the possibility of increased infections with infliximab should be further evaluated.[39] Anti-TNF therapy seems to show promise for some patients with acute and chronic GVHD, although mortality rates for steroid-resistant disease remain high. On the basis of the reports presented herein, infliximab appears to be most effective for skin and GI tract manifestations and less effective for liver involvement and high-grade acute disease for those patients who have not responded to previous treatments. It does not appear to offer improvements over standard treatments in previously untreated patients.

There are no human studies available to resolve the important issue of whether infliximab may be associated with reduced transplant efficacy as confirmed in animals following inhibition of transmembrane TNF-α.

Stevens–Johnson Syndrome and Toxic Epidermal Necrolysis

Stevens–Johnson syndrome (SJS) and toxic epidermal necrolysis (TEN) are rare, acute, life-threatening mucocutaneous diseases characterized by widespread sloughing of the epidermis and of the mucous membranes. Mortality is high and increases with more extensive skin detachment. Although its exact role is not completely clear, TNF-α appears to be important in the pathogenesis of TEN. Various studies have found that blister fluid from patients with TEN has an elevated concentration of TNF-α compared with fluid from patients with thermal burns.[40–42] It has been proposed that TNF-α may contribute to epidermal necrosis both indirectly, through recruitment of T cells and macrophages, and directly, through facilitation of keratinocyte apoptosis.[43,44] Others suggest, however, that the TNF-α found in blister fluid is produced by keratinocytes as a defensive response to T-cell invasion.[45] Interestingly, thalidomide, which is thought to act, at least in part, through inhibition of TNF-α in other disorders, was shown to be detrimental in the treatment of TEN in a randomized, controlled trial.[46] Patients in the thalidomide-treated group had higher levels of blister fluid and serum TNF-α than did control patients, possibly indicating that thalidomide caused a paradoxical increase of TNF-α in these patients. Others have suggested that thalidomide's stimulatory effect on T cells may have led to the deterioration observed in the treated patients.[47]

The first case of TEN treated satisfactorily with a single dose of infliximab (5 mg/kg) was published in 2002.[48] Since then, 5 more cases have been reported,[49–51] all with a satisfactory response. The most recent publication reported 3 cases with characteristics compatible with exanthematous pustulosis and TEN that had not responded to corticosteroids or suspension of the drug responsible for the symptoms. However, in these cases a single dose of infliximab led to a rapid and significant improvement.[51]

Further research is clearly needed to elucidate the role of TNF-α in therapy for TEN and to determine whether TNF antagonists will have efficacy beyond these case reports.

ETANERCEPT

Etanercept (Enbrel, Amgen and Wyeth, Thousand Oaks, CA) is a recombinant fusion protein comprising domains of the 75-kDa human TNF receptor and human IgG, which inhibits the activity of TNF-α. It binds primarily to soluble TNF-α as well as to TNF-β (lymphotoxin). Binding of etanercept prevents TNF from binding to its receptor, thereby effectively blocking its physiologic functions.[52] Unlike infliximab, it does not fix complement, cause antibody-dependent cytotoxicity, or trigger T-cell apoptosis.[53]

Indications

Etanercept is approved for use in moderate-to-severe RA, polyarticular-course juvenile RA, ankylosing spondylitis, psoriatic arthritis, and chronic moderate-to-severe plaque psoriasis.

Dosage

Recommended dosage for RA, ankylosing spondylitis, and psoriatic arthritis is 25 mg administered subcutaneously twice weekly for the entire year. For plaque-type psoriasis patients; the dosing is 50 mg twice weekly for the first 12 weeks followed by a "step-down" to 25 mg twice weekly for another 12 weeks or 25 mg twice weekly for 24 weeks.

Side Effects

Injection site reactions occurring in up to 40% of patients were the most commonly reported adverse events in initial psoriasis clinical trials. The rate of development of anti-etanercept antibodies has been less than 10% and has not been observed to lead to decreased efficacy.[54–56]

Long-term data from clinical trials in many patients receiving etanercept for other indications, such as RA, found infrequent cases of tuberculosis, a possible increased risk of certain neurological disorders in patients taking etanercept, rare cases of pancytopenia, and congestive heart failure.[14]

ETANERACEPT IN DERMATOLOGIC EMERGENCIES

Autoimmune Blistering Diseases: CP

One report has been published of the successful use of etanercept for the treatment of CP. The case involved a patient with CP affecting the oral cavity, with disease resistant to multiple previous treatments.[57] Etanercept, 25 mg twice weekly, was added to the existing regimen of prednisone 60 mg daily. The patient received 6 doses of etanercept. No new blister formation was observed after the third dose, and clinical remission persisted through 8 months of follow-up. During this time, the prednisone dosage was tapered to 1 mg daily.

Bullous Pemphigoid

BP is a subepidermal autoimmune blistering disorder characterized by autoantibodies against BP Ag 1 and 2. BP is usually considered a benign bullous disease, particularly compared with PV, yet it can be lethal, especially in elderly patients or in those with higher daily steroid dosage at discarge. In BP, TNF levels are elevated in both serum and blister fluid and correlate with the severity of disease.[58–62] TNF is thought to mediate the recruitment of neutrophils and eosinophils seen in the inflammatory infiltrate of BP lesions and stimulate the production of other inflammatory cytokines and chemokines.[59] Yet, there has only been one case report of a patient with concurrent BP and psoriasis who was successfully maintained on a regimen of etanercept after initial treatment with prednisone.[63] Etanercept allowed for the successful tapering of prednisone without a rebound of the patient's psoriasis or a flare of the BP.

Acute GVHD

Etanercept has also shown promise in the treatment of acute GVHD. One case report has been published of an 11-year-old girl who achieved complete remission of steroid-refractory acute GVHD with etanercept treatment.[64] In a phase II study of etanercept in combination with the interleukin-2 receptor antibody daclizumab for the treatment of steroid-refractory acute GVHD in 21 patients, the overall response rate was 67% (38% complete response, 29% partial response).[65] Similarly, in a pilot study on the use of etanercept in combination with tacrolimus and methylprednisolone as initial therapy for 20 patients with stage II or III acute GVHD, 75% of patients had a complete response within 4 weeks of initiating treatment.[66]

Chronic GVHD

A study that describes 10 patients with steroid-dependent chronic GVHD treated with etanercept reported more than 50% alleviation of symptoms in 5 of 8 patients who were able to be evaluated and steroid dose reduction in

6 patients.[37] Etanercept was administered at 25 mg twice weekly for 4 weeks and then once weekly for the subsequent 4 weeks; all patients were receiving concurrent steroids, and 4 patients were started on a regimen of mycophenolate mofetil with etanercept.

Two patients died before completion of the study (1 of relapsed malignancy, 1 of thrombotic thrombocytopenic purpura), and 1 patient died of infection after relapse of chronic GVHD that occurred after study completion.

RITUXIMAB

Rituximab (Rituxan; Genentech, South San Francisco, CA) is a chimeric murine–human monoclonal antibody to CD20, which induces depletion of B cells in vivo.[67] In 1997, rituximab became the first monoclonal antibody approved for treatment of malignancy. Rituximab's cytotoxicity is mediated by several mechanisms, including antibody-dependent cytotoxicity, complement-mediated lysis, and direct disruption of signaling pathways and triggering of apoptosis. The contribution of each mechanism remains unclear, and different mechanisms may predominate in the treatment of different diseases.[68,69] Rituximab results in depletion of normal as well as malignant B cells, leading to investigation of its use in autoimmune disorders, including systemic lupus erythematosus (SLE), RA, autoimmune thrombocytopenia and hemolytic anemia, antineutrophil cytoplasmic antibody-positive vasculitis, and autoimmune neuropathies.[70,71]

Indications

Rituximab is indicated for use in non-Hodgkin lymphoma (NHL) and active RA not responsive to one or more TNF antagonist therapies. It is also currently approved for the treatment of relapsed or refractory, low-grade or follicular, CD20[+] B-cell lymphoma.[72]

Dosage

The initial approved dosing regimen was four weekly infusions of 375 mg/m[2].

Side Effects

CD20 is a B-cell specific antigen expressed on the surface of B lymphocytes throughout differentiation from the pre-B cell to the mature B-cell stage, but not on plasma cells or stem cells.[67,73] Because plasma cells and hematopoietic precursors are spared, immunoglobulin levels do not fall dramatically and B cells typically begin to return to the circulation within 6 months of therapy.[74,75] Hence the incidence of serious adverse effects with rituximab is relatively low. Infusion reactions are the most common adverse effects. In most cases, these are mild and occur only with the first infusion.[74,76] In a recent study of rituximab for the treatment of RA, infections occurred in 35% of patients in the rituximab group compared with 28% of the placebo group. Serious infections occurred in 2% of the rituximab group compared with 1% of the placebo group.[77] Human antichimeric antibodies (HACAs) developed in less than 1% of patients treated for lymphoma.[78] The incidence may be higher, however, in patients treated for autoimmune disease. In a study of rituximab for SLE, 6 of 18 patients developed detectable HACAs; no patients had adverse events related to this development.[79]

RITUXIMAB IN DERMATOLOGIC EMERGENCIES PV

Rituximab treatment for PV was first attempted based on its success in other autoimmune disorders and the hypothesis that depletion of B cells would result in a decrease in production of the disease-causing autoantibodies.[80] The correlation of decreases in PV autoantibody levels with clinical improvement in most of the patients in whom these levels were reported would seem to support this theory.[80–83] This theory also seems to suggest that most PV autoantibodies are produced by CD20[+] B-cell clones susceptible to rituximab. Alternatively, it has been suggested that, although both plasma cells and memory B cells may produce PV autoantibodies, plasma cells, which are CD20 negative and thus resistant to the effects of rituximab, may predominantly produce the less pathogenic IgG1 dsg 3 antibodies whereas the memory B cells produce the IgG4 antibodies responsible for disease.

This alternative theory might explain the clinical improvement in the face of persistently elevated PV antibody titers observed in one patient and the improvement preceding decreased titers in a second patient.[84,85] Furthermore, in SLE patients, for whom clinical improvement after rituximab is regularly correlated with B-cell depletion but not to any decrease in other serologic markers or autoantibody levels, it is postulated that disruption of antibody-independent activities of B cells, including presentation of autoantigens, costimulation of T cells, and regulation of leukocytes and dendritic cells, are central to rituximab's effect on the disease.[79] Thus the critical effects of rituximab in PV may expand beyond decreasing autoantibody production to inhibiting B-cell–dependent activation of T cells. The successful use of rituximab in more than 20 individual cases of treatment-resistant PV including a case of refractory childhood PV and also two cases of pemphigus foliaceus has been reported.[80–94] In all cases, the standard course of 375 mg/m[2] given IV for 4 weekly doses was administered initially. B-cell depletion after treatment was seen in all cases in which it was measured. In most cases, the response to rituximab was rapid, with improvement noted within the first 2–4 weeks. There is one report of a delayed response, where improvement was not noted for 3 months and clinical remission was not achieved until 11 months after the first infusion.

Rituximab was well tolerated in most of the cases reported, consistent with the observations made in lymphoma and other autoimmune disorders; however, four cases of serious infections were reported, including pneumonia, a relapse of septic arthritis of the hip,[85] sepsis,[84] and fatal *Pneumocystis carinii* (now renamed *Pneumocystis jiroveci*) pneumonia.[91] These events may indicate that close surveillance of PV patients undergoing rituximab treatment is warranted until the incidence of infectious complications in this patient population is better understood.

Paraneoplastic Pemphigus

Paraneoplastic pemphigus (PNP) usually presents with painful mucosal ulcerations and polymorphous skin lesions, which usually progress to blistering eruptions on the trunk and extremities. A wide variety of both benign and malignant tumors are found in these patients. Most reported patients die from their underlying tumors, whereas others may die from bronchiolitis obliterans. Before 2005, there were 5 reported cases of PNP treated with rituximab. Three case reports describe significant improvement in oral and cutaneous lesions after rituximab[95–97] and two reports describe less successful treatment, especially with regard to mucosal lesions.[98,99] Rituximab in a patient with PNP with underlying NHL was treated with rituximab and, not surprisingly, the patient improved, given the indication for treatment of NHL with rituximab.[100]

The mechanism of action in PNP is likely similar to that in PV. In addition, most of the treated patients experienced at least partial remission of the underlying neoplasm, and this remission may have contributed to the observed improvement.

Chronic GVHD

The use of rituximab in the treatment of chronic GVHD has been reported in 4 series of patients. The largest series is a phase I/II trial featuring 21 patients with steroid-refractory disease.[101] Cutaneous findings included both sclerodermatous and lichenoid changes. Patients were treated with one, two, or three cycles of 4 weekly infusions of rituximab at a dose of 375 mg/m². Patients were allowed to continue stable doses of other immunosuppressive medications throughout the trial. The overall clinical response rate was 70%, including 2 complete responses. Cutaneous and musculoskeletal manifestations of GVHD were more amenable to treatment with rituximab than were mucous membrane and hepatic manifestations. The other 3 series showed similar findings.[102–104] Experimental evidence has indicated that T cells and natural killer cells play a central role in the pathogenesis of chronic GVHD.[105] Evidence for the involvement of B cells has also been accumulating. In one mouse model of chronic GVHD, an expansion of host B cells directed by CD41 T cells is a critical step in the development of disease.[104,106,107] It has been shown that fibrosis in the tight-skin mouse, a model for systemic sclerosis, is mediated by hyperactive B cells that overexpress CD19 and overproduce interleukin-6 (IL-6).[108] This process may also be active in the sclerodermatous change seen in chronic GVHD.[102] Patients with chronic GVHD develop autoantibodies similar to those seen in patients with autoimmune disease.[102,105,109] Antibodies to Y chromosome–encoded minor histocompatibility antigens are generated after sex-mismatched transplantation, and the presence of these antibodies has been correlated to the occurrence of GVHD.[110,111] In the trial discussed previously, there were four male recipients of female grafts.[101] All four of these patients had autoantibodies before treatment that became undetectable after rituximab. The autoantibodies disappearance correlated with a clinical response. The success of rituximab in these 4 series provides further evidence for the role of B cells in chronic GVHD. These studies have also raised the question of whether rituximab may be useful in localized or systemic scleroderma, and trials are currently under way in these diseases.

IV IMMUNOGLOBULIN

IV immunoglobulin (IVIG) comes in several formulations, including Carimune (ZLB Behring LLC, King of Prussia, PA), Flebogamma (Instituto Grifols, SA, Barcelona, Spain), Gammagard (Baxter, Deerfield, IL), Gammar (Aventis Behring, King of Prussia, PA), Gamunex (Talecris Biotherapeutics, Research Triangle Park, NC), Octagam (Octapharma, Lachen, Switzerland), Panglobulin (ZLB Behring LLC), Polygam (Baxter), Gamimune (Talecris Biotherapeutics), Iveegam (Oesterreichisches Institut fuer Hemoderivate GmbH. OIH), Sandoglobulin (Novartis, Basel, Switzerland), and Venoglobulin (Alpha Therapeutic Corporation, Grifols USA, Los Angeles, CA). The mechanism of action of IVIG is not fully understood and likely differs depending on the disease. The following mechanisms have been proposed: lowering the levels of deleterious autoantibodies through idiotypic antibodies contained in IVIG;[112,113] accelerating the catabolism of pathogenic IgG by saturating neonatal Fc receptors (FcRns) with exogenous IgG;[114,115] inhibiting the pathogenic activation of T lymphocytes by antibodies to CD4 and other T-cell receptors;[116,117] inhibiting complement-mediated damage;[118] interfering with the production, release, and function of inflammatory cytokines including interleukins-2, -3, -4, -5, -6, and -10, TNF-α, and granulocyte–macrophage colony-stimulating factor;[119–123] inhibiting the differentiation and maturation of dendritic cells, thereby reducing the activation of harmful T cells;[124] increasing sensitivity to corticosteroids;[125] and inhibition of thromboxane A₂ and endothelin, and increased prostacyclin secretion.[126]

Indications

Indications are primary and secondary immunodeficiencies (i.e., common variable immunodeficiency), X-linked agammaglobulinemia, severe combined immunodeficiency, Wiskott–Aldrich syndrome, acute and chronic immune thombocytopenic purpura, human immunodeficiency virus (HIV) in children, chronic lymphocytic leukemia, Kawasaki disease, Guillain–Barré syndrome, and GVHD prophylaxis in patients receiving allogeneic bone-marrow transplantation.

Dosage

IVIG is composed of human plasma derived from pools of 1000–15,000 donors.[126] The purified immunoglobulin is stabilized with glucose, maltose, sucrose, mannitol, sorbitol, glycine, or albumin. IVIG is made up of more than 90% IgG and small amounts of IgM and IgA. Generally, IVIG is given at a dose of 2 g/kg over 3–5 days, but can be given over 2 days in younger patients with normal renal and cardiovascular function. The total amount of immunoglobulins that are infused with a 2 g/kg dose is enormous; serum IgG will increase approximately fivefold.[127]

Side Effects

Infusion-related side effects occur in less than 10% of patients and are generally mild and self-limiting.[127] These side effects include headache, myalgias, flushing, fever, chills, fatigue, nausea or vomiting, low backache, chest discomfort, hypotension and hypertension, tachycardia, and skin eruptions such as eczematous reactions, urticaria, lichenoid reactions, pruritus of the palms, and petechiae.[127,128] Premedication with acetaminophen, nonsteroidal antiinflammatory agents, antihistamines, or low-dose IV corticosteroids may help avoid other infusion-related adverse events. Myalgias, chills, and chest discomfort may occur during the first hour and respond to halting the infusion for 30 minutes and then resuming it at a slower rate. Postinfusion fatigue, fever, or nausea may occur and last for 24 hours. More serious, but rare, adverse events include thromboembolic events; therefore, caution should be used in patients with risk factors for thromboembolism, immobilized patients, and patients with hyperviscosity syndromes. The U.S. Food and Drug Administration has identified high infusion rates and high doses as potential risk factors for thromboembolism in patients at risk.[129] Hemolytic anemia may result from blood group antibodies. Neutropenia is common, transient (lasting 2–14 days), and usually benign.[130-132] Some clinicians [132] hypothesize that this may be a result of antineutrophil antibodies contained in IVIG or from induction of neutrophil apoptosis. Transfusion-related acute lung injury is characterized by severe respiratory distress occurring 1–6 hours after the infusion. Aseptic meningitis,[129,133] occurs in 11% of patients receiving IVIG, particularly patients with a history of migraines.[134] It usually presents with headache, meningismus, and photophobia. Severe anaphylactic reactions may occur in patients with IgA deficiency. Acute tubular necrosis, which is usually reversible, may occur in individuals with preexisting renal disease and/or diabetes mellitus and in the elderly population.[135] Acute tubular necrosis has been associated with IVIG products containing high concentrations of sucrose.[134]

As with all blood products, there is a risk of transmission of viruses and prions. IVIG is screened for hepatitis B and C, HIV, and syphilis, and donors are carefully selected. Additional methods to remove viruses include physical inactivation with heat and chemical inactivation with solvents, low pH detergents, and caprylate. Caprylate and nanofiltration may also remove prions.[136] Transmission of hepatitis B virus and HIV has not been reported.[134] Transmission of hepatitis C virus has been reported and was likely a result of inadequate viral inactivation steps. The introduction of improved viral inactivation techniques, such as incubation at pH 4 and solvent–detergent treatment, should minimize this risk.[137] In addition, there remains the risk of transmission of currently unidentified infectious agents.

IVIG IN DERMATOLOGIC EMERGENCIES

PV

IVIG has been shown to be effective in the treatment of PV in numerous studies. IVIG lowers antibody titers to dsg 1 and dsg 3, often making them undetectable.[138–143] In the two largest studies, which are from one institution, 42 patients were treated with IVIG (2 g/kg every 4 weeks) until control was achieved, as defined by healing of old lesions and no new lesions.[139,141] The interval between IVIG treatments was then gradually increased to every 16 weeks. Prednisone and immunosuppressive agent (ISA) were tapered off during this time in all patients; IVIG was then used as monotherapy. Treatment with IVIG led to a clinical remission in all patients. In another study,[141] control was achieved after a mean of 4.5 months, prednisone was tapered off after a mean of 4.8 months, and ISAs were tapered off after a mean of 2.9 months. Both studies were prospective, but uncontrolled.

There have been an additional two case series and six case reports of the successful treatment of 23 patients with PV with IVIG.[142,144–150] A juvenile case of PV had excellent response to IVIG.[151]

In France, 12 patients with PV were treated with IVIG, and 8 were in complete remission at the end of treatment.[152] In Mexico, a patient with refractory PV was treated with IVIG and healing of her mucosal and cutaneous lesions was seen in 3 weeks;[153] however, IVIG was not always successful; nine case reports of treatment failures from other institutions have been reported.[154–157] In one case, the patient received only one cycle of IVIG.[156]

Pemphigus Foliaceus

Pemphigus foliaceus (PF) is an autoimmune blistering disorder characterized by autoantibodies to dsg 1. Sami and colleagues[158] conducted a prospective study of 8 patients with severe (body surface area >30%) steroid-resistant PF. Patients were treated with IVIG (2 g/kg every 4 weeks) until they were completely healed. The interval between IVIG treatments was then gradually lengthened to every 16 weeks. All patients attained clinical control after a mean of 4 months. Prednisone was tapered off in a mean of 2.9 months; IVIG was used as monotherapy thereafter.

Eleven patients with PF were treated with IVIG (2 g/kg every 4 weeks) until they were completely healed.[159] The interval between IVIG treatments was then gradually lengthened to every 16 weeks. All patients cleared after an average of 5.3 months of therapy. Prednisone was tapered off in a mean of 4.5 months and other ISAs after a mean of 2.6 months; IVIG was used as monotherapy thereafter. All 11 patients maintained remission after discontinuation of IVIG for a mean follow-up time of 18.6 months. A case of eyelid PF was also responsive to IVIG.

Overall, there are three published case series[158–160] and two case reports[161,162] of the successful use of IVIG in the treatment of PF. IVIG lowers antibody titers to dsg 1, often making them undetectable.[158] In all, at least 26 patients were treated successfully with IVIG for PF.[158–160,163]

Bullous Pemphigoid

There are two published case series[141,162,164] and three case reports ($n = 5$)[144,148,157] reporting the successful use of IVIG in the treatment of BP. There have been two reported treatment failures.[157] IVIG lowers autoantibody titers to both BP Ag 1 and Ag 2.[164]

In the only prospective study[141] 15 patients were treated with BP with IVIG (2 g/kg every 4 weeks). The interval between IVIG treatments was then gradually lengthened to every 16 weeks after patients cleared. All 15 patients cleared after a mean of 2.9 months and were able to discontinue prednisone after a mean of 3.3 months. IVIG was used as monotherapy thereafter. All 15 patients achieved sustained remission with a mean duration of follow-up off IVIG of 22.9 months.

Cicatricial Pemphigoid

CP was treated with IVIG, leading to improvement in the disease in more than 78 patients.[158,165–174] One patient had no response.[157] IVIG has been shown to lower titers of β4-integrin and α6-integrin in patients with CP.[165,166]

IVIG was effective in the treatment of CP in several prospective studies from one institution.[158,165,166,171,173,175,176] These patients were initially treated with corticosteroids and other ISAs, which were tapered off in all cases. Remission was generally attained in 4–5 months, and treatment with IVIG led to prolonged remissions that persisted after treatment with IVIG was discontinued. There have been two additional case reports of treatment successes and one treatment failure from other institutions.[157,169,172]

One study of 16 patients with stage 2 ocular CP compared IVIG with standard treatment with corticosteroids and ISAs.[176] Randomization was based on whether insurance would pay for IVIG. Eight patients (group A) were treated with IVIG (2 g/kg every 2–4 weeks) until control was achieved. The interval between IVIG treatments was then gradually lengthened to every 16 weeks, and corticosteroids and other ISAs were tapered off. The other 8 patients (group B) were treated with corticosteroids and other ISAs. The median times to remission for groups A and B were 4 and 8.5 months, respectively. There were no recurrences for group A, whereas 5 of 8 patients in group B experienced a recurrence. No patients in group A experienced progression, whereas 4 of 8 patients in group B progressed to stage 3.

In summary, large, multicenter, randomized, controlled studies of IVIG for the treatment of autoimmune bullous diseases have not been performed; nevertheless, the results of the studies presented here suggest that IVIG can be considered as a viable treatment option for patients with PV, PF, BP, and CP who are resistant to conventional therapy, have experienced complications as a result of conventional therapy, or for whom conventional therapy is contraindicated. In most cases, patients were treated in conjunction with corticosteroids or other ISAs, which could often be tapered or discontinued. Maintenance infusions are generally required to maintain remission, although the interval between treatments can be lengthened to 16 weeks. Some patients have maintained prolonged remissions after treatment with IVIG, and indeed a consensus statement on the use of IVIG in the treatment of autoimmune mucocutaneous blistering diseases has been published.[129] The authors recommend a starting dose of 2 g/kg every 3–4 weeks until control can be achieved. Thereafter, the interval between treatments can be lengthened in 2-week intervals to 16 weeks. For patients with aggressive ocular CP it appears that more frequent IVIG treatments every 2 weeks are required to gain control. Because the vast majority of the literature on the use of IVIG for autoimmune bullous diseases was generated at a single institution, additional reports of large case series by other authors are encouraged, as a retrospective series published by the Mayo Clinic failed to obtain such strikingly positive results.[157]

Stevens–Johnson Syndrome and Toxic Epidermal Necrolysis

Patients with SJS–TEN may have a high mortality rate. The average reported mortality of patients with TEN in large series ranges between 25% and 35%.[177–181] The mortality of patients with SJS is lower.[178] Current treatment options are limited to supportive care in intensive care and burn units. Treatment with corticosteroids and other immunosuppressives is controversial and may result in higher incidences of complications secondary to sepsis.

The mechanism of action of IVIG in the treatment of TEN is not fully understood, but may partially be explained by the observation of Viard and colleagues[182] that antibodies present in IVIG block Fas-mediated keratinocyte apoptosis in vitro. Because of the low prevalence of TEN, randomized controlled studies have not been performed. The evidence for and against IVIG in the treatment of SJS and TEN consists of two open-label, prospective studies and a number of retrospective case series and case reports.[182–209] In addition, there has been one report of the successful use of IVIG (2.4 g/kg given over 3 days) as prophylaxis for a patient with recurrent episodes of SJS from IV contrast.[210] Particularly in regard to case reports, one should not forget the possibility of a selection bias toward reporting favorable results.

IVIG has been reportedly used in at least 162 cases of TEN,[183–186,209,211–214] with improved survival in the majority of patients. IVIG and plasmapheresis used in 5 patients with severe TEN had a mortality of 20%, compared with the 66% mortality as predicted by a severity-of-illness score for TEN (SCORTEN).[211] In an Asian series, 8 patients with TEN and 4 with overlap TEN–SJS demonstrated a 91.6% survival after treatment with IVIG.[212]

In a German study of 9 patients, 5 were treated with IVIG. The rate of mortality was 20% in the IVIG group compared with 50% in the non-IVIG group.[215] In 38 Korean patients, 14 received IVIG, and a trend of lower actual rate of mortality compared with predicted rate was discovered.[190]

A pediatric case of a 2-year-old-girl with TEN–SJS overlap was treated successfully with IVIG.[209] Another pediatric series from India of 10 patients had a rate of mortality of 0% when using low-dose IVIG to treat TEN.[216] A review of published case series found 156 patients treated with IVIG for TEN or SJS. The data reviewed, however, did not significantly demonstrate efficacy for IVIG.[217] Conversely, a 2006 review notes that 6 of 8 studies demonstrate benefit of IVIG at doses greater than 2 g/kg for TEN.[218]

Although caution should be used because comparison across studies is difficult as a result of differences in severity of disease, patient characteristics, efficacy variables, and outcome measures. Of the 11 studies, 8 concluded that IVIG was beneficial in the treatment of TEN, although in only one of the studies using a comparator group was a statistically significant result achieved.[185] Shortt and colleagues[186] concluded that IVIG was not beneficial in their retrospective series; although patients receiving IVIG experienced a lower mortality compared with historic control subjects, the difference was not statistically significant. There was also a trend toward less progression of skin sloughing in the IVIG-treated group compared with historic control subjects. A prospective, open-label study[184] and a retrospective study[192] also did not find IVIG to be beneficial in the treatment of TEN. The study by Bachot and colleagues[184] included patients with SJS. The study by Brown and colleagues[192] was confounded by the fact that 67% of the patients treated with IVIG also received concomitant corticosteroids. Brown and colleagues also used lower doses of IVIG than did most other studies (mean dose 1.6 g/kg). This finding is important, because Prins and colleagues[183] found a higher mortality with lower doses (mean 2.7 g/kg in survivors vs. 2 g/kg in those who died) in their retrospective review. Moreover, the number of days from onset of symptoms to treatment was 9.2 in the IVIG group versus 5.6 in the historic control group, although this difference was not statistically significant. Again, Prins and colleagues[183] found a higher mortality when treatment was delayed (6.8 days in survivors vs. 10.2 days in those who died). Because several studies did not include a comparator group, a compilation of mortality benefit from IVIG across studies is not possible.

Because of the lack of controlled, prospective, multicenter trials, strong conclusions regarding the effectiveness of IVIG in the treatment of TEN cannot be reached. Moreover, because IVIG is a biologic substance, there is variation in the final product between manufacturers and batch to batch that could affect results.[219] For example, if interruption of Fas-mediated cell death by antibodies in IVIG is the mechanism of its action in TEN, then batches that are lacking these antibodies will not be successful. Thus, the variability of different batches can account for the difference in results attained by Prins and colleagues[183] and Trent and colleagues,[185] who used multiple brands of IVIG and attained positive results, with Bachot and colleagues[184] and Shortt and colleagues,[186] who used one brand (Tegeline and Gamimune N, respectively) and did not attain positive results. The brand used in the study by Brown and colleagues[192] was not stated. Furthermore, Tegeline contains sucrose, which may be nephrotoxic. Bachot and colleagues[184] noted that mortality in their patients treated with IVIG mostly occurred in elderly patients with preexisting renal dysfunction.

Although the results from the majority of case series support the use of IVIG in the treatment of TEN and TEN–SJS overlap. Because randomized, controlled, multicenter studies are lacking, treatment with IVIG cannot be considered the standard of care in these cases.

Angioedema with Hypereosinophilia

Orson[220] treated a 54-year-old man with angioedema and hypereosinophilia with prednisone (40 mg/d) and IVIG (400 mg/kg every 3 weeks). The patient had a marked decrease in symptoms and eosinophil count after 6 weeks, and prednisone was tapered off in 6 months. Interestingly, when the brand of IVIG was changed from Panglobulin to Gamimune N, the patient's illness recurred. Retreatment with Panglobulin led to remission again. This case report emphasizes the biologic variability that may exist between brands of IVIG.

REFERENCES

1. Rapp SR, Feldman SR, Exum ML, et al. Psoriasis causes as much disability as other major medical diseases. J Am Acad Dermatol. 1999;41:401–7.

2. Henseler T, Christophers E. Disease concomitance in psoriasis. J Am Acad Dermatol. 1995;32:982–6.

3. Graves JE, Nunley K, Heffernan MP. Off-label uses of biologics in dermatology: rituximab, omalizumab, infliximab, etanercept, adalimumab, efalizumab, and alefacept (part 2 of 2). J Am Acad Dermatol. 2007;56:55–79.

4. Wasserman MJ, Weber DA, Guthrie JA, et al. Infusion-related reactions to infliximab in patients with rheumatoid arthritis in a clinical practice setting: relationship to dose, antihistamine pretreatment, and infusion number. J Rheumatol. 2004;31:1912–17.

5. Cheifetz A, Smedley M, Martin S, et al. The incidence and management of infusion reactions to infliximab: a large center experience. Am J Gastroenterol. 2003;98:1315–24.

6. Bendtzen K, Geborek P, Svenson M, et al. Treatment of rheumatoid arthritis (RA) with anti-TNF-alpha antibody (Remicade). Individual monitoring of bioavailability and immunogenicity–secondary publication. Ugeskr Laeger. 2007;169:420–3.

7. Baert F, Vermeire S, Noman M, et al. Management of ulcerative colitis and Crohn's disease. Acta Clin Belg. 2004;59:304–14.

8. Baert F, Noman M, Vermeire S, et al. Influence of immunogenicity on the long-term efficacy of infliximab in Crohn's disease. N Engl J Med. 2003;348:601–8.

9. Bendtzen K, Geborek P, Svenson M, et al. Individualized monitoring of drug bioavailability and immunogenicity in rheumatoid arthritis patients treated with the tumor necrosis factor alpha inhibitor infliximab. Arthritis Rheum. 2006;54:3782–9.

10. Vermeire S, Noman M, Van Assche G, et al. Autoimmunity associated with anti-tumor necrosis factor alpha treatment in Crohn's disease: prospective cohort study. Gastroenterology. 2003;125:32–9.

11. Farrell RJ, Alsahli M, Jeen YT, et al. Intravenous hydrocortisone premedication reduces antibodies to infliximab in Crohn's disease: a randomized controlled trial. Gastroenterology. 2003;124:917–24.

12. Hamilton CD. Infectious complications of treatment with biologic agents. Curr Opin Rheumatol. 2004;16:393–8.

13. Enayati PJ, Papadakis KA. Association of anti-tumor necrosis factor therapy with the development of multiple sclerosis. J Clin Gastroenterol. 2005;39:303–6.

14. Mohan N, Edwards ET, Cupps TR, et al. Demyelination occurring during anti tumor necrosis factor alpha therapy for inflammatory arthritides. Arthritis Rheum. 2001;44:2862–9.

15. Thomas CW, Jr., Weinshenker BG, Sandborn WJ. Demyelination during anti-tumor necrosis factor alpha therapy with infliximab for Crohn's disease. Inflamm Bowel Dis. 2004;10:28–31.

16. Tran TH, Milea D, Cassoux N, et al. Optic neuritis associated with infliximab. J Fr Ophtalmol. 2005;28:201–4.

17. Wolfe F, Michaud K. Lymphoma in rheumatoid arthritis: the effect of methotrexate and anti-tumor necrosis factor therapy in 18 572 patients. Arthritis Rheum. 2004;50:1740–51.

18. Chakravarty EF, Michaud K, Wolfe F. Skin cancer, rheumatoid arthritis, and tumor necrosis factor inhibitors. J Rheumatol. 2005;32:2130–5.

19. Askling J, Fored CM, Brandt L, et al. Risks of solid cancers in patients with rheumatoid arthritis and after treatment with tumour necrosis factor antagonists. Ann Rheum Dis. 2005;64:1421–6.

20. Cush JJ. Unusual toxicities with TNF inhibition: heart failure and drug-induced lupus. Clin Exp Rheumatol. 2004;22:Suppl 35:S141–7.

21. Wolfe F, Michaud K. Heart failure in rheumatoid arthritis: rates, predictors, and the effect of anti-tumor necrosis factor therapy. Am J Med. 2004;116:305–11.

22. Jacobi A, Shuler G, Hertl M. Rapid control of therapy refractory pemphigus vulgaris by treatment with the tumour necrosis factor-alpha inhibitor infliximab. Br J Dermatol. 2005;153:448–9.

23. Pardo J, Mercader P, Mahiques L, et al. Infliximab in the management of severe pemphigus vulgaris. Br J Dermatol. 2005;153:222–3.

24. Lee SJ, Li Z, Sherman B, Foster CS. Serum levels of tumor necrosis factor-alpha and interleukin-6 in ocular cicatricial pemphigoid. Invest Ophthalmol Vis Sci. 1993;34:3522–5.

25. Heffernan MP, Bentley DD. Successful treatment of mucous membrane pemphigoid with infliximab. Arch Dermatol. 2006;142:1268–70.

26. Jacobsohn DA. Novel therapeutics for the treatment of graft versus host disease. Expert Opin Investig Drugs. 2002;11:1271–80.

27. Couriel D, Saliba R, Hicks K, et al. Tumor necrosis factor-alpha blockade for the treatment of acute GVHD. Blood. 2004;104:649–54.

28. Couriel D, Hicks K, Ipolotti C. Infliximab for the treatment of graft-versus-host disease in allogenic transplant recipients: an update. Blood. 2000;46:400a.

29. Ross WA. Treatment of gastrointestinal acute graft versus host disease. Curr Treat Options Gastroenterol. 2005;8:249–58.

30. Patriarca F, Sperotto A, Damiani D, et al. Infliximab treatment for steroid-refractory acute graft-versus-host disease. Haematologica. 2004;89:1352–9.

31. Jacobsohn DA, Hallick J, Anders V, et al. Infliximab for steroid-refractory acute GVHD: a case series. Am J Hematol. 2003;74:119–24.

32. Kobbe G, Schneider P, Rohr U, et al. Treatment of severe steroid refractory acute graft versus host disease with infliximab, a chimeric human/mouse anti TNF alpha antibody. Bone Marrow Transplant. 2001;28:47–9.

33. Yamane T, Yamamura R, Aoyama Y, et al. Infliximab for the treatment of severe steroid refractory acute graft-versus-host disease in three patients after allogeneic hematopoietic transplantation. Leuk Lymphoma. 2003;44:2095–7.

34. Magalhaes-Silverman M, Lee CK, Hohl R, et al. Treatment of steroid refractory acute graft versus host disease with infliximab. Blood. 2001;98:5208a.

35. Rodriguez V, Anderson PM, Trotz BA, et al. Use of infliximab-daclizumab combination for the treatment of acute and chronic graft-versus-host disease of the liver and gut. Pediatr Blood Cancer. 2007;49:212–15.

36. Antin JH, Chen AR, Couriel DR, et al. Novel approaches to the therapy of steroid-resistant acute graft-versus-host disease. Biol Blood Marrow Transplant. 2004;10:655–68.

37. Chiang KY, Abhyankar S, Bridges K, et al. Recombinant human tumor necrosis factor receptor fusion protein as complementary treatment for chronic graft-versus-host disease. Transplantation. 2002;73:665–7.

38. Reidi I, Knoche J, Tanner AR, et al. Salvage therapy with infliximab for patients with severe acute and chronic GVHD abstract. Blood. 2001;98(Suppl):399a.

39. Marty FM, Lee SJ, Fahey MM, et al. Infliximab use in patients with severe graft-versus-host disease and other emerging risk factors of non-Candida invasive fungal infections in allogeneic hematopoietic stem cell transplant recipients: a cohort study. Blood. 2003;102:2768–76.

40. Correia O, Delgado L, Barbosa IL, et al. Increased interleukin 10, tumor necrosis factor alpha, and interleukin 6 levels in blister fluid of toxic epidermal necrolysis. J Am Acad Dermatol. 2002;47:58–62.

41. Paquet P, Nikkels A, Arrese JE, et al. Macrophages and tumor necrosis factor alpha in toxic epidermal necrolysis. Arch Dermatol. 1994;130:605–8.

42. Paquet P, Pierard GE. Soluble fractions of tumor necrosis factor-alpha, interleukin-6 and of their receptors in toxic epidermal necrolysis: a comparison with second-degree burns. Int J Mol Med. 1998;1:459–62.

43. Paquet P, Paquet F, Al Saleh W, et al. Immunoregulatory effector cells in drug-induced toxic epidermal necrolysis. Am J Dermatopathol. 2000;22:413–17.

44. Paul C, Wolkenstein P, Adle H, et al. Apoptosis as a mechanism of keratinocyte death in toxic epidermal necrolysis. Br J Dermatol. 1996;134:710–14.

45. Nassif A, Moslehi H, Le Gouvello S, et al. Evaluation of the potential role of cytokines in toxic epidermal necrolysis. J Invest Dermatol. 2004;123:850–5.

46. Wolkenstein P, Latarjet J, Roujeau JC, et al. Randomised comparison of thalidomide versus placebo in toxic epidermal necrolysis. Lancet. 1998;352:1586–9.

47. Klausner JD, Kaplan G, Haslett PA. Thalidomide in toxic epidermal necrolysis. Lancet. 1999;353:324.

48. Fischer M, Fiedler E, Marsch WC, Wohlrab J. Antitumour necrosis factor-alpha antibodies (infliximab) in the treatment of a patient with toxic epidermal necrolysis. Br J Dermatol. 2002;146:707–9.

49. Al-Shouli S, Abouchala N, Bogusz MJ, et al. Toxic epidermal necrolysis associated with high intake of sildenafil and its response to infliximab. Acta Derm Venereol. 2005;85:534–5.

50. Hunger RE, Hunziker T, Buettiker U, et al. Rapid resolution of toxic epidermal necrolysis with anti-TNF-alpha treatment. J Allergy Clin Immunol. 2005;116:923–4.

51. Meiss F, Helmbold P, Meykadeh N, et al. Overlap of acute generalized exanthematous pustulosis and toxic epidermal necrolysis: response to antitumour necrosis factor-alpha antibody infliximab: report of three cases. J Eur Acad Dermatol Venereol. 2007;21:717–19.

52. Mohler KM, Torrance DS, Smith CA, et al. Soluble tumor necrosis factor (TNF) receptors are effective therapeutic agents in lethal endotoxemia and function simultaneously as both TNF carriers and TNF antagonists. J Immunol. 1993;151:1548–61.

53. Yamauchi PS, Gindi V, Lowe NJ. The treatment of psoriasis and psoriatic arthritis with etanercept: practical considerations on monotherapy, combination therapy, and safety. Dermatol Clin. 2004;22:449–59, ix.

54. Bathon JM, Martin RW, Fleischmann RM, et al. A comparison of etanercept and methotrexate in patients with early rheumatoid arthritis. N Engl J Med. 2000;343:1586–93.

55. Nanda S, Bathon JM. Etanercept: a clinical review of current and emerging indications. Expert Opin Pharmacother. 2004;5:1175–86.

56. Weinblatt ME, Kremer JM, Bankhurst AD, et al. A trial of etanercept, a recombinant tumor necrosis factor receptor: Fc fusion protein, in patients with rheumatoid arthritis receiving methotrexate. N Engl J Med. 1999;340:253–9.

57. Sacher C, Rubbert A, Konig C, et al. Hunzelmann N. Treatment of recalcitrant cicatricial pemphigoid with the tumor necrosis factor alpha antagonist etanercept. J Am Acad Dermatol. 2002;46:113–15.

58. Ameglio F, D'Auria L, Bonifati C, et al. Cytokine pattern in blister fluid and serum of patients with bullous pemphigoid: relationships with disease intensity. Br J Dermatol. 1998;138:611–14.

59. D'Auria L, Cordiali Fei P, Ameglio F. Cytokines and bullous pemphigoid. Eur Cytokine Netw. 1999;10:123–34.

60. D'Auria L, Mussi A, Bonifati C, et al. Increased serum IL-6, TNF-alpha and IL-10 levels in patients with bullous pemphigoid: relationships with disease activity. J Eur Acad Dermatol Venereol. 1999;12:11–15.

61. Giacalone B, D'Auria L, Bonifati C, et al. Decreased interleukin-7 and transforming growth factor-beta1 levels in blister fluids as compared to the respective serum levels in patients with bullous pemphigoid. Opposite behavior of TNF-alpha, interleukin-4 and interleukin-10. Exp Dermatol. 1998;7:157–61.

62. Rhodes LE, Hashim IA, McLaughlin PJ, Friedmann PS. Blister fluid cytokines in cutaneous inflammatory bullous disorders. Acta Derm Venereol. 1999;79:288–90.

63. Yamauchi PS, Lowe NJ, Gindi V. Treatment of coexisting bullous pemphigoid and psoriasis with the tumor necrosis factor antagonist etanercept. J Am Acad Dermatol. 2006;54 Suppl:S121–2.

64. Andolina M, Rabusin M, Maximova N, Di Leo G. Etanercept in graft-versus-host disease. Bone Marrow Transplant. 2000;26:929.

65. Wolff D, Roessler V, Steiner B, et al. Treatment of steroid-resistant acute graft-versus-host disease with daclizumab and etanercept. Bone Marrow Transplant. 2005;35:1003–10.

66. Uberti JP, Ayash L, Ratanatharathorn V, et al. Pilot trial on the use of etanercept and methylprednisolone as primary treatment for acute graftversus-host disease. Biol Blood Marrow Transplant. 2005;11:680–7.

67. Reff ME, Carner K, Chambers KS, et al. Depletion of B cells in vivo by a chimeric mouse human monoclonal antibody to CD20. Blood. 1994;83:435–45.

68. Johnson PW, Glennie MJ. Rituximab: mechanisms and applications. Br J Cancer. 2001;85:1619–23.

69. Olszewski AJ, Grossbard ML. Empowering targeted therapy: lessons from rituximab Oncology (Williston Park). 2005;19:297–306; discussion 306, 308, 317–33.

70. Looney RJ, Anolik J, Sanz I. B cells as therapeutic targets for rheumatic diseases. Curr Opin Rheumatol. 2004;16: 180–5.

71. Silverman GJ, Weisman S. Rituximab therapy and autoimmune disorders: prospects for anti-B cell therapy. Arthritis Rheum. 2003;48:1484–92.

72. Grillo-Lopez AJ. Rituximab: an insider's historical perspective. Semin Oncol. 2000;27 Suppl:9–16.

73. Stashenko P, Nadler LM, Hardy R, Schlossman SF. Characterization of a human B lymphocyte-specific antigen. J Immunol. 1980;125:1678–85.

74. Maloney DG, Grillo-Lopez AJ, White CA, et al. IDEC-C2B8 (Rituximab) anti-CD20 monoclonal antibody therapy in patients with relapsed low-grade non-Hodgkin's lymphoma. Blood. 1997;90:2188–95.

75. Maloney DG, Liles TM, Czerwinski DK, et al. Phase I clinical trial using escalating single-dose infusion of chimeric anti-CD20 monoclonal antibody (IDEC-C2B8) in patients with recurrent B-cell lymphoma. Blood. 1994;84:2457–66.

76. Hainsworth JD. Safety of rituximab in the treatment of B cell malignancies: implications for rheumatoid arthritis. Arthritis Res Ther. 2003;Suppl 4;S12–16.

77. Emery P, Fleischmann R, Filipowicz-Sosnowska A, et al. The efficacy and safety of rituximab in patients with active rheumatoid arthritis despite methotrexate treatment: results of a phase IIB randomized, double-blind, placebo-controlled, dose ranging trial. Arthritis Rheum. 2006;54:1390–400.

78. McLaughlin P, Grillo-Lopez AJ, Link BK, et al. Rituximab chimeric anti-CD20 monoclonal antibody therapy for relapsed indolent lymphoma: half of patients respond to a four-dose treatment program. J Clin Oncol. 1998;16:2825–33.

79. Looney RJ, Anolik JH, Campbell D, et al. B cell depletion as a novel treatment for systemic lupus erythematosus: a phase I/II dose-escalation trialrituximab. Arthritis Rheum. 2004;50:2580–9.

80. Salopek TG, Logsetty S, Tredget EE. Anti-CD20 chimeric monoclonal antibody (rituximab) for the treatment of recalcitrant, life-threatening pemphigus vulgaris with implications in the pathogenesis of the disorder. J Am Acad Dermatol. 2002;47:785–8.

81. Dupuy A, Viguier M, Bedane C, et al. Treatment of refractory pemphigus vulgaris with rituximab (anti-CD20 monoclonal antibody). Arch Dermatol. 2004;140:91–6.

82. Goebeler M, Herzog S, Brocker EB, Zillikens D. Rapid response of treatment-resistant pemphigus foliaceus to the anti-CD20 antibody rituximab. Br J Dermatol. 2003;149:899–901.

83. Herrmann G, Hunzelmann N, Engert A. Treatment of pemphigus vulgaris with anti-CD20 monoclonal antibody (rituximab). Br J Dermatol. 2003;148:602–3.

84. Cooper HL, Healy E, Theaker JM, Friedmann PS. Treatment of resistant pemphigus vulgaris with an anti-CD20 monoclonal antibody (Rituximab). Clin Exp Dermatol. 2003;28:366–8.

85. Espana A, Fernandez-Galar M, Lloret P, et al. Long-term complete remission of severe pemphigus vulgaris with monoclonal anti-CD20 antibody therapy and immunophenotype correlations. J Am Acad Dermatol. 2004;50:974–6.

86. Virgolini L, Marzocchi V. Anti-CD20 monoclonal antibody (rituximab) in the treatment of autoimmune diseases. Successful result in refractory pemphigus vulgaris: report of a case. Haematologica. 2003;88:ELT24.

87. Arin MJ, Engert A, Krieg T, Hunzelmann N. Anti-CD20 monoclonal antibody (rituximab) in the treatment of pemphigus. Br J Dermatol. 2005;153:620–5.

88. Belgi AS, Azeez M, Hoyle C, Williams RE. Response of pemphigus vulgaris to anti-CD20 antibody therapy (rituximab) may be delayed. Clin Exp Dermatol. 2006;31:143.

89. Esposito M, Capriotti E, Giunta A, et al. Long lasting remission of pemphigus vulgaris treated with rituximab. Acta Derm Venereol. 2006;86:87–9.

90. Kong HH, Prose NS, Ware RE, Hall RP 3rd. Successful treatment of refractory childhood pemphigus vulgaris with anti-CD20 monoclonal antibody (rituximab). Pediatr Dermatol. 2005;22:461–4.

91. Morrison LH. Therapy of refractory pemphigus vulgaris with monoclonal anti-CD20 antibody (rituximab). J Am Acad Dermatol. 2004;51:817–19.

92. Niedermeier A, Worl P, Barth S, et al. Delayed response of oral pemphigus vulgaris to rituximab treatment. Eur J Dermatol. 2006;16:266–70.

93. Schmidt E, Herzog S, Brocker EB, et al. Long-standing remission of recalcitrant juvenile pemphigus vulgaris after adjuvant therapy with rituximab. Br J Dermatol. 2005;153:449–51.

94. Wenzel J, Bauer R, Bieber T, Tuting T. Successful rituximab treatment of severe pemphigus vulgaris resistant to multiple immunosuppressants. Acta Derm Venereol. 2005;85: 185–6.

95. Ahmed AR, Avram MM, Duncan LM. Case records of the Massachusetts General Hospital. Weekly clinicopathological exercises. Case 23–2003. A 79-year-old woman with gastric lymphoma and erosive mucosal and cutaneous lesions. N Engl J Med. 2003;349:382–91.

96. Borradori L, Lombardi T, Samson J, et al. Anti-CD20 monoclonal antibody (rituximab) for refractory erosive stomatitis secondary to CD20(+) follicular lymphoma-associated paraneoplastic pemphigus. Arch Dermatol. 2001;137:269–72.

97. Heizmann M, Itin P, Wernli M, et al. Successful treatment of paraneoplastic pemphigus in follicular NHL with rituximab: report of a case and review of treatment for paraneoplastic pemphigus in NHL and CLL. Am J Hematol. 2001;66:142–4.

98. Rossum MM, Verhaegen NT, Jonkman MF, et al. Follicular non-Hodgkin's lymphoma with refractory paraneoplastic pemphigus: case report with review of novel treatment modalities. Leuk Lymphoma. 2004;45:2327–32.

99. Schadlow MB, Anhalt GJ, Sinha AA. Using rituximab (anti-CD20 antibody) in a patient with paraneoplastic pemphigus. J Drugs Dermatol. 2003;2:564–7.

100. Barnadas M, Roe E, Brunet S, et al. Therapy of paraneoplastic pemphigus with rituximab: a case report and review of literature. J Eur Acad Dermatol Venereol. 2006;20:69–74.

101. Cutler C, Miklos D, Kim HT, et al. Rituximab for steroid-refractory chronic graft-vs.-host disease. Blood. 2006;108:756–62.

102. Canninga-van Dijk MR, Van Der Straaten HM, Fijnheer R, et al. Anti-CD20 monoclonal antibody treatment in 6 patients with therapy-refractory chronic graft-versus-host disease. Blood. 2004;104:2603–6.

103. Okamoto M, Okano A, Akamatsu S, et al. Rituximab is effective for steroid-refractory sclerodermatous chronic graft-versus-host disease. Leukemia. 2006;20:172–3.

104. Ratanatharathorn V, Ayash L, Reynolds C, et al. Treatment of chronic graft-versus-host disease with anti-CD20 chimeric monoclonal antibody. Biol Blood Marrow Transplant. 2003;9:505–11.

105. Gilliam AC. Update on graft versus host disease. J Invest Dermatol. 2004;123:251–7.

106. Murphy WJ. Revisiting graft-versus-host disease models of autoimmunity: new insights in immune regulatory processes. J Clin Invest. 2000;106:745–7.

107. Shustov A, Luzina I, Nguyen P, et al. Role of perforin in controlling B-cell hyperactivity and humoral autoimmunity. J Clin Invest. 2000;106:R39–47.

108. Saito E, Fujimoto M, Hasegawa M, et al. CD19-dependent B lymphocyte signaling thresholds influence skin fibrosis and autoimmunity in the tight-skin mouse. J Clin Invest. 2002;109:1453–62.

109. Rouquette-Gally AM, Boyeldieu D, Prost AC, Gluckman E. Autoimmunity after allogeneic bone marrow transplantation. A study of 53 long-term-surviving patients. Transplantation. 1988;46:238–40.

110. Miklos DB, Kim HT, Miller KH, et al. Antibody responses to H-Y minor histocompatibility antigens correlate with chronic graft-versus-host disease and disease remission. Blood. 2005;105:2973–8.

111. Miklos DB, Kim HT, Zorn E, et al. Antibody response to DBY minor histocompatibility antigen is induced after allogeneic stem cell transplantation and in healthy female donors. Blood. 2004;103:353–9.

112. Rossi F, Kazatchkine MD. Anti idiotypes against autoantibodies in pooled normal human polyspecifinc IG. J Immunol. 1989;143:4104–9.

113. Dwyer JM. Manipulating the immune system with immune globulin. N Engl J Med. 1992;326:107–11.

114. Yu Z, Lennon VA. Mechanism of intravenous immune globulin therapy in antibody-mediated autoimmune diseases. N Engl J Med. 1999;340:227–8.

115. Masson PL. Elimination of infectious antigens and increase of IgG catabolism as possible modes of action of IVIg. J Autoimmun. 1993;6:683–9.

116. Hurez V, Kaveri SV, Mouhoub A, et al. Anti-CD4 activity of normal human immunoglobulin G for therapeutic use (intravenous immunoglobulin, IVIg). Ther Immunol. 1994;1:269–77.

117. Toyoda M, Zhang XM, Petrosian A, et al. Inhibition of allospecific responses in the mixed lymphocyte reaction by pooled human gamma-globulin. Transpl Immunol. 1994;2:337–41.

118. Basta M, Fries LF, Frank MM. High doses of intravenous immunoglobulin do not affect the recognition phase of the classical complement pathway. Blood. 1991;78:700–2.

119. Toyoda M, Zhang X, Petrosian A, et al. Modulation of immunoglobulin production and cytokine mRNA expression in peripheral blood mononuclear cells by intravenous immunoglobulin. J Clin Immunol. 1994;14:178–89.

120. Abe Y, Aesushi H, Masazumi M, Kimura S. Anticytokine nature of natural human immunoglobulin: one possible mechanism of the clinical effect of intravenous immunoglobulin therapy. Immunol Rev. 1994;129:5–19.

121. Andersson UG, Bjork L, Skansen-Saphir U, Andersson JP. Down-regulation of cytokine production and interleukin-2 receptor expression by pooled human IgG. Immunology. 1993;79:211–16.

122. Amran A, Renz H, Lack G, et al. Suppression of cytokine-dependent human T-cell proliferation by intravenous immunoglobulin. Clin Immunol Immunopathol. 1994;73:180–6.

123. Ross C, Svenson M, Hansen MB, et al. High avidity IFN-neutralizing antibodies in pharmacologically prepared IgG (intravenous immunoglobulin). Eur J Immunol. 1995;95:1974–8.

124. Bayry J, Lacroix-Desmazes S, Carbonneil C, et al. Inhibition of maturation and function of dendritic cells by intravenous immunoglobulin. Blood. 2003;101:758–65.

125. Kazatchkine MD, Kaveri SV. Immunomodulation of autoimmune and inflammatory diseases with intravenous immune globulin. N Engl J Med. 2001;345:747–5.

126. Fazekas Z, Kantor I, Lebwohl M. A patient with pityriasis rubra pilaris responds to therapy with alefacept. J Am Acad Dermatol. 2006;54:AB198 (poster abstract).

127. Dalakas MC. The use of intravenous immunoglobulin in the treatment of autoimmune neuromuscular diseases: evidence-based indications and safety profile. Pharmacol Ther. 2004;102:177–93.

128. Vecchietti G, Kerl K, Prins C, et al. Severe eczematous skin reaction after high-dose intravenous immunoglobulin infusion. Report of 4 cases and review of the literature. Arch Dermatol. 2006;142:213–17.

129. Ahmed AR, Dahl MV. Consensus statement on the use of intravenous immunoglobulin therapy in the treatment of autoimmune mucocutaneous blistering diseases. Arch Dermatol. 2003;139:1051–9.

130. Matsuda M, Hosoda W, Sekijima Y, et al. Neutropenia as a complication of high-dose intravenous immunoglobulin therapy in adult patients with neuroimmunologic disorders. Clin Neuropharmacol. 2003;26:306–11.

131. Berkovitch M, Dolinski G, Tauber T, et al. Neutropenia as a complication of intravenous immunoglobulin (IVIG) therapy in children with immune thrombocytopenic purpura: common and non-alarming. Int J Immunopharmacol. 1999;21;411–15.

132. Niebanck AE, Kwiatkowski JL, Raffini LJ. Neutropenia following IVIG therapy in pediatric patients with immune-mediated thrombocytopenia. J Pediatr Hematol Oncol. 2005;27:145–7.

133. Jolles S, Hill H. Management of aseptic meningitis secondary to intravenous immunoglobulin. BMJ. 1998;316:936.

134. Dahl MV, Bridges AG. Intravenous immune globulin: fighting antibodies with antibodies. J Am Acad Dermatol. 2001;45:775–83.

135. Sati HI, Ahya R, Watson HG. Incidence and associations of acute renal failure complicating high-dose intravenous immunoglobulin therapy. Br J Haematol. 2001;113:556–7.

136. Roifman CM, Schroeder H, Berger M, et al. Comparison of the efficacy of IGIV-C, 10% (caprylate/chromatography) and IGIV-SD, 10% as replacement therapy in primary immune deficiency: a randomized double-blind trial. Int Immunopharmacol. 2003;3:1325–33.

137. Yap PL. The viral safety of intravenous immune globulin. Clin Exp Immunol. 1996;104 Suppl:35–42.

138. Herzog S, Schmidt E, Goebeler M, et al. Serum levels of autoantibodies to desmoglein 3 in patients with therapy-resistant pemphigus vulgaris successfully treated with adjuvant intravenous immunoglobulins. Acta Derm Venereol. 2004;84:48–52.

139. Sami N, Bhol KC, Ahmed RA. Influence of intravenous immunoglobulin therapy on autoantibody titers to desmoglein 3 and desmoglein 1 in pemphigus vulgaris. Eur J Dermatol. 2003;13:377–81.

140. Sami N, Qureshi A, Ruocco E, Ahmed AR. Corticosteroid-sparing effect of intravenous immunoglobulin therapy in patients with pemphigus vulgaris. Arch Dermatol. 2002;138:1158–62.

141. Ahmed AR. Intravenous immunoglobulin therapy in the treatment of patients with pemphigus vulgaris unresponsive to conventional immunosuppressive treatment. J Am Acad Dermatol. 2001;45:679–90.

142. Bystryn JC, Jiao D, Natow S. Treatment of pemphigus with intravenous immunoglobulin. J Am Acad Dermatol. 2002;47:358–63.

143. Sami N, Bhol KC, Beutner EH, et al. Diagnostic features of pemphigus vulgaris in patients with bullous pemphigoid: molecular analysis of autoantibody profile. Dermatology. 2002;204:108–17.

144. Harman KE, Black MM. High-dose intravenous immune globulin for the treatment of autoimmune blistering diseases: an evaluation of its use in 14 cases. Br J Dermatol. 1999;140:865–74.

145. Sibaud V, Beylot-Barry M, Doutre MS, Beylot C. Successful treatment of corticoid-resistant pemphigus with high-dose intravenous immunoglobulins. Ann Dermatol Venereol. 2000;127:408–10.

146. Colonna L, Cianchini G, Frezzolini A, et al. Intravenous immunoglobulins for pemphigus vulgaris: adjuvant or first choice therapy. Br J Dermatol. 1998;138:1102–3.

147. Wever S, Zillikenz D, Broker EB. Successful treatment of pemphigus vulgaris by pulsed intravenous immunoglobulin therapy. Br J Dermatol. 1996;135:862–3.

148. Beckers RC, Brand A, Vermeer BJ, Boom BW. Adjuvant high-dose intravenous gammaglobulin in the treatment of pemphigus and bullous pemphigoid: experience in six patients. Br J Dermatol. 1995;133:289–93.

149. Humbert P, Derancourt C, Aubin F, Agache P. Effects of intravenous gammaglobulin in pemphigus. J Am Acad Dermatol. 1990;22:326.

150. Bewley AP, Keefe M. Successful treatment of pemphigus vulgaris by pulsed intravenous immunoglobulin therapy. Br J Dermatol. 1996;135:128–9.

151. Szep Z, Danilla T, Buchvald D. Treatment of juvenile pemphigus vulgaris with intravenous immunoglobulins. Cas Lek Cesk. 2005;144:700–3.

152. Levy A, Doutre MS, Lesage FX, et al. Treatment of pemphigus with intravenous immunoglobulin. Ann Dermatol Venereol. 2004;131:957–61.

153. Nieves Renteria A, Ochoa Fierro JG, Martinez Ordaz VA, Fernández del Castillo MA. Treatment with high doses of intravenous immunoglobulin in a case of complicated pemphigus vulgaris. Rev Alerg Mex. 2005;52:39–41.

154. Jolles S, Hughes J, Rustin M. Therapeutic failure of high-dose intravenous immunoglobulin in pemphigus vulgaris. J Am Acad Dermatol. 1999;40:499–500.

155. Messer G, Sizmann N, Feucht H, Meurer M. High-dose intravenous immunoglobulins for immediate control of severe pemphigus vulgaris. Br J Dermatol. 1995;133:1014–16.

156. Tappeiner G, Steiner A. High-dosage intravenous gamma globulin: therapeutic failure in pemphigus and pemphigoid. J Am Acad Dermatol. 1989;20:684–5.

157. Wetter DA, Davis MD, Yiannias JA, et al. Effectiveness of intravenous immunoglobulin therapy for skin disease other than toxic epidermal necrolysis: a retrospective review of Mayo Clinic experience. Mayo Clin Proc. 2005;80:41–7.

158. Sami N, Bhol KC, Ahmed AR. Influence of IVIg therapy on auto antibody titers to desmoglein 1 in patients with pemphigus foliaceus. Clin Immunol. 2002;105:192–8.

159. Ahmed AR, Sami N. Intravenous immunoglobulin therapy for patients with pemphigus foliaceus unresponsive to conventional therapy. J Am Acad Dermatol. 2002;46:42–9.

160. Sami N, Qureshi A, Ahmed AR. Steroid sparing effect of intravenous immunoglobulin therapy in patients with pemphigus foliaceus. Eur J Dermatol. 2002;12:174–8.

161. Toth GG, Jonkman MF. Successful treatment of recalcitrant penicillamine-induced pemphigus foliaceus by low-dose intravenous immunoglobulins. Br J Dermatol. 1999;141:583–5.

162. Godard W, Roujeau JC, Guillot B, et al. Bullous pemphigoid and intravenous gammaglobulin. Ann Intern Med. 1985;103:964–5.

163. Daoud YJ, Foster CS, Ahmed R. Eyelid skin involvement in pemphigus foliaceus. Ocul Immunol Inflamm. 2005;13:389–94.

164. Sami N, Ali S, Bhol KC, Ahmed AR. Influence of intravenous immunoglobulin therapy on autoantibody titres to BP Ag1 and BP Ag2 in patients with bullous pemphigoid. J Eur Acad Dermatol Venereol. 2003;17:641–5.

165. Yeh SW, Usman AQ, Ahmed AR. Profile of autoantibody to basement membrane zone proteins in patients with mucous membrane pemphigoid: long-term follow up and influence of therapy. Clin Immunol. 2004;112:268–72.

166. Sami N, Bhol KC, Ahmed AR. Treatment of oral pemphigoid with intravenous immunoglobulin as monotherapy. Long-term follow-up: influence of treatment on antibody titers to human alpha6 integrin. Clin Exp Immunol. 2002;129:533–40.

167. Foster CS, Ahmed AR. Intravenous immunoglobulin therapy for ocular cicatricial pemphigoid: a preliminary study. Ophthalmology. 1999;106:2136–43.

168. Jolles S. High-dose intravenous immunoglobulin (hdIVIg) in the treatment of autoimmune blistering disorders. Clin Exp Immunol. 2002;129:385–9.

169. Urcelay ML, McQueen A, Douglas WS. Cicatricial pemphigoid treated with intravenous immunoglobulin. Br J Dermatol. 1997;137:477–8.

170. Letko E, Bhol K, Foster SC, Ahmed RA. Influence of intravenous immunoglobulin therapy on serum levels of anti-beta 4 antibodies in ocular cicatricial pemphigoid: a correlation with disease activity: a preliminary study. Curr Eye Res. 2000;21:646–54.

171. Ahmed AR, Colon JE. Comparison between intravenous immunoglobulin and conventional immunosuppressive therapy regimens in patients with severe oral pemphigoid: effects on disease progression in patients nonresponsive to dapsone therapy. Arch Dermatol. 2001;137:1181–9.

172. Leverkus M, Gerogi M, Nie Z, et al. Cicatricial pemphigoid with circulating IgA and IgG autoantibodies to the central portion of the BP180 ectodomain: beneficial effect of adjuvant therapy with high-dose intravenous immunoglobulin. J Am Acad Dermatol. 2002;46:116–22.

173. Sami N, Letko E, Androudi S, et al. Intravenous immunoglobulin therapy in patients with ocular-cicatricial pemphigoid: a long-term follow-up. Ophthalmology. 2004;111:1380–2.

174. Daoud Y, Amin KG, Mohan K, Ahmed AR. Cost of intravenous immunoglobulin therapy versus conventional immunosuppressive therapy in patients with mucous membrane pemphigoid: a preliminary study. Ann Pharmacother. 2005;39:2003–8.

175. Kumari S, Bhol KC, Rehman F, et al. Interleukin 1 components in cicatricial pemphigoid: role in intravenous immunoglobulin therapy. Cytokine. 2001;14:218–24.

176. Letko E, Miserocchi E, Daoud YJ, et al. A nonrandomized comparison of the clinical outcome of ocular involvement in patients with mucous membrane (cicatricial) pemphigoid between conventional immunosuppressive and intravenous immunoglobulin therapies. Clin Immunol. 2004;111:303–10.

177. Revuz J, Penso D, Roujeau JC, et al. Toxic epidermal necrolysis: clinical findings and prognosis factors in 87 patients. Arch Dermatol. 1987;123:1160–5.

178. Roujeau JC, Guillaume JC, Fabre JP, et al. Toxic epidermal necrolysis (Lyell syndrome): incidence and drug etiology in France, 1981–1985. Arch Dermatol. 1990;126:37–42.

179. Schopf E, Stuhmer A, Rzany B, et al. Toxic epidermal necrolysis and Stevens-Johnson syndrome: an epidemiologic study from West Germany. Arch Dermatol. 1991;127:839–42.

180. Bastuji-Garin S, Zahedi M, Guillaume JC, Roujeau JC. Toxic epidermal necrolysis (Lyell syndrome) in 77 elderly patients. Age Ageing. 1993;22:450–6.

181. Mockenhaupt M, Norgauer J. Cutaneous adverse drug reactions. Stevens-Johnson syndrome and toxic epidermal necrolysis. ACI International. 2002;14:143–50.

182. Viard I, Wehrli P, Bullani R, et al. Inhibition of toxic epidermal necrolysis by blockade of CD95 with human intravenous immunoglobulin. Science. 1998;282:490–3.

183. Prins C, Kerdel FA, Padilla RS, et al. TEN-IVIG Study Group, et al. Treatment of toxic epidermal necrolysis with high-dose intravenous immunoglobulins: multicenter retrospective analysis of 48 consecutive cases. Arch Dermatol. 2003;139:26–32.

184. Bachot N, Revuz J, Roujeau JC. Intravenous immunoglobulin treatment for Stevens-Johnson syndrome and toxic epidermal necrolysis: a prospective noncomparative study showing no benefit on mortality or progression. Arch Dermatol. 2003;139:33–6.

185. Trent JT, Kirsner RS, Romanelli P, Kerdel FA. Analysis of intravenous immunoglobulin for the treatment of toxic epidermal necrolysis using SCORTEN: the University of Miami experience. Arch Dermatol. 2003;139:39–43.

186. Shortt R, Gomez M, Mittman N, Cartotto R. Intravenous immunoglobulin does not improve outcome in toxic epidermal necrolysis. J Burn Care Rehabil. 2004;25:246–55.

187. Stella M, Cassano P, Bollero D, et al. Toxic epidermal necrolysis treated with intravenous high-dose immunoglobulins: our experience. Dermatology. 2001;203:45–9.

188. Campione E, Marulli GC, Carrozzo AM, et al. High-dose intravenous immunoglobulin for severe drug reactions: efficacy in toxic epidermal necrolysis. Acta Derm Venereol. 2003;83:430–2.

189. Tristani-Firouzi P, Petersen MF, Saffle JR, et al. Treatment of toxic epidermal necrolysis with intravenous immunoglobulin in children. J Am Acad Dermatol. 2002;47:548–52.

190. Kim KJ, Lee DP, Suh HS, et al. Toxic epidermal necrolysis: analysis of clinical course and SCORTEN-based comparison of mortality rate and treatment modalities in Korean patients. Acta Derm Venereol. 2005;85:497–502.

191. Al-Mutairi N, Arun J, Osama NE, et al. Prospective, noncomparative open study from Kuwait of the role of intravenous immunoglobulin in the treatment of toxic epidermal necrolysis. Int J Dermatol. 2004;43:847–51.

192. Brown KM, Siliver GM, Halerz M, et al. Toxic epidermal necrolysis: does immunoglobulin make a difference? J Burn Care Rehabil. 2004;25:81–8.

193. Morici MV, Galen WK, Shetty AK, et al. Intravenous immunoglobulin therapy for children with Stevens-Johnson syndrome. J Rheumatol. 2000;27:2494–7.

194. Metry DW, Jung P, Levy ML. Use of intravenous immunoglobulin in children with Stevens-Johnson syndrome and toxic epidermal necrolysis: seven cases and review of the literature. Pediatrics. 2003;112:1430–6.

195. Yip LW, Thong BY, Tan AW, et al. High-dose intravenous immunoglobulin in the treatment of toxic epidermal necrolysis: a study of ocular benefits. Eye. 2005;19:846–53.

196. Amato GM, Travia A, Ziino O. The use of intravenous high-dose immunoglobulins (IVIG) in a case of Stevens-Johnson syndrome. Pediatr Med Chir. 1992;14:555–6.

197. Moudgil A, Porat S, Brunnel P, Jordan SC. Treatment of Stevens-Johnson syndrome with pooled human intravenous immuneglobulin. Clin Pediatr. 1995;34:48–51.

198. Sanwo M, Nwadiuko R, Beall G. Use of intravenous immunoglobulin in the treatment of severe cutaneous drug reactions in patients with AIDS. J Allergy Clin Immunol. 1996;98:1112–5.

199. Phan TG, Wong RC, Crotty K, Adelstein S. Toxic epidermal necrolysis in acquired immunodeficiency syndrome treated with intravenous gammaglobulin. Australas J Dermatol. 1999;40:153–7.

200. Magina S, Lisboa C, Goncalves E, et al. A case of toxic epidermal necrolysis treated with intravenous immunoglobin. Br J Dermatol. 2000;142:191–2.

201. Straussberg R, Harel L, Ben-Amitai D, et al. Carbamazepine-induced Stevens-Johnson syndrome treated with IV steroids and IVIG. Pediatr Neurol. 2000;22:231–3.

202. Brett AS, Philips D, Lynn AW. Intravenous immunoglobulin therapy for Stevens-Johnson syndrome. South Med J. 2001;94:342–3.

203. Samimi SS, Siegfried E. Stevens-Johnson syndrome developing in a girl with systemic lupus erythematosus on high-dose corticosteroid therapy. Pediatr Dermatol. 2002;19:52–5.

204. Simeone F, Rubio ER. Treatment of toxic epidermal necrolysis with intravenous immunoglobulin. J La State Med Soc. 2003;155:266–9.

205. Sidwell RU, Swift S, Yan CL, et al. Treatment of toxic epidermal necrolysis with intravenous immunoglobulin. Int J Clin Pract. 2003;57:643–5.

206. Tan A, Tan HH, Lee CC, Ng SK. Treatment of toxic epidermal necrolysis in AIDS with intravenous immunoglobulins. Clin Exp Dermatol. 2003;28:269–71.

207. Mayorga C, Torres MJ, Corzo JL, et al. Improvement of toxic epidermal necrolysis after the early administration of a single high dose of intravenous immunoglobulin. Ann Allergy Asthma Immunol. 2003;91:86–91.

208. Kalyoncu M, Cimsit G, Cakir M, Okten A. Toxic epidermal necrolysis treated with intravenous immunoglobulin and granulocyte colony-stimulating factor. Indian Pediatr. 2004;41:392–5.

209. Arca E, Kose O, Erbil AH, et al. A 2-year-old girl with Stevens-Johnson syndrome toxic epidermal necrolysis treated with intravenous immunoglobulin. Pediatr Dermatol. 2005;22:317–20.

210. Hebert AA, Bogle MA. Intravenous immunoglobulin prophylaxis for recurrent Stevens-Johnson syndrome. J Am Acad Dermatol. 2004;50:286–8.

211. Lissia M, Figus A, Rubino C. Intravenous immunoglobulins and plasmapheresis combined treatment in patients with severe toxic epidermal necrolysis: preliminary report. Br J Plast Surg. 2005;58:504–10.

212. Tan AW, Thong BY, Yip LW, et al. High-dose intravenous immunoglobulins in the treatment of toxic epidermal necrolysis: an Asian series. J Dermatol. 2005;32:1–6.

213. Nasser M, Bitterman-Deutsch O, Nassar F. Intravenous immunoglobulin for treatment of toxic epidermal necrolysis. Am J Med Sci. 2005;329:95–8.

214. Neff P, Meuli-Simmen C, Kempf W, et al. Lyell syndrome revisited: analysis of 18 cases of severe bullous skin disease in a burns unit. Br J Plast Surg. 2005;58:73–80.

215. Spornraft-Ragaller P, Theilen H, Gottschlich GS, Ragaller M. Treatment of toxic epidermal necrolysis experience with 9 patients with consideration of intravenous immunoglobulin. Hautarzt. 2006;57:185–94.

216. Mangla K, Rastogi S, Goyal P, et al. Efficacy of low dose intravenous immunoglobulins in children with toxic epidermal necrolysis: open uncontrolled study. Indian J Dermatol Venereol Leprol. 2005;71:398–400.

217. Faye O, Roujeau JC. Treatment of epidermal necrolysis with high dose intravenous immunoglobulins (IVIg): clinical experience to date. Drugs. 2005;65:2085–90.

218. French LE, Trent JT, Kerdel FA. Use of intravenous immunoglobulin in toxic epidermal necrolysis and Stevens-Johnson syndrome: our current understanding. Int Immunopharmacol. 2006;6:543–9.

219. Wolff K, Tappeiner G. Treatment of toxic epidermal necrolysis: the uncertainty persists but the fog is dispersing. Arch Dermatol. 2003;139:85–6.

220. Orson FM. Intravenous immunoglobulin therapy suppresses manifestations of the angioedema with hypereosinophilia syndrome. Am J Med Sci. 2003;326:94–7.

CHAPTER 5

Critical Care: Stuff You Really, Really Need to Know

Haim Shmilovich

Arie Roth

ALL PHYSICIANS should be experienced in the practices and procedures of Basic Life Support (BLS) and Advanced Cardiopulmonary Life Support (ACLS). Outside the hallowed hospital walls, "Is there a doctor in the house?" means you! Within the hospital, the fundamental equipment and staff are on hand, but it is the responsibility of the nearest available physician to get it right and at maximum speed. The dermatology ward is no stranger to life-threatening events: This chapter is intended as a brief refresher course for the situations that cannot wait.

The ultimate goal of resuscitation is to maintain cerebral perfusion until and after cardiopulmonary functions are restored. Most adult cardiac arrests are due to ventricular arrhythmias for which early defibrillation is critical. The emphasis is on stabilizing the patient on site so that he or she can survive to get to an intensive care unit (ICU). The critically ill patients already on the ward are still not out of trouble, because they are usually being treated with many medications, leaving them vulnerable to adverse drug reactions, toxicity, and side effects, which themselves occur more frequently in these patients due to altered hemodynamics and metabolism. The high rate and rapid initiation of complications necessitate careful monitoring of vital signs and frequent physical examinations and laboratory tests. A high index of suspicion and close attention to changing symptoms and parameters are mandatory for preventing and/or treating any newly emerging medical problem. Routine care of a critically ill patient involves continuous assessment of symptoms, physical examination, hemodynamics, monitoring the need for changing the dose and/or route of administration of drugs, and constant vigilance in terms of the supportive care that is being administered.

Sedatives and analgesics are commonly administered to the critically ill patient. The clinician must recognize the diverse and often unpredictable effects of critical illness on the pharmacokinetics and pharmacodynamics of sedatives and analgesics. Failure to do so may lead to inadequate or excessive sedation. Bear in mind that sedatives and analgesics may cause prolonged alterations in mental status and may mask the development of coincident complications of critical illness.

The provision of resuscitation is based on medical guidelines, written by expert panels from many disciplines. They provide clear-cut instructions on the measures to be taken for treating life-threatening situations while allowing alterations in individual cases. First and foremost, the physician must rapidly and correctly recognize the nature of the emergent situation. To standardize treatment during resuscitation, a number of algorithms have been developed that were based on large studies and on laboratory and clinical evidence. These have been compiled into the BLS and ACLS guidelines published and updated regularly.[1,2] The most significant recent changes were made to simplify cardiopulmonary resuscitation (CPR) instructions and increase the number of chest compressions delivered per minute while reducing the number of interruptions in chest compressions during CPR. After delivering two rescue breaths, the rescuer begins chest compressions immediately. A universal recommendation is to provide a single compression-to-ventilation ratio of 30:2. An important recommendation is that all rescue efforts – including insertion of an advanced airway, administration of medications, and reassessment of the patient – be performed in a way that minimizes interruption of chest compressions. *The most important determinant of survival from sudden cardiac arrest (SCA) is the presence of a trained rescuer who is ready, willing, able, and equipped to act.*

Unlike other medical interventions, CPR can be initiated without a physician's order, based on implied consent for emergency treatment. A physician's order, however, is necessary to withhold CPR. The decision to terminate resuscitative efforts rests with the treating physician in the hospital and is based on consideration of many factors, including time to CPR, time to defibrillation, comorbid disease, prearrest state, and initial arrest rhythm. Witnessed collapse, bystander CPR, and a short interval from collapse to the arrival of professionals improve the chances of a successful resuscitation. Local ethical and cultural norms must be considered when beginning and ending a resuscitation attempt: It behooves the physician to know what they are. Patients or families may ask physicians to provide care that is inappropriate. Physicians are not obliged to provide such care when there is scientific and social consensus against such treatment. One example is the administration of CPR for patients with the clear-cut signs of irreversible death. Whereas health care providers are not obliged to provide CPR if no benefit from CPR and ACLS can be expected, few criteria can accurately predict the futility of CPR. In light of this uncertainty, all patients in cardiac arrest should receive resuscitation, unless the patient has a valid Do Not Attempt Resuscitation (DNR) order, if the patient has the standard signs of irreversible death, or if no physiological benefit can be expected because vital functions have deteriorated despite maximal therapy.

BASIC LIFE SUPPORT

BLS includes recognition of life-threatening situations (such as SCA, heart attack, pulmonary embolism [PE], stroke, anaphylaxis, and foreign body airway obstruction [FBAO]) and the provision of rapid and effective CPR and defibrillation. SCA is a leading cause of death. Four critical points are important for the purpose of resuscitation: early recognition of the emergency situation, early CPR, early delivery of a shock, and early ACLS followed by postresuscitation care. The algorithm of BLS consists of the mnemonic *ABC*: *A* for airway, *B* for breathing, and *C* for circulation/compression. When a person lies unresponsive and without movement, check the airway and open it by the head tilt–chin lift maneuver. If the patient isn't breathing, give two breaths. If there is a pulse, give breaths at a rate of 10–12 per minute and recheck the pulse every 2 minutes. If there is no central pulse, give a ratio of chest compressions to breaths of 30:2. The chest compressions should be on the lower half of the sternum at a rate of 100 per minute. It is important not to interrupt the chest compressions until the return of spontaneous rhythm/circulation (ROSC) or the arrival of a defibrillator: Chest compressions are preferable to ventilation when there is a single rescuer.

Supplementary oxygen should be used when available. When the victim has an advanced airway in place during CPR, two rescuers should no longer deliver cycles of CPR (compressions interrupted by pauses for ventilation). Instead, the compressing rescuer should administer continuous chest compressions at a rate of 100 per minute without pausing for ventilation. The rescuer delivering ventilation should provide 8 breaths per minute. If the rhythm can be altered by shock (e.g., a rapid heart rhythm), administer one shock with the highest energy and continue CPR immediately for five more cycles of 30:2. Recheck pulse and continue with shocks and CPR. If there is no pulse or the rhythm had not been suitable for applying shock, continue

CPR and begin ACLS consisting of definitive breathing with intubation and the use of medications.

All BLS providers should be trained to provide defibrillation because ventricular fibrillation (VF) is the most common rhythm found in adults with witnessed, nontraumatic SCA. For these victims, survival rates are highest when immediate bystander CPR is provided and defibrillation occurs within 3–5 minutes. The rescuer should intervene if the choking victim has signs of severe FBAO. These include signs of poor air exchange and increased breathing difficulty, such as a silent cough, cyanosis, or inability to speak or breathe. Do not interfere with the patient's spontaneous coughing and breathing efforts. Chest thrusts, back slaps, and abdominal thrusts are permissible and effective for relieving severe FBAO in conscious adults. If the adult victim with FBAO becomes unresponsive, the rescuer should carefully support the patient to the ground, and then begin CPR.[3,4]

CARDIAC ARREST

Cardiac arrest, defined as the sudden complete loss of cardiac output and therefore blood pressure, is the leading cause of death in the developed world. The mechanism of cardiac arrest in victims of trauma, drug overdose, drowning, and in many children is asphyxia. CPR with both compressions and rescue breaths is critical for resuscitation of these victims. In the majority of cases, the underlying etiology of arrest is myocardial ischemia in the setting of coronary artery disease. Conversely, cardiac arrest is the initial presentation of myocardial ischemia in approximately 20% of patients. A wide variety of other processes can lead to cardiac arrest, including septic shock, electrolyte abnormalities, hypothermia, PE, and massive trauma.

Survival from cardiac arrest remains low, even after the introduction of electrical defibrillation and CPR more than 50 years ago. In the best cases (witnessed VF arrest with rapid defibrillation), survival to hospital discharge is about 35%, although overall out-of-hospital arrest survival is usually much lower, about 15%. Several studies have documented the effects of time to defibrillation and the effects of bystander CPR on survival from SCA. For every minute that passes between collapse and defibrillation, survival rates from witnessed VF-SCA decrease by 10% if no CPR is provided. If bystanders provide immediate CPR, many adults in VF can survive with intact neurological function, especially if defibrillation is performed within about 5 minutes after SCA. CPR prolongs VF (the window of time during which defibrillation can occur) and provides a small amount of blood flow that may maintain some oxygen to the heart and brain. Basic CPR alone, however, is unlikely to eliminate VF and restore a perfusing rhythm. Even after successful resuscitation from cardiac arrest, most patients die within 48 hours despite aggressive intensive care treatment.

CPR is important both before and after shock delivery. When performed immediately after collapse from VF-SCA, CPR can double or triple the victim's chance of survival. CPR should be provided uninterruptedly until a defibrillator is available. After about 5 minutes of VF with no treatment, outcome may be better if defibrillation is preceded by a period of CPR with effective chest compressions that deliver some blood to the coronary arteries and brain. CPR is also important immediately after shock delivery: Most victims demonstrate asystole or pulseless electrical activity (PEA) for several minutes after defibrillation, and CPR can convert these rhythms to a perfusing rhythm. Most victims of SCA demonstrate VF, which is characterized by chaotic rapid complexes that cause the heart to tremble so that it is unable to pump blood effectively. Bear in mind that many SCA victims can survive if bystanders act immediately while VF is still present, but successful resuscitation is unlikely when the rhythm deteriorates to asystole.

During cardiac arrest, basic CPR and early defibrillation are of primary importance, and drug administration is of secondary importance. After beginning CPR and defibrillation, rescuers can insert an advanced airway, establish intravenous (IV) access, and consider drug therapy. If spontaneous circulation does not return after defibrillation and peripheral venous drug administration, the provider may consider placement of a central line through the subclavian vein. When dealing with a pulseless arrest rhythm, begin BLS and CPR and call for help immediately. Attach defibrillator leads. VF or ventricular tachycardia (VT) are shockable rhythms. Give one shock (maximum energy) and continue five cycles of CPR with ACLS. Check again for rhythm and, if appropriate, give shock medications until return of a pulse. These medications are epinephrine (adrenaline) 1 mg IV every 3–5 minutes for 3 doses, or a single dose of vasopressin 40 U IV. After a second cycle of shocks–medications without response, consider the administration of amiodarone 300 mg IV, lidocaine IV at 1–1.5 mg/kg, and/or magnesium 1–2 g IV. If asystole is diagnosed, continue CPR while giving epinephrine or vasopressin as already mentioned, and consider atropine 1 mg IV every 3–5 minutes up to 3 doses. Check routinely for pulse or shockable rhythms and proceed accordingly, all the while bearing in mind that chest compressions must not be interrupted until ROSC. In adults with a prolonged arrest, shock delivery may be more successful after a period of effective chest compressions. There is insufficient evidence to recommend routine administration of fluids to treat cardiac arrest, but fluids should be infused if hypovolemia is suspected.[5–9]

Finally, it is important to search for and treat possible reversible etiologies which are summarized as "6h's and 5t's": *h*ypovolemia, *h*ypoxia, *h*ydrogen ion (acidosis), *h*ypo/*h*yperkalemia, *h*ypoglycemia, *h*ypothermia, *t*oxins, *t*amponade, *t*ension pneumothorax, *t*hrombosis (coronary or pulmonary), and *t*rauma.

ASYSTOLE AND PULSELESS ELECTRICAL ACTIVITY

PEA encompasses a heterogeneous group of pulseless rhythms. Pulseless patients with electrical activity have associated mechanical contractions, but these contractions are too weak to produce a blood pressure detectable by palpation or noninvasive blood pressure monitoring. PEA is often caused by reversible conditions (the 6h's and 5t's) and can be treated if those conditions are identified and corrected. Patients who have either asystole or PEA will not benefit from defibrillation attempts. The focus of resuscitation is to perform high-quality CPR with minimal interruptions and to identify reversible causes or complicating factors. Providers should insert an advanced airway. Rescuers should minimize interruptions in chest compressions while inserting the airway and should not interrupt CPR while establishing IV access. If the rhythm check confirms asystole or PEA, resume CPR immediately. A vasopressor (epinephrine or vasopressin) may be administered at this time. Epinephrine can be administered approximately every 3–5 minutes during cardiac arrest; one dose of vasopressin may be substituted for either the first or second epinephrine dose. For a patient in asystole or slow PEA, consider atropine. Do not interrupt CPR to deliver any medication. Give the drug as soon as possible after the rhythm check. After drug delivery and approximately five cycles (or about 2 minutes) of CPR, recheck the rhythm. If a shockable rhythm is present, deliver a shock. If no rhythm is present or if there is no change in the appearance of the electrocardiogram (ECG), immediately resume CPR. If an organized rhythm is present, try to palpate a pulse. If no pulse is present, continue CPR. If a pulse is present, the provider should identify the rhythm and treat accordingly. If the patient appears to have an organized rhythm with a good pulse, begin postresuscitative care.

SYMPTOMATIC BRADYARRHYTHMIA OR TACHYARRHYTHMIA

Cardiac arrhythmias are a common cause of sudden death. ECG monitoring should be established as soon as possible for all patients who collapse suddenly or have symptoms of coronary ischemia or infarction. In general, if bradycardia produces signs and symptoms (acute alteration of mental status, ongoing severe ischemic chest pain, congestive heart failure, and hypotension) that persist despite adequate airway and breathing, prepare to provide pacing. For symptomatic high-degree atrioventricular (AV) block (second-degree AV block Mobitz type II and third-degree AV block) provide transcutaneous pacing without delay. If the tachycardic patient is unstable with severe signs and symptoms related to tachycardia, prepare for immediate cardioversion. If the patient with tachycardia is stable, determine if he or she has a narrow-complex or wide-complex tachycardia and then tailor therapy accordingly. In a patient with a heart rate lower than 60 beats per minute, which is inadequate for the clinical situation, check for airway and breathing and provide supplementary oxygen. Check vital signs, establish an IV access, and try to diagnose the bradyarrhythmia. If there are signs of adequate perfusion, observe and monitor the patient for the possibility of reversible causes with either later improvement or continuing deterioration. If there are signs of poor perfusion, call a cardiologist and begin to prepare for transcutaneous pacing, while considering atropine 0.5 mg IV for a total dose of 3 mg, and if the atropine is ineffective, begin to pace. Also consider epinephrine or dopamine by continuous drip while waiting for pacing. Use a temporarily external pacemaker if one is available. In conjunction with all of the above, identify and treat contributing factors (the 6h's and 5t's).

Atropine remains the first-line drug for acute symptomatic bradycardia. An initial dose of 0.5 mg, repeated as needed to a total of 3 mg, is effective in the treatment of symptomatic bradycardia. Transcutaneous pacing is usually indicated if the patient fails to respond to atropine, although second-line drug therapy with medications such as dopamine or epinephrine may be successful. Atropine will not suffice for infranodal blocks; they require a pacemaker. Other medications to consider are epinephrine (adrenaline), dopamine, or glucagon in the case of beta blocker or calcium channel blocker toxicity. Transcutaneous pacing is a class I intervention for any symptomatic bradycardia. It should be started immediately for patients who are unstable, particularly those with high-degree AV block.

After defibrillation and stabilization of the patient, the next step is to treat the factors that may have precipitated the tachycardia, if possible, such as fever, pulmonary emboli, hyperthyroidism, or acute myocardial infarction (MI). Supraventricular tachycardias (SVTs) with the pathophysiology of reentry will respond to carotid massage and/or adenosine 6-mg IV administration with abrupt cessation of the tachycardia. Other SVTs will necessitate slowing of the ventricular response by slowing the AV node conduction with IV medications such as beta blockers and/or calcium channel blockers and by trying to convert the rhythm to sinus rhythm if the tachyarrhythmia is not of long duration and there is a minimal risk of thromboembolism. Wide-complex tachycardias are often hemodynamically unstable and necessitate defibrillation. If the patient is stable (systolic blood pressure greater than 90 mm Hg, no angina pectoris, no altered mentation or signs of hypoperfusion), one can try IV medications. If there is the possibility of VT (note: any regular wide-complex tachycardia in an elderly person with a history of prior MI has a more than 80% chance of being VT), a trial of amiodarone or lidocaine is recommended. Amiodarone is given as a loading dose of 150 mg over 15 minutes and then in a 1200-mg maintenance drip over 24 hours. Lidocaine is given as a loading dose of

1–1.5 mg/kg slow push and then a maintenance drip of 2 g/day. If the diagnosis of VT is not possible, a trial of procainamide 20 mg every 1 minute should be considered until the tachycardia responds.

Although synchronized cardioversion is preferred for treatment of an organized ventricular rhythm, it is not possible for some arrhythmias. The many QRS configurations and irregular rates that comprise polymorphic VT make it difficult or impossible to reliably synchronize to a QRS complex. In addition, the patient with persistent polymorphic VT will probably not maintain perfusion/pulses for very long, so any attempt to distinguish between polymorphic VT with or without pulses quickly becomes doubtful. A good rule of thumb is that if your eye cannot synchronize to each QRS complex, neither can the defibrillator. If there is any doubt whether monomorphic or polymorphic VT is present in the unstable patient, do not delay shock delivery to perform detailed rhythm analysis – provide high-energy unsynchronized shocks. After shock delivery, be prepared to provide immediate CPR and follow the ACLS Pulseless Arrest Algorithm if pulseless arrest develops.

MEDICATION IN ACLS AND OTHER CARDIAC EMERGENT CASES

Epinephrine

Epinephrine produces beneficial effects in patients during cardiac arrest, primarily because of its adrenergic receptor-stimulating (vasoconstrictor) properties, which increase coronary and cerebral perfusion pressure during CPR. The value and safety of the β-adrenergic effects of epinephrine are controversial because they may increase myocardial work and reduce subendocardial perfusion. It is appropriate to administer a 1-mg dose of epinephrine IV every 3–5 minutes during adult cardiac arrest. If IV access is delayed or cannot be established, epinephrine may be given by the endotracheal route at a dose of 2–2.5 mg.

Vasopressin

Vasopressin is a nonadrenergic peripheral vasoconstrictor that also causes coronary and renal vasoconstriction. There are no significant differences between vasopressin and epinephrine for ROSC, 24-hour survival, or survival to hospital discharge. Because vasopressin effects have not been shown to differ from those of epinephrine in cardiac arrest, one dose of vasopressin 40 U IV may replace either the first or second dose of epinephrine in the treatment of pulseless arrest.

Atropine

Atropine reverses cholinergic-mediated decreases in heart rate, systemic vascular resistance, and blood pressure. It can be considered for asystole or PEA. The recommended dose of atropine for cardiac arrest is 1 mg IV, which can be repeated every 3–5 minutes (maximum total of 3 doses or 3 mg) if asystole persists.

Amiodarone

IV amiodarone affects sodium, potassium, and calcium channels as well as α- and β-adrenergic blocking properties. It can be considered for the treatment of VF or pulseless VT unresponsive to shock delivery, CPR, and a vasopressor. It improves survival rates and defibrillation response when given for VF or hemodynamically unstable VT.

Lidocaine

Lidocaine is an alternative antiarrhythmic of long-standing familiarity with fewer immediate side effects than may be encountered with other antiarrhythmics. Lidocaine, however, has no proven short-term or long-term efficacy in cardiac arrest. It should be considered an alternative treatment to amiodarone. The initial dose is 1–1.5 mg/kg IV. If VF/pulseless VT persists, additional doses of 0.5–0.75 mg/kg IV push may be administered at 5- to 10-minute intervals, to a maximum dose of 3 mg/kg.

Magnesium

Magnesium can effectively terminate torsades de pointes (irregular/polymorphic VT associated with prolonged QT interval). It is not likely to be effective in terminating irregular/polymorphic VT in patients with a normal QT interval. The acute treatment is 1- to 2-g IV loading dose and a maintenance dose of 3–5 g/day. Care must be taken in renal failure and congestive heart failure, where those dosages should be halved, and serum magnesium level should be monitored.

Adenosine

Adenosine is an endogenous purine nucleoside that briefly depresses AV node and sinus node activity. It is recommended for defined, stable, narrow-complex AV nodal or sinus nodal reentry tachycardias. Adenosine will not terminate arrhythmias, such as atrial flutter, atrial fibrillation, or atrial or ventricular tachycardias, because these arrhythmias are not caused by reentry involving the AV or sinus node. Adenosine has a short half-life. Its acute dose is 6 mg IV while monitoring the ECG. If there is no response within 3–5 minutes, a repeat dose of 12 mg IV should be tried, and then a third one by the same rules. Each dose of adenosine should be flushed with 20 cc of saline.

Calcium Channel Blockers: Verapamil and Diltiazem

Verapamil and diltiazem are nondihydropyridine calcium channel blocking agents that slow conduction and increase refractoriness in the AV node. These actions may terminate reentrant arrhythmias and control ventricular response rate in patients with a variety of atrial tachycardias. These medications are indicated for stable, narrow-complex, reentry mechanism tachycardias (reentry SVT) if rhythm remains uncontrolled or unconverted by adenosine or vagal maneuvers, for stable, narrow-complex, automaticity mechanism tachycardias if the rhythm is not controlled or converted by adenosine or vagal maneuvers, and for controlling the rate of ventricular response in patients with atrial fibrillation or atrial flutter. IV verapamil 2.5–5 mg is effective for terminating narrow-complex reentry SVT, and it may also be used for rate control in atrial fibrillation. Verapamil should be given only to patients with narrow-complex reentry SVT or arrhythmias known with certainty to be of supraventricular origin. It should not be given to patients with impaired ventricular function or heart failure.

Diltiazem seems to be equivalent in efficacy to verapamil. It is administered at a dose of 20 mg IV over 2 minutes, and repeated after 15 minutes at a dose of 25 mg. Verapamil and, to a lesser extent, diltiazem may decrease myocardial contractility and critically reduce cardiac output in patients with severe left ventricular dysfunction.

β-Adrenergic Blockers

Beta blocking agents (atenolol, metoprolol, labetalol, propranolol, esmolol) reduce the effects of circulating catecholamines and decrease heart rate and blood pressure. They also have various cardioprotective effects for patients with ACS. For acute tachyarrhythmias, these agents are indicated for rate control for narrow-complex tachycardias that originate from either a reentry mechanism (reentry SVT) or an automatic focus uncontrolled by vagal maneuvers and adenosine in the patient with preserved ventricular function, and to control the rate in atrial fibrillation and atrial flutter in the patient with preserved ventricular function. Commonly used drugs in the acute situation are propranolol 1 mg IV and metoprolol 5 mg IV. They can later be converted to oral propranolol 10 mg three times per day or oral metoprolol 25 mg twice a day, respectively. Side effects related to β-blockade include bradycardias, AV conduction delays, and hypotension. Cardiovascular decompensation and cardiogenic shock after β-adrenergic blocker therapy are infrequent complications. Contraindications to the use of β-adrenergic blocking agents include second- or third-degree heart block, hypotension, severe congestive heart failure, and lung disease associated with bronchospasm. These agents may be harmful for patients with atrial fibrillation or atrial flutter associated with known preexcitation (Wolff–Parkinson–White [WPW]) syndrome.

Procainamide

Procainamide suppresses both atrial and ventricular arrhythmias by slowing conduction in myocardial tissue.

Procainamide is superior to lidocaine in terminating spontaneously occurring VT when given in doses of 100 mg IV every 5–10 minutes as tolerated, not to exceed 1000 mg. Procainamide may be considered in stable monomorphic VT in patients with preserved ventricular function, control of heart rate in atrial fibrillation or atrial flutter in patients with preserved ventricular function, acute control of heart rhythm in atrial fibrillation or atrial flutter in patients with known preexcitation (WPW) syndrome and preserved ventricular function, and for AV reentrant, narrow-complex tachycardias, such as reentry SVT if rhythm is uncontrolled by adenosine and vagal maneuvers in patients with preserved ventricular function.

OTHER EMERGENCIES

Foreign Body Airway Obstruction

Death from FBAO is an uncommon but preventable cause of death. Most reported cases of FBAO in adults are caused by impacted food and occur while the victim is eating. Because recognition of airway obstruction is the key to successful outcome, it is important to distinguish this emergency from fainting, heart attack, seizure, or other conditions that may cause sudden respiratory distress, cyanosis, or loss of consciousness. When FBAO produces signs of severe airway obstruction, rescuers must act quickly to relieve the obstruction. If mild obstruction is present and the victim is coughing forcefully, do not interfere with his or her spontaneous coughing and breathing efforts. Attempt to relieve the obstruction only if signs of severe obstruction develop: The cough becomes silent, respiratory difficulty increases and is accompanied by stridor, or the victim becomes unresponsive. For responsive adults and children at least 1 year old with severe FBAO, case reports show the feasibility and effectiveness of back blows or "slaps," abdominal thrusts, and chest thrusts. Although these maneuvers are feasible and effective for relieving severe FBAO in conscious adults and children at least 1 year of age, for simplicity in training, we recommend that the abdominal thrust be applied in rapid sequence until the obstruction is relieved. If abdominal thrusts are not effective, the rescuer may consider chest thrusts. It is important to note that abdominal thrusts are not recommended for infants younger than 1 year because the thrusts themselves may cause injuries. Chest thrusts should be used for obese patients if the rescuer is unable to encircle the victim's abdomen. If the choking victim is in the late stages of pregnancy, the rescuer should use chest thrusts instead of abdominal thrusts. If the adult victim with FBAO becomes unresponsive, the rescuer should carefully support the patient to the ground and then begin CPR. A health care provider should use a finger sweep only when the provider can see solid material obstructing the airway of an unresponsive patient.

Pulmonary Embolism

PE is a life-threatening condition. The embolus usually derives from the deep veins of the leg or pelvis. Critically ill and bedridden patients are at high risk. Other common risk factors include thrombophilia and cancer. The main clues of an existing PE are dyspnea, tachypnea, tachycardia, low saturation, and sometimes pleuritic chest pain, in the above settings. The gold standard for diagnosis is computed tomographic (CT) angiography. The patient should be treated with oxygen and anticoagulation (e.g., subcutaneous [SC] enoxaparin 1 mg/kg twice a day, reduced to once daily if renal function is impaired). In severe life-threatening cases assessed clinically and/or echocardiographically, the treatment should be fibrinolysis (IV streptokinase 250,000 U bolus maintained at 100,000 U/h for up to 48–72 hours). To prevent PE, critically ill patients should be treated with anticoagulation prophylaxis while bedridden (SC enoxaparin 1 mg/kg once daily or SC heparin 5000–7500 U twice or thrice daily). Recurrent PE or contraindications to anticoagulation will necessitate the usage of an inferior vena caval filter.

Pulmonary Edema

Pulmonary edema is a life-threatening condition caused by both cardiogenic and noncardiogenic etiologies, such as acute MI, acute heart failure, hypertensive crisis, pulmonary emboli, or infections. The etiology must be sought and treated, in parallel with the administration of diuretics, vasodilators, and morphine, as needed. Recommended doses are IV furosemide 40 mg (or 60 mg in renal failure), IV nitroglycerin 1 mg/h and uptitrated as blood pressure permits (contraindicated if systolic blood pressure is <90 mm Hg), and IV morphine 3 mg, repeated as needed. A continuous positive airway pressure (CPAP) device and sometimes intubation will be needed until the patient is stabilized.

Myocardial Infarction

MI is primarily the consequence of atherothrombotic disease of the coronary arteries. Atherosclerosis of the coronary arteries is a common phenomenon in the vast majority of the population, and its occurrence coincides with "atherosclerotic risk factors," for example, smoking, diabetes mellitus, hypertension, hyperlipidemia, and family history of premature coronary disease. Atherosclerotic plaques can disrupt blood flow caused by mechanical or inflammatory factors, and they can erode and rupture so that a thrombus evolves rapidly on top of them, thus atherothrombosis. Other etiologies of MI include embolization or spasm of the coronary artery. Many patients suffering an acute MI die instantly because of acute complications, such as malignant ventricular arrhythmia or mechanical failure of the heart. Others who reach the hospital need to be treated immediately to open the occluded coronary artery, either medically with thrombolytics or mechanically with percutaneous coronary intervention (PCI). Afterward, the patient must take medications for secondary prevention (aspirin, beta blockers, angiotensin-converting enzyme [ACE] inhibitors) and aggressively treat any modifiable risk factor.

A patient with risk factors and/or a prior coronary event who presents with typical chest pain must immediately be given chewable aspirin 300 mg, IV heparin 80 U/kg, and sublingual nitrate if his or her blood pressure is normal. An ECG must be immediately performed and interpreted: If it shows classical signs of ST elevation MI, the patient has to be prepared for immediate PCI. If the ECG is normal, the patient needs to be monitored, undergo repeat ECG, and have blood drawn for measuring troponin levels at 4–6 hours from the beginning of pain: A high troponin level means a non-ST elevation MI, and a normal value means acute coronary syndrome (ACS) or unstable angina pectoris (UAP). Either way, based on clinical and hemodynamic parameters and on noninvasive tests, a diagnostic coronary angiography will need to be performed to evaluate the need for revascularization.

Stroke

Stroke is the number 3 killer and a leading cause of severe, long-term disability. Fibrinolytic therapy administered within the first hours of the onset of symptoms contains neurological injury and improves outcome in selected patients with acute ischemic stroke. The window of opportunity is, however, extremely limited. Effective therapy requires early detection of the signs of stroke, appropriate evaluation and testing, and rapid delivery of fibrinolytic agents to eligible patients. The goal of stroke care is to minimize brain injury and maximize patient recovery. When there is suspicion of stroke, the goal of care is to perform the initial assessment within 10 minutes, performing and interpreting a CT scan within 25 minutes, and administering fibrinolytics to selected patients within 3 hours of the onset of symptoms. If the stroke patient is not eligible for fibrinolytic therapy and there is no suspicion of a hemorrhagic stroke (either by CT or clinically/anamnestically, such as no head trauma, no anticoagulation therapy, no uncontrolled hypertension or arteriovenous malformations), then the immediate treatment is high-dose aspirin. A rapid assessment of consciousness and neurological status is performed using the Glasgow Coma Scale, which is based on three parameters: eye movement, motor assessment, and verbal assessment. The scores range from 3 (poorest) to 15 (best). Any stroke victim with a score less than 8 needs airway protection with endotracheal intubation.

Patients with acute stroke are at risk for respiratory compromise from aspiration, upper airway obstruction, hypoventilation, and neurogenic pulmonary edema. The combination of poor perfusion and hypoxemia will exacerbate and extend ischemic brain injury, and has been associated with worse outcome from stroke. The administration of supplementary oxygen is mandatory.

A 12-lead ECG does not take priority over the CT scan, but it may identify a recent acute MI or arrhythmias (atrial fibrillation) as the cause of an embolic stroke. There is general agreement to recommend cardiac monitoring during the initial evaluation of patients with acute ischemic stroke to detect atrial fibrillation and potentially life-threatening arrhythmias. Management of hypertension in the stroke patient is controversial. For patients eligible for fibrinolytic therapy, however, control of blood pressure is required to reduce the potential risk of bleeding. If a patient who is otherwise eligible for treatment with tissue plasminogen activator (tPA) has elevated blood pressure, try to lower it to <185/<110 mm Hg. Because the maximum interval from onset of stroke until effective treatment of stroke with tPA is limited, most patients with sustained hypertension above these levels cannot be treated with IV tPA. Fibrinolytic administration is not recommended if the patient's neurological signs appear to be clearing spontaneously and approaching baseline.

As with all medications, fibrinolytics have potential adverse effects. The physician must verify that there are no exclusion criteria, consider the risks and benefits to the patient, and be prepared to monitor and treat any potential complications. The major complication of IV tPA for stroke is symptomatic intracranial hemorrhage.

Hypertensive Crisis

Marked elevation of blood pressure to levels greater than 200/120 mm Hg requires immediate attention. The urgency and the method of treatment are not dictated solely by the absolute level of blood pressure but also according to the patient's clinical status. The treatment is urgent if the patient is encephalopathic, pregnant with toxemia, or suffering from acute myocardial ischemia, aortic dissection, or acute stroke. Malignant hypertension is a clinical diagnosis manifested by systolic blood pressure greater than 220 mm Hg and/or diastolic blood pressure greater than 130 mm Hg with hemorrhagic retinopathy, papilledema, and other end-organ involvement, such as renal failure and encephalopathy. Clinically, the patient is likely to have pulmonary edema, in which case the treatment of choice will combine a diuretic (IV furosemide 40 mg) with a vasodilator (e.g., as nitroglycerin 1 mg/h and uptitrated or nitroprusside 0.3–10 µg/kg/min). Other maintenance therapies constitute thiazides (oral chlorothiazide 12.5 mg once daily), ACE inhibitors (e.g., oral enalapril 10 mg twice daily), central acting drugs (oral aldimine 250 mg twice daily), and alpha (oral doxazosin 1–8 mg once daily), beta (oral metoprolol 25 mg twice daily), and/or calcium blockers (oral amlodipine 5 mg once daily). The aim of urgent treatment is to lower the blood pressure by not more than 25% so as not to impair cerebral blood flow. Practically, the drug regimen should contain IV furosemide 40 mg push and IV nitroglycerin 20 mg/100 mg saline (beginning 2 cc/h rate, uptitrated as needed). Consider a beta blocker (also exerting alpha-blocking effects) such as labetalol at an initial IV dose of 20 mg injected over 2 minutes and additional injections of 40 or 80 mg every 10 minutes as needed up to a total dose of 300 mg. Another possibility is an agent with direct vasodilator properties, such as nitroprusside with a starting dosage of 0.1 g/kg/min and increased as necessary and as tolerated.

Shock

Shock is a syndrome of low blood pressure and inadequate end-organ perfusion. Its main etiologies are cardiogenic, septic, hemorrhagic, and anaphylactic. Cardiogenic shock must be considered in a patient with a history of heart disease who presents with chest pain and low blood pressure with peripheral hypoperfusion. In such a patient, the shock is most probably due to acute MI and/or acute heart failure. As such, treatment will constitute revascularization with either PCI or coronary artery bypass grafting and inotropic drugs (e.g., IV dopamine 400 mg/500 cc saline in an initial rate of 5 cc/h, or IV dobutamine 500 mg/500 cc saline, in an initial rate of 5 cc/h). Septic shock is probable in a patient with fever, chills, and infection; the patient must be treated with fluids, antibiotics, and glucocorticoids for adrenal insufficiency. Patients who have lost blood must be treated with blood transfusion. Anaphylactic shock is due to drugs or toxins, and the immediate treatment is SC adrenaline 0.1 mg and the usual supportive treatment.

SPECIAL PROCEDURES

Endotracheal Intubation

The endotracheal tube confirms a patent airway, permits suctioning of airway secretions, enables delivery of a high concentration of oxygen, provides an alternative route for the administration of some drugs, facilitates delivery of a selected tidal volume, and, with the use of a cuff, may protect the airway from aspiration. Endotracheal intubation attempts by unskilled providers can produce complications such as trauma to the oropharynx, interruption of compressions and ventilations for unacceptably long periods, and hypoxemia from prolonged intubation attempts or failure to recognize tube misplacement or displacement. Indications for emergency endotracheal intubation are the inability of the rescuer to adequately ventilate the unconscious patient with a bag and mask and the absence of airway protective reflexes (coma or cardiac arrest).

During CPR, the rescuers should minimize the number and duration of interruptions in chest compressions, with the goal of limiting interruptions to no more than 10 seconds except as needed for interventions, such as placement of an advanced airway. Interruptions needed for intubation can be minimized if the intubating rescuer is prepared to begin the intubation attempt as soon as the compressing rescuer pauses in administering compressions. The compressions should be interrupted for only as long as the intubating rescuer needs to visualize the vocal cords and insert the tube. The compressing rescuer should be prepared to resume chest compressions immediately after the tube is passed through the vocal cords. If more than one intubation attempt is required, the rescuers should provide a period of adequate ventilation and oxygenation and chest compressions between attempts. If endotracheal intubation is performed for the patient with a perfusing rhythm, use pulse oximetry and ECG monitoring continuously during intubation attempts and interrupt the attempt to provide oxygenation and ventilation if needed.

Even when the endotracheal tube is seen to pass through the vocal cords and tube position is verified by chest expansion and auscultation during positive-pressure ventilation, rescuers should obtain additional confirmation of placement by using an end-tidal CO_2 or esophageal detection device. The most important caveats for rescuers performing CPR after insertion of the advanced airway are to be sure the advanced airway is correctly placed and to not cease CPR efforts.

Complications of endotracheal intubation are associated with improper endotracheal tube positioning. Esophageal and right main stem bronchus intubation should be suspected if hypoxemia, hypoventilation, or cardiac decompensation occurs. Abdominal distension, lack of breath sounds over the thorax, and regurgitation of stomach contents indicate esophageal intubation. In emergency settings when standard endotracheal intubation cannot be performed, needle cannulation of the cricothyroid membrane can be performed as a stopgap before providing a more definitive airway.

Central Venous Catheterization

Central venous catheterization is the insertion of an indwelling catheter to a large central vein, mostly the subclavian or internal jugular veins. It is mainly indicated for better fluid therapy, drug administration, and parenteral nutrition, and for monitoring of the central venous pressure. The only contraindication against its use is an existing coagulopathy.

Postresuscitation Support

The management of successfully resuscitated patients should focus on the treatment of the underlying disease process and the maintenance of electrical, hemodynamic, and respiratory stability. All patients require careful repeated assessment and should be initially monitored in an ICU. Few randomized, controlled clinical trials have dealt specifically with supportive care following cardiopulmonary–cerebral resuscitation from cardiac arrest; nevertheless, postresuscitation care has significant potential to improve early mortality caused by hemodynamic instability and multiorgan failure and later mortality/morbidity resulting from brain injury.

The initial objectives of postresuscitation care are to optimize cardiopulmonary function and systemic perfusion, especially perfusion to the brain, and to continue care in an appropriately equipped critical care unit. Attempts are made to identify the precipitating causes of the arrest, and measures are instituted to prevent recurrence and improve long-term, neurologically intact survival.

Induced Hypothermia

Both permissive hypothermia (allowing a mild degree of hypothermia >33°C that often develops spontaneously after arrest) and active induction of hypothermia may play a valuable role in postresuscitation care. In two randomized, clinical trials,[10,11] induced hypothermia resulted in improved outcome in adults who remained comatose after initial resuscitation from cardiac arrest. Complications associated with cooling can include coagulopathy and arrhythmias, particularly with an unintentional drop below target temperature. There was some increase in the number of cases of pneumonia and sepsis in the hypothermia-induction group. Cooling may also increase hyperglycemia. These authors concluded that mild hypothermia may be beneficial to neurological outcome and is likely to be well tolerated without significant risk of complications.

Glucose Control

The postresuscitation patient is likely to develop electrolyte abnormalities that may be detrimental to recovery. Many studies have documented a strong association between high blood glucose after resuscitation from cardiac arrest and poor neurological outcomes. Tight control of blood glucose using insulin reduced hospital mortality rates in critically ill patients who required mechanical ventilation. Signs of hypoglycemia are less apparent in comatose patients, so clinicians must monitor serum glucose closely to avoid hypoglycemia when treating hyperglycemia. On the basis of findings of improved outcomes in critically ill patients, when glucose levels are maintained in the normal range, it makes sense to maintain strict glucose control during the postresuscitation period.

Organ-Specific Evaluation and Support

After ROSC, patients may remain comatose or have decreased responsiveness for a variable period of time. If spontaneous breathing is absent or inadequate, mechanical ventilation via an endotracheal tube or other advanced airway device may be required. Hemodynamic status may be unstable when there are abnormalities of cardiac rate, rhythm, systemic blood pressure, and organ perfusion. Clinicians must prevent, detect, and treat hypoxemia and hypotension, because these conditions can exacerbate brain injury. It is essential to determine the baseline postarrest status of each organ system and support impaired organ function as needed.

Respiratory System

Respiratory dysfunction is not uncommon after ROSC. Some patients will remain dependent on mechanical ventilation and will need an increased inspired concentration of oxygen. They should undergo a full physical examination as well as a chest x-ray to verify appropriate endotracheal tube depth of insertion and to identify any cardiopulmonary complications of resuscitation. Mechanical ventilatory support should be adjusted based on the patient's blood gas values, respiratory rate, and work of breathing. As the patient's spontaneous ventilation becomes more efficient, the level of respiratory support may be decreased until spontaneous respiration returns. If the patient continues to require high inspired oxygen concentrations, providers should determine if the cause is pulmonary or cardiac and take measures accordingly. There is some debate as to the length of time that patients who require ventilatory support should remain sedated. To date, there is little evidence to guide therapeutic scheduling and inadequate data to recommend for or against the use of a defined period of sedation or neuromuscular blockade after cardiac arrest. Use of neuromuscular blocking agents should be kept to a minimum because they preclude thorough neurological assessments during the first 12–72 hours after ROSC.

Sustained hypocapnia may reduce cerebral blood flow. After cardiac arrest, restoration of blood flow results in an initial hyperemic blood flow response, followed by a more prolonged period of low blood flow. During this latter period of late hypoperfusion, there may be a mismatch between blood flow and oxygen requirement. If the patient is hyperventilated at this stage, cerebral vasoconstriction may further decrease cerebral blood flow and increase cerebral ischemia and ischemic injury. There is no evidence that hyperventilation protects the brain or other vital organs from further ischemic damage after cardiac arrest.

In summary, although there are no data to support targeting a specific arterial $PaCO_2$ level after resuscitation from cardiac arrest, data extrapolated from patients with brain injury support ventilation to reach normocarbic levels. Routine hyperventilation is detrimental.[12]

Cardiovascular System

Both the ischemia/reperfusion of cardiac arrest and electrical defibrillation can cause transient myocardial stunning and dysfunction that can last many hours but may improve with vasopressors. Cardiac biomarker levels may be increased in association with global ischemia caused by absent or decreased coronary blood flow during cardiac arrest and CPR. Increased cardiac biomarkers may also indicate acute MI as the cause of cardiac arrest.

Hemodynamic instability is common after cardiac arrest, and early death caused by multiorgan failure is associated with a persistently low cardiac index during the first 24 hours after resuscitation. Thus, after successful resuscitation, clinicians should evaluate the patient's ECG, radiographs, and laboratory analyses of serum electrolytes and cardiac biomarkers. Performing an ECG within the first 24 hours after arrest is useful to guide ongoing management. Patients who are resuscitated following out-of-hospital cardiac arrest may have significant early but reversible myocardial dysfunction and low cardiac output, followed by later vasodilation. Hemodynamic instability usually responds to fluid administration and vasoactive support. Invasive monitoring may be necessary to measure blood pressure accurately and to determine the most appropriate combination of medications to optimize blood flow and distribution. The provider should titrate volume administration and vasoactive (e.g., norepinephrine), inotropic (e.g., dobutamine), and vasodilator (e.g., milrinone) drugs that are given to support blood pressure, cardiac index, and systemic perfusion. Both cardiac arrest and sepsis are thought to involve multiorgan ischemic injury and microcirculatory dysfunction. Goal-directed therapy with volume and vasoactive drug administration has been effective in improving survival from sepsis. The greatest survival benefit is due to a decreased incidence of acute hemodynamic collapse, a challenge also seen in the postresuscitation setting. Relative adrenal insufficiency may develop following the stress of cardiac arrest, but the use of early corticosteroid supplementation in such patients to improve either hemodynamics or outcome is unproven and requires further evaluation. Although SCA may be precipitated by cardiac arrhythmia, it is unclear if antiarrhythmics are beneficial or detrimental in the postresuscitation period. Thus, there is insufficient evidence to recommend for or against prophylactic administration of antiarrhythmic drugs to patients who have survived cardiac arrest from any cause. It may be reasonable, however, to continue an infusion of an antiarrhythmic drug that was associated with ROSC. Also, given the cardioprotective effects of beta blockers in the context of ischemic heart disease, the use of beta blockers in the postresuscitation setting seems prudent if there are no contraindications.

Central Nervous System

A healthy brain and a functional patient are the primary goals of cardiopulmonary–cerebral resuscitation. Following ROSC, cerebral blood flow is reduced after a brief initial period of hyperemia (the "no-reflow phenomenon") as a result of microvascular dysfunction. This reduction occurs even when cerebral perfusion pressure is normal. Neurological support for the unresponsive patient should include measures to optimize cerebral perfusion pressure by maintaining a normal or slightly elevated mean arterial pressure and reducing intracranial pressure if it is elevated. Because hyperthermia and seizures increase the oxygen requirements of the brain, hyperthermia must be controlled and therapeutic hypothermia should be considered.[13]

PROGNOSTIC FACTORS

The period after resuscitation is often stressful to medical staff and family members as questions arise about the patient's ultimate prognosis. Ideally, a clinical assessment, laboratory test, or biochemical marker would reliably predict the outcome during or immediately after cardiac arrest. Unfortunately, no such predictors are available. Determination of prognosis based on initial physical examination findings can be difficult, and coma scores may be less predictive than individual motor and brainstem reflexes found in the first 12–72 hours after arrest.

Five clinical signs that were found to strongly predict death or poor neurological outcome, with 4 of the 5 predictors detectable at 24 hours after resuscitation are absent corneal reflex at 24 hours, absent pupillary response at 24 hours, absent withdrawal response to pain at 24 hours, no motor response at 24 hours, and no motor response at 72 hours. An electroencephalogram performed >24–48 hours after resuscitation also has been shown to provide useful predictive information and can help define prognosis.[10]

Other Complications

Sepsis is a potentially fatal postresuscitation complication. Patients with sepsis will benefit from goal-directed therapy. Renal failure and pancreatitis, although often transient, should be ruled out.

MONITORING

Blood pressure

Blood pressure can be monitored either noninvasively or invasively, and it is fundamental for hemodynamic assessment. When intraarterial monitoring is in place during the resuscitative effort (in an intensive care setting), the clinician should try to maximize arterial diastolic pressures to achieve an optimal coronary perfusion pressure.

Pulses

Arterial pulses should be palpated during chest compressions to assess the effectiveness of compressions. No studies have shown the validity or clinical utility of checking pulses during ongoing CPR. Carotid pulsations during CPR do not indicate the efficacy of coronary blood flow or myocardial or cerebral perfusion during CPR.

Arterial Blood Gases

Arterial blood gas monitoring during cardiac arrest is not a reliable indicator of the severity of tissue hypoxemia, hypercarbia (and therefore the adequacy of ventilation during CPR), or tissue acidosis. It provides the foundation for the assessment of respiratory function.

Oximetry

During cardiac arrest, pulse oximetry will not function because pulsatile blood flow is inadequate in peripheral tissue beds, which are also constricted. It is, however, commonly used in emergency departments and critical care units for monitoring patients who are not in arrest because it provides a simple, continuous method of tracking oxyhemoglobin saturation. Normal pulse oximetry saturation, however, does not ensure adequate systemic oxygen delivery.

End-Tidal CO$_2$ Monitoring

End-tidal CO$_2$ monitoring is a safe and effective noninvasive indicator of cardiac output during CPR and may be an early indicator of ROSC in intubated patients. CO$_2$ continues to be generated throughout the body during cardiac arrest. In the patient with ROSC, continuous or intermittent monitoring of end-tidal CO$_2$ provides assurance that the endotracheal tube is maintained in the trachea. End-tidal CO$_2$ can guide ventilation, especially when correlated with the PaCO$_2$ from an arterial blood gas measurement.

Sedatives

Sedatives and analgesics used commonly in the care of critically ill patients often exhibit pharmacokinetics and pharmacodynamics that are significantly different than those that are exhibited in studies of their use in other settings. Knowledge of these differences is crucial to designing a sedation protocol for the critically ill patient. Intravascular catheters, endotracheal intubation, suctioning, immobility, and underlying illnesses all may cause pain in the critically ill patient. Most patients require IV narcotics at least initially (IV morphine 3 mg or IV dolestine 12.5 mg). Thus, adequate sedation begins with adequate analgesia. Regional pain control techniques, such as with epidural catheter–administered anesthetics or opiates, can be highly effective at achieving pain control in the postoperative patient. The evaluation of sedation adequacy can be performed only at the bedside and is facilitated by use of validated sedation scales, along with a protocol for the systematic assessment and administration of sedatives and analgesics. Most postarrest patients require larger doses of sedatives in the initial 48 hours. Thus, the level of sedation must be reassessed continuously and a protocol for downward titration of sedation applied. If continuous administration is used, daily sedative interruption is recommended to prevent drug accumulation, to allow the performance of a neurological examination, and to permit reassessment of the need for sedation. An example of a sedative is oxazepam 10 mg thrice daily.

REFERENCES

1. 2005 American Heart Association guidelines for cardiopulmonary resuscitation and emergency cardiovascular care. Circulation. 2005;112 Supplement I:IV-1–IV-45.
2. International Liaison Committee on Resuscitation. 2005 International consensus on cardiopulmonary resuscitation and emergency cardiovascular care science with treatment recommendations. Resuscitation. 2005;67:157–341.
3. Washington University School of Medicine Department of Medicine, Green GB, Harris, IS, et al. (editors). The Washington manual of medical therapeutics. 31st ed. (spiral-bound). Philadelphia: Lippincott, Williams & Wilkins, 2004;1–15;536–44.
4. Gabbott D, Smith G, Mitchell S, et al. Cardiopulmonary resuscitation standards for clinical practice and training in the UK. Resuscitation. 2005;64:13–19.
5. Wik L, Hansen TB, Fylling F, et al. Delaying defibrillation to give basic cardiopulmonary resuscitation to patients with out-of-hospital ventricular fibrillation: a randomized trial. JAMA. 2003;289:1389–95.
6. Van Alem A, Sanou B, Koster R. Interruption of CPR with the use of the AED in out of hospital cardiac arrest. Med Ann Emerg Med. 2003;42:449–57.
7. Eftestol T, Sunde K, Steen PA. Effects of interrupting precordial compressions on the calculated probability of defibrillation success during out-of-hospital cardiac arrest. Circulation. 2002;105:2270–3.
8. Van Alem AP, Vrenken RH, de Vos R, et al. Use of automated external defibrillator by first responders in out of hospital cardiac arrest: prospective controlled trial. BMJ. 2003;327:1312.
9. Peberdy MA, Kaye W, Ornato JP, et al. Cardiopulmonary resuscitation of adults in the hospital: a report of 14720 cardiac arrests from the National Registry of Cardiopulmonary Resuscitation. Resuscitation. 2003;58:297–308.
10. Sandroni C, Nolan J, Cavallaro F, Antonelli M. In-hospital cardiac arrest: incidence, prognosis and possible measures to improve survival. Intensive Care Med. 2007;33:237–45.

11. Boddicker KA, Zhang Y, Zimmerman MB, et al. Hypothermia improves defibrillation success and resuscitation outcomes from ventricular fibrillation. Circulation. 2005;111: 3195–201.

12. Stocchetti N, Maas AI, Chieregato A, van der Plas AA. Hyperventilation in head injury: a review. Chest. 2005;127:1812–27.

13. Berk JL, Sampliner JE, editors. Handbook of critical care. 3rd ed. Boston: Little, Brown and Company; 1989;153–213.

CHAPTER 6

Acute Skin Failure: Concept, Causes, Consequences, and Care

Robert A. Norman

Gwynn Coatney

PHYSICIANS AND health care professionals working at hospitals and in acute care facilities strive to prevent and treat organ failure on a daily basis. The skin is one organ system that is usually overlooked when considering organ failure. The concept of skin failure is not well circulated in the medical world but is an important topic that should be addressed. The potential for a severe prognosis and increased morbidity and mortality is a significant reason why skin failure needs to be addressed.

WHAT IS SKIN FAILURE?

Failure of any organ system occurs when its normal tasks and functions can no longer be performed. The same goes for the integument, which is the largest organ of the body. The skin plays many important roles. It acts as a physical barrier against trauma and aids in the prevention of foreign materials, including bacteria, from entering the body. Conversely, this barrier also prevents loss of body fluids and essential nutrients, such as protein and iron. Normally functioning skin also serves in temperature regulation, detection of sensation, toxin excretion, and vitamin D synthesis and as an immune modulator. When this organ loses the ability to maintain temperature control; when it can no longer retain the balance of fluids, electrolytes, and nutrition; and/or when it fails as a mechanical barrier, skin failure has occurred.[1]

ACUTE VERSUS CHRONIC AND END-STAGE SKIN FAILURE

Acute skin failure has a rapid onset and occurs simultaneously with a critical illness or event. Any medical condition that results in the patient suffering from severe hypotension, hypovolemia, or organ failure, could also develop acute skin failure. Chronic skin failure has a slower, steadier presentation and occurs during an ongoing disease state. This type of skin failure is more prevalent in elderly patients with multiple comorbidities. End-stage skin failure occurs at the end of life and is associated with increased morbidity

and mortality of the patient. The most common example is the decubitus ulcer, also called a pressure ulcer or bed sore.[2]

CAUSES OF ACUTE SKIN FAILURE

Acute skin failure has many etiologies (Table 6.1). The most common and the best known may be thermal burns. Acute medical conditions or illnesses can also lead to acute skin failure. Hypoperfusion of the skin can occur when other organ systems, such as the cardiovascular or renal system, become severely dysfunctional or fail. Blood, along with essential nutrients and oxygen, is then shunted to the core organs, and the peripheral skin becomes impoverished of its blood supply. The end result is that the skin and underlying tissue begin to fail.

Common dermatologic conditions such as eczema and psoriasis can develop into acute skin failure if the cases are severe or if there is extensive involvement of the integument. Erythrodermic or generalized pustular psoriasis is an example of what could potentially become a severe case.

TABLE 6.1: Causes of Acute Skin Failure

No. Principle causes for acute skin failure

1. Erythroderma
  a. Primary (idiopathic)
  b. Dermatitis (atopic, seborrheic, contact dermatitis)
  c. Psoriasis, pityriasis, rubra pilaris
  d. Exfoliative drug eruption
  e. Disorders of keratinization (lamellar ichthyosis, bullous and nonbullous ichthyosiform erythroderma)
  f. Cutaneous T-cell lymphoma
  g. Graft versus host disease
2. Stevens–Johnson syndrome, toxic epidermal necrolysis
3. Acute generalized pustular psoriasis
4. Immunobullous disorders: Pemphigus vulgaris and pemphigus foliaceus
5. Infections: Staphylococcal scalded skin syndrome, febrile viral exanthemas

Reproduced, with permission, from Ref. 7.

TABLE 6.2: A Severity of Illness Score for Toxic Epidermal Necrolysis (SCORTEN)

1. Age	>40 y
2. Concurrent illness	Presence of malignancy
3. Epidermal detachment	>30%
4. Serum urea-nitrogen level	>28 mg/dL > 10 mmol/L
5. Blood glucose level	>252 mg/dL >14 mmol/L
6. Serum bicarbonate level	<20 mEq/L < 20 mmol/L
7. Heart rate	>120 bpm

Reproduced, with permission, from Ref. 7.

Significant dermatologic diseases such as toxic epidermal necrolysis (TEN), Stevens–Johnson syndrome (SJS), cutaneous T-cell lymphoma, exfoliative drug reaction eruptions, infections such as staphylococcal scalded skin syndrome or viral exanthemas, pemphigus vulgaris, and graft versus host disease can also cause acute skin failure.[1,3]

RISK FACTORS

There are several components that can increase the possibility of acute skin failure or make the prognosis more severe.

With increased age the skin becomes thinner and has decreased elasticity and increased fragility. Elderly skin also has decreased vascularity that may result in slower repair and healing. Additionally, sun damage and smoking effectuate premature aging of the skin.

The percentage of surface area in failure is directly proportional to the amount of fluid and nutrients lost. An increased fluid and nutrition loss also elevates the risk of infection and raises the risk of poor prognosis.

Patients who have incontinence of their bowel or bladder are more likely to develop skin failure. Constant exposure of feces and urine to the skin causes an increased need for cleansing. When the skin is cleaned with soap or alcohol, the top layers are debrided; this debridement may cause thinning and an increase in the skin's pH, which makes the skin more susceptible to bacterial infection and breakdown.

Multiple comorbidities or immunocompromised patients further complicate acute skin failure. In a patient with concurrent skin failure and heart disease, there is an increase in cardiac output and blood volume needed for circulation, which can ultimately lead to heart failure. A significant loss of fluids and electrolytes can precipitate renal failure.[4,5]

MANAGEMENT

Acute skin failure is considered to be a dermatologic emergency, and should be managed in an intensive care setting (Table 6.2). Some literature suggests that treatment should be conducted in a burn unit. Special attention should be paid to patients who are at an increased risk.

TABLE 6.3: Definite Indications of Antibiotic Use

1. High bacterial count (single strain) from skin/catheter sample of urine
2. Sudden hypothermia in a relatively stabilized patient
3. Confused mental status, anxiety, and excitement
4. Symptoms of infections pertaining to a particular system, e.g., pneumonia/urinary tract infection

Reproduced, with permission, from Ref. 7.

The body's ability to regulate temperature is lost when skin fails. Hyperthermia is seen in patients who have decreased function or blockage of their sweat ducts. An increase in dermal blood flow occurs with severely damaged skin, causing radiant heat expenditure resulting in hypothermia. Hypothermia can be the initial sign of septic shock in the infected patient. Therefore, temperature should be maintained at 30–32°C.

When the stratum corneum is destroyed, the amount of fluid lost through this physical barrier is greatly increased. In a patient with 50% body surface involvement, fluid loss can exceed 4–5 L/day. It is important to quickly replace intravascular fluid loss (Table 6.3). Normal saline is the first-line treatment, but human albumin and fresh frozen plasma are other treatment options. Urine output and body weight should be measured daily to monitor fluid balance.

Infection is common in acute skin failure and can lead to sepsis and even death. Bacterial culture sensitivity should be tested at the initial presentation and throughout the hospital course to treat with appropriate systemic antibiotics (Table 6.4). Topical antiseptics may also be applied to the affected areas.

There can be long-term complications as a result of acute skin failure (Table 6.5), which is just another reason why patients should be treated quickly and aggressively. The underlying etiology should be treated specifically. For

TABLE 6.4: Long-Term Complications of Acute Skin Failure

No.	Organ involved	Complications
1.	Eye	Ectropion, entropion, corneal, scarring, symblepharon, secondary sicca syndrome
2.	Mucosal involvement: Esophagus Urethra Vagina	Dysphagia resulting from stricture Stricture and phimosis Synechiae
3.	Skin	Pigmentary changes (hypo- and hyperpigmentation), contracture
4.	Hair	Scarring alopecia
5.	Nail	Beau's lines, splinter hemorrhage, distal onycholysis, dystrophy, complete shedding of nail

Reproduced, with permission, from Ref. 7.

TABLE 6.5: Important Parameters to be Monitored in Patients with Acute Skin Failure

Clinical	Biochemical	Hematological	Microbiological
Pulse rate	Blood and urine	Total and differential white blood cell count	Bacteriology of skin lesions
Respiratory rate	Sugar	Platelet count	Urine culture
Level of consciousness	Urea/creatinine	Albumin	
Urine output	Serum electrolytes		
Gastric emptying	Phosphorus		

Reproduced, with permission, from Ref. 7.

example, systemic steroids should be used to treat pemphigus vulgaris and biologic agents for psoriasis.[6,7]

TEN is a major cause of acute skin failure. SCORTEN is a scoring system used to assess the risk factors associated with the morbidity and mortality of TEN (Table 6.6). The majority of TEN cases are related to chemicals systemically administered as drug therapy – in particular, antibacterial sulfonamides, anticonvulsants, allopurinol, pyrazolone derivatives, and, less frequently, other nonsteroidal antiinflammatory drugs (NSAIDs).[8] The SCAR (severe cutaneous adverse reactions) study included 245 patients with TEN and SJS in Europe. The study confirmed the "classical culprit" drugs: antibacterial sulfonamides (cotrimoxazole); aromatic anticonvulsants (phenobarbital, phenytoin, carbamazepine); some antimicrobials (aminopenicillins, quinolones, cephalosporins); some NSAIDs (tenoxicam, piroxicam), chlormezanone,

and allopurinol.[9] Although most of these drugs are therapeutic and the overall risk is low, if there are early signs of SCAR, then these drugs are the likely suspects and should be stopped and be avoided completely in the future. The person should wear a medical alert bracelet with the name of the drug.

CONCLUSIONS

The complications that stem from acute skin failure are serious and potentially fatal. Other factors to consider are the patient's age and the presence of multiple comorbidities. Acute skin failure can be caused by many etiologies, and it should be managed aggressively to ensure a positive prognosis. Patients should be immediately hospitalized and treated with the same level of care as patients suffering from heart or kidney failure.

TABLE 6.6: Fluid Electrolyte Replacement and Nutrition in Patients with Acute Skin Failure

	IV fluid	Nasogastric feeding
	Human albumin (diluted in NS 40 g/L) 1 mL/kg Body weight per % BSA	
Initial 24 h +	Saline 0.7 mL/kg	1500–2000 mL (providing normal 1500–2000 calories)
	Body weight per % BSA	
Thereafter	To be guided by previous day's output	Progressive increase of nasogastric/oral supplementation
	Gradual decrease of IV fluids	Increase by 500 cal/d, up to 3500–4000 cal/d
Electrolytes	Supplementation of potassium phosphate in initial 24 h	
Hypokalemia (alkalosis ruled out)	Inj. potassium chloride 40 mmol/L in 5% dextrose–saline/5% dextrose/NS, 6–8 nightly	Milk, fruit juice, honey, potassium chloride syrup
Hyponatremia	NS (500 mL/d) supply normal daily requirement. Further deficit can be replaced by extra amount of NS	

BSA, bovine serum albumin; IV, intravenous; NS, normal saline. Reproduced, with permission, from Ref. 7.

REFERENCES

1. Irvine C. "Skin failure"-a real entity: discussion paper. J R Soc Med. 1991;84:412–13.
2. Parish LC, Witkowski JA, Crissey JT. The decubitus ulcer in clinical practice. New York: Springer Verlag; 1997. pp. 1–241.
3. Witkowski JA, Parish LC. The decubitus ulcer and destructive behavior. Int J Dermatol. 2000;39:894–6.
4. Roujeau JC. Toxic epidermal necrolysis (Lyell syndrome): more than "acute skin failure." Intensive Care Med. 1992; 18:4–5.
5. Benbow M. Back to basics-skin and wounds. J Com Nurs. 2007;21:34–8.
6. Col Vaishampayan SS, Brig Sharma YK, Col Das AL, Lt Col Verma R. Emergencies in dermatology: acute skin failure. MJAFI. 2006;62:56–9.
7. Inamadar AC, Palit A. Acute skin failure: concept, causes, consequences and care. Indian J Dermatol Venereol Leprol. 2005;71:379–85.
8. Heimbach DM, Engrav LH, Marvin JA, et al. Toxic epidermal necrolysis: a step forward in treatment. JAMA. 1987;257:2171–5.
9. Roujeau JC, Kelly JP, Naldi L, et al. Medication use and the risk of Stevens-Johnson syndrome or toxic epidermal necrolysis. N Engl J Med. 1995;333:1600–7.

CHAPTER 7

Cutaneous Symptoms and Neonatal Emergencies

Daniel Wallach

Pierre-Henri Jarreau

EMERGENCIES ARE frequent in neonatal medicine as the physiological fragility of the newborn induces rapid deterioration of general condition in many circumstances, including initially localized infections. In a broad sense, one could argue that the majority of cutaneous abnormalities found in a newborn requires a rapid diagnosis[1,2] for adequate management and relevant parental information.

Among neonatal emergencies, a few situations imply cutaneous symptoms, either as a predominant feature or as one of the elements of a complex clinical situation. The goal of this chapter is to provide dermatologists with the clinical knowledge of the main cutaneous neonatal problems requiring rapid diagnosis or intervention.

Taking care of these babies, whatever their cutaneous problem, generally requires a hospitalization in a neonatal unit and thus involves a neonatal team. Indeed, the consequences of the initial condition as well as of the loss of the cutaneous barrier may be severe and require supportive care, which depends on neonatologists.

To facilitate the identification of these problems, we will classify them according to the clinical presentation. We must point out that, whatever the cutaneous condition, when called to see a neonate, the physician must have always in mind infection as a possible diagnosis. Infection may be the cause of the cutaneous symptoms, or appear as a complication of an initially noninfectious skin disorder.

BULLOUS ERUPTIONS

Staphylococcal Infections

Newborns are exquisitely sensitive to the infection by *Staphylococcus aureus* strains that produce exfoliatin because of the immaturity of the epidermal barrier and of the renal elimination of toxins. *S. aureus* infections are acquired postnatally and must be prevented by adequate hygiene and antisepsis of the nurseries, mothers, medical staff, and all persons in contact with newborns. General hygiene of the facilities, "surgical" hand washing, meticulous care of the nipple area of breastfeeding mothers, and nontoxic antiseptic care of the umbilicus (aqueous chlorhexidine) are mandatory parts of this prevention.

Neonatal staphylococcal infection starts as a localized superficial lesion located in the umbilical area, around folds, and/or in the diaper or periorificial areas: yellow crusts, erythema, and oozing, small pustules.

Bullous impetigo is the localized form of the epidermal bullous disease caused by the exfoliatin secreted by some phage II group *S. aureus* strains. Lesions appear as flat, flaccid bullae, rapidly ruptured, leaving round erosions or crusts. If untreated, these localized infections may lead to the following types of complications:

- cellulitis, fasciitis, abscesses, lymphadenitis;
- osteomyelitis, arthritis, septic pleuritis, pneumonia, septicemia, by hematogenous spread;
- a toxinic generalized skin disease called SSSS (staphylococcal scalded skin syndrome), resembling toxic epidermal necrolysis.

SSSS starts as a bright, scarlatiniform, erythematous rash, predominating in periflexural and periorificial areas. Rapidly, the superficial part of the epidermis is shed, as an extensive peeling or superficial blistering, with a positive Nikolsky sign (Figure 7.1). This desquamation phase lasts 2–4 days, and is followed by complete healing, without scarring. Complications may include dehydration, hypothermia, and generalized sepsis.

SSSS is caused by some strains of phage group II *S. aureus*. The portal of entry is a superficial infection: cutaneous wound (umbilicus, circumcision, puncture), nasopharynx, conjunctiva. Epidermolytic toxins are disseminated through the bloodstream and exert a proteolytic activity on desmoglein 1, leading to an exfoliation at the subcorneal level of the epidermis (similar to superficial pemphigus).

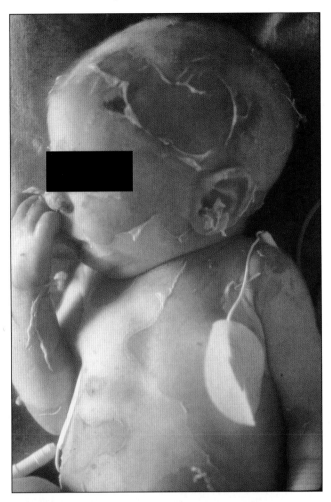

FIGURE 7.1: *Staphylococcal scalded skin syndrome.*

Differential diagnosis includes all neonatal bullous eruptions. The onset after a few days helps differentiating infection blisters form epidermolysis bullosa (EB). Burns, ichthyosis bullosa, or toxic epidermolysis may be considered.

SSSS has a good prognosis, provided the following measures are taken:

- intravenous antibiotics: methicillin, oxacillin, cloxacillin, or vancomycin in case of resistance to β-lactams. Fusidic acid, mupirocin, or retapamulin may be used for the topical treatment of localized staphylococcal infections.
- isolation in an incubator;
- nontraumatic skin care, including the use of emollients (sterile petrolatum, paraffin oil); the shedding epidermis must be conserved as a "biologic dressing."

Epidermolysis Bullosa

EB is a group of rare genetic diseases characterized by an increased fragility to mechanical trauma (mechanobul-lous diseases), resulting in an epidermal detachment. EB includes numerous subtypes of variable severity, including severe, lethal, or incapacitating forms. Each of these subtypes is due to a genetic defect in one of the many molecules involved in the cohesion between the epidermis and the dermis. They are classified by mode of inheritance, clinical features, histopathology, and more recently molecular defect.

The Newborn with EB

When no prior history is known, the birth of a child with EB is a difficult problem that is better dealt with in a neonatal intensive care unit (NICU), in cooperation with a reference center.

Trauma- or friction-induced blisters are the hallmark of EB. These blisters are initially located on the areas of presentation in the case of vaginal delivery, and are induced by handling by the obstetrician, midwife, and neonatal staff. Later, hands, feet, and the diaper area will be the most involved areas.

The child must be placed in an incubator (it is important to avoid overheating), and the general principles of care are similar to those for premature infants, whose skin is also fragile.

A precise subtype diagnosis is difficult or impossible during the first week, and the course is difficult to predict. It is advisable to be cautious in the indications given to the parents. In addition to the support by the medical staff, useful information and psychological support may be provided by groups such as the Dystrophic Epidermolysis Bullosa Research Association (DEBRA).

A skin biopsy will be helpful to establish a precise diagnosis. The biopsy must be taken on a normal appearing, recently rubbed area to induce splitting. Conventional histology, antigenic mapping, and electron microscopy by a specialized center will allow a subtype diagnosis, which is important both for the patient himself or herself and for future prenatal diagnoses. Deoxyribonucleic acid (DNA) mutations may be identified in the blood cells of the child and his or her parents.

THE MAIN EB SUBTYPES

EB Simplex

The most common EB type, called the Koebner type, is an autosomal dominant, relatively mild disease. It is caused by mutations of keratins 5 and 14. The bullae are intraepidermal and heal without scarring. Even in the case of neonatal onset, nails and mucosae are uninvolved, there is no extracutaneous manifestation, and the prognosis is good with progressive improvement.

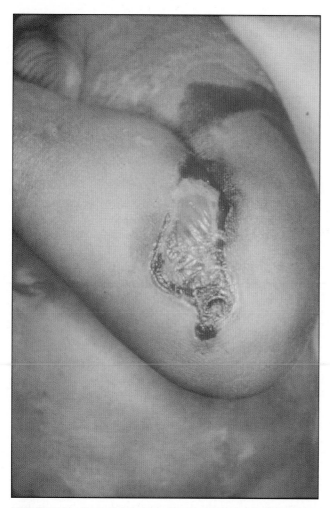

FIGURE 7.2: *Superficial ulceration in junctional epidermolysis bullosa.*

The Dowling–Meara variant, which is more severe, is characterized by a herpetiform pattern of the blisters (mimicking nonmechanical bullae). An autosomal recessive variant, clinically more severe and associated with muscular dystrophy, is caused by mutations of the protein plectin.

Junctional EB

The Herlitz type of junctional EB is a rare, severe, often lethal disease. It is an autosomal recessive disorder, due to mutations of laminin 5, which induces splitting at the level of the lamina lucida.

Bullae and large erosive areas heal very slowly after birth (Figure 7.2). The formation of granulating tissue following blisters around the nails is characteristic. There is a severe mucosal involvement, with oral blisters; respiratory, digestive, and urinary lesions; and ocular complications. Failure to thrive, anemia, and (later) severe dental problems cause many distressing and life-threatening local and systemic complications. Patients with Herlitz disease die early in childhood from one of these complications or from sepsis.

Variants of junctional EB include a form with pyloric atresia, which may be revealed by polyhydramnios. Urologic complications may also be present. This form is due to a defect in the α-6 β-4 integrin.

Dystrophic EB

Dystrophic EB is due to mutations of the COL7A1 gene, coding for collagen VII, a major component of anchoring fibrils. Blisters in the superficial dermis heal poorly, with scars and many possible complications.

Dominant dystrophic EB (Cockayne–Touraine type) is a relatively mild disease, although blistering may be present at birth. Atrophic scars and milia are frequent (hands, feet, knees).

Recessive dystrophic EB (Hallopeau–Siemens type) is a severe disease. Extensive blistering since birth leads to large nonhealing ulcerations, atrophic scars, and/or joint contractures. On the hands and feet, repeated blistering and abnormal scarring end in a "mitten-like" deformation, functional limitation, and severe handicap. Oral ulcerations and digestive involvement are frequent. Children face multiple nutritional deficiencies, growth failure, and ocular and urinary complications and are susceptible to infection (and later to squamous cell carcinomas). The management of a child with recessive dystrophic EB requires a trained specialized multidisciplinary team.

Principles of Management

No therapy is able to correct the skin fragility. Hopes of genetic therapy stand in the future. Recently, hematopoietic stem cell therapy has been successfully performed in severe forms, general medical and psychological support is most important. Reference centers and specialized associations exist in many countries.

During the neonatal period, hospitalization in a NICU is necessary for control of the general and cutaneous conditions. The main principles of management of a newborn with EB are[3] special attention to the avoidance of all trauma to the skin, use of bland emollients and nonadhesive dressings, protection of all fragile areas, feeding with special bottles in case of oral lesions, and attention to all the numerous possible complications, including pain, bacterial infection, dehydration, and undernutrition.

OTHER NEONATAL BULLOUS DISORDERS

Other Skin Fragility Syndromes

In addition to the many subtypes of EB, other genetic disorders may start with a neonatal bullous eruption: peeling skin syndrome and/or[4] transient bullous dermolysis of the newborn.[5]

Kindler syndrome, a rare disorder with poikiloderma and photosensitivity in childhood, may induce traumatic blisters in the neonatal period.[6] It is due to mutations in the gene coding for kindlin-1, a protein linking actin filaments to the extracellular matrix.

Neonatal Syphilis

Congenital syphilis has disappeared where effective prophylaxis is performed in pregnant women. In other situations, it may still be observed. The first sign is usually rhinitis, an unusual symptom in newborns. Many types of cutaneous eruptions may be seen, including a characteristic bullous eruption on the palms and soles. Congenital syphilis is a systemic infection with hepatic, bone, and neurologic manifestations. Spirochetes can be found in the lesions. Serological tests are reactive. Parenteral penicillin G is the first-line treatment.

Porphyria

Congenital erythropoietic porphyria, or Gunther disease, is due to the absence of uroporphyrinogen III synthase. Children suffer from extreme photosensitivity, which may induce blistering on exposed areas and skin fragility, starting in the neonatal period.

Autoimmune Bullous Diseases

Transient neonatal blistering may be caused by the transplacental transmission of maternal autoantibodies. The diagnosis is usually easy, but the affected mother may (rarely) have an inactive disease.

The maternal disease is usually pemphigoid gestationis (herpes gestationis), an autoimmune subepidermal bullous disease associated with pregnancy.[7] Newborns from mothers with pemphigus vulgaris may suffer from neonatal blisters and mucosal lesions.[8]

VESICULAR/PUSTULAR ERUPTIONS

Neonatal Sepsis

Neonatal sepsis is a worldwide problem and a leading cause of mortality in newborns. Prevention and treatment strategies have been discussed.[9] Cutaneous symptoms are not infrequent in neonatal sepsis, but the majority are nonspecific.[10] Therefore, a diagnosis of sepsis must systematically be suspected and appropriate biological examinations performed. The availability of superficial lesions, however, may be helpful for the bacteriological identification of the causing organism.

Listeriosis

Listeria monocytogenes is a rare cause of maternal–fetal infection. Affected mothers, contaminated by food, develop a

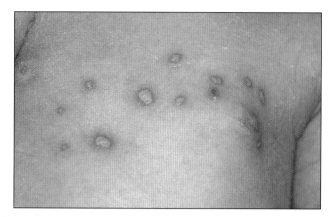

FIGURE 7.3: *Neonatal herpes simplex. (Photo courtesy of Alain Taïeb, MD, Bordeaux, France.)*

flu-like febrile illness before onset of labor. Infants appear septicemic with a multisystemic involvement. Cutaneous lesions are present at birth. A macular–papular generalized rash, with petechiae, progresses to vesicles, then pustules. Gram-positive rods can be found in the pustules. Immediate antibiotic treatment is needed, using ampicillin and an aminoglycoside.

Herpes Simplex Infection

Neonatal herpes is usually acquired perinatally from an infected mother. The more frequent cause is primary herpes simplex virus (HSV)2 infection, but HSV1 and recurrences may also infect the newborn. The dermatologist may diagnose neonatal herpes by clinical examination showing isolated or grouped 1- to 3-mm vesicles with a slight surrounding erythema (Figure 7.3) on the skin or, more rarely, the oral mucosa.

The diagnosis may be rapidly confirmed by Tzanck smear, polymerase chain reaction, or immunofluorescence. The treatment is intravenous acyclovir, 20 mg/kg every 8 hours.

There are three forms of neonatal herpes simplex infection:

- Superficial herpes simplex infection (50% of cases): There is no extracutaneous dissemination, and the prognosis is good.
- Encephalitis (40% of cases). Cutaneous lesions may not be present. The prognosis is severe, with possible sequelae despite antiviral treatment.
- Disseminated herpes (10%). Newborns appear septicemic, with fever, neurological signs, and multisystemic involvement (lung, liver, eye). Cutaneous lesions are present in half the cases. Even with treatment, mortality is high and survivors often suffer from ocular and neurological sequelae.

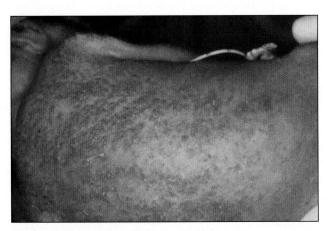

FIGURE 7.4: *Invasive candidal dermatitis.*

Varicella

Congenital varicella, acquired in utero from a maternal varicella between the 13th and the 20th week of pregnancy, is rare.[11] It may result in limb abnormalities and/or ocular and neurological involvement. The cutaneous lesions are irregular scars (sometimes zosteriform), atrophic areas, and/or hemorrhagic blisters.

Perinatal varicella is a severe disease, occurring when the mother presents varicella between 5 days before and 2 days after delivery. The newborn has a disseminated, vesicular rash, as well as a visceral varicella (lung, liver). Specific immunoglobulins may prevent or lessen the severity of neonatal varicella.[12] Acyclovir and supportive therapy are needed. The varicella vaccine should eradicate this severe disease.

Congenital Candidosis

Newborns may have localized *Candida* infections: oral thrush, perianal diaper dermatitis, and/or nail infection with paronychia.

Congenital cutaneous candidosis is acquired in utero from a candidal chorioamniotitis. It is manifest at birth or shortly after, as a generalized rash, made of dozens of small erythematous papules that rapidly progress to vesicles and pustules, followed by superficial desquamation. Respiratory infection can be found, but systemic dissemination is rare, in contrast with systemic candidosis, which may include skin lesions. A parenteral antifungal therapy is required if there is evidence of pneumonia or birth weight is less than 1500 g.

Invasive fungal dermatitis is a severe candidal infection occurring in only extremely premature babies (birth weight <1000 g). The fungi (organisms other than *Candida albicans* may be responsible) invade the body through the skin, because of the absence of an efficient epidermal barrier. This disseminated dermatitis starts a few days after birth, as an erythematous crusty eruption, with erosions and pustules (Figure 7.4). As in all forms of superficial candidiasis,

fungal filaments are easily found in the lesions. Parenteral antifungal therapy and supportive care are necessary.

Scabies

The incubation period of scabies is approximately 15 days, and a newborn may be contaminated by the cutaneous contact of an infested individual. The newborn does not express pruritus. The skin lesions are a papular–vesicular eruption, with small nodules predominating around the axillae, vesicles, or pustules on the palms and soles. Burrows may be seen by the naked eye, and dermoscopy may identify the intraepidermal mite. The contaminating person is usually rapidly found.

First-line treatment for neonatal scabies is a scabicide product containing pyrethroids. Care must be taken in the decontamination of the linen, the treatment of contact individuals, and the avoidance of repeated or toxic treatments.

Infantile acropustulosis is a rare pustulosis of infants, predominating on the hands and feet. It must not be mistaken for scabies, but may follow an efficiently treated scabies.

Incontinentia Pigmenti

All of the preceding vesicular–pustular conditions of neonates are of an infectious nature. Incontinentia pigmenti is an X-linked dominant genetic disorder, occurring almost only in girls.[13] It is due to mutations of the NEMO gene, located in X q 28. Inflammatory vesicles in a blaschkoid pattern are the first clinical manifestation of incontinentia pigmenti. Papular, keratotic, then pigmentary lesions may follow or coexist. Eosinophils are found in the vesicles, and there is at the same time a blood hypereosinophilia. Incontinentia pigmenti is usually a benign, limited disorder, but may include neurological (epilepsy, mental retardation), ocular, and dental abnormalities requiring specialized consultations. A genetic consultation is also advised.

OTHER NEONATAL ERUPTIONS

Macular–Papular Eruptions

Bacterial neonatal infections (neonatal sepsis) are multisystemic. A macular–papular rash may be observed, but is not indicative of any etiological agent.[10]

Purpuras

Apart from traumatic purpura resulting from a difficult delivery, purpura in a newborn is always an emergency. The main causes are platelet abnormalities, coagulation defects, and infections.

Protein C and protein S deficiency may cause neonatal purpura fulminans. Infections may include purpura

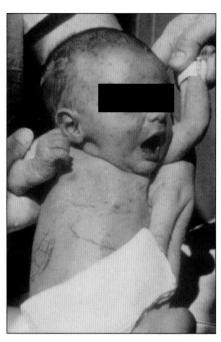

FIGURE 7.5: *Bluish nodular eruption ("blueberry muffin baby") during a cytomegalovirus infection. (Photo courtesy of Odile Enjolras, MD, Paris, France.)*

by many mechanisms, including thrombocytopenia and extramedullary erythropoiesis.

TORCH Syndrome

TORCH is an acronym designating a clinical condition that can be caused by several congenital infections: **T**oxoplasmosis, **O**ther infections, **R**ubella, **C**ytomegalovirus, and **H**erpes.

Clinical manifestations include petechial purpura, jaundice, and cutaneous nodules of erythropoiesis (blueberry muffin baby) (Figure 7.5).[14] The systemic consequences of the infections may be very severe.

Lupus Erythematosus

Neonatal lupus erythematosus (NLE) is due to the transplacental transfer of some antinuclear antibodies (anti-Ro–SSA, more rarely anti-LA–SSB). Mothers may be asymptomatic or suffering from a connective tissue disease. The autoantibodies are pathogenic for the skin and the cardiac conducting tissue. Cutaneous NLE consists of annular papulosquamous lesions, located on the upper part of the face and scalp. They disappear in a few weeks. NLE may also cause congenital heart block and, rarely, liver disease and hematologic manifestations.

Nodular Eruptions

Subcutaneous fat necrosis of the newborn is a benign panniculitis occurring in newborns with some risk factors.[15]

Subcutaneous nodules, starting shortly after birth, are located on the upper back, shoulders, and arms. They resolve in a few weeks, and their main complication is hypercalcemia.

NEONATAL ERYTHRODERMA

Erythroderma, in other words, generalized erythema and desquamation, can occur in newborns.[16] This must be differentiated from toxinic erythema (SSSS), generalized mastocytosis (skin infiltration, bullae), and ichthyosis bullosa (erythema, hyperkeratosis, bullae).

The main causes of neonatal erythroderma are immunodeficiencies (including Omenn syndrome); inflammatory dermatoses such as psoriasis, seborrheic dermatitis (Leiner disease), or atopic dermatitis; some metabolic disorders; and inherited ichthyoses. Erythroderma is a state of subacute cutaneous insufficiency, and affected newborns are at risk of superinfections as well as metabolic complications due to proteic, aqueous, and ionic transepidermal losses. They require intensive neonatal care, careful investigation, and follow-up. Cutaneous management is based on emollients and prevention of infection.

Inherited ichthyoses are a group of genetic skin diseases characterized by excessive desquamation. Some of these disorders can be present at birth. The clinical presentation is a neonatal erythroderma, or a *collodion baby*.

The collodion baby is a striking phenotype: The baby seems to be surrounded by a shiny, erythematous envelope resembling cellophane or collodion. Tension around the eyes and the mouth gives rise to eclabion and ectropion (Figure 7.6). The collodion-like envelope soon fissures and desquamates. Collodion babies are at risk of dehydration, hypothermia, and infection from an inefficient skin barrier and they must be kept in incubators. Skin care is based on abundant emollients and prevention of infection. Systemic toxicity of any topical must be considered. Collodion babies must be differentiated from the desquamation of postmature newborns, and from the collodion-like hyperkeratotic aspect of some ectodermal dysplasias. Although the majority of collodion babies have variants of congenital ichthyosis,[17] some cases rapidly recover, with perfectly normal skin. It is impossible to predict the prognosis during the first days or weeks after birth.

Netherton syndrome is characterized by a special form of ichthyosis (ichthyosis linearis circumflexa), trichorrhexis invaginata, and atopic dermatitis. This syndrome is due to mutations of the gene SPINK 5, which codes for a protease inhibitor called LEKTI. Affected children may be erythrodermic at birth (Figure 7.7). In this condition, the epidermal barrier is greatly impaired and there is a risk of hypernatremic dehydration, as well as systemic intoxication from absorbed topical drugs. The same risk exists, to a lesser degree, in all erythrodermic infants and, as said, in collodion babies.

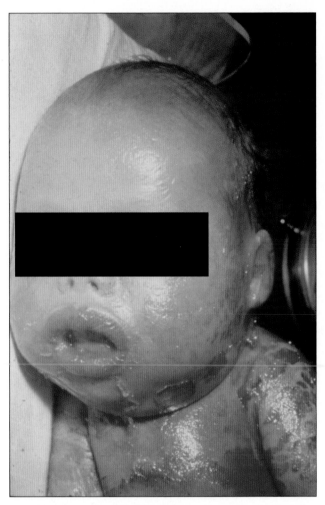

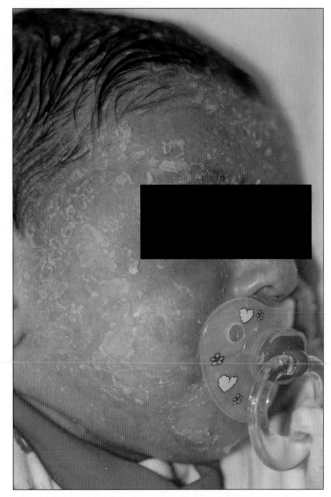

FIGURE 7.6: *Collodion baby. (Photo courtesy of Claudine Blanchet-Bardon, MD, Paris, France.)*

FIGURE 7.7: *Neonatal erythroderma of Netherton syndrome.*

CONGENITAL CUTANEOUS TUMORS

Hemangiomas

Hemangiomas usually become visible after a few weeks. At birth, they may be mistaken for capillary angiomas. White vasoconstriction areas may herald the development of a hemangioma.

Hemangioma-related emergencies may result from a rapid increase in size, associated with thrombocytopenia (Kasabach–Merritt syndrome), from diffuse hemangiomatosis with visceral involvement, or from ulcerations of periorificial hemangiomas.

Congenital hemangiomas[18] can even be diagnosed prenatally. They realize violaceous superficial tumors (Figure 7.8). Some regress rapidly. If the diagnosis of hemangioma cannot be ascertained clinically, a biopsy is necessary.

Hamartomas

Localized cutaneous malformations are visible at birth. Epidermal nevi, melanocytic nevi, and other hamartomas,

must be diagnosed rapidly. The two areas of concern are the needed workup, the specialized medical–surgical management, and the psychological support to the parents.

Infantile myofibromatosis appears at birth as cutaneous nodules that may be solitary or multiple. Skin lesions may regress spontaneously, but visceral lesions may be fatal.

Mastocytosis

Mastocytosis is a benign infiltration of the skin by mast cells. Several forms exist, which may be present at birth. Darier's sign is a useful clinical clue: The gentle rubbing of the lesion induces an urticarial papulation. The rubbing must be done on a very small area, to avoid generalized flushing.

Mastocytoma is a round elevated nodule, usually solitary.

Diffuse cutaneous mastocytosis presents as large, thick, orange or brown plaques (Figure 7.9). Urtication or bulla formation may be the consequence of pressure or friction by clothes.

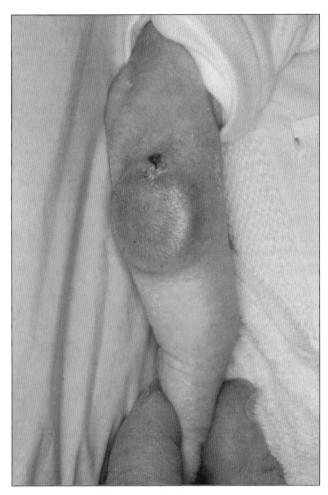

FIGURE 7.8: *Congenital hemangioma.*

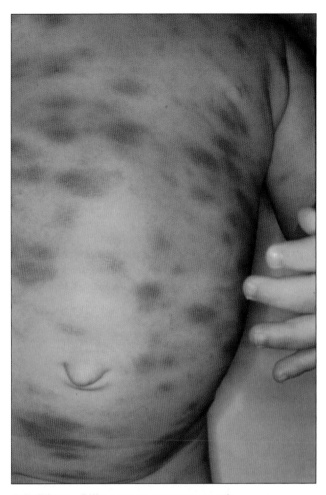

FIGURE 7.9: *Diffuse cutaneous mastocytosis.*

Urticaria pigmentosa is the name given to papular mastocytosis, which develops later in infancy.

Neoplastic Diseases

Langerhans cell histiocytosis (LCH) is a polymorphous disorder. It cannot be considered as an emergency, but it is important to suspect LCH when a newborn has papular–crusty, sometimes purpuric lesions in the folds, the scalp, and/or the diaper area (Letterer–Siwe disease). Visceral and/or bone involvement, as well as diabetes insipidus, may be present. A nodular form of LCH is regressive (Hashimoto–Pritzker syndrome).

Neuroblastoma may be present at birth. Cutaneous metastases appear as firm, bluish nodules (Figure 7.10), which may blanch on palpation. Histological examination will differentiate these lesions from leukemia or nonneoplastic causes of "blueberry muffin" lesions.

Leukemia is rarely congenital. Purpuric and nodular lesions appear in the context of a systemic leukemia. Biopsy and blood examinations provide the precise diagnosis.

Rhabdomyosarcoma is a malignant tumor that can be congenital. It appears as a shiny, red to purple firm tumor.

Usual locations are the head and neck and the perineal area.

Congenital melanoma is a rare occurrence. It may present as a nodule on a giant congenital melanocytic nevus.

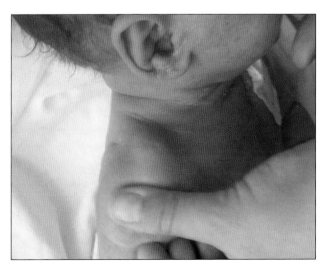

FIGURE 7.10: *Subcutaneous metastasis of neuroblastoma. (Photo courtesy of Aïcha Salhi, MD, Algiers, Algeria.)*

In all these cases of neonatal cutaneous tumors, the diagnosis relies on the histological examination of a biopsy, which may be considered as urgent. Special stains may be necessary.

APLASIA CUTIS

Aplasia cutis is a congenital absence of skin, on a limited area. The majority of cases are small, round atrophic patches of the scalp, near the vertex, with no associated anomaly.

There are in fact many other situations, including associations with EB (Bart syndrome), malformative syndromes, and chromosomal defects.[19]

Some cases of aplasia cutis are large congenital ulcerations requiring careful wound care. Large ulcerations of the scalp may involve the underlying structures, with the risk of lethal hemorrhages of the venous system. Radiologic imaging and surgery may be necessary.

PREMATURITY AS A CUTANEOUS EMERGENCY

The main function of the skin is to constitute a barrier between the organism and the environment. This function is carried out by the stratum corneum, which is formed during the last trimester of gestation. Premature babies (born before the 37th week) lack an efficient epidermal barrier and are at risk of dehydration, hypothermia, infection, and systemic toxicity of topicals. The procedures of neonatal medicine, including the care in heat- and hydration-controlled incubators, aim at alleviating the consequences of the functional insufficiency of the immature skin.[20]

REFERENCES

1. Eichenfield LF, Frieden IJ, Esterly NB. Textbook of neonatal dermatology. Philadelphia: WB Saunders; 2001.
2. Taieb A, Enjolras E, Vabres P, Wallach D. Dermatologie néonatale. Paris: Vigot Maloine; 2009.
3. Lin AN. Management of patients with epidermolysis bullosa. Dermatol Clin. 1996;14:381–7.
4. Levy SB, Goldsmith LA. The peeling skin syndrome. J Am Acad Dermatol. 1982;7:606–13.
5. Fassihi H, Diba VC, Wessagowit V, et al. Transient bullous dermolysis of the newborn in three generations. Br J Dermatol. 2005;153:1058–63.
6. Fassihi H, Wessagowit V, Jones C, et al. Neonatal diagnosis of Kindler syndrome. J Dermatol Sci. 2005;39:183–5.
7. Aoyama Y, Asai K, Hioki K, et al. Herpes gestationis in a mother and newborn: immunoclinical perspectives based on a weekly follow-up of the enzyme-linked immunosorbent assay index of a bullous pemphigoid antigen noncollagenous domain. Arch Dermatol. 2007;143:1168–72.
8. Campo-Voegeli A, Muñiz F, Mascaró JM, et al. Neonatal pemphigus vulgaris with extensive mucocutaneous lesions from a mother with oral pemphigus vulgaris. Br J Dermatol. 2002;147:801–5.
9. Vergnano S, Sharland M, Kazembe P, et al. Neonatal sepsis: an international perspective. Arch Dis Child Fetal Neonatal Ed. 2005;90:F220–4.
10. Olivier-Martin M, Wallach D, Bordier C, et al. Les signes cutanés des infections bactériennes néonatales. Arch Fr Pediatr. 1985;42:471–82.
11. Enders G, Miller E, Cradock-Watson J, et al. Consequences of varicella and herpes zoster in pregnancy: prospective study of 1739 cases. Lancet. 1994;343:1548–51.
12. Heuchan AM, Isaacs D. The management of varicella-zoster virus exposure and infection in pregnancy and the newborn period. Australasian Subgroup in Paediatric Infectious Diseases of the Australasian Society for Infectious Diseases. Med J Aust. 2001;174:288–92.
13. Hadj-Rabia S, Froidevaux D, Bodak N, et al. Clinical study of 40 cases of incontinentia pigmenti. Arch Dermatol. 2003;1399:1163–70.
14. Epps RE, Pittelkow MR, Su WPD. TORCH syndrome. Semin Dermatol. 1995;14:179–86.
15. Mahé E, Girszyn N, Hadj-Rabia S, et al. Subcutaneous fat necrosis of the newborn: a systematic evaluation of risk factors, clinical manifestations, complications and outcome of 16 children. Br J Dermatol. 2007;156:709–15.
16. Pruszkowski A, Bodemer C, Fraitag S, et al. Neonatal and infantile erythrodermas: a retrospective study of 51 patients. Arch Dermatol. 2000;136:875–80.
17. Paller AS. Disorders of cornification (ichthyosis). In: Eichenfield LF, Frieden IJ, Esterly NB, editors. Textbook of neonatal dermatology. Philadelphia:WB Saunders; 2001. pp. 276–93.
18. Mulliken JB, Enjolras O. Congenital hemangiomas and infantile hemangioma: missing links. J Am Acad Dermatol. 2004;50:875–82.
19. Frieden IJ. Aplasia cutis congenita: a clinical review and proposal for classification. J Am Acad Dermatol. 1986;14:646–60.
20. Williams ML. Skin of the premature infant. In: Eichenfield LF, Frieden IJ, Esterly NB, editors. Textbook of neonatal dermatology. Philadelphia: WB Saunders; 2001. pp. 46–61.

CHAPTER 8

Necrotizing Soft-Tissue Infections, Including Necrotizing Fasciitis

Ronni Wolf

Yalçin Tüzün

Batya B. Davidovici

SKIN AND SKIN structures are among the most frequent sites of human bacterial infection and account for ~10% of hospital admissions in the United States.[1]

The terminology used for infections of skin and skin structures is often confusing. "Primary" skin infections occur in otherwise normal skin and are usually caused by group A streptococci or *Staphylococcus aureus*. Infections are called "secondary" when they complicate chronic skin conditions (e.g., eczema or atopic dermatitis).

A second classification system divides skin and skin-structure infections into "uncomplicated" or "complicated," the latter defined as involving abnormal skin or wound infections occurring in a compromised host or requiring substantial surgical intervention.

A more important and, for our purposes, relevant distinction with essential management implications subdivides soft-tissue infections into "non-necrotizing" and "necrotizing" processes. This chapter reviews only the necrotizing soft-tissue infections (NSTIs) – the ones that pose real emergencies that are rapidly progressive, destructive, and highly lethal.

NSTIs can be defined as infections of any of the layers within the soft-tissue compartment (dermis, subcutaneous tissue, superficial fascia, deep fascia, or muscle) that are associated with necrotizing changes. NSTIs are typically not associated with abscesses, although they can originate from an untreated or inadequately drained abscess.

The incidence of NSTIs in the United States, as recently established from insurance databases from various states, is 0.04 cases per 1000 person-years.[2] This number is high enough to predict that surgeons, family physicians, internists, and dermatologists will encounter at least one patient during their practice, but too low for these doctors to acquire any real degree of familiarity with the disease. Distinguishing NSTIs from non-NSTIs and establishing the diagnosis of these infections is probably the greatest challenge in managing them. Early diagnosis and aggressive

surgical debridement of these often fatal and crippling diseases will save patients' lives and reduce morbidity. It is for this reason that familiarity with the clinical characteristics, diagnostic tools, and principles of management is so important when dealing with affected individuals.

Necrotizing fasciitis (NF) is categorized as type 1, 2, or 3, depending on the causative organisms.[3] Type 1 NF is mostly a mixed infection from aerobic and anaerobic bacteria, including Group A β-hemolytic *streptococci* (GAS), *S. aureus*, *Klebsiella* species, *Enterococci*, *Escherichia coli*, and *Clostridium* and *Bacteroides* species. The infecting organisms are often introduced at sites of surgery or trauma, and the lesions are often found in perineal and abdominal areas.

Type 2 NF is caused by GAS, possibly with a coinfection by *S. aureus*, and primarily affects the extremities. Type 3 NF is associated with *Vibrio vulnificus*, which enters the subcutaneous tissues via puncture wounds from fish or marine insects.

Another similar classification[1] distinguishes among the following subgroups of NF:

1. Polymicrobial fasciitis (type I),

2. Fournier gangrene,

3. Synergistic necrotizing "cellulitis" with fasciitis and myonecrosis,

4. Streptococcal gangrene (type II), and

5. Fasciitis caused by *V. vulnificus* and other *vibrio* species.

Myonecrosis is further subdivided into crepitant myonecrosis and noncrepitant myonecrosis.

It should be noted, however, that anatomical boundaries are not necessarily respected by invasive pathogens and one form of infection can rapidly progress to another (e.g., cellulitis can progress to fasciitis and myonecrosis and vice versa).

CLINICAL PRESENTATION AND LABORATORY AIDS REQUIRED FOR DIAGNOSIS

We will briefly describe an actual case that emphasizes the essence of early diagnosis.

One of us (RW) was called for a consultation in the rheumatology clinic to examine a 26-year-old woman with systemic lupus erythematosus due to severe pain at the hip area. The affected skin was erythematous and – we willl get ahead of ourselves here – it had a giveaway color, something between pink and violet, a color that, once you see, you will never miss. She was febrile but appeared to be in good physical condition, and had come for consultation independently. We prescribed ampicillin with clavulinic acie and instructed her to return the following week. Instead, she presented on the same evening to the emergency room because of worsening of the pain that was now unbearable. Because nothing in her clinical situation seemed to have changed, the consultant dermatologist ordered an x-ray, which showed no bone or joint involvement, so he discharged her with the same medication. She returned to the emergency room on the following morning and died one day later from septic shock (the result of cultures was GAS) and multiorgan failure. What we want to emphasize in this tragic case is the paucity of dermatologic symptoms and the absence of systemic symptoms except for severe localized pain. There were no signs of either sepsis or shock, when the patient was first seen by us.

It is our experience that too many cases of NF are misdiagnosed as non-NSTIs, and vice versa. This is also the experience of others. In a large case series[4] of NF, only 14.6% of the patients were correctly diagnosed or suspected as having NF on admission. The majority of the patients were diagnosed as having cellulitis (58.4%) or abscesses (18%). Similar numbers were recorded on the case report forms of 42 cases of GAS NF at the Florida Department of Health.[5] Only 9.5% were correctly diagnosed as having NF, and 4.8% were diagnosed as suffering from invasive GAS disease or toxic shock syndrome (also an acceptable diagnosis), but 31% of the patients had an admitting diagnosis of cellulitis and 24% of sepsis. The reason for this misdiagnosis is, in our opinion, the enormous dread of discovering that our patient is suffering from "flesh-eating disease" together with the erroneous expectation that the clinical signs should be suitably dramatic.

Clinicians should be aware that the pathological process involved in NF takes place very deeply – in other words, at the level of the fascial planes and even deeper – thus sparing the top layers of the skin at the earliest stages. This is unlike cellulitis, which involves the dermis and subcutaneous tissues early on, and much different from erysipelas, the most superficial infection. Consequently, clinical signs (e.g., the color, hemorrhagic bullae, and necrotic skin ulcers) are more prominent in the more superficial skin infections and less noticeable in the deeper ones. Erysipelas would appear

TABLE 8.1: Signs and Symptoms of NF

Symptom/Physical finding	% of patients
Pain	>97%
Erythema	~100%
Swelling	~75%
Fever	40%–70%
Skin necrosis	30%–45%
Blistering	20%–40%
Crepitus	12%–25%
X-ray findings	~20%

to the inexperienced clinician as being more serious than cellulitis, and cellulitis more alarming than NF. It cannot be emphasized enough that the very early stage of NF, the time when we strive to make the correct diagnosis, is characterized by mild symptoms that provide no clues of the seriousness and grave prognosis of the disease. Most of the patients we saw were febrile (but in apparent good health) and came for consultation independently with no need for special transportation. This experience is also the experience of others.[6] The affected dermal area characteristically had the typical rose–violet color. One symptom that no report misses is the disproportionately severe pain at the site of involvement. Another clue to diagnosis is the tenderness extending beyond the apparent area of involvement. The explanation for this phenomenon is the rapid spread of the infection along the deep fascia, faster than in the epidermis.

An additional cause and possible explanation for misdiagnosis or delay in diagnosing NF is the search for specific findings that are either not as common as previously thought, or, more important, are signs that become apparent only later in the evolution of the disease. These signs include the presence of crepitus on physical examination or soft-tissue air on plain x-ray, hemorrhagic and gangrenous bullae and ulcers, and the appearance of compartment syndrome (one of the favorite signs of the orthopedic surgeons). Pathognomonic as all these signs may be, waiting for them to emerge would lead to a regrettable and unfortunate postponement in arriving at the correct diagnosis. According to some large, retrospective case series[4,6–8] and reviews,[9] the most common symptom of NF is pain (>97%), and the most common clinical findings on admission are erythema, tenderness, and warm skin on palpation (>90%–100%). Much less common and inconsistent symptoms are fever and tachycardia (40%–70%), bullae/vesicle formation (20%–40%), and discoloration (20%–40%). Still less common are crepitations (12%–25%), x-ray findings (~20%), skin necrosis, and hypotension, which are also late signs (Table 8.1).

Although we do not doubt the claims that crepitus, blistering, or radiographic evidence of soft-tissue gas are found in more than 80% of patients on admission,[10] we believe that these are not the early signs that the clinician should look for. Indeed, it is not uncommon for NF patients to progress with alarming rapidity through the early, intermediate, and late presentations within hours of initial insult, so they present with "hard signs" on admission. These cannot and should not be considered early signs. Indeed, although the previously mentioned symptoms are the ones apparent at admission, it does not mean that they are the earliest ones.

KEYS TO EARLY DIAGNOSIS

- Do not look for the "hard signs," such as necrosis, crepitation, x-ray findings, or compartment syndrome. These are late signs and, in any event, are present in the minority of patients.
- Do not expect to see a severely ill patient with signs of septic shock. NF patients are often in apparently good health and walk into your clinic just like ordinary otherwise fit patients.
- Look for severe disproportionate pain and the typical color of the erythema: They are, in our opinion, the most reliable signs that should raise suspicion of NF.
- Tenderness usually extends beyond the area of skin involvement.

TREATMENT

The treatment of NF involves the principles of treatment of any kind of surgical infection: source control, antimicrobial therapy, support (hemodynamic, nutritional) and monitoring. NF is an excellent example of the important role of source control. When treatment is based only on antimicrobial therapy and support, mortality approaches 100%.[11,12] Antibiotics have not been shown to halt the infection in NF when pre- and postantibiotic series are compared.[12] It is clear that early and complete debridement is essential for effective treatment of NF. Concomitantly, appropriate broad-spectrum antibiotic coverage combined with adequate organ support and close monitoring helps patients during the acute phase of the disease, but, again, it is only the complete debridement of infected tissue that controls the infection and allows for future recovery.

Wide debridement of all necrotic and poorly perfused tissue at the time of initial presentation is clearly the most important step. The debridement is extended until skin and subcutaneous tissue cannot be elevated off the deep fascia by a gentle forward pushing maneuver. Healthy, viable, bleeding tissue should be present at the edges of the excision site, and aggressive resuscitation should accompany the perioperative period. Poorly perfused tissue is a nidus for continued bacterial proliferation. The anesthesiologist plays a critical role in the initial management of hemodynamic instability. Because NF fuels the progression of the septic state, one may not be able to completely stabilize the patient hemodynamically before surgery, and delay may lead to a fatal outcome. After the initial debridement has been done, management in an intensive care unit is recommended, and scheduled debridements should be performed as necessary.

Physiologic support combined with close monitoring in an intensive care unit setting is mandatory. Appropriate nutritional (enteral or parenteral) support administered as early as possible cannot be overemphasized. The magnitude of protein and fluid loss from the large wounds associated with NF is tremendous. In general, patients with severe tissue loss should receive twice their basal caloric requirements.[7,11] Aggressive fluid resuscitation and blood component therapy is often required during the perioperative period.

It is not uncommon to see patients with NF develop organ failure, such as acute renal failure (~30%), adult respiratory distress syndrome (~30%), multiorgan system dysfunction (20%), infectious complications, and others,[10] all of which require careful monitoring and prompt treatment.

As for the role of antibiotics in NF, we refer to the Infectious Disease Society of America guidelines.[13] Antimicrobial therapy must be directed at the pathogens and used in appropriate doses until repeated operative procedures are no longer needed, until the patient has demonstrated obvious clinical improvement, and until fever has been absent for 48–72 hours.

ANTIMICROBIALS

Mixed infection: Ampicillin-sulbactam or piperacillin-tazobactam + clindamycin + ciprofloxacin. Alternatively, meropenem, ertapenem, cefotaxime + metronidazole or clindamycin

GAS infection (type II NF): Penicillin + clindamycin

S. aureus infection: Nafcillin, oxacillin, cefazolin, vancomycin (for resistant strains), clindamycin

Clostridium infection: Clindamycin or penicillin

Until recently, therapy directed against methicillin-resistant *S. aureus* (MRSA) was not recommended in standard guides, presumably because of the rarity of this pathogen as a cause of NF. Over the past few years, community-associated infections caused by MRSA (CA-MRSA), the majority involving skin and soft tissues, have become common in multiple areas in the United States and worldwide. CA-MRSA should no longer be regarded as a strictly nosocomial pathogen.[14] MRSA is now the most common pathogen isolated in the emergency department from skin and soft-tissue infections.[15] Recently, 14 cases of NF associated with CA-MRSA were identified among 843 patients whose wound cultures grew MRSA,[16] and wound cultures were monomicrobial for MRSA in 12 of them. Although all these patients survived, serious complications were common, including prolonged stays in the intensive care unit, the need for mechanical ventilation and reconstructive surgery, septic shock, nosocomial infections, and endophthalmitis. The main lesson from this and other reports is that we should include antibiotics with good activity against CA-MRSA in the currently recommended therapy for NF.[16,17] Vancomycin is still the preferred antibiotic for empirical coverage and definitive therapy, but whether it should remain so is questionable. It is a less effective anti-staphylococcal agent than the penicillins, and increased use will further exacerbate problems with vancomycin-resistant enterococci and staphylococci.[17] Newer effective antibiotics, such as linezolid and teicoplanin, represent appropriate empirical therapeutic options.[14]

Single-organism NF is also increasingly recognized as a manifestation of *Klebsiella* infections[18–20] probably due to the emergence of the highly virulent K1 capsular serotype, the predominant serotype of potentially lethal disseminated infection with this pathogen in Asia, including NF.[18] Single-organism NF due to *Klebsiella* species is strongly associated with predisposing conditions, such as diabetes mellitus, and has a propensity for metastatic dissemination resulting in multiple sites of infection.[20]

Hyperbaric oxygen as an adjunctive treatment has been advocated by different groups that argue for a decrease in the number of debridements and an associated decrease in mortality.[7,21,22] Results from this therapeutic strategy are contradictory, and no real epidemiologically based studies have been performed to elucidate the effect of this form of therapy. Certainly, hyperbaric oxygen therapy should not jeopardize standard therapy for NF. Hyperbaric oxygen is not available at all institutions and is hardly standard equipment of ordinary intensive care units; thus patients would have to be transported to the chamber at least 3 times per day, which may expose them to risk of contamination and may limit the ability to perform close monitoring and timely debridements while they are in the chamber.

Another adjuvant treatment that has been used is intravenous immunoglobulin (IVIG). The value of this form of therapy is difficult to assess given the small number of patients that had ever been treated with this method, the differences in methodologies and, particularly, the diversity between batches of the different companies.[23] The use of IVIG has been advocated mainly for GAS infections. Information on the efficacy of IVIG in GAS bacteremia can be found in a publication of the Canadian Streptococcal Study Group.[24] They compared survival in 21 consecutive patients with streptococcal toxic shock syndrome who had been given IVIG to that of 32 control patients who did not receive the therapy. Sixty-seven percent of the treated patients survived compared with only 34% of the control patients. A double-blind, placebo-controlled trial from northern Europe showed no significant improvement in survival for the IVIG group.[25] We suggest adopting the conclusion of the Infectious Disease Society of America[13] "...that additional studies of the efficacy of IVIG are necessary before a recommendation can be made..." We vigorously disagree with those clinicians who suggest that this therapy "may allow an initial non-operative or minimally invasive approach."[26] No therapy should tempt the surgeon to postpone surgery or to perform less mutilating and, consequently, less effective surgery.

PROGNOSIS AND FACTORS THAT AFFECT OUTCOME

Many attempts have been made to understand the factors affecting mortality from NF. The fortunate rarity of the disease and the multiple factors that influence the outcome (such as causative agent, site of infection, and host factors) have paradoxically hampered the establishment of an effective scoring system. Objective estimation of the probability of death from NF would have provided an explicit basis for clinical decisions, aided in the understanding of the relative contribution of these specific prognostic criteria, and reduced the reliance on clinical intuition.

The mortality rates for NF vary considerably, ranging between less than 10% and as high as 75%. The larger, more robust, retrospective case series have narrowed these rates to between 25% and 40%.[27] What is clear, however, is that the prognosis has improved considerably over the past two decades as a result of early recognition and improved supportive multidisciplinary measures.

In a recently published retrospective analysis of 99 patients with NF treated in three tertiary care hospitals in Ontario, Canada,[28] the overall mortality was 20%. Sixteen patients underwent amputation or suffered organ loss. There was a strong positive association between a patient's age and mortality, with the risk of death increasing by 4% every year. Apart from age, streptococcal toxic shock syndrome and immunocompromised status were independent predictors of mortality. There was also a significant association between diabetes and negative outcome. The anatomic sites of infection did not reach a level of significance in predicting outcome, with the exception of perineal infection, which was significantly associated with a negative outcome. Interestingly, the hyperbaric oxygen therapy group had a higher mortality rate than did the nonhyperbaric oxygen therapy group.[28]

NSTI CAUSED BY *V. VULNIFICUS*

Although *V. vulnificus* infections had probably occurred in ancient times (the first fatal infection was possibly reported by Hippocrates in the 5th century BCE),[29] it was not until the reporting of the first case in 1987 (in Taiwan)[30] that an increased prevalence became apparent. Recent findings suggest that the reason might be associated with global warming and prolongation of warmer weather and warmer water temperature.[31] *V. vulnificus* is considered one of the most dangerous waterborne bacterial pathogens, with a case fatality rate that may reach 50% for *V. vulnificus* septicemia. Notably, *V. vulnificus* is estimated to account for 95% of all seafood-related deaths in the United States.[32]

Microbiology and Epidemiology

V. vulnificus is a naturally occurring, gram-negative, halophilic bacterium of the noncholera group that is a free-living inhabitant of estuaries and marine environments throughout the world. *Vibrio* species have been found in warm coastal waters ranging in temperature from 9°C to 21°C in geographically diverse regions that include the Gulf of Mexico, South America, Asia (Thailand, Taiwan, Hong Kong), and Australia.[33] The bacterium is frequently found in oysters, crustaceans, and shellfish (according to various reports, up to 50% of oysters and up to 11% of crabs are cultured positive during summer).[34]

Clinical Manifestations

The disease manifestations caused by *V. vulnificus* depend on the route of infection, with three recognized syndromes: 1) primary septicemia, which is classically linked to the consumption of raw oysters; 2) wound infection resulting from cellulitis caused by direct inoculation of the microorganism, which may result in tissue necrosis and secondary bacteremia (usually involving the exposure of chafed skin to salty water containing the microorganism or injuries associated with the cultivation and/or preparation of seafood); and 3) gastrointestinal illness, characterized by vomiting, diarrhea, or abdominal pain. Pneumonia and endometritis have also been reported. Skin lesions appear within 24–48 hours of exposure. The disease process begins with localized tenderness followed by erythema, edema, and indurated plaques. A purplish discoloration develops in the center of the lesions and then undergoes necrosis, eventually forming hemorrhagic bullae or ulcers. These clinical manifestations occur in nearly 90% of patients and are most common on the lower extremities. Noteworthy, these symptoms are different from those described earlier for NF because the infection usually starts superficially and is accompanied by cellulitis. In a survey from Israel,[35] for example, 57 of 62 cases of NSTI caused by *V. vulnificus* developed cellulitis, and only 4 had NF.

The disease occurs mostly in immunocompromised host–associated diseases. In a recent study of 67 patients,[36] 27 (40%) had hepatic disease, 17 (25.4%) had chronic renal insufficiency, and 12 (17.9%) exhibited adrenal insufficiency.

The diagnosis of NSTI caused by *V. vulnificus* is difficult because the symptoms of sepsis caused by *V. vulnificus* are not different from those of any other form of sepsis. This infection should be suspected in patients with a

rapidly progressive inflammation of the skin and soft tissues following recent exposure to contaminated seawater or raw seafood, and possibly one of the associated predisposing diseases. Definitive diagnosis is made by identifying the bacteria from cultures. Gram-negative bacteria can be seen on Gram's staining.

Treatment

Soft-tissue infection by *V. vulnificus* represents a true surgical emergency. Early recognition and prompt aggressive debridement of all necrotic tissue are critical for survival and improve the rate of survival. The cause of death in most cases is multiorgan failure, acute respiratory distress syndrome, or overwhelming sepsis. With appropriate early surgical intervention, mortality varies from 8.7% to 50%, depending on a number of variables.[36] Without surgical intervention, the disease is usually fatal because antibiotics alone are ineffective against the large soft-tissue bacterial inocula resulting from the invasive nature of these infections and because of the widespread obliterative vasculitis, vascular necrosis, and thrombosis of the supplying vessels that hinder the penetration of antibiotics to the affected area. As with other types of NSTIs and NF, debridement must be aggressive, all necrotic tissue with overlying skin should be excised deeply and beyond the necrotic area, and all necrotic fascia and fat should be removed until healthy viable tissue is evident. A second examination should be done within 24 hours to assess the progression of the condition and check the need for further debridement.[36]

In addition to aggressive surgical debridement, efficient and early presurgical antimicrobial treatment is essential for management of *V. vulnificus* infection. Antimicrobial use should be initiated as soon as the diagnosis is considered likely. The combination of cefotaxime and minocycline demonstrated a better outcome than monotherapy with either drug alone.[36] This combination is also better than first- or second-generation cephalosporin. More recently, the newer fluoroquinolones have been demonstrated to be as effective as the combination cefotaxime plus minocycline in vitro and in vivo.[37] The combination of quinolone plus cefotaxime showed a superior in vitro efficacy than either drug alone or the combination of minocycline plus cefotaxime.[37]

All other measures to be taken are the same as for other types of NF.

REFERENCES

1. DiNubile MJ, Lipsky BA. Complicated infections of skin and skin structures: when the infection is more than skin deep. J Antimicrob Chemother. 2004;53 Suppl 2:ii37–ii50.
2. Ellis Simonsen SM, van Orman ER, Hatch BE, et al. Cellulitis incidence in a defined population. Epidemiol Infect. 2006; 134:293–9.

3. Salcido RS. Necrotizing fasciitis: reviewing the causes and treatment strategies. Adv Skin Wound Care. 2007;20:288–93.

4. Wong CH, Chang HC, Pasupathy S, et al. Necrotizing fasciitis: clinical presentation, microbiology, and determinants of mortality. J Bone Joint Surg Am. 2003;85-A:1454–60.

5. Mulla ZD. Group A streptococcal necrotizing fasciitis: reducing the risk of unwarranted litigation. Am J Emerg Med. 2005;23:578–9.

6. Wang YS, Wong CH, Tay YK. Staging of necrotizing fasciitis based on the evolving cutaneous features. Int J Dermatol. 2007;46:1036–41.

7. Childers BJ, Potyondy LD, Nachreiner R, et al. Necrotizing fasciitis: a fourteen-year retrospective study of 163 consecutive patients. Am Surg. 2002;68:109–16.

8. Singh G, Sinha SK, Adhikary S, et al. Necrotising infections of soft tissues–a clinical profile. Eur J Surg. 2002;168:366–71.

9. Cunningham JD, Silver L, Rudikoff D. Necrotizing fasciitis: a plea for early diagnosis and treatment. Mt Sinai J Med. 2001;68:253–61.

10. Elliott DC, Kufera JA, Myers RA. Necrotizing soft tissue infections. Risk factors for mortality and strategies for management. Ann Surg. 1996;224:672–83.

11. Anaya DA, Dellinger EP. Necrotizing soft-tissue infection: diagnosis and management. Clin Infect Dis. 2007;44:705–10.

12. Burge TS. Necrotizing fasciitis–the hazards of delay. J R Soc Med. 1995;88:342P–343P.

13. Stevens DL, Bisno AL, Chambers HF, et al. Practice guidelines for the diagnosis and management of skin and soft-tissue infections. Clin Infect Dis. 2005;41:1373–406.

14. Maltezou HC, Giamarellou H. Community-acquired methicillin-resistant Staphylococcus aureus infections. Int J Antimicrob Agents. 2006;27:87–96.

15. Moran GJ, Krishnadasan A, Gorwitz RJ, et al. Methicillin-resistant S. aureus infections among patients in the emergency department. N Engl J Med. 2006;355:666–74.

16. Miller LG, Perdreau-Remington F, Rieg G, et al. Necrotizing fasciitis caused by community-associated methicillin-resistant Staphylococcus aureus in Los Angeles. N Engl J Med. 2005;352:1445–53.

17. Chambers HF. Community-associated MRSA–resistance and virulence converge. N Engl J Med. 2005;352:1485–7.

18. Kohler JE, Hutchens MP, Sadow PM, et al. Klebsiella pneumoniae necrotizing fasciitis and septic arthritis: an appearance in the Western hemisphere. Surg Infect (Larchmt). 2007;8:227–32.

19. Liu YM, Chi CY, Ho MW, et al. Microbiology and factors affecting mortality in necrotizing fasciitis. J Microbiol Immunol Infect. 2005;38:430–5.

20. Wong CH, Kurup A, Wang YS, et al. Four cases of necrotizing fasciitis caused by Klebsiella species. Eur J Clin Microbiol Infect Dis. 2004;23:403–7.

21. Jallali N, Withey S, Butler PE. Hyperbaric oxygen as adjuvant therapy in the management of necrotizing fasciitis. Am J Surg. 2005;189:462–6.

22. Riseman JA, Zamboni WA, Curtis A, et al. Hyperbaric oxygen therapy for necrotizing fasciitis reduces mortality and the need for debridements. Surgery. 1990;108:847–50.

23. Kaul R, McGeer A, Low DE, et al. Population-based surveillance for group A streptococcal necrotizing fasciitis: clinical features, prognostic indicators, and microbiologic analysis of seventy-seven cases. Ontario Group A Streptococcal Study. Am J Med. 1997;103:18–24.

24. Kaul R, McGeer A, Norrby-Teglund A, et al. Intravenous immunoglobulin therapy for streptococcal toxic shock syndrome–a comparative observational study. The Canadian Streptococcal Study Group. Clin Infect Dis. 1999;28:800–7.

25. Darenberg J, Ihendyane N, Sjolin J, et al. Intravenous immunoglobulin G therapy in streptococcal toxic shock syndrome: a European randomized, double-blind, placebo-controlled trial. Clin Infect Dis. 2003;37:333–40.

26. Muller AE, Oostvogel PM, Steegers EA, Dorr PJ. Morbidity related to maternal group B streptococcal infections. Acta Obstet Gynecol Scand. 2006;85:1027–37.

27. Carter PS, Banwell PE. Necrotising fasciitis: a new management algorithm based on clinical classification. Int Wound J. 2004;1:189–98.

28. Golger A, Ching S, Goldsmith CH, et al. Mortality in patients with necrotizing fasciitis. Plast Reconstr Surg. 2007;119:1803–7.

29. Baethge BA, West BC. Vibrio vulnificus: did Hippocrates describe a fatal case? Rev Infect Dis. 1988;10:614–15.

30. Yuan CY, Yuan CC, Wei DC, Lee AM. Septicemia and gangrenous change of the legs caused by marine vibrio, V. vulnificus–report of a case.. Taiwan Yi Xue Hui Za Zhi. 1987;86:448–51.

31. Paz S, Bisharat N, Paz E, et al. Climate change and the emergence of Vibrio vulnificus disease in Israel. Environ Res. 2007;103:390–6.

32. Oliver JD, Bockian R. In vivo resuscitation, and virulence towards mice, of viable but nonculturable cells of Vibrio vulnificus. Appl Environ Microbiol. 1995;61:2620–3.

33. Strom MS, Paranjpye RN. Epidemiology and pathogenesis of Vibrio vulnificus. Microbes Infect. 2000;2:177–88.

34. Tamplin M, Rodrick GE, Blake NJ, Cuba T. Isolation and characterization of Vibrio vulnificus from two Florida estuaries. Appl Environ Microbiol. 1982;44:1466–70.

35. Bisharat N, Agmon V, Finkelstein R, et al. Clinical, epidemiological, and microbiological features of Vibrio vulnificus biogroup 3 causing outbreaks of wound infection and bacteraemia in Israel. Israel Vibrio Study Group. Lancet. 1999;354:1421–4.

36. Kuo YL, Shieh SJ, Chiu HY, Lee JW. Necrotizing fasciitis caused by Vibrio vulnificus: epidemiology, clinical findings, treatment and prevention. Eur J Clin Microbiol Infect Dis. 2007;26:785–92.

37. Kim DM, Lym Y, Jang SJ, et al. In vitro efficacy of the combination of ciprofloxacin and cefotaxime against Vibrio vulnificus. Antimicrob Agents Chemother. 2005;49:3489–91.

CHAPTER 9

Life-Threatening Bacterial Skin Infections

Richard B. Cindrich

Donald Rudikoff

DERMATOLOGISTS are often called on to diagnose severe life-threatening skin infections in the emergency department, hospital wards, and in their clinical practices. The observational skills of the dermatologic specialist enable him or her to differentiate conditions that are potentially fatal from those that may look horrific but are not life threatening. This chapter provides essential information on serious infections, many of which are not usually discussed in depth in most dermatologic texts. These include periorbital (preseptal) and orbital cellulitis, malignant external otitis, meningococcemia, Rocky Mountain spotted fever (RMSF), Mediterranean spotted fever, anthrax, tularemia, and infections with *Vibrio vulnificus*, *Aeromonas hydrophila* and *Chromobacterium violaceum*. It is hoped that prompt recognition of these infections by the clinician will reduce morbidity and possibly be lifesaving.

PERIORBITAL (PRESEPTAL) CELLULITIS AND ORBITAL CELLULITIS

Background

Eyelid infections presenting with erythema and edema are not uncommon in children and adults and in some cases can cause serious sequelae. Involvement of the orbit with bacterial infection can result in severe damage to the eye, cavernous sinus thrombosis, and death. Preseptal cellulitis is an infection of the eyelids and surrounding skin anterior to the orbital septum (Figure 9.1).[1] This layer of fibrous tissue arises from the periosteum of the orbit and extends into the eyelids.[2] Infection posterior to the septum is referred to as orbital cellulitis. Although less common than preseptal cellulitis, it is a much more worrisome condition with the potential for major sequelae. It is essential when confronted with a patient with eyelid infection to distinguish orbital cellulitis from preseptal infection and other entities that may present similarly. Whereas preseptal cellulitis often can be managed in an outpatient setting, orbital cellulitis requires hospitalization, intravenous (IV) antibiotics, and sometimes surgical intervention. Immediate ophthalmological consultation is essential and, because the process

may derive from sinus infection, otolaryngological consultation is often helpful.

Clinical and Laboratory Aids Required for Diagnosis

Distinction between preseptal and orbital cellulitis in patients with periorbital inflammation is the major priority. Patients with preseptal cellulitis complain of pain, symptoms of conjunctivitis, epiphora, and blurred vision and display eyelid and periorbital erythema and edema that may be so severe that they cannot open the eye.[3] Although edema may frustrate examination, the visual acuity, light reflexes, and range of motion of the globe should be assessed. Unlike preseptal cellulitis, orbital cellulitis presents with some degree of ophthalmoplegia, pain on eye movement, and/or proptosis. The latter condition may also compromise the optic nerve causing vision loss, abnormal papillary reflexes, and disk edema. Computed tomography with contrast should be undertaken when physical examination is impeded by obtundation or patient age to rule out abscess formation, if orbital cellulitis is suspected.

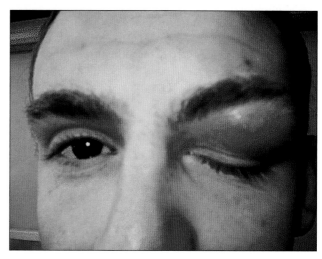

FIGURE 9.1: *Left preseptal cellulitis. Reproduced with permission from the BMJ Publishing Group. Br J Ophthalmol. 2007; 91:1723–4.*

Orbital cellulitis can be caused by penetrating trauma but is almost always a consequence of sinusitis. Most commonly, the ethmoid sinus is involved in extension across the lamina papyracea. Blood cultures and complete blood counts (CBCs) should be done in all patients but do not reliably differentiate between the two conditions. Leukocytosis with left shift will be present in most patients with either condition. Bacteremia is infrequent but more common in young children. Cultures should be obtained from the eyelid, or any conjunctival or lacrimal sac discharge.[3]

Preseptal cellulitis occurs as a consequence of facial infection, trauma, insect bites, or herpetic lesion. It also may occur as a result of bacteremia in children younger than 36 months. In this setting, prior to the introduction and routine use of conjugated *Hemophilus* vaccine, the most common pathogen was *Hemophilus influenzae* but it is now *Streptococcus pneumoniae*. The intact orbital septum usually prevents posterior spread of preseptal cellulitis in adults, but in children such spread can occur. Clinical evidence of trauma, insect bites, herpes infection, dacryocystitis, or sinus infection should be sought in all patients presenting with eyelid and periorbital inflammation.

Therapy

Oral antimicrobial coverage for *Staphylococcus aureus* and group A *Streptococci* is usually sufficient in uncomplicated cases of preseptal cellulitis in adults. Typical regimens include oral amoxicillin/clavulanic acid, a first-generation cephalosporin, or intramuscular ceftriaxone. Younger children should be admitted to the hospital and additionally receive antibiotic coverage for *S. pneumoniae* with an agent such as cefuroxime. Local prevalence of methicillin-resistant *S. aureus* and penicillin-resistant *S. pneumoniae* in the community should be considered in deciding initial antibiotic coverage pending the receipt of culture results. An evidence-based literature review to determine whether children with simple preseptal periorbital cellulitis should be treated with IV or oral antibiotics failed to find any evidence that either approach was superior.[4] The authors noted that, in one hospital series, four pediatric patients with preseptal cellulitis developed intracranial, epidural abscess or empyema.[5]

Suspected cases of orbital cellulitis should be admitted to the hospital for IV antibiotic treatment. Consultation with ophthalmology and otolaryngology should be obtained on an emergency basis. Following culture collection, antibiotic therapy should be initiated with coverage of Streptococcus species, *S. aureus*, anaerobes, nontypable *Hemophilus*, and *Moraxella catarrhalis*.

Course and Prognosis

Preseptal cellulitis usually has an excellent prognosis if recognized early and treated aggressively. Duration of therapy is dependent on response and extent of infection. If improvement does not occur in 24–48 hours, a resistant organism or orbital infection should be suspected. Treatment should be continued for about 10 days.

For orbital cellulitis, IV antibiotics should be continued until the infection is well controlled and consideration given to oral therapy to complete a course of 3–4 weeks. Venous sinus thrombosis is a potential complication of orbital cellulitis as venous drainage of the orbit is through the cavernous sinus.

MALIGNANT EXTERNAL OTITIS

Background

Malignant (necrotizing) external otitis is an invasive infection of the external auditory canal and skull base most commonly occurring in elderly individuals with diabetes mellitus (86%–90%) and in patients with acquired immunodeficiency syndrome.[6,7] It is caused by *Pseudomonas aeruginosa* in more than 98% of cases. Case reports have implicated other bacteria in some cases including *S. aureus*, *Proteus mirabilis*, and others. *Aspergillus fumigatus* has been implicated in cases of fungal malignant external otitis. Occasional pediatric cases of malignant otitis externa have been reported, particularly in adolescents with diabetes and children with immune dysfunction as a result of leukemia, malnutrition, and/or solid tumors.[8] Children with the disease may display fever, leukocytosis, and pseudomonas bacteremia and develop facial nerve palsy more often than adults may. Rare cases have been reported in infancy. Malignant external otitis may be complicated by facial nerve palsy, meningitis, brain abscess, and dural sinus thrombophlebitis and may be fatal.

Clinical and Laboratory Aids Required for Diagnosis

Patients with malignant otitis externa typically present with ear pain and drainage, and frequently they will have failed therapy with topical agents. They may also give a history of recent irrigation for impacted cerumen. Pain may extend to the temporomandibular joint and be exacerbated by chewing. A predisposing immunocompromising condition, diabetes most commonly, is usually present.

On physical examination, granulation tissue is noted in the auditory canal at the bony cartilaginous junction.[9] Drainage is present, but the tympanic membrane is usually undamaged.

Therapy

Following culture, therapy should be initiated with antibiotics covering Pseudomonas species. Until recently, oral therapy with ciprofloxacin 750 mg twice daily with or without the addition of rifampin has been advocated as the treatment of choice.[10,11] Due to increasing use of fluoroquinolones, resistance of Pseudomonas species to ciprofloxacin has been increasing with anywhere from 20% to 30% of isolates being reported as resistant.[12–14] Hospital admission and IV antibiotic therapy with a third-generation cephalosporin such as ceftazidime with anti-Pseudomonas activity is indicated when there is a history of recent fluoroquinolone use, high community rates of ciprofloxacin-resistant Pseudomonas, or when clinical severity warrants close observation. The use of hyperbaric oxygen has been advocated to improve outcomes in malignant external otitis, but an analysis of published studies failed to find sufficient evidence in controlled studies for its use.[15]

Course and Prognosis

Osteomyelitis of the skull base with involvement of vital structures is the most serious complication of malignant otitis externa.[16] Cranial nerve neuropathy, especially of the facial nerve, may occur. The earliest series in the literature reporting on elderly diabetic patients with late-stage disease who underwent extensive surgery as primary therapy had a mortality rate of approximately 50%.[17] Because of the high mortality with surgery, the use of synergistic combinations of semisynthetic penicillins and aminoglycosides was introduced to control pseudomonas; subsequently, third-generation cephalosporins such as ceftazidime were shown to have similar efficacy.[18–20] Later, ciprofloxacin at a dosage of 1.5 g/d used over an average of 10 weeks showed superior efficacy with a reduction of mortality from approximately 30% to 2%–3%; however, this result was prior to recent increases in ciprofloxacin resistance.[10,18] Premature termination of treatment may result in recurrence rates of 15%–20%.[21] Prolonged treatment is more likely to be associated with adverse drug reactions in patients receiving β-lactam antibiotics than in those treated with ciprofloxacin.[22] In a recent study, facial nerve involvement previously cited as a poor prognostic indicator did not adversely affect survival.[16,23]

MENINGOCOCCEMIA

Background

Meningococcemia, with or without meningitis, is one of the most serious emergencies in medicine. The causative organism, *Neisseria meningitidis*, has the ability to cause outbreaks as well as sporadic cases of invasive meningococcal disease with devastating consequences often progressing rapidly to purpura fulminans, shock, and death. Large-scale outbreaks occurred in the United States in the 1940s associated with military deployments, but disease rates have remained relatively stable for the past 20 years, at 1.0–1.5 per 100,000 population.[24] Despite advances in treatment, approximately 10% of affected patients die from the disease,

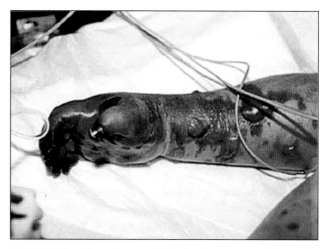

FIGURE 9.2: *Necrotic purpuric bullae in a 5-year-old boy with meningococcemia who developed purpura fulminans. Source: DermAtlas, Johns Hopkins University; 2000–2009 (meningococcemia_1_031001), Andreas Eliades, MD.*

and another 10%–20% are left with severe sequelae such as hearing loss and limb amputation.[25] Affecting primarily the pediatric population, the highest rates of both meningitic and nonmeningitic meningococcal disease occur in infants younger than 1 year.[26] Approximately one third of all cases of sporadic meningococcal disease occur in adults, and one half of these present without rash or meningitis.[27] Given the high morbidity and mortality of meningococcal infections, rapid institution of antibiotic therapy and supportive care are advocated by most authorities. Preadmission parenteral antibiotics (benzylpenicillin, ceftriaxone, chloramphenicol) have been suggested for patients presenting to a physician's office with signs of invasive meningococcal disease. Assuredly, no physician wants to miss the diagnosis of meningococcemia. The diagnosis of patients presenting with typical signs of acute meningitis is often straightforward. It is the patient who does not appear ill on initial presentation who represents a major diagnostic challenge.[28] To not miss the diagnosis, it has been suggested that, in any acutely febrile patient, it is prudent to ask, "Why is this patient seeking help now?" then "Could this patient have meningococcemia?"[28]

Clinical and Laboratory Aids Required for Diagnosis

Early clinical clues to meningococcemia include a hemorrhagic (petechial or purpuric) eruption; a blanching macular or maculopapular rash appearing in the first 24 hours; true rigors; severe pain in the extremities, neck, and back; vomiting; headache; and rapid evolution of illness.[28] The lesions of acute meningococcemia are indurated, gun metal gray patches of purpura that display an irregular (infarctive) pattern (Figure 9.2).[29] These may occur anywhere on the skin and can develop bullae and ulcerate. A transient blanching erythematous maculopapular eruption may arise before the appearance of purpura.[29] In a study of children and adolescents with invasive meningococcal disease, the first classical sign to emerge was rash, which at the onset was nonspecific and only developed into a petechial (and then a largely hemorrhagic) eruption over several hours.[30] In this study, fever was the first symptom noted in children younger than 5 years. Headache was the first symptom in patients older than 5 years; 94% developed fever at some point, and irritability was a prominent symptom in younger children.[30] Three important features were identified as signs of early meningococcal disease in children and adolescents: leg pain, cold hands and feet, and abnormal skin color (pallor or mottling).[30] Eruption, meningism, and impaired consciousness occurred later.

Therapy

The prompt initiation of IV antibiotic therapy is essential in patients with suspected meningococcal disease. Recommended treatment regimens include a 5- to 7-day course of: (1) penicillin G, 500,000 U/kg/d in six divided doses; (2) ceftriaxone, 100 mg/kg/d in one or two divided doses; or (3) cefotaxime, 200 mg/kg/d in three divided doses.[31,32] Recently, intermediate resistance of some meningococci to penicillin has been reported from Europe. In a Portuguese study, one quarter (24.6%) of the isolates showed moderate resistance to penicillin.[33] A study from Scotland found an absence of "high-level" resistance to penicillin among meningococci and an 8.3% prevalence of moderate resistance.[34] Although there is some indication that a small number of strains in the United States display intermediate resistance to penicillin, the U.S. Centers for Disease Control and Prevention (CDC) has not recommended routine susceptibility testing of meningococcal isolates.[35] Treatment of meningitis in children is aimed at the most likely pathogen based on epidemiologic information.[36] Because of the significant prevalence of penicillin-resistant *S. pneumoniae*, empirical treatment of meningitis in children 1 month old or older should include vancomycin plus cefotaxime or ceftriaxone.[36]

Course and Prognosis

In general, the mortality rate for meningococcal septicemia exceeds that of meningococcal meningitis. Reported mortality from meningococcemia ranges from 18% to 53% whereas that of meningococcal meningitis has in the past 15–20 years hovered around 10%.[31,37] Among adults with single episodes of community-acquired meningitis, risk factors for death included older age ($\geq$60 years), obtunded mental state on admission, and seizures within the first 24 hours.[38] In a study of 3335 meningococcal deaths in the United States, 58% of deaths occurred among persons younger than 25 years. Mortality was increased in infants, young adults (15–24 years old), and older adults (older than

74 years).[39] Neurological sequelae following meningococcal disease occurred in 10%–20% of patients.[40]

A number of treatment modalities have been used to improve the prognosis of meningococcal disease. There is controversy as to whether corticosteroids improve prognosis, but many groups use them routinely.

A subgroup analysis of patients with meningococcal meningitis treated with corticosteroids showed a nonsignificant favorable trend in mortality.[41]

ROCKY MOUNTAIN SPOTTED FEVER

Background

RMSF is one of the most virulent human infections ever identified; 5%–10% of individuals infected die, and many others suffer sequelae such as amputation, deafness, or permanent learning disability.[42] RMSF occurs throughout the continental United States, Canada, Mexico, Central America, and parts of South America. During the period 1997–2002, there were 2.2 cases per 1 million per year in the United States, and more than one half (56%) of cases were reported from only five states: North Carolina, South Carolina, Texas, Oklahoma, and Arkansas.[43] Although cases are reported throughout the year, most occur from May through January with a peak in July, August, and September (46% of 2298 cases in 2006).[44] During 2006, more than half of cases were reported from the South Atlantic region with 962 cases (42% of total U.S. cases) from North Carolina. Arkansas and Tennessee accounted for 13% and 11.5% of cases, respectively. RMSF is most common in boys and men and Caucasians, and although children younger than 10 years were the group at highest risk in previous studies, in 2003 the highest age-specific incidence was in persons 40–64 years old.[45]

Clinical and Laboratory Aids Required for Diagnosis

The initial symptoms of RMSF include sudden onset of fever, chills, and headache, associated with malaise and myalgias. Anorexia, nausea, vomiting, and photosensitivity are also commonly seen. Because eruption may not be evident at the time a patient first presents for evaluation, clinicians should still maintain a high index of suspicion for the diagnosis in patients with a history of outdoor activities. History of a tick bite is elicited in only one half of patients with RMSF. Sixty to 70 percent of patients with RMSF present with the classic triad of fever (94%), headache (86%), and eruption (85%) 1–2 weeks after tick exposure.[46] However, this occurs in only 3% of cases in the first 3 days of illness.[47] Fever usually exceeds 38.9°C (102°F), and the majority of patients develop an eruption within 3–5 days following its onset.[46] Children with RMSF present with fever (98%), eruption (97%), nausea and/or vomiting (73%), and headache (61%).[48] The eruption is

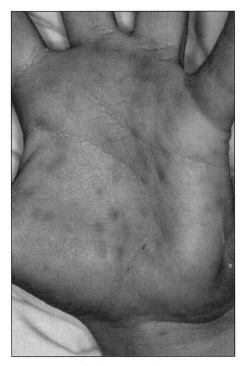

FIGURE 9.3: *Rocky Mountain spotted fever with red, partially blanching papules on the palms. Source: DermAtlas, Johns Hopkins University; 2000–2009 (rmsf_2_010907), Bernard Cohen, MD.*

maculopapular before the appearance of petechiae and may be easily missed, especially in dark-skinned individuals.[49] Blanching erythematous macules, 1–5 mm in diameter, initially arise on the wrists and ankles and spread to the palms and soles (Figure 9.3).[29,47] The eruption of erythematous macules on the wrists, ankles, palms, and soles is followed by centripetal spread to the arms, legs, and trunk (Figure 9.4). In 24–48 hours, petechiae and purpuric macules develop that may superficially resemble meningococcemia.[29]

Bilateral periorbital edema, suffusion of the conjunctivae, and edema of the hands and feet are highly sug-

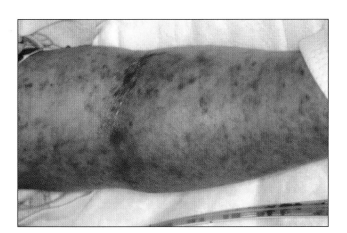

FIGURE 9.4: *Rocky Mountain spotted fever. Diffuse petechiae, purpura, and edema. Source: DermAtlas, Johns Hopkins University; 2000–2009 (rmsf_5_010907), Bernard Cohen, MD.*

gestive of RMSF in the appropriate clinical setting. The severe headache (which patients may describe as the worst they have ever experienced) may mimic meningitis with meningismus in 18% of patients.[46,47,50] The headache is usually frontal and is often associated with restlessness; severe myalgias of the abdomen, back, and legs; nausea; vomiting; and abdominal pain. Patients may display amnesia, psychiatric symptoms, and transient hearing loss.

CBC and a comprehensive metabolic panel should be done when considering rickettsial disease. White cell count in RMSF is usually normal, but increased numbers of immature band forms are often seen. Thrombocytopenia, mild elevations of hepatic transaminases, and hyponatremia also can occur.

Blood cultures and examination of a peripheral smear are useful in ruling out other conditions that mimic RMSF. The presence of morula in the peripheral smear in either monocytes or granulocytes suggests human monocytic ehrlichiosis (HME) or human granulocytic anaplasmosis (HGA), respectively. Leukopenia with elevations of liver transaminases and thrombocytopenia further suggest HGA and HME. HGA is transmitted through the *Ixodes scapularis* tick, which does not transmit *Rickettsia rickettsii*, whereas HME is transmitted to humans through the lone star tick or *Amblyomma americanum* and possibly other tick species. Blood cultures are useful in assessing bacterial infections, particularly meningococcal infection the early signs of which can be difficult to distinguish from RMSF. Cerebrospinal fluid in RMSF usually shows a pleocytosis (usually with <100 cells per milliliter) with neutrophilic or lymphocytic predominance. Protein is elevated, but glucose remains normal. Gram-negative diplococci with neutrophilic predominance and low glucose clearly favor meningococcal infection; however, there remains considerable overlap, and empiric coverage for meningococcus is frequently unavoidable. Serological testing and immunohistochemical or polymerase chain reaction (PCR) analysis of skin biopsy specimens can also confirm the diagnosis.

In a study of RMSF in children by Buckingham[48] laboratory findings were nonspecific and similar to those that might occur, for example, in viral syndromes such that "no constellation of clinical and laboratory abnormalities has adequate sensitivity for their absence to exclude the diagnosis of RMSF in a child."[48]

Because of the rapid progression of infection, empiric therapy should not be withheld awaiting laboratory confirmation.

Treatment

Doxycycline is the drug of choice for treatment of both adults and children with presumptive or proven RMSF. Even though the use of tetracyclines in young children has been discouraged because of the potential for tooth discoloration, this effect is dose related and does not necessarily preclude the use of this agent.[51] One course of doxycycline in young children for presumed RMSF, a potentially life-threatening disease, has not been shown to cause clinically significant staining of permanent teeth.[52] Moreover, doxycycline effectively treats ehrlichiosis, which may be confused with RMSF. Chloramphenicol is the preferred agent for treating RMSF occurring during pregnancy.[53]

Patients with RMSF should be admitted to the hospital and observed closely and treated for altered mental status or any organ dysfunction. Patients in more advanced stages of disease warrant admission to an intensive care unit for aggressive supportive measures.

Course and Prognosis

Appropriate treatment of patients with RMSF is often delayed for a number of reasons including lack of tick-exposure history; occurrence of illness at times of year when tick activity is not at its peak; absence or delayed appearance of eruption; symptoms other than the classic triad of fever, eruption, and headache; and lack of headache.[48,54–58] Of interest, presentation to a health care provider early in the course of the disease has been associated with delay in the initiation of specific antirickettsial therapy.[48,58] For example, in one study by Buckingham,[48] children were seen by medical providers after a median of 2 days of symptoms but did not receive specific antirickettsial treatment until after a median of 7 days of symptoms. In fact, 2 of the 3 children who died in that study, although seen early on, were not given appropriate treatment. Also in that study, more than one third of patients spent time in an intensive care unit, 16% received mechanical ventilation, and 17% received pressors.

Before the introduction of effective antirickettsial agents, 13% of children with RMSF died.[51] Despite the availability of specific therapy and improved supportive medical care, the case fatality rate in children younger than 10 years is still 2%–3%. Several clinical and laboratory variables have been associated with fatal outcome including increased age; male sex; neurological involvement; elevated levels of creatinine, aspartate aminotransferase, and bilirubin; decreased levels of serum sodium; and decreased platelet count.[59] The development of acute renal failure increased the odds ratio of dying 17-fold in one study.[59] The presence of a deficiency of the enzyme glucose-6-phosphate dehydrogenase (G6PD) may portend a more fulminant course because of the development of hemolysis.[60]

Even with recovery, patients may suffer ongoing neuromotor impairment at the time of discharge from the hospital; this impairment may persist in some patients,[61] particularly if neurologic compromise, especially coma, occurs during the acute phase of the illness. Persistent sequelae include dysarthria, difficulty reading, impaired memory, deafness, and paresthesias. Gangrene can necessitate amputation of digits or entire extremities.

MEDITERRANEAN SPOTTED FEVER

Background

Mediterranean fever (Boutonneuse fever) has been described in many countries under a variety of names. It is caused by *Rickettsia conorii* and its subspecies, and the vector is the brown dog tick *Rhipicephalus sanguineus*. Although usually a benign, uncomplicated disease with recovery the norm, it may sometimes be severe and fatal.[62] The mortality rate is usually estimated at approximately 2.5%, but a fatality rate of up to 5.6% has been reported in affected hospitalized patients in Israel, France, and Portugal.[63] The disease tends to be more severe in the elderly population and in patients with cirrhosis, chronic alcoholism, and G6PD deficiency.[64] In Beja, a Portuguese southern district, a case fatality rate of 32.3% was reported in hospitalized patients with Mediterranean spotted fever.[65] The risk of dying was associated with diabetes, uremia, vomiting, and dehydration. A subspecies of *R. conorii* (*israelensis*), the cause of Israeli spotted fever, has been isolated from patients in Sicily and Portugal and may be associated with more severe disease. The disease has been reported throughout the Mediterranean basin, sub-Saharan Africa, India, around the Black Sea, and in the eastern part of Russia close to Japan. Diagnosis peaks in August in endemic areas of France and Spain suggest that larvae and nymph forms are important in disease spread. The peak activity of adult ticks occurs several months earlier during the spring. Reports of Mediterranean spotted fever throughout the year and from colder areas removed from the Mediterranean imply that *R. sanguineus* can survive in the microclimates of homes and kennels.

Clinical and Laboratory Aids Required for Diagnosis

The incubation period of Mediterranean spotted fever is approximately 7 days. Disease onset is abrupt and typically begins with high fever, flu-like symptoms, a black eschar (tache noire) at the site of the tick bite, and a maculopapular eruption. The tache noir is said to be present in approximately 74% of cases but is uncommon in the Israeli form. Eruption is described as maculopapular but may be purpuric in 10% of cases. Laboratory studies are often nonspecific with thrombocytopenia, leukocyte count abnormalities, both lymphopenia and leukocytosis, and elevated hepatic enzyme levels.

Early diagnosis of Mediterranean spotted fever can be achieved using immunofluorescence or immunohistochemical studies of skin biopsy material or by PCR.[66,67] Both techniques require experienced personnel and may have limited availability.

Serologic studies provide retrospective confirmation of the diagnosis. Antibodies to rickettsiae may not be detectable until 7–10 days after infection is clinically manifest. An acute blood sample should be collected early in the course of the disease, and a second specimen should be obtained 2 weeks later. If a fourfold increase in antibody titer is not observed, collection of a third sample after 4–6 weeks should be considered. Specific diagnosis may not be made until the patient has recovered or died.

Treatment

Treatment should be initiated as soon as the diagnosis is suspected. Doxycycline is the drug of choice and is given for a 7-day course of therapy or until the patient is afebrile for 3 days. Doxycycline has been shown to effectively treat Mediterranean spotted fever with a 1-day course of therapy.[68] Doxycycline is contraindicated in pregnancy and not usually recommended for use in children younger than 8 years with the exception of patients with RMSF. Chloramphenicol is also an effective antibiotic agent and had previously been used in pregnancy. Aplastic anemia occurs in 10 of 40,000 patients treated with chloramphenicol, and gray baby syndrome (comprising abdominal distension, pallor, cyanosis, and vasomotor collapse usually leading to death) has been described in neonates treated with this drug. Although there has been no report of an infant exposed in utero having developed gray baby syndrome or aplastic anemia, few obstetricians and pediatricians are comfortable with its prescription. In vitro studies of clarithromycin and azithromycin have suggested effectiveness of these antibiotics in treatment of *R. conorii* infection. Clinical trials suggest that these agents provide a safe and effective alternative for treatment of children younger than 8 years with Mediterranean spotted fever.[69,70] Fluoroquinolones also have been shown in vitro to be effective against *R. conorii*.[71]

Course and Prognosis

In general, Mediterranean spotted fever has a good prognosis if appropriately treated. Risk factors for more severe disease include diabetes, G6PD deficiency, older age, cirrhosis, and alcoholism. Delay in initiation of appropriate antibiotic coverage is also frequently cited as a risk factor for poor prognosis; however, a retrospective study in the Beja district of southern Portugal, which experienced a 32.3% case fatality rate for hospitalized patients in 1997, did not bear this out. Diabetes, vomiting, volume depletion, and uremia were significantly correlated with risk of dying.

Treatment of severe illness induced by *R. conorii* may require more than chemotherapeutic elimination of the etiologic agent. The multiorgan manifestations of endothelial damage and increased vascular permeability may necessitate admission to an intensive care unit for monitoring of central pressures and airway management. Additional antibiotic coverage may be required to cover bacterial leakage from a compromised gut or from aspiration.

ANTHRAX

Background

Anthrax is primarily a disease of wild and domestic animals (cattle, sheep, and goats) caused by the spore-forming bacterium *Bacillus anthracis*. Human disease results from exposure to infected animals or tissue from infected animals. This exposure occurs after cutaneous inoculation or inhalation of spores or after ingestion of infected material. *B. anthracis* can exist as a stable spore form for years and can be weaponized as a bioterrorism agent. This weaponization occurred in the United States in 2001 when powder containing anthrax was placed in letters and disseminated via the U.S. Postal Service.

Although the cutaneous form of anthrax is usually considered the least severe presentation, it can result in fatality if not adequately treated. A rare complication, malignant edema, is characterized by severe edema, induration, multiple bullae, and shock.[72] Involvement of the face, neck, and chest may require intubation and corticosteroids to prevent asphyxiation. In a series of 28 cases of cutaneous anthrax reported in 2003 from Turkey, two patients (8%) died from anthrax sepsis.[73] A recent study from the Artibonite Valley of Haiti reported 87 cases of cutaneous anthrax over a 4-year period.[74] Seven of 87 patients (8%) died, 4 from asphyxiation after facial and neck edema compressed the trachea, causing airway obstruction. Two patients died of symptoms associated with concurrent gastrointestinal anthrax. Anthrax can cause a severe, usually fatal meningoencephalitis from both the cutaneous and inhalational routes.[72,75]

Clinical and Laboratory Aids Required for Diagnosis

The diagnosis of anthrax is usually straightforward when it occurs in a typical occupational or environmental setting involving exposure to infected animals or contaminated animal products, such as hides, wool, hair, or ivory tusks.[76] In the past, urban cases of anthrax were usually associated with imported products such as shaving brushes, and recently two cases were reported in Connecticut in a drum maker and his child after exposure to contaminated goat hides imported from Guinea.[77–79]

The primary lesion of cutaneous anthrax is a painless papule that usually develops approximately 7 days (range = 1–12 days) after inoculation of infected material.[80] It most commonly occurs on the head, neck, or arms and develops a central vesicle or bulla that becomes hemorrhagic as the lesion enlarges. The classic black central eschar is often surrounded by erythema and sometimes extreme edema (Figure 9.5). The presence of a primary pustular lesion should suggest another diagnosis. Multiple lesions sometimes occur, and there may be tender regional lymphadenopathy and systemic symptoms of fever, chills, and fatigue.[80] Anthrax may occur on the eyelid and be associated

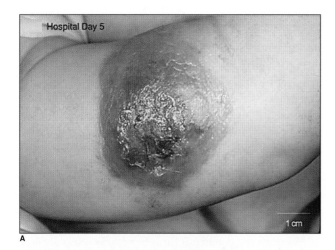

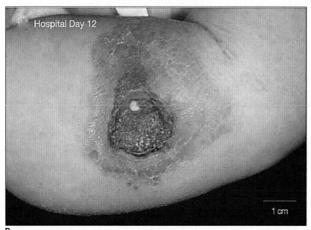

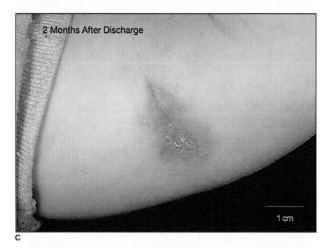

FIGURE 9.5: Cutaneous anthrax in a 7-month-old infant. Progression of lesions: A. hospital day 5, B. hospital day 12, C. 2 months after discharge. Used with permission. JAMA. 2002; 287:869–74. Copyright © (2002). American Medical Association. All rights reserved.

with preseptal cellulitis, and severe edema resulting from a primary lesion on the neck (bull neck) may result in asphyxiation (Figure 9.6).[74,81]

Cutaneous anthrax should be differentiated from insect bites, brown recluse spider bite (almost always painful),

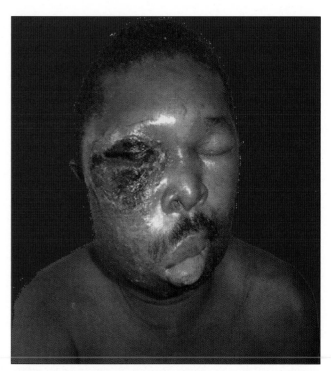

FIGURE 9.6: Facial cutaneous anthrax with massive edema. Am J Trop Med Hyg. 2007; 77:806–11.

tularemia, the tache noir of rickettsial diseases, cat scratch disease, ecthyma gangrenosum, orf, and staphylococcal or streptococcal ecthyma.

When dealing with a patient with suspected cutaneous anthrax, universal precautions should be followed. The American Academy of Dermatology recommendations include swabbing exudates using a dacron- or rayon-tipped swab (cotton should not be used) to obtain material for Gram stain and culture.[80] Vesicular fluid is optimal for isolation of the organism. If only an eschar is present, the edge should be lifted and swabs inserted to obtain fluid. Two skin biopsies are advocated, one for histological examination including special stains and immunohistochemistry and the other for culture.[82] Treatment should be instituted while awaiting results. Serology and PCR assay may be available through governmental agencies such as the CDC.[83]

Treatment

Uncomplicated localized cutaneous anthrax should be treated with oral ciprofloxacin 500 mg twice daily or doxycycline 100 mg twice daily.[84] Usual duration of treatment is 7–10 days, but in the context of a bioterrorism attack, the CDC recommends a 60-day course of treatment because of the increased likelihood of exposure to aerosolized anthrax. For children, the CDC recommends oral ciprofloxacin 10–15 mg/kg every 12 hours, not to exceed 1 g/d or doxycycline. For children up to 8 years old (or those older than 8 years weighing <45 kg), the CDC recommends a doxycycline dosage of 2.2 mg/kg every 12 hours. The dosage of doxycycline for children older than 8 years and weighing at least 45 kg is 100 mg every 12 hours. The CDC has also recommended the use of ciprofloxacin and doxycycline in pregnant woman although these agents traditionally have been avoided in pregnancy.

Cutaneous anthrax occurring on the head and neck and cases with systemic involvement or severe edema should be treated with the IV antibiotic regimens recommended for inhalational anthrax. A multidrug regimen is recommended in suspected cases of bioterrorism because antibiotic resistance may have been engineered into weaponized anthrax. The initial treatment protocol recommended for inhalational bioterrorism-associated anthrax is ciprofloxacin 400 mg IV every 12 hours *or* IV doxycycline 100 mg every 12 hours plus one or two additional agents. IV therapy can be switched to oral treatment when clinically warranted. Additional agents that have activity against *B. anthracis* include penicillin, ampicillin, imipenem, clindamycin, clarithromycin, rifampin, chloramphenicol, and vancomycin. Inhalational anthrax and severe cutaneous disease in children are treated with IV ciprofloxacin 10–15 mg/kg every 12 hours (not to exceed 1 g/d in children) or IV doxycycline. Children younger than 8 years and those 8 years old or older but who weigh less than 45 kg are treated with IV doxycycline 2.2 mg/kg every 12 hours. Children older than 8 years and who weigh more than 45 kg should receive doxycycline 100 mg every 12 hours. One or two additional antibiotics are added to this regimen in this protocol.

Course and Prognosis

Prognosis of anthrax depends on the type of exposure. Many sources quote a mortality rate of up to 20% in untreated cutaneous anthrax, 25%–75% for gastrointestinal anthrax, and 80% or more for inhalational anthrax. In one series, four patients (5.6% of patients) with cutaneous anthrax developed meningoencephalitis, and three died.[85] Less commonly cutaneous anthrax can progress to septicemia and shock.[86] Fulminant inhalational anthrax is usually fatal, but initiation of antibiotics or anthrax antiserum therapy during the prodromal phase can improve survival.[87]

TULAREMIA

Background

Tularemia is a zoonotic disease with worldwide distribution caused by *Francisella tularensis*, a fastidious, gram-negative organism.[88,89] It has been speculated that tularemia was the cause of the biblical plague of the Philistines.[90] The Old Testament warns in Leviticus 11:6 and 11:8, "And the hare is unclean to you. Of their flesh ye shall not eat, and their carcasses ye shall not touch."[91] Transmission to humans occurs by several mechanisms, most commonly direct or indirect inoculation of the skin from infected animal tissues, body fluids, or pelts.[92] The animals implicated in transmission of tularemia depend on the geographic area. In the United States, jackrabbits, cottontail rabbits, beavers, muskrats, meadow voles, and sheep are usually implicated. The disease may also be spread by arthropod vectors such as deerflies, mosquitoes, and several varieties of ticks.

Interest in tularemia has been heightened in recent years because of its potential for use as an agent of bioterrorism. The organism is highly virulent in susceptible hosts. A low infectious dose of 10–50 organisms can establish infection in an open wound or if aerosolized and inhaled. The two subspecies of *F. tularensis* commonly associated with human disease are *F. tularensis tularensis* and *F. tularensis holarctica*. The *tularensis* subspecies is found only in North America and is the more virulent of the two.

The type of disease that develops reflects the route of infection. Ulceroglandular disease, the most common presentation, follows exposure of broken skin to contaminated animal material and occurs on the upper extremities in more than 75% of patients.[93] Lesions on the lower extremities, abdomen, back, or head usually result from exposure to ticks or deerflies.

Clinical and Laboratory Aids Required for Diagnosis

Dermatologists are most likely to encounter patients with ulceroglandular, glandular, or perhaps oculoglandular tularemia. A typical patient will present with the abrupt onset of fever, chills, malaise, and fatigue after an incubation period of 1–10 days (average of 3 days).[92] The most common presenting complaint is of enlarged, tender, localized lymphadenopathy with overlying erythema. The initial skin lesion may be present at the time of presentation or shortly thereafter and is a painful, red papule that undergoes necrosis leaving a tender ulcer with a raised border (Figure 9.7).[94] Cutaneous ulcers range in size from 0.4 to 3.0 cm and are usually solitary. Multiple lesions can sometimes occur and are usually caused by exposure to more than one animal.[93] The primary lesion may evolve over the course of the disease. In a recent Swedish study, primary lesions were described as "encrusted" in one third of cases and "ulcerous" or "pustular" each in about 20% of cases. "Papular" primary lesions were noted in 13% and "macular" or "vesicular" lesions each occurred in approximately 3%–4% of cases. Indeed, cases of tularemia have been initially misdiagnosed as herpes simplex or herpes zoster infection.[95] Secondary skin eruptions including erythema nodosum have been reported in patients with tularemia. In the previously mentioned Swedish study, almost 30% of patients displayed a secondary skin eruption apart from any primary lesions or erythema overlying enlarged lymph nodes. Such eruptions were most commonly papular or maculopapular. Erythema

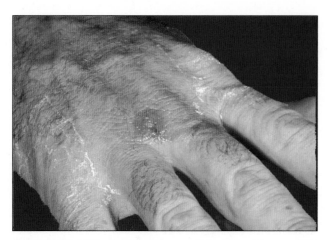

FIGURE 9.7: *Tularemia–cutaneous ulcer. From Oyston PCF, et al. Tularaemia: bioterrorism defence renews interest in Francisella tularensis. Nat Rev Microbiol. 2004; 2:967–8.*

nodosum occurred in 3% of patients, all girls and women. Suppuration of involved lymph nodes may occur. In glandular disease, lymphadenopathy occurs in the absence of a primary lesion.

Ulceroglandular tularemia must be differentiated from other causes of ulceroglandular disease including *Bartonella henselae* (cat scratch fever), *Yersinia pestis* (plague), *Spirillum minus* (spirillary rat bite fever), and other bacterial adenitis. Other diagnostic considerations are anthrax, herpes simplex, chancroid, syphilis, and mycobacterial disease.[96]

Oculoglandular disease resulting from direct or indirect exposure of the conjunctivae to infectious material presents with conjunctivitis, chemosis, lacrimation, photosensitivity, lid edema, and conjunctival ulceration accompanied by tender lymphadenopathy in the preauricular, submandibular, and cervical regions. Pharyngeal disease occurs when the primary exposure is within the oral cavity with contaminated foods or water. Typhoidal tularemia is distinct from the other forms in that it is not accompanied by adenopathy and the portal of entry may not be identifiable. This form usually affects persons with some degree of immune compromise and may have a rapid and fulminant course. A pneumonic form also exists in which the pulmonary findings are the most prominent feature.

Tularemia should be suspected when typical clinical findings occur in a patient with an occupational or recreational exposure to animals in an endemic area. Diagnosis outside of an endemic area requires a high index of suspicion.[96] The incubation period is usually approximately 3–5 days, and onset of disease is often abrupt. Fever, chills, malaise, sore throat, and headache are frequent, and pulse–temperature dissociation may occur in 42% of cases. Persistent fever, greater than 101°F, is common over the course of several days. Routine laboratory testing is nonspecific. Leukocytosis may or may not be present. Thrombocytopenia, elevation of transaminases and creatine kinase, and myoglobinuria may also be present.

The organism can be isolated from wound drainage, lymph aspirates, sputum, and blood. Stringent precautions should be taken when handling specimens to prevent infection in hospital and laboratory personnel. *Francisella* is a biosafety level 3 pathogen, and the laboratory should be warned if it is suspected. Relay of specimens to government health departments for processing may be the best option for both expertise in culture and availability of PCR or fluorescent antibody testing. Confirmation of infection is usually made with increasing titers of antibodies in acute and convalescent sera.

Treatment

Streptomycin is the preferred drug for treatment of tularemia. Because it may not be readily available, gentamicin is commonly used with good results. β-lactam antibiotics and macrolides are not effective and should not be used. Fluoroquinolines provide effective coverage, as do tetracyclines. A study from Spain showed ciprofloxacin to be superior to both streptomycin and doxycycline in that it had the lowest percentage of primary treatment failures; however, this study was nonrandomized and retrospective. If the condition of the patient merits hospitalization, IV therapy with streptomycin or gentamicin is indicated. Stable patients may be treated with oral antibiotics with ciprofloxacin or doxycycline, with ciprofloxacin being the preferred oral agent for confirmed tularemia.

Course and Prognosis

Suppuration of large or flocculent lymph nodes is a common complication. Large nodes should be aspirated to prevent this complication. Another possible sequela to infection with tularemia is a prolonged period of fatigue that may persist several weeks even following adequate antibiotic treatment.

Prior to the introduction of streptomycin in the 1950s, patients often suffered from lingering symptoms and the case mortality for ulceroglandular disease was about 5%.[97] Death rates from all forms of tularemia in the antibiotic era are about 4% but were as high as 33% prior to the use of streptomycin.[94]

V. VULNIFICUS INFECTION

Background

V. vulnificus is not only the most virulent food-borne pathogen in the United States but is a source of invasive, potentially life-threatening wound infections.[98] Most cases in the United States occur in individuals with cirrhosis who eat undercooked oysters from the Gulf of Mexico, but cases of *V. vulnificus* have been reported from Japan, Taiwan, Korea, Brazil, Mexico, Germany (from the Baltic

Sea), Denmark, Spain, Israel, and Australia.[99–109] A severe outbreak occurred in Israel in fish market workers from handling infected tilapia.[108]

V. vulnificus is present in shallow sea and estuarial waters especially during the warm summer months. The gram-negative, comma-shaped organism is found in oysters, crustaceans, and shellfish.[100]

The main risk factors for developing *V. vulnificus* infection are consumption of raw or inadequately cooked oysters or shellfish, exposure of a preexisting open wound to contaminated sea water, injury to the skin while in contact with infected water, and handling contaminated marine species (as in fish handlers). Wound infections are most likely serious in persons with underlying chronic liver disease or other predisposing factors who engage in water recreational activities. Also at risk are victims of natural disasters such as tsunamis and flooding after hurricanes. Eighteen wound-associated *Vibrio* cases were reported in several states in victims of Hurricane Katrina of which 14 (82%) were *V. vulnificus* and 3 were *V. parahaemolyticus.* Five (28%) patients with wound-associated *Vibrio* infections died, three from *V. vulnificus* and two from *V. parahaemolyticus.*

Because early, specific antibiotic therapy, aggressive wound management, and supportive measures can reduce mortality, it is incumbent on physicians to be familiar with the recognition of *V. vulnificus* infection.

Clinical and Laboratory Aids Required for Diagnosis

Infection with *V. vulnificus* should be suspected in any patient presenting with cellulitis or sepsis after exposure to brackish or salt water or with a history of recent ingestion of raw or undercooked seafood, mainly raw oysters. The presence of hemorrhagic bullae complicating cellulitis in a patient with a history of liver disease or diabetes should further suggest the diagnosis (Figure 9.8).[110] A small study comparing the clinical aspects of necrotizing fasciitis caused by *Vibrio* with that caused by Streptococci pointed out several significant differences. All cases of *Vibrio* infection occurred during summer months in patients with underlying chronic liver dysfunction and were probably caused by raw seafood consumption.[111] In this study, Streptococcus-induced necrotizing fasciitis occurred in winter, and only one patient had chronic liver disease. In patients with *Vibrio*-induced disease, edema and subcutaneous bleeding (ecchymosis and purpura) were seen early on, but cutaneous necrosis didn't occur. In patients with streptococcal disease, subcutaneous bleeding was rare and necrosis was common.

Blood and wound cultures should be obtained immediately in all patients with suspected *Vibrio* infection. Gram stain of exudative material may suggest the pathogen and reinforce clinical suspicion. Progression of infection can be rapid and fulminant, so that expediency in workup

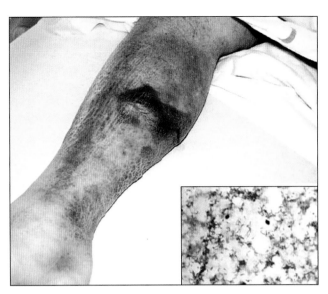

FIGURE 9.8: Vibrio vulnificus *infection with hemorrhagic cellulitis. Inset: Gram-negative rods seen on Gram stain. Falcon LM, et al. Hemorrhagic cellulitis after consumption of raw oysters. N Engl J Med. 2005; 353:1604.*

and prompt initiation of antibiotic therapy are essential. Soft-tissue infection with *V. vulnificus* has a propensity to rapidly progress to necrotizing fasciitis. Clinical findings may include edema, patchiness, erythema, and tenderness. Hemorrhagic bullae or compartment syndrome may already be apparent at the time of presentation.

Treatment

Prompt initiation of antibiotic therapy and surgical debridement are the cornerstones in the management of *Vibrio* infections. When there is suspicion of this pathogen, antibiotic treatment should be started with a third-generation cephalosporin and a tetracycline. The combination of third-generation cephalosporins, commonly ceftriaxone or ceftazidime, with tetracycline, minocycline, or doxycycline have shown synergy. Recent studies with fluoroquinones have shown these agents to be as effective as the cephalosporin–tetracycline combination in vitro and in murine models. Because of the rarity of the infection, it is unlikely that a blinded clinical trial will be carried out. Surgical consultation should be obtained and appropriate debridement of necrotic tissue done on an emergency basis. Fasciotomy may be needed, and if infection has progressed amputation may be required to remove the devitalized limb and control systemic sepsis.

Course and Prognosis

Prognosis is significantly better with early intervention and timely initiation of antibiotic coverage. Patients in whom the severity of infection is not immediately recognized or those who present later in the course of infection do not do as well. Overall, 40% of *V. vulnificus* infections are fatal, with case fatality rates of approximately 50% from primary septicemia and 15%–20% for wound infections.[112,113] Persons most at risk are those with chronic alcoholic liver disease, hepatitis B or C, hemochromatosis, renal insufficiency, or adrenal insufficiency.[100]

A. HYDROPHILA INFECTION

Background

Aeromonas species are gram-negative rods usually found in fresh or brackish water and soil, but also have been isolated from chlorinated drinking water and even from hospital water supplies.[114,115] They cause disease in fish and other cold-blooded aquatic animals, mammalian species, and humans.[116] Human infection occurs through contact with contaminated fresh or brackish water and soil giving rise to cellulitis within 8–48 hours. *A. hydrophila* is the species most commonly associated with soft-tissue infection.

The clinical presentation is similar to that of *V. vulnificus* soft-tissue infection and similarly gives rise to sepsis primarily in patients with underlying cirrhosis or malignancy.[117]

Clinical and Laboratory Aids Required for Diagnosis

The most important clue suggesting *A. hydrophila* infection is a history of soft-tissue injury associated with exposure to fresh water or soil. Posttraumatic wound infections caused by *Aeromonas* may be clinically indistinguishable from cellulitis due to *Streptococcus pyogenes* or *S. aureus*, so limiting empiric therapy to these organisms will likely miss the pathogen. Infection with *A. hydrophila* occurs in a variety of settings. In recreational activities involving fresh water (such as boating, swimming, or wading), abrasions or lacerations may become infected, and in commercial situations (such as in fisheries), wounds may be exposed to contaminated fresh water. Infections of burns with *Aeromonas* have been reported after submersion or dousing of the injured part with water and after rolling the victim in soil to extinguish flames. Motor vehicle, machinery, or boating accidents may also expose people to wound contamination with *Aeromonas* in a culture bed of devitalized tissue. Although *Aeromonas* bacterial counts are often similar in marine environments to those in fresh water, infection from sea water, for some unknown reason, usually doesn't occur. *Aeromonas* cellulitis also may develop in skin grafts or flaps in which leeches were utilized to relieve venous congestion.[118] *Aeromonas* species are resident flora in the foregut of leeches aiding them in the digestion of heme.

Initial evaluation should include Gram stain of exudates or aspirates and bacterial culture. Depending on the extent of the disease, leukocytosis and fever may be present. In a study of a community outbreak of *Aeromonas* cellulitis following a mud football tournament, 26 cases of soft-tissue infection were catalogued with 22 of 26 persons presenting with nonlesional symptoms including eruption, malaise, fever, rigors, headache, nausea, sore throat, or earache. Many authors make note of an odd fishy or sweet, sickly, foul odor.[119,120]

Therapy

A combination of surgical and medical therapy is most often required. The tendency of *Aeromonas* to form subcutaneous abscesses may not be clinically apparent, and early surgical consultation is advised.[119] Incision and drainage may be curative in some cases. The *Aeromonas* species are β-lactamase producers and often resistant to penicillin, ampicillin, carbenicillin, first-generation cephalosporins, ticarcillin, vancomycin, and clindamycin.[120] Susceptibility to piperacillin, ticarcillin–clavulanate, and tetracyclines is variable. Fluoroquinolones and trimethoprim–sulfamethoxazole are usually effective, but reports of decreasing susceptibility of strains emphasize the need to follow response to therapy closely and adjust antimicrobial therapy with the guidance of microbiological sensitivities.

Course and Prognosis

Aeromonas infection has a guarded prognosis. Bacteremia and septicemia are more common in patients with underlying cirrhosis and malignancy and portend a worse outcome. In contrast, cases of septicemia have been reported in otherwise healthy individuals.[121] In a study from Taiwan, the crude fatality rate of monomicrobial *Aeromonas* bacteremia was 30% within 2 weeks after the onset of infection.[117] Some patients with myonecrosis from *Aeromonas* infection require limb amputation.[122]

C. VIOLACEUM INFECTION

Background

C. violaceum is a gram-negative rod that occurs as a ubiquitous saprophyte of soil and water in tropical and subtropical areas.[123] It is an uncommon pathogen in humans (<150 cases in the literature), but has a high fatality rate. Cases have been reported from Asia, Australia, Africa, the United States, and South America.[123,124] Most cases in the United States are reported from Florida. Human infection usually begins with cellulitis and skin abscesses that rapidly progress to sepsis and abscesses of internal organs. U.S. cases have been related to wading in pools of rain water or muddy ditches, walking barefoot, following trauma, and swimming in fresh water.[125]

Clinical and Laboratory Aids Required for Diagnosis

C. violaceum infection can be rapidly fatal. The most crucial factor in determining survival is the recognition that the bacterium may be present and to cover for it

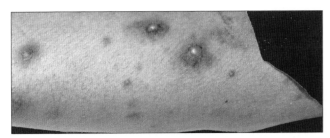

FIGURE 9.9: Chromobacterium violaceum *infection. Multiple hemorrhagic and pustular blebs. Photo courtesy of Virat Sirisanthana, MD, Faculty of Medicine, Chiang Mai University, Chaing Mai, Thailand. Used with permission.*

empirically. The infection is found in tropical and subtropical regions and usually occurs in the summer months. There is a predilection for patients with chronic granulomatous disease, deficiency of polymorphonuclear leukocyte G6PD, and neutrophil dysfunction; however, fulminant disease has been reported repeatedly in patients with no apparent immune dysfunction.[126] Localized infection with regional lymphadenopathy occurs after contamination of damaged skin exposed to soil or stagnant water. Systemic infection can occur following aspiration or ingestion of contaminated material.

The usual presentation is with fever, hepatic abscess, and skin lesions, although preseptal and orbital cellulitis has been reported as well as osteomyelitis, meningitis, and brain abscess. Skin lesions may consist of multiple nodules, hemorrhagic and pustular blebs with surrounding erythema, abscesses, cellulitis, and purpura scattered over the face, body, and extremities (Figure 9.9).[127,128] The palms and soles may be affected (Figure 9.10). Ecthyma gangrenosum also has been reported.[129] Leukocytosis with left shift may be the only laboratory abnormality. Liver enzymes, platelet counts, and sedimentation rates may or may not be abnormal early in the course of infection. Culture of the organism confirms the diagnosis. Material from wound drainage, blood, conjunctival exudates, and abscess drainage or aspirant should immediately be sent for culture and susceptibility testing.

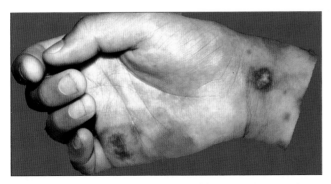

FIGURE 9.10: Chromobacterium violaceum *infection. Pustular blebs and purpura of the palm. Photo courtesy of Virat Sirisanthana, MD, Faculty of Medicine, Chiang Mai University, Chaing Mai, Thailand. Used with permission.*

C. violaceum is generally known to be resistant to first-generation cephalosporins and penicillins. Third-generation cephalosporins, ureidopenicillins, tetracyclines, and aminoglycosides have demonstrated mixed effectiveness. The organism is generally sensitive to trimethoprim sulfamethoxazole, gentamicin, ciprofloxacin, and imipenem. The frequency of hepatic abscess formation has prompted some authors to advocate ultrasound examination of the liver and spleen in all persons from whom *C. violaceum* has been cultured followed by surgical drainage of any abscesses visualized.

Course and Prognosis

Anyone found to be infected with *C. violaceum* should be evaluated for underlying immunodeficiency.[129] IV antibiotic therapy should be continued until all foci of infection have been cleared. As the organism has been known to recur following apparent resolution of infection, consideration of an extended course of oral antibiotic therapy is appropriate. Survival is dependent on the early recognition of the infection with initiation of effective antibiotic therapy. Recognition of the potential of this organism to form abscesses in multiple sites is important. The fatality rate of all cases with known outcome was 65% in 1998. Improvements in antibiotics and medical management have decreased the fatality rate of 81% (from 1939 through 1979) to 41% (from 1980 through 1994).[3] Under the best of circumstances, the prognosis with this infection remains guarded.

CONCLUSION

We have described the clinical presentation and treatment of several infections with which the dermatologist and other specialists should be familiar. Most of these are relatively uncommon so physicians may not include them in their differential diagnoses. For that reason, knowledge of their often dramatic clinical presentations is essential as it will allow early diagnosis and the initiation of prompt therapy, which may be lifesaving.

REFERENCES

1. Carlisle RT, Fredrick GT. Preseptal and orbital cellulitis. Hosp Physician. 2006; 42:15–19.
2. Givner LB. Periorbital versus orbital cellulitis. Pediatr Infect Dis J. 2002; 21:1157–8.
3. Sobol AL, Hutcheson KA. Cellulitis, preseptal. WebMD; 2008 [updated April 4, 2008; cited 2008 June 29, 2008]; Available from: http://www.emedicine.com/oph/topic206.htm.
4. Al-Nammari S, Roberton B, Ferguson C. Towards evidence based emergency medicine: best BETs from the Manchester Royal Infirmary. Should a child with preseptal periorbital cellulitis be treated with intravenous or oral antibiotics? Emerg Med J. 2007; 24:128–9.
5. Reynolds DJ, Kodsi SR, Rubin SE, Rodgers IR. Intracranial infection associated with preseptal and orbital cellulitis in the pediatric patient. J AAPOS. 2003; 7:413–17.

6. Rubin Grandis J, Branstetter BF 4th, Yu VL. The changing face of malignant (necrotising) external otitis: clinical, radiological, and anatomic correlations. Lancet Infect Dis. 2004; 4:34–9.

7. Weinroth SE, Schessel D, Tuazon CU. Malignant otitis externa in AIDS patients: case report and review of the literature. Ear Nose Throat J. 1994; 73:772–4, 7–8.

8. Rubin J, Yu VL, Stool SE. Malignant external otitis in children. J Pediatr. 1988; 113:965–70.

9. Grandis JR, Curtin HD, Yu VL. Necrotizing (malignant) external otitis: prospective comparison of CT and MR imaging in diagnosis and follow-up. Radiology. 1995; 196:499–504.

10. Levenson MJ, Parisier SC, Dolitsky J, Bindra G. Ciprofloxacin: drug of choice in the treatment of malignant external otitis (MEO). Laryngoscope. 1991; 101:821–4.

11. Rubin J, Stoehr G, Yu VL, et al. Efficacy of oral ciprofloxacin plus rifampin for treatment of malignant external otitis. Arch Otolaryngol Head Neck Surg. 1989; 115:1063–9.

12. Bernstein JM, Holland NJ, Porter GC, Maw AR. Resistance of Pseudomonas to ciprofloxacin: implications for the treatment of malignant otitis externa. J Laryngol Otol. 2007; 121:118–23.

13. Berenholz L, Katzenell U, Harell M. Evolving resistant pseudomonas to ciprofloxacin in malignant otitis externa. Laryngoscope. 2002; 112:1619–22.

14. Carfrae MJ, Kesser BW. Malignant otitis externa. Otolaryngol Clin North Am. 2008; 41:537–49, viii–ix.

15. Phillips JS, Jones SE. Hyperbaric oxygen as an adjuvant treatment for malignant otitis externa. Cochrane Database Syst Rev. 2005(2):CD004617.

16. Soudry E, Joshua BZ, Sulkes J, Nageris BI. Characteristics and prognosis of malignant external otitis with facial paralysis. Arch Otolaryngol Head Neck Surg. 2007; 133:1002–4.

17. Chandler JR. Malignant external otitis. Laryngoscope. 1968; 78:1257–94.

18. Lucente FE, Parisier SC. James R. Chandler: "Malignant external otitis." (Laryngoscope. 1968; 78:1257–94). Laryngoscope. 1996; 106:805–7.

19. Kimmelman CP, Lucente FE. Use of ceftazidime for malignant external otitis. Ann Otol Rhinol Laryngol. 1989; 98:721–5.

20. Meyers BR, Mendelson MH, Parisier SC, Hirschman SZ. Malignant external otitis. Comparison of monotherapy vs combination therapy. Arch Otolaryngol Head Neck Surg. 1987; 113:974–8.

21. Singh A, Al Khabori M, Hyder MJ. Skull base osteomyelitis: diagnostic and therapeutic challenges in atypical presentation. Otolaryngol Head Neck Surg. 2005; 133:121–5.

22. Shichmanter R, Miller EB, Landau Z. Adverse drug reactions due to prolonged antibiotic therapy for malignant external otitis. Eur J Intern Med. 2004; 15:441–5.

23. Mani N, Sudhoff H, Rajagopal S, et al. Cranial nerve involvement in malignant external otitis: implications for clinical outcome. Laryngoscope. 2007; 117:907–10.

24. Rosenstein NE, Perkins BA. Update on Haemophilus influenzae serotype b and meningococcal vaccines. Pediatr Clin North Am. 2000; 47:337–52, vi.

25. Healy CM, Baker CJ. The future of meningococcal vaccines. Pediatr Infect Dis J. 2005; 24:175–6.

26. Jackson LA, Wenger JD. Laboratory-based surveillance for meningococcal disease in selected areas, United States, 1989–1991. MMWR CDC Surveill Summ. 1993; 4;42:21–30.

27. Stephens DS, Hajjeh RA, Baughman WS, et al. Sporadic meningococcal disease in adults: results of a 5-year population-based study. Ann Intern Med. 1995; 123:937–40.

28. Yung AP, McDonald MI. Early clinical clues to meningococcaemia. Med J Aust. 2003; 178:134–7.

29. Braverman IM. Skin signs of systemic disease. 2nd ed. Philadelphia: WB Saunders; 1981, p. 816.

30. Thompson MJ, Ninis N, Perera R, et al. Clinical recognition of meningococcal disease in children and adolescents. Lancet. 2006; 4;367:397–403.

31. Kirsch EA, Barton RP, Kitchen L, Giroir BP. Pathophysiology, treatment and outcome of meningococcemia: a review and recent experience. Pediatr Infect Dis J. 1996; 15:967–78; quiz 79.

32. Milonovich LM. Meningococcemia: epidemiology, pathophysiology, and management. J Pediatr Health Care. 2007; 21:75–80.

33. Ferreira E, Dias R, Canica M. Antimicrobial susceptibility, serotype and genotype distribution of meningococci in Portugal, 2001–2002. Epidemiol Infect. 2006; 134:1203–7.

34. Kyaw MH, Clarke SC, Christie P, et al. Invasive meningococcal disease in Scotland, 1994 to 1999, with emphasis on group B meningococcal disease. J Clin Microbiol. 2002; 40:1834–7.

35. Jackson LA, Tenover FC, Baker C, et al. Prevalence of Neisseria meningitidis relatively resistant to penicillin in the United States, 1991. Meningococcal Disease Study Group. J Infect Dis. 1994; 169:438–41.

36. Rosenstein NE, Perkins BA, Stephens DS, et al. Meningococcal disease. N Engl J Med. 2001; 344:1378–88.

37. Swartz MN. Bacterial meningitis–a view of the past 90 years. N Engl J Med. 2004; 351:1826–8.

38. Durand ML, Calderwood SB, Weber DJ, et al. Acute bacterial meningitis in adults. A review of 493 episodes. N Engl J Med. 1993; 328:21–8.

39. Sharip A, Sorvillo F, Redelings MD, et al. Population-based analysis of meningococcal disease mortality in the United States: 1990–2002. Pediatr Infect Dis J. 2006; 25:191–4.

40. Gondim FA, Singh MK. Meningococcal meningitis. WebMD; 2007 [updated 2007; cited July 18, 2008]; Available from: http://www.emedicine.com/neuro/topic210.htm.

41. van de Beek D, de Gans J, McIntyre P, Prasad K. Corticosteroids for acute bacterial meningitis. Cochrane Database Syst Rev. 2007(1):CD004405.

42. Dumler JS, Walker DH. Rocky Mountain spotted fever–changing ecology and persisting virulence. N Engl J Med. 2005; 353:551–3.

43. Chapman AS, Murphy SM, Demma LJ, et al. Rocky Mountain spotted fever in the United States, 1997–2002. Ann N Y Acad Sci. 2006; 1078:154–5.

44. McNabb SJ, Jajosky RA, Hall-Baker PA, et al. Summary of notifiable diseases–United States, 2006. MMWR Morb Mortal Wkly Rep. 2008; 55:1–92.

45. Hopkins RS, Jajosky RA, Hall PA, et al. Summary of notifiable diseases–United States, 2003. MMWR Morb Mortal Wkly Rep. 2005; 52:1–85.

46. Lacz NL, Schwartz RA, Kapila R. Rocky Mountain spotted fever. J Eur Acad Dermatol Venereol. 2006; 20:411–7.

47. Dantas-Torres F. Rocky Mountain spotted fever. Lancet Infect Dis. 2007; 7:724–32.

48. Buckingham SC, Marshall GS, Schutze GE, et al. Clinical and laboratory features, hospital course, and outcome of Rocky Mountain spotted fever in children. J Pediatr. 2007; 150: 180–4.

49. Cunha BA. Clinical features of Rocky Mountain spotted fever. Lancet Infect Dis. 2008; 8:143–4.

50. Bleck TP. Central nervous system involvement in Rickettsial diseases. Neurol Clin. 1999; 17:801–12.

51. Abrahamian FM. Consequences of delayed diagnosis of Rocky Mountain spotted fever in children–West Virginia, Michigan, Tennessee, and Oklahoma, May–July 2000. Ann Emerg Med. 2001; 37:537–40.

52. Lochary ME, Lockhart PB, Williams WT, Jr. Doxycycline and staining of permanent teeth. Pediatr Infect Dis J. 1998; 17:429–31.

53. Markley KC, Levine AB, Chan Y. Rocky Mountain spotted fever in pregnancy. Obstet Gynecol. 1998; 91:860.

54. Dalton MJ, Clarke MJ, Holman RC, et al. National surveillance for Rocky Mountain spotted fever, 1981–1992: epidemiologic summary and evaluation of risk factors for fatal outcome. Am J Trop Med Hyg. 1995; 52:405–13.

55. Helmick CG, Bernard KW, D'Angelo LJ. Rocky Mountain spotted fever: clinical, laboratory, and epidemiological features of 262 cases. J Infect Dis. 1984; 150:480–8.

56. Hattwick MA, Retailliau H, O'Brien RJ, et al. Fatal Rocky Mountain spotted fever. JAMA. 1978; 240:1499–503.

57. Cohen JI, Corson AP, Corey GR. Late appearance of skin rash in Rocky Mountain spotted fever. South Med J. 1983; 76:1457–8.

58. Kirkland KB, Wilkinson WE, Sexton DJ. Therapeutic delay and mortality in cases of Rocky Mountain spotted fever. Clin Infect Dis. 1995; 20:1118–21.

59. Conlon PJ, Procop GW, Fowler V, et al. Predictors of prognosis and risk of acute renal failure in patients with Rocky Mountain spotted fever. Am J Med. 1996; 101:621–6.

60. Walker DH, Kirkman HN. Rocky Mountain spotted fever and deficiency in glucose-6-phosphate dehydrogenase. J Infect Dis. 1980; 142:771.

61. Bergeron JW, Braddom RL, Kaelin DL. Persisting impairment following Rocky Mountain spotted fever: a case report. Arch Phys Med Rehabil. 1997; 78:1277–80.

62. Textbook of military medicine. Part III, Disease and the environment. Falls Church, VA: Office of the Surgeon General, Dept. of the Army, U.S. of America; 1993.

63. Keysary A, Potasman I, Itzhaki A, et al. Clusters of Mediterranean spotted fever in Israel. Vector Borne Zoonotic Dis. 2007; 7:143–6.

64. Brouqui P, Parola P, Fournier PE, Raoult D. Spotted fever rickettsioses in southern and eastern Europe. FEMS Immunol Med Microbiol. 2007; 49:2–12.

65. de Sousa R, Nobrega SD, Bacellar F, Torgal J. Mediterranean spotted fever in Portugal: risk factors for fatal outcome in 105 hospitalized patients. Ann N Y Acad Sci. 2003; 990:285–94.

66. Raoult D, de Micco C, Gallais H, Toga M. Laboratory diagnosis of Mediterranean spotted fever by immunofluorescent demonstration of Rickettsia conorii in cutaneous lesions. J Infect Dis. 1984; 150:145–8.

67. Dujella J, Morovic M, Dzelalija B, et al. Histopathology and immunopathology of skin biopsy specimens in Mediterranean spotted fever. Acta Virol. 1991; 35:566–72.

68. Bella F, Espejo E, Uriz S, et al. J. Randomized trial of 5-day rifampin versus 1-day doxycycline therapy for Mediterranean spotted fever. J Infect Dis. 1991; 164:433–4.

69. Cascio A, Colomba C, Antinori S, et al. Clarithromycin versus azithromycin in the treatment of Mediterranean spotted fever in children: a randomized controlled trial. Clin Infect Dis. 2002; 34:154–8.

70. Cascio A, Colomba C, Di Rosa D, et al. Efficacy and safety of clarithromycin as treatment for Mediterranean spotted fever in children: a randomized controlled trial. Clin Infect Dis. 2001; 33:409–11.

71. Raoult D, Gallais H, De Micco P, Casanova P. Ciprofloxacin therapy for Mediterranean spotted fever. Antimicrob Agents Chemother. 1986; 30:606–7.

72. Dixon TC, Meselson M, Guillemin J, Hanna PC. Anthrax. N Engl J Med. 1999; 341:815–26.

73. Demirdag K, Ozden M, Saral Y, et al. Cutaneous anthrax in adults: a review of 25 cases in the eastern Anatolian region of Turkey. Infection. 2003; 31:327–30.

74. Peck RN, Fitzgerald DW. Cutaneous anthrax in the Artibonite Valley of Haiti: 1992–2002. Am J Trop Med Hyg. 2007; 77:806–11.

75. Meyer MA. Neurologic complications of anthrax: a review of the literature. Arch Neurol. 2003; 60:483–8.

76. Swartz MN. Recognition and management of anthrax–an update. N Engl J Med. 2001; 345:1621–6.

77. Test shaving brush of anthrax victim: Health department to seek today for germ which killed Michael F. Farley. New York Times. 1921 October 10.

78. Anthrax is spread by street vendors: Bellevue experts find dreaded germs in cheap shaving brushes bought from peddlers. New York Times. 1922 January 22.

79. Cutaneous anthrax associated with drum making using goat hides from west Africa–Connecticut, 2007. MMWR Morb Mortal Wkly Rep. 2008; 57:628–31.

80. Carucci JA, McGovern TW, Norton SA, et al. Cutaneous anthrax management algorithm. J Am Acad Dermatol. 2002; 47:766–9.

81. Artac H, Silahli M, Keles S, et al. A rare cause of preseptal cellulitis: anthrax. Pediatr Dermatol. 2007; 24: 330–1.

82. Shieh WJ, Guarner J, Paddock C, et al. The critical role of pathology in the investigation of bioterrorism-related cutaneous anthrax. Am J Pathol. 2003; 163:1901–10.

83. Bode E, Hurtle W, Norwood D. Real-time PCR assay for a unique chromosomal sequence of Bacillus anthracis. J Clin Microbiol. 2004; 42:5825–31.

84. Update: Investigation of bioterrorism-related anthrax and interim guidelines for exposure management and antimicrobial therapy, October 2001. MMWR Morb Mortal Wkly Rep. 2001; 50:909–19.

85. Maguina C, Flores Del Pozo J, Terashima A, et al. Cutaneous anthrax in Lima, Peru: retrospective analysis of 71 cases, including four with a meningoencephalic complication. Rev Inst Med Trop Sao Paulo. 2005; 47:25–30.

86. Doganay M, Bakir M, Dokmetas I. A case of cutaneous anthrax with toxaemic shock. Br J Dermatol. 1987; 117:659–62.

87. Holty JE, Bravata DM, Liu H, et al. Systematic review: a century of inhalational anthrax cases from 1900 to 2005. Ann Intern Med. 2006; 144:270–80.

88. Eliasson H, Back E. Tularaemia in an emergent area in Sweden: an analysis of 234 cases in five years. Scand J Infect Dis. 2007; 39:880–9.

89. Tularemia transmitted by insect bites–Wyoming, 2001–2003. MMWR Morb Mortal Wkly Rep. 2005; 54:170–3.

90. Trevisanato SI. The biblical plague of the Philistines now has a name, tularemia. Med Hypotheses. 2007; 69:1144–6.

91. The holy scriptures according to the Masoretic text. Philadelphia: The Jewish Publication Society of America; 1955, p. 144.

92. Myers JP, Baird IM. Case report. Tularemia in Ohio: report of two cases and clinical review. Am J Med Sci. 1981; 282:148–52.

93. Evans ME, Gregory DW, Schaffner W, McGee ZA. Tularemia: a 30-year experience with 88 cases. Medicine (Baltimore). 1985; 64:251–69.

94. Penn RL. Fransicella tularensis. In: Mandell GL, Douglas RG, Bennett JE, editors. Principles and practice of infectious diseases. 2nd ed. New York: Wiley; 1985; pp. 2060–8.

95. Byington CL, Bender JM, Ampofo K, et al. Tularemia with vesicular skin lesions may be mistaken for infection with herpes viruses. Clin Infect Dis. 2008; 47:e4–6.

96. Guffey MB, Dalzell A, Kelly DR, Cassady KA. Ulceroglandular tularemia in a nonendemic area. South Med J. 2007; 100:304–8.

97. Weinberg AN. Commentary: Wherry WB, Lamb BH. Infection of man with Bacterium tularense (J Infect Dis 1914; 15:331–40). J Infect Dis. 2004; 189:1317–20.

98. Oliver JD. Wound infections caused by Vibrio vulnificus and other marine bacteria. Epidemiol Infect. 2005; 133:383–91.

99. Inoue Y, Ono T, Matsui T, et al. Epidemiological survey of Vibrio vulnificus infection in Japan between 1999 and 2003. J Dermatol. 2008; 35:129–39.

100. Kuo YL, Shieh SJ, Chiu HY, Lee JW. Necrotizing fasciitis caused by Vibrio vulnificus: epidemiology, clinical findings, treatment and prevention. Eur J Clin Microbiol Infect Dis. 2007; 26:785–92.

101. Park SD, Shon HS, Joh NJ. Vibrio vulnificus septicemia in Korea: clinical and epidemiologic findings in seventy patients. J Am Acad Dermatol. 1991; 24:397–403.

102. de Araujo MR, Aquino C, Scaramal E, et al. Vibrio vulnificus infection in Sao Paulo, Brazil: case report and literature review. Braz J Infect Dis. 2007; 11:302–5.

103. Porras-Cortes G, Viana JJ, Chavez-Mazari B, Sierra-Madero J. [Vibrio vulnificus in Mexico: a case report and review of the literature]. Rev Invest Clin. 1994; 46:495–8.

104. Frank C, Littman M, Alpers K, Hallauer J. Vibrio vulnificus wound infections after contact with the Baltic Sea, Germany. Euro Surveill. 2006; 11:E0608171.

105. Ruppert J, Panzig B, Guertler L, et al. Two cases of severe sepsis due to Vibrio vulnificus wound infection acquired in the Baltic Sea. Eur J Clin Microbiol Infect Dis. 2004; 23:912–15.

106. Dalsgaard A, Frimodt-Moller N, Bruun B, et al. Clinical manifestations and molecular epidemiology of Vibrio vulnificus infections in Denmark. Eur J Clin Microbiol Infect Dis. 1996; 15:227–32.

107. Torres L, Escobar S, Lopez AI, et al. Wound infection due to Vibrio vulnificus in Spain. Eur J Clin Microbiol Infect Dis. 2002; 21:537–8.

108. Paz S, Bisharat N, Paz E, et al. Climate change and the emergence of Vibrio vulnificus disease in Israel. Environ Res. 2007; 103:390–6.

109. Ralph A, Currie BJ. Vibrio vulnificus and V. parahaemolyticus necrotising fasciitis in fishermen visiting an estuarine tropical northern Australian location. J Infect. 2007; 54:e111–14.

110. Tyring SK, Lee PC. Hemorrhagic bullae associated with Vibrio vulnificus septicemia. Report of two cases. Arch Dermatol. 1986; 122:818–20.

111. Fujisawa N, Yamada H, Kohda H, et al. Necrotizing fasciitis caused by Vibrio vulnificus differs from that caused by streptococcal infection. J Infect. 1998; 36:313–16.

112. CDC. Fact Sheet: Vibrio Vulnificus. 2005 [updated 2005; cited May 10, 2008]; Available from: http://www.cdc.gov/nczved/dfbmd/disease_listing/vibriov_gi.html.

113. Bross MH, Soch K, Morales R, Mitchell RB. Vibrio vulnificus infection: diagnosis and treatment. Am Fam Physician. 2007; 76:539–44.

114. Millership SE, Chattopadhyay B. Aeromonas hydrophila in chlorinated water supplies. J Hosp Infect. 1985; 6:75–80.

115. Millership SE, Stephenson JR, Tabaqchali S. Epidemiology of Aeromonas species in a hospital. J Hosp Infect. 1988; 11:169–75.

116. Zhiyong Z, Xiaoju L, Yanyu G. Aeromonas hydrophila infection; clinical aspects and therapeutic options. Rev Med Microbiol. 2002; 13:151–62.

117. Ko WC, Lee HC, Chuang YC, et al. Clinical features and therapeutic implications of 104 episodes of monomicrobial Aeromonas bacteraemia. J Infect. 2000; 40:267–73.

118. Lineaweaver WC, Hill MK, Buncke GM, et al. Aeromonas hydrophila infections following use of medicinal leeches in replantation and flap surgery. Ann Plast Surg. 1992; 29:238–44.

119. Gold WL, Salit IE. Aeromonas hydrophila infections of skin and soft tissue: report of 11 cases and review. Clin Infect Dis. 1993; 16:69–74.

120. Kienzle N, Muller M, Pegg S. Aeromonas wound infection in burns. Burns. 2000; 26:478–82.

121. Adamski J, Koivuranta M, Leppanen E. Fatal case of myonecrosis and septicaemia caused by Aeromonas hydrophila in Finland. Scand J Infect Dis. 2006; 38:1117–19.

122. Smith JA. Aeromonas hydrophila: analysis of 11 cases. CMAJ. 1980; 122:1270–2.

123. de Siqueira IC, Dias J, Ruf H, et al. Chromobacterium violaceum in siblings, Brazil. Emerg Infect Dis. 2005; 11:1443–5.

124. Huffam SE, Nowotny MJ, Currie BJ. Chromobacterium violaceum in tropical northern Australia. Med J Aust. 1998; 168:335–7.

125. Midani S, Rathore M. Chromobacterium violaceum infection. South Med J. 1998; 91:464–6.
126. Macher AM, Casale TB, Fauci AS. Chronic granulomatous disease of childhood and Chromobacterium violaceum infections in the southeastern United States. Ann Intern Med. 1982; 97:51–5.
127. Teoh AY, Hui M, Ngo KY, et al. Fatal septicaemia from Chromobacterium violaceum: case reports and review of the literature. Hong Kong Med J. 2006; 12:228–31.
128. Sirisanthana V. Fever with hemorrhagic and pustular blebs in 13 year old boy. Chiang Mai, Thailand: Department of Pediatrics, Faculty of Medicine, Chiang Mai University; 2008 [updated 2008; cited 2008]; Available from: http://www.med.cmu.ac.th/dept/pediatrics/06-interest-cases/ic-1-case1/case-1-chromo.htm.
129. Brown KL, Stein A, Morrell DS. Ecthyma gangrenosum and septic shock syndrome secondary to Chromobacterium violaceum. J Am Acad Dermatol. 2006; 54(5 Suppl):S224–8.

CHAPTER 10

Bacteremia, Sepsis, Septic Shock, and Toxic Shock Syndrome

Geeta Patel

Ryan Hawley

Noah Scheinfeld

IN THE EMERGENCY department, intensive care unit, and primary care setting, dermatological conditions rank as one of the most common disease presentations. It is often a challenge for physicians to differentiate routine skin ailments from more serious, life-threatening conditions that require immediate intervention. This chapter highlights some dermatologic emergencies that plague physicians daily and initially may present with cutaneous manifestations. Septic shock and toxic shock syndrome (TSS) are potentially fatal medical emergencies that manifest with dermatologic signs, making a good understanding of dermatology a crucial step in rapid and early diagnosis of these two emergencies. As part of a clinical continuum, the terms bacteremia, sepsis, and septic shock have for many years been confused due to the inaccurate usage of terminology associated with such infections. In 1991, the American College of Chest Physicians and the Society of Critical Care Medicine convened a Consensus Conference to standardize terminology and provide a framework for physicians to accurately identify the body's systemic response to infection. These quantifiable definitions work on a clinical continuum established by clinical and laboratory findings. Unfortunately, to date there is no single definitive census for the standard of care and defined illness; the 1992 consensus is commonly accepted and reputable for defining disease for this topic and will be used as a guideline for this chapter (Table 10.1).

BACTEREMIA, SEPSIS, SEPTIC SHOCK, AND TSS

Bacteremia

Bacteremia refers to the presence of viable bacteria in blood.[1] To gain access to the circulation, bacteria and their toxins must penetrate through protective mechanisms such as anatomic barriers (skin), the nonspecific immune system, and the specific immune system. Bacteremia can range from a benign asymptomatic course to a more continual infection that can progress to septic shock or TSS. Bacteremia can

be described as primary (direct invasion of blood stream, as in intravenous [IV] drug use) or secondary (infection at another site complicated by microorganisms invading the bloodstream, as in pneumonia or soft-tissue infections).[2] It can present as:

- Transient Bacteremia – short periods (minutes to hours) of viable bacteria in blood usually with normal flora pathogens. Common during toothbrushing, routine dental work, and menstruation. It is usually cleared by the reticuloendothelial system.

- Intermittent Bacteremia – recurrent episodes of viable bacteria from extravascular abscesses, spreading cellulitis,

TABLE 10.1: Definitions from 1992 Consensus Conference

Term	Definition
Infection	Inflammatory response to the presence of microorganisms or the invasion of normally sterile host tissue by those organisms
Bacteremia	Presence of viable bacteria in blood
SIRS	Systemic inflammatory response to a variety of severe clinical insults manifested by two or more of the following conditions: (1) temperature $>38°C$ or $<36°C$; (2) heart rate >90 bpm; (3) respiratory rate >20 breaths per minute or PaCO <32 mm Hg; or (4) white blood cell count $>12,000$/cu mm, $<4,000$/cu mm, or $>10\%$ immature (band) forms
Sepsis	SIRS and documented or suspected infection
Severe sepsis	Sepsis associated with organ dysfunction, hypoperfusion, or hypotension
Septic shock	Sepsis with hypotension despite adequate fluid resuscitation along with the presence of perfusion abnormalities

Adapted from (1).
SIRS, systemic inflammatory response syndrome.

TABLE 10.2: Community-Acquired and Hospital-Acquired Bacteremia

	Gram-negative pathogens	Normal flora of:
Community-acquired bacteremia	E. coli	Small and large intestine
and	K. pneumoniae	Large intestine
hospital-acquired bacteremia	P. aeruginosa	Small and large intestine
	Gram-positive pathogens	
	S. aureus	Anterior nares, skin, eye, upper respiratory tract, large intestine
	S. pneumoniae	Upper respiratory tract, eye, oral cavity
	E. faecalis	Small intestine

or body infections such as septic arthritis, peritonitis, or an empyema.

● Continuous Bacteremia – usually occurring when infection is intravascular, such as with infected endothelium seen in infective endocarditis or with infected hardware as with an indwelling catheter.

There is a continuous increase in the incidence of bacteremia-associated mortality worldwide, mainly attributed to the increased usage of invasive devices and invasive procedures, increased usage of aggressive drug therapy that results in immunodeficiency, increasing population of critically ill patients due to advancements in life support, and advances in the development of highly sensitive diagnostic tools.[3] Bacteremia can be community acquired or nosocomial in inheritance. Table 10.2 displays the most common pathogens seen in patients with documented bacteremia.

In studies documenting bacteremia, *Escherichia coli* was the most frequently isolated pathogen among older patients with community-acquired bacteremia. In contrast, *Staphylococcus aureus* was the most frequently isolated pathogen among younger adults with community-acquired bacteremia. S. aureus was the most common pathogen causing nosocomial bacteremia, regardless of age.[4] The most common source of bacteremia is the urinary tract, with suspected cases followed by pneumonia and central venous catheter (femoral > subclavian) and wound infection.[5] Many factors determine whether bacteremia will progress to sepsis, septic shock, or TSS. Elderly patients have an increased tendency to develop severe sepsis due to bacteremia compared to younger patients.[4,6] Some other factors that can aid in the progression to sepsis or septic shock are the immunocompetence of the patient, the

virulence and number of pathogens in the blood, and the timing and nature of a therapeutic intervention.

Sepsis

Sepsis can be a life-threatening infection and is characterized as a systemic response manifested by two of the following with evidence of infection:[1]

● Temperature >38°C or <36°C;

● Heart rate >90 beats per minute; or

● White blood cell count >12,000 mcL, <4,000 mcL or >10% immature (band) forms.

Due to the potential for rapid progression to severe sepsis or septic shock, sepsis is considered a true medical emergency, and thus rapid diagnosis is crucial to decrease morbidity and mortality. Sepsis is the leading cause of death in critically ill patients and among the top 10 overall causes of death in patients in the United States.[7] Sepsis develops in 750,000 people annually, with 435,000 cases progressing to septic shock and more than 215,000 cases leading to death.[8,9] There is a higher incidence in men than in women and in nonwhite persons than in white persons.[10] Although the median age of patients with a sepsis-related hospital discharge diagnosis is approximately 60 years, the incidence is high among infants (>500 cases/100,000 population per year), with low-birth-weight newborns experiencing particularly high risk.[11] Sepsis incidence and sepsis-related mortality decrease after the first year of life and then increase steadily with increasing age.[8] Approximately 80% of cases of sepsis progressing to severe sepsis in adults occurred in individuals who were already hospitalized for another reason.[12,13]

Sepsis is a clinical syndrome that can be caused by a variety of microorganisms (i.e., virus, bacteria, fungus, or parasites), although typically gram-negative and gram-positive bacteria account for most cases. In 30%–50% of septic cases, a definite microbial etiology was not found.[13–15] It should be noted that sepsis is defined as an immune response to microorganisms, and the number of organisms necessary to launch such a response varies depending on the patient's immune response to bacterial antigens.

Septic Shock

Septic shock is the clinical extension of sepsis with the addition of hypotension and secondary hypoperfusion of tissue refractory to fluid administration, thus substantially increasing the mortality rate.[1] Sepsis is usually reversible, whereas patients with septic shock often succumb despite aggressive therapy. Septic shock represents the most severe host response to infection. These patients do not display normal hemodynamic response to administered fluid bolus, and thus have persistent perfusion abnormalities, including tissue and organ hypoperfusion manifesting as lactic acidosis, oliguria, and/or acute alteration in mental status.[16] These findings should yield high suspicion for multiple organ dysfunction syndrome (MODS), the most worrisome consequence of septic shock and most likely to result in mortality if not recognized and corrected early. Septic shock is the major cause of death in intensive care units; the mortality rate is as high as 50%–80% depending on the patient population.[8] Septic shock and MODS are the most common causes of death in patients with sepsis.[12] The incidence has increased owing to an increased number of patients who are immunocompromised, the increased use of invasive devices, and the growing elderly population.

Septic shock is part of the continuum associated with the systemic inflammatory response syndrome (SIRS). Although any microorganism may cause septic shock, it is most often associated with gram-negative bacteria such as *E. coli*, *Klebsiella pneumoniae*, *Pseudomonas*, and *Serratia*. Gram-positive bacteria such as *S. aureus* can also cause septic shock and, in past years, have led to outbreaks of TSS. Lower respiratory infections, abdominal infections, urinary tract infections, and soft-tissue infections are the nidus in, respectively, 35%, 21%, 13%, and 7% percent of documented cases of septic shock.[17,18] Common factors or conditions that are associated with septic shock include diabetes mellitus, malnutrition, alcohol abuse, cirrhosis, respiratory infections, hemorrhage, cancer, and surgery.[19]

Toxic Shock Syndrome

TSS is a rare, often life-threatening illness that develops suddenly after an infection and can rapidly progress, affecting many organ systems and requiring prompt recognition and medical treatment. It was first described in 1978 in seven children with *S. aureus* infections.[20] After an epidemic in 1981, TSS has been typically associated with tampon use in healthy menstruating women. Due to physician and public awareness, the incidence of TSS has since declined in this population group, with the majority of documented cases now reporting men, neonates, and nonmenstruating women with TSS.[21] A similar but more threatening TSS-like syndrome, streptococcal TSS, has emerged. It is associated with invasive and noninvasive Streptococcal infections and has a rapidly progressive course and a high case-fatality rate. TSS is the result of infection by *Streptococcus pyogenes* or *S. aureus* bacteria.[22,23] These pathogenic bacteria typically comprise a small percentage of the host's normal flora and usually do not cause severe disease. TSS occurs when these bacteria have an optimal environment for replication and toxin production that can enter the bloodstream and cause a severe immune reaction in immunosuppressed and/or immunocompetent persons. The host's immune response to bacterial toxins causes the symptoms associated with TSS.

Staphylococcal TSS came to prominence in 1980–1981, when numerous cases were associated with the introduction of superabsorbent tampons for use during menstrua-

tion.[21,24] The disease is characterized by a fulminant onset, often in previously healthy persons. The diagnosis is based on clinical findings that include high fever (>38.9°C), headache, vomiting, diarrhea, myalgias, and an erythematous eruption characterized as a sunburn. TSS often develops from a site of colonization rather than infection.[25–27]

Streptococcal TSS carries a mortality rate of 30% or higher, despite aggressive and timely medical therapy. Streptococcal TSS is epidemiologically distinct from other invasive infections in that younger and healthier populations are commonly affected.[22,28] Group A β-hemolytic streptococcal (GAS) TSS may often originate in the skin of young, healthy patients at a site of local trauma. In 5%–10% of cases, there may be accompanying necrotizing fasciitis. Bacteremia has been shown to be a key component in a large majority of severe GAS infections.[29] TSS can occur as a consequence of GAS sinusitis, cellulitis, peritonitis, and tracheitis and as a complication of varicella infections.[30,31]

TSS is separated into two distinct categories: menstrual and nonmenstrual. Both menstrual and nonmenstrual TSS had higher incidence in white women. Although most cases of TSS are related to menstruation, nonmenstrual cases have increased and now account for approximately one third of all cases. These nonmenstrual cases have been associated with localized infections, surgery, or insect bites. Patients with nonmenstrual TSS have a higher mortality rate than do those with menstrual TSS.[27]

PATHOPHYSIOLOGY

Sepsis is the endpoint of a multifaceted process that begins with an infection. The initial host response is to mobilize inflammatory cells, neutrophils and macrophages, to the site of infection. These inflammatory cells then release circulating molecules that trigger a cascade of other inflammatory mediators that result in a coordinated host response. If these mediators are not appropriately regulated, sepsis will occur. In the setting of ongoing toxin release, a persistent inflammatory response occurs with ongoing mediator activation, cellular hypoxia, tissue injury, shock, multiorgan failure, and (potentially) death. Much of the damage inflicted on the septic host is attributable to microbial toxins and the host's response to them.[32–34]

In sepsis and septic shock, microbial antigens contain pathogen-associated molecular patterns that bind to the host protein's pattern recognition receptors, called Toll-like receptors (TLRs), directing the activation of antibody-mediated immunity. Mutations associated with TLRs have been implicated in hyporesponsive antibody-mediated immunity, thus increasing certain patients' susceptibility to developing septic shock from gram-negative bacteria.[35,36]

One important microbial toxin in the pathogenesis of sepsis is lipopolysaccharide (LPS). LPS is the major structural component of the outer membrane of gram-negative bacteria. It is essential for cell viability for virtually all gram-negative bacterial pathogens.[37] LPS has no intrinsic toxic properties by itself.[38] The toxicity of LPS is related to the host response to this antigen (such an antigen is also termed a superantigen). Similar pathogen-associated molecular pattern mediators (superantigens) exist in gram-positive bacteria, lipoteichoic acid, that induce a potentially harmful host response during sepsis.

LPS binds to LPS-binding protein, creating an LPS–LPS-binding protein complex. This complex binds to the receptor located on the CD14 molecule that is found on monocytes, macrophages, and neutrophils. Peptidoglycans of gram-positive bacteria and LPS of gram-negative bacteria bind to TLR-2 and TLR-4, respectively. Given their central role in the recognition of microbes, TLRs are likely to have a crucial role in sepsis: TLRs are on the one hand essential for the early detection of pathogens, but on the other hand cause excessive inflammation after uncontrolled stimulation. TLR-2 and TLR-4 binding activates intracellular signal transduction pathways, which increase transcription of cytokines such as tumor necrosis factor-α (TNF-α), interleukin-1β (IL-1β), interleukin-6 (IL-6), and interleukin-10 (IL-10).[39,40] TNF-α, IL-1β, and IL-6 are proinflammatory cytokines that activate an immune response but also cause both direct and indirect host cellular injury such as endothelial damage and eventually capillary leakage. LPS and TNF-α probably promote intravascular coagulation initially by inducing blood monocytes to express tissue factor, by initiating the release of plasminogen activator inhibitor type 1, and by inhibiting the expression of thrombomodulin and plasminogen activator by vascular endothelial cells. IL-10 is an antiinflammatory cytokine that inactivates macrophages, as well as altering of monocyte function, decreasing antigen presenting activity, and reducing production of proinflammatory cytokines, and is underexpressed in the Th2-mediated immune response.[35,40,41]

In TSS, the staphylococcal and streptococcal toxins are able to function as superantigens, which are proteins that simultaneously bind nonspecifically to T-cell receptors (TCRs) and major histocompatibility complex (MHC) class II molecules.[42] Toxic shock syndrome toxin 1 (TSST-1), the best characterized of the toxins, binds to the MHC class II molecule.[43] These toxins are known as superantigenic because they activate CD4 T-cell populations at a level that is at least five orders of magnitude greater than conventional antigens.[44] Superantigens are not processed by antigen-presenting cells. They bind directly to MHC class II molecules expressed on antigen-presenting cells and cross-link with a large number of T cells that bear common Vβ chains and their TCRs. High concentrations of lymphokines and monokines result and induce TSS. Immune activation induced by superantigens potentiates the host response to other microbial mediators, including bacterial endotoxin.[45] The large numbers of effector CD4+ T cells resulting from this nonspecific proliferation begin stimulating monocytes to secrete several cytokines, including TNF-α and IL-1. The secretion of these cytokines

(instead of the localized secretion that normally occurs during infection) is the major determinant for morbidity associated with staphylococcal and streptococcal TSS.

CLINICAL AND LABORATORY AIDS REQUIRED FOR DIAGNOSIS

To diagnose bacteremia, sepsis, septic shock, or TSS as early as possible, it is necessary to recognize historical, clinical, and laboratory findings that are indicative of infection and organ dysfunction.[17] A thorough physical examination is vital for the identification of the source of infection. Patients with bacteremia and often sepsis present a diagnostic challenge to clinicians owing to nonspecific, and sometimes nonexistent early clinical manifestations. The diagnosis must rely on a strong clinical suspicion supported by the presence of several of the signs of sepsis if possible. Two populations in which a high index of suspicion for bacteremia and sepsis should remain despite lack of clinical features are infants/children and the elderly population.[5,46,47] Criteria for establishing diagnosis are within the definitions of bacteremia, sepsis, and septic shock, thus one must consider the diagnosis if a patient meets the criteria set forth from the 1992 consensus.[1]

BACTEREMIA, SEPSIS, AND SEPTIC SHOCK

Symptoms that suggest the onset of sepsis are often nonspecific and include sweats, chills or rigors, breathlessness, nausea and vomiting or diarrhea, and headache.[48] Fever, often accompanied by shaking chills, is the most common clinical manifestation of bacteremia and sepsis. In a study reported by Kreger and colleagues[49] and Vincent,[50] fever (temperature > 37.6°C) was seen in 82% of patients. Hypothermia (temperature < 36.4°C) was seen in 13% of bacteremic patients. Although the most common sign of bacteremic and septic patients is fever, a significant percentage of patients who present with bacteremia are also found to be hypothermic. Age, renal insufficiency, corticosteroid or antipyretic administration, and malignancy all increase the likelihood that a patient will not mount a febrile response. Mental status changes may occur in patients with bacteremia or sepsis. Changes may range from mild anxiety or restlessness to profound confusional states. Change in mental state is an important clinical finding in elderly patients who may exhibit few other early signs of disease. Tachypnea and altered mental status were more common among patients older than 75 years than among younger patients, whereas tachycardia and hypoxemia were less common among older patients. The hemodynamic instability of the young population with sepsis is of clinical importance. This effect is due to younger patients' ability to regulate blood pressure via vasoconstriction, leading to rapid onset of hypotension in this population.[51]

A number of dermatologic manifestations have been described in patients with bacteremia, sepsis, septic shock,

TABLE 10.3: Tissue Involvement by Gram-Negative Microbial Pathogens

Name	Suggestive of:	Description	Histologic findings
Palpable purpura[56,57,58]	*N. meningitidis; H. influenzae; R. rickettsii; S. aureus*	>3 mm, elevated, nonblanching, erythematous to violaceous plaques or nodules; dependent areas such as legs and feet are common areas; appears 12–36 h after onset of illness	Angiocentric inflammation with endothelial cell swelling fibrinoid necrosis and a neutrophilic cellular infiltrate around and within blood vessel walls Deposits of immunoglobulins and complement in blood vessel walls
Petechiae[56,59,60,61]	Infective endocarditis 2° to bacteremia; *N. meningitidis; E. coli;* other gram-negative bacteria	<3 cm, range from erythematous to violaceous; commonly found on lower legs but can also be found on the conjunctiva and palate; appears 12–36 h after onset of illness	Vascular thrombosis; perivascular hemorrhage
Ecthyma gangrenosum[52,53,54,55]	*P. aureus; A. hydrophila;* gram-negative bacteria; *V. vulnificus*	Painless, round, erythematous macules; they become indurated and progress to hemorrhagic bluish bullae; lesions later slough to form a deep gangrenous ulcer with a gray–black eschar and a surrounding erythematous halo; process evolves rapidly over a period of 12–24 h; usually found between umbilicus and knees but may occur anywhere on the body	Bacterial invasion of the media and adventitia of vein walls deep in the dermis Sparing of the intima and lumen Minimal inflammation
Acrocyanosis[62,63]	Septic shock DIC	Blueness of hands and feet with preserved pinkness in mucous membranes	
Hemorrhagic bullous[64,65]	*V. vulnificus* (contact with seafood)	Erythematous painful swollen limb (lower > upper) with bilateral hemorrhagic plaques and bullae; develops 36 h after onset	Noninflammatory bulla, epidermal necrosis, hemorrhage, and bacteria in dermal vessels
Cellulitis[66,67]	*S. aureus* *S. pyogenes* *S. pneumoniae* Gram-negative bacilli	Not raised, and demarcation from uninvolved skin is indistinct; tissue feels hard on palpation and is extremely painful; cellulitis extends into subcutaneous tissues	

DIC, disseminated intravascular coagulation.

and/or TSS. Skin may be the primary site of disease manifestation. To diagnose bacteremia, sepsis, or septic shock from cutaneous lesions, one must look at the overall picture in addition to the definition of the infection established in the 1992 consensus. Cutaneous lesions that occur as a result of bacterial infection can be divided into three categories:

- direct bacterial involvement of the skin and underlying soft tissues (e.g., cellulitis, erysipelas, and fasciitis);
- lesions that occur as a consequence of sepsis, hypotension, and disseminated intravascular coagulation (DIC; e.g., acrocyanosis and necrosis of peripheral tissues); and
- lesions secondary to intravascular infections (e.g., microemboli and/or immune complex vasculitis).

Recognition of certain characteristic lesions can greatly assist etiologic diagnosis. Musher distinguished three patterns of tissue involvement by gram-negative microbial pathogen:[52]

1. Cellulitis and thrombophlebitis are associated with intense local inflammation. Bacteria implicated in case reports include *Campylobacter fetus*, *Vibrio* species, and *Aeromonas hydrophila*. Only a few bacteria are present in the affected tissues, however, making definitive diagnosis by Gram stain difficult as most biopsied lesions will contain very few organisms. For this reason, much better results may be obtained from culturing.

2. When the inflammatory response is impaired, usually by neutropenia, ecthyma gangrenosum or bullous lesions may occur; *Pseudomonas aeruginosa* is the most commonly isolated microorganism.

3. In symmetrical peripheral gangrene associated with DIC, fibrin thrombi are seen in small vessels, but neither inflammatory cells nor bacteria are found.

TABLE 10.4: Clinical Signs and Symptoms of Sepsis and Septic Shock

System	Clinical symptoms
CNS[68,69]	Confusion
	Focal signs, seizures, and cranial nerve palsies are rare
	Encephalopathy (may be associated with a poor prognosis)
	Diffuse weakness
Endocrine	Hypotension
	Hypoglycemia or hyperglycemia
	Adrenal insufficiency
Cardiovascular	Tachycardia
Pulmonary	Hyperventilation
Renal	Oliguria
GI	Nausea/Vomiting/Diarrhea
	Ileus
	Upper GI bleeding from stress ulcers
Hepatic	Jaundice

CNS, central nervous system; GI, gastrointestinal.

Although often considered pathognomonic for *P. aeruginosa* bacteremia, ecthyma gangrenosum also has been observed in patients whose blood cultures grew *Klebsiella*, *Serratia*, *A. hydrophila*, or *E. coli*. Almost all patients with

ecthyma gangrenosum are neutropenic at the time the lesions develop and are associated with lesions of skin or mucous membranes that rapidly worsen and evolve into nodular patches marked by hemorrhage, ulceration, and necrosis.[52–55]

Ischemic changes (dusky or pallid color, coldness, loss of pulses) usually occur in the hands and feet, where they may follow thrombosis of small to medium-size arteries. Such ischemic changes are usually seen in septic shock. Inflammation-induced coagulopathy and vasoconstriction both contribute to their pathogenesis (Table 10.3).[62,63]

Table 10.4 displays other common clinical signs and symptoms of sepsis and septic shock.

Laboratory Findings

Table 10.5 displays common laboratory findings seen in sepsis and septic shock.

TOXIC SHOCK

History and physical examination are vital in the identification of a presumptive source of TSS. Whereas septic shock has hypotension and subsequent organ failure, toxic shock is characterized as coinciding hypotension with

TABLE 10.5: Laboratory Findings in Sepsis and Septic Shock

Laboratory study	Findings	Comments
White blood cell count	Leukocytosis or leucopenia	Stress response, increased margination of neutrophils in sepsis; toxic granulation may be seen; occasionally, bacteria may be found in the peripheral blood smear
Platelet	Thrombocytopenia	Look for evidence of fragmentation hemolysis in the peripheral blood smear; thrombocytopenia may or may not be accompanied by disseminated intravascular coagulation
Glucose	Hyperglycemia or hypoglycemia	Acute stress response, inhibition of gluconeogenesis
Clotting factors	Prolonged prothrombin time, activated partial thromboplastin time, low fibrinogen levels, and evidence of fibrinolysis	Coagulopathy often seen with systemic endotoxin release
Liver enzymes	Elevated alkaline phosphatase, bilirubin, and transaminases; low albumin	–
Blood cultures	Bacteremia or fungemia	The presence of positive blood culture does not make the diagnosis, and its absence does not exclude the diagnosis
Plasma lactate	Mild elevations (>2.2 mmol/L)	Hypermetabolism, anaerobic metabolism, inhibition of pyruvate dehydrogenase
C-reactive protein	Elevated	Acute-phase reactant, sensitive but not specific for sepsis
Arterial blood gas	Respiratory alkalosis (early); metabolic acidosis (late)	Measurements of O_2 content and mixed venous O_2 saturation useful in management
Serum phosphate	Hypophosphatemia	Inversely correlated with high levels of inflammatory cytokines

TABLE 10.6: Major Criteria for Diagnosis of S. Aureus TSS

1. *Fever*: Temperature ≥38.9°C (102°F)
2. *Eruption*: Diffuse macular erythroderma ("sunburn" eruption)
3. *Hypotension*: Systolic blood pressure (BP) ≤90 mm Hg (adults) or less than fifth percentile for age (children <16 years old); or orthostatic hypotension (orthostatic drop in diastolic BP by 15 mm Hg, orthostatic dizziness, or orthostatic syncope)
4. *Involvement of at least three of the following organ systems*:
   a. Gastrointestinal (vomiting or diarrhea at onset of illness)
   b. Muscular (severe myalgias or serum creatine phosphokinase level at least twice the upper limit of normal)
   c. Mucous membranes (vaginal, oropharyngeal, conjunctival hyperemia)
   d. Renal (blood urea nitrogen or creatinine level at least twice upper limit of normal or pyuria)
   e. Hepatic
   f. Hematologic (thrombocytopenia)
   g. Central nervous system
5. *Desquamation*: 1–2 weeks after onset of illness (typically palms/fingers, soles/toes)
6. *Evidence against alternative diagnosis*: Negative results of cultures of blood, throat, or cerebrospinal fluid (if performed); no increase in titers of antibody to the agents of Rocky Mountain spotted fever, leptospirosis, and rubeola (if obtained)
   Probable Diagnosis:
   • Desquamation and 3 other major criteria
   • All 5 major criteria in the absence of desquamation

TSS, toxic shock syndrome.

organ failure. TSS caused by *S. aureus* and TSS caused by *S. pyogenes* are both characterized by an acute illness with fever, sudden-onset hypotension, rapidly accelerated renal failure, and multisystem organ failure. Clinical definitions of staphylococcal and streptococcal TSS are described in Tables 10.6 and 10.7, respectively. Both types of syndrome also have differences that can help differentiate them on clinical appearance. Table 10.8 highlights those differences. The presence of fever, vomiting, watery diarrhea, myalgias, and conjunctival hyperemia are suggestive of *S. aureus* TSS whereas soft-tissue infections such as cellulitis, abscess, or necrotizing fasciitis with increased pain commonly occur with streptococcal TSS. Both can form without an identifiable source of infection.

Staphylococcal TSS

Staphylococcal TSS should be suspected in any individual with a sudden onset of a fever (>38.9°C) with chills, malaise, vomiting or diarrhea, myalgias, dizziness, syncope, beefy edematous mucous membranes, and/or conjunctival hyperemia.

In addition to signs and symptoms, there may be a history of superabsorbant tampon use, recent surgery, diaphragm contraception, or indwelling foreign body. On physical examination, the patient appears ill and has a fever >38.9°C. There may be clinical evidence of hypotension, peripheral edema, and muscle tenderness. If an infected wound is the source of TSS, the clinical presentation will be out of proportion to the wound presentation. Skin

TABLE 10.7: Major Criteria for Diagnosis of S. Pyogenes TSS

1. *Isolation of group A β-hemolytic streptococci*
   (a) from a normally sterile site (e.g., blood, cerebrospinal fluid, peritoneal fluid, tissue biopsy specimen)
   (b) from a nonsterile site (e.g., throat, sputum, vagina)
2. *Hypotension*: systolic blood pressure <90 mm Hg in adults or lower than the fifth percentile for age in children
3. Two or more of the following signs:
   • renal impairment: creatinine level >177 μmol/L (≥2 mg/dL) for adults or two times or more the upper limit of normal for age
   • coagulopathy: platelet count < ≤100,000/mcL or disseminated intravascular coagulation
   • hepatic involvement: ALT, AST, or total bilirubin levels two times or more the upper limit of normal for age
   • adult respiratory distress syndrome
   • generalized erythematous macular eruption that may desquamate
   • soft-tissue necrosis, including necrotizing fasciitis or myositis, or gangrene
An illness fulfilling criteria 1(a), 2, and 3 can be defined as a definite case. An illness fulfilling criteria 1(b), 2, and 3 can be defined as probable case if no other cause for the illness is identified.

TSS, toxic shock syndrome; ALT, alanine aminotransferase; AST, aspartate aminotransferase.

TABLE 10.8: Differences in Staphylococcal and Streptococcal TSS

Characteristics	Staphylococcal TSS	Streptococcal TSS
Predisposing factors	Tampons, burns, wounds	Varicella, wounds
Site of infection	Superficial (i.e., impetigo, burns, diaper rash, genital tract)	Deep (i.e., blunt trauma, necrotizing fasciitis, myositis, septic joint)
Abrupt onset of pain	Rare	Common
Eruption	Very common	Less common
Vomiting/Diarrhea	Very common	Less common
Increased creatinine kinase	Rare	Common in fasciitis
Bacteremia	<5%	60%
Desquamation	7–14 days	Less common
Mortality	3%–5%	5%–10%

TSS, toxic shock syndrome.

examination shows that there is a flexurally accentuated diffuse nonpruritic, blanching macular–papular erythroderma, described as "sunburn." The distribution always involves the extremities, with erythematous palms and soles. Erythema of the mucous membranes is commonly observed as well. The eruption may be subtle and is often missed in heavily pigmented patients or when the patient is examined in a poorly illuminated room. The eruption fades in approximately 3 days, but sheet-like desquamation of the hands and feet occurs in all patients 5–12 days after the eruption disappears. Some patients also may develop reversible alopecia and nail shedding. In menstrual TSS, edema and erythema of the inner thigh and perineum with a normal uterine and adnexal examination may be noted. In nonmenstrual TSS, another focus of infection may be present.

Laboratory findings reflect dysfunction of several organ systems. Laboratory abnormalities included as criteria for diagnosing TSS are elevated creatinine phosphokinase, acute renal insufficiency, sterile pyuria, elevated liver function tests, and thrombocytopenia. Some laboratory findings that are not included in the criteria for TSS but can commonly be seen are electrolyte abnormalities (hypophosphatemia and hypocalcemia), leukocytosis, and decreased serum albumin and total protein due to capillary leakage. The prothrombin, international normalized ratio, and partial thromboplastin times may be elevated, with or without thrombocytopenia. Laboratory abnormalities usually return to normal within 7–10 days of disease onset. Cultures of material from the vagina or cervix are usually positive for *S. aureus*. Blood cultures are negative in 85% of patients with TSS, but must still be obtained.

Streptococcal TSS occurs in all age groups without a predisposing factor. A hallmark feature of *S. pyogenes* TSS is pain that is severe and abrupt in onset. The pain is usually preceded by tenderness. Symptoms that remain the hallmark in staphylococcal TSS (such as fever, chills, myalgias, vomiting, and diarrhea) are present in less than 20% of streptococcal cases. Most cases present with fever and a localized soft-tissue infection that can progress to necrotizing fasciitis or myositis and require surgical debridement or even amputation. Laboratory data on streptococcal TSS cases are similar to those on staphylococcal TSS. Symptoms of streptococcal TSS are nonspecific. Physicians should have clinical suspicion in children and in persons with chronic underlying illness. Clues to suggest streptococcal TSS are localized severe pain as opposed to myalgia, skin lesion, or history of trauma at site of pain.

THERAPY

Successful management of bacteremia requires elimination of the offending pathogen by the timely administration of antibiotics and removal of the source of infection. Bacteremia should be treated if one obtains 2–4 positive blood cultures; sensitivity is dependent on the volume of blood cultured, with 30–40 mL per session being recommended for optimal results. One must draw at least 10 mL of blood for culture by venipuncture with at least 10 mL through each lumen of a central vascular catheter when one is present. Empiric antimicrobial therapy of bacteremia and sepsis depends upon localizing the site of infection to a particular organ, which determines the pathogenic flora in the septic process. The usual pathogens are determined by the organ or infection site, are predictable, and are the basis for the selection of appropriate empiric antimicrobial therapy. Coverage should be directed against the most common pathogens and does not need to be excessively broad or contain unnecessary activity against uncommon pathogens. If multiple drugs are used initially, the regimen should be modified and coverage narrowed based on the results of culture and sensitivity testing.

When sepsis is identified, treatment should be started immediately. To aid in uniform and consistent management, two sets of severe sepsis bundles were defined by

TABLE 10.9: Sepsis Bundles

Sepsis resuscitation bundle

1. Serum lactate measured
2. Blood cultures obtained before antibiotics administered
3. Improve time to broad-spectrum antibiotics
4. In the event of hypotension or lactate >4 mmol/L (36 mg/dL):
   a. deliver an initial minimum of 20 mL/kg of crystalloid (or colloid equivalent)
   b. apply vasopressors for ongoing hypotension
5. In the event of persistent hypotension despite fluid resuscitation or lactate >4 mmol/L (36 mg/dL):
   a. achieve central venous pressure of 8–12 mm Hg
   b. achieve central venous oxygen saturation of ≥70%

Sepsis management bundle
1. Administer low-dose steroids
2. Administer drotrecogin alfa (activated)
3. Maintain adequate glycemic control
4. Prevent excessive inspiratory plateau pressures

the 2002 Surviving Sepsis Campaign: the sepsis resuscitation bundle and the sepsis management bundle (Tables 10.9 and 10.10). The resuscitation bundle should be implemented within the initial 6 hours after patient admission to the hospital. It is also recommended to implement the sepsis management bundle as soon as possible but within the first 24 hours.[70]

For TSS, hemodynamic stabilization and antimicrobial therapy are the initial goals of treatment. Immediate and aggressive management of hypovolemic shock is critical. Thus, fluid resuscitation with crystalloid or colloidal solution is important in the mainstay of treatment. Tampons or other packing material should be promptly removed. It is often difficult to determine initially whether *Streptococcus* or *Staphylococcus* is the offending bacterium, so coverage for both is necessary. Suggested regimens include penicillin plus clindamycin, erythromycin, or ceftriaxone plus clindamycin. Patients with suspected methicillin-resistant staphylococcal TSS should be treated with IV vancomycin 1 g every 12 hours for 10–15 days, with dose adjustment based on creatinine clearance. Patients with streptococcal TSS require hospitalization for care, usually initially in an intensive care setting. Patients with streptococcal TSS should be treated with both IV penicillin G, 3–4 million units every 4 hours, and IV clindamycin, 600–900 mg every 8 hours for 10–15 days, followed by oral therapy. Double antibiotic coverage is the standard of care for streptococcal TSS because this infection is characterized by extremely large numbers of stationary bacteria and penicillin alone is not effective in this scenario.

PROGNOSIS

Severe sepsis and septic shock are associated with case-fatality ratios of approximately 30% and 50%, respectively. Outcome is significantly (and most profoundly) influenced by the patient's underlying disease. Bacteremia with certain microbes (e.g., *S. aureus*) may also be independently related to mortality in multivariate analyses. Of the many studied

TABLE 10.10: Suggested Initial Drug Therapy Based on Presumed Source

Source	Antibiotic treatment	Comment
Community-acquired pneumonia	Erythromycin[a] and third-generation cephalosporin[b] OR First- or second-generation cephalosporin[c] plus aminoglycoside[d]	Gram-negative bacteria cause 10%–20% of community-acquired pneumonias requiring hospitalization; *H. influenzae, K. pneumoniae,* and others implicated; consider *Legionella* species if patient is elderly or immunosuppressed
Hospital-acquired pneumonia	Antipseudomonal β-lactam[e] plus aminoglycoside[d]	Must treat for more resistant organisms including *P. aeruginosa*
Urinary tract infections	Ampicillin[a] plus aminoglycoside[d]	Combination also covers enterococci
Intraabdominal or biliary tract infections	β-Lactam inhibitor[f] plus aminoglycoside OR Imipenem plus aminoglycoside	Use against enteric gram-negative bacteria and anaerobes
Neutropenic patients	Antipseudomonal β-lactam[e] plus aminoglycoside[d]	Add vancomycin for *Staphylococcus* species if intravascular catheter is present
Unknown source	Imipenem or β-lactam inhibitor[f] plus aminoglycoside[d]	Add vancomycin if gram-positive infection is a consideration

Data from Stein JH, ed. Internal Medicine, 5th edition. St. Louis, Mosby-Year Book, 1998.

[a] Others: Ampicillin 1–2 g every 4–6 h; erythromycin 0.5–1 g every 6 h; ticarcillin clavulanate 3.1 g every 4–8 h; vancomycin 1 g every 12 h.
[b] Cefotaxime 1–2 g every 6–8 h; ceftriaxone 1–2 g every 24 h; ceftazidime 1–2 g every 8 h.
[c] Cefazolin 1 g every 8 h; cephalothin 1–2 g every 4–6 h; cefuroxime 1 g every 8 h.
[d] Gentamicin, tobramycin 3–5 mg/kg/d divided every 8 h; amikacin 15 mg/kg/d divided every 8 h. Must adjust for renal dysfunction.
[e] Piperacillin, mezlocillin, ticarcillin 3 g every 4 h; ceftazidime 1–2 g every 8 h; imipenem 500 mg every 6 h.
[f] Ticarcillin clavulanate 3.1 g every 4–6 h; piperacillin/tazobactam 3 g every 4–6 h.

biologic markers, plasma IL-6 levels and a high IL-10/TNF-α ratio may correlate best with risk of dying. None of these measurements warrants routine use.

The mortality rate in patients with staphylococcal TSS is 5%–15%, whereas that for streptococcal toxic shock syndrome may be 5 times higher.

REFERENCES

1. Bone RC, Balk RA, Cerra FB, et al. Definition for sepsis and organ failure and guidelines for the use of innovative therapies in sepsis. Chest. 1992; 101:1644–55.
2. Strusbaugh LJ, Joseph CL. Epidemiology and prevention of infections in residents of long term care facilities In: Mayhall CG 3rd, editor. Hospital epidemiology and infection control. Philadelphia: Lippincott Williams & Wilkins; 2004. p. 1869.
3. Brun-Buisson C, Doyon F, Carlet J. Bacteremia and severe sepsis in adults: a multicenter prospective survey in ICUs and wards of 24 hospitals. French Bacteremia-Sepsis Study Group. Am J Respir Crit Care Med. 1996; 154:617–24.
4. Girard TD, Ely EW. Bacteremia and sepsis in older adults. Clin Geriatr Med. 2007; 23:633–47.
5. Greenberg BM, Atmar AL, Stager CE, Greenberg SB. Bacteraemia in the elderly: predictors of outcome in an urban teaching hospital. J Infect. 2005; 50:288–95.
6. Lee CC, Chen SY, Chang IJ, et al. Comparison of clinical manifestations and outcome of community-acquired bloodstream infections among the oldest old, elderly, and adult patients. Medicine. 2007; 86:138–44.
7. National Center for Health Statistics. Leading causes of death. Center for Disease Control; 2008 [cited 2 May 2008]. Available at: http://www.cdc.gov/nchs/FASTATS/lcod.htm.
8. Angus DC, Linde-Zwirble WT, Lidicker J, et al. Epidemiology of severe sepsis in the United States: analysis of incidence, outcome, and associated costs of care. Crit Care Med. 2001; 29:1303–10.
9. Dellinger RP. Cardiovascular management of septic shock. Crit Care Med. 2003; 31:946–55.
10. Martin GS, Mannino DM, Eaton S, Moss M. The epidemiology of sepsis in the United States from 1979 through 2000. N Engl J Med. 2003; 348:1546–54.
11. Watson RS, Carcillo JA, Linde-Zwirble WT, et al. The epidemiology of severe sepsis in children in the United States. Am J Respir Crit Care Med. 2003; 167:695–701.
12. Alberti C, Brun-Buisson C, Goodman SV, et al. Influence of systemic inflammatory response syndrome and sepsis on outcome of critically ill infected patients. Am J Respir Crit Care Med. 2003; 168:77–84.
13. Sands KE, Bates DW, Lanken PN, et al. Epidemiology of sepsis syndrome in 8 academic medical centers. JAMA. 1997; 278;234–40.
14. Brun-Buisson C, Doyon F, Carlet J, et al. Incidence, risk factors, and outcome of severe sepsis and septic shock in adults: a multicenter prospective study in intensive care units. JAMA. 1995; 274:968–74.
15. Catenacci MH, King K. Severe sepsis and septic shock: improving outcomes in the emergency department. Emerg Med Clin N Am. 2008; 26:603–23.
16. Harris RL, Muscher DM, Bloom K, et al. Manifestations of sepsis. Arch Intern Med. 1987; 147:1895–906.
17. Talan DA, Moran GJ, Abrahamian FM. Severe sepsis and septic shock in the emergency department. Infect Dis Clin N Am. 2008; 22:1–31.
18. Cunha BA. Sepsis and septic shock: selection of empiric antimicrobial therapy. Crit Care Clin. 2008; 24:313–34.
19. Picard KM, O'Donoghue SC, Young-Kershaw DA, Russell KJ. Development and implementation of a multidisciplinary sepsis protocol. Crit Care Nurse. 2006; 26:43–54.
20. Todd J, Fishaut M, Kapral F, Welch T. Toxic-shock syndrome associated with phage-group 1 staphylococci. Lancet. 1978; ii:1116–18.
21. Reingold AL, Dan BB, Shands KN, Broome CV. Toxic shock syndrome not associated with menstruation. Lancet. 1982; i:1–4.
22. Hoge CW, Schwartz B, Talkington DF, et al. The changing epidemiology of invasive group A streptococcal infections and the emergence of streptococcal toxic shock-like syndrome: a retrospective population-based study. JAMA. 1993; 269:384–9.
23. The Working Group on Severe Streptococcal Infections. Defining the group A streptococcal toxic shock syndrome: rationale and consensus definition. JAMA. 1993; 269:390–1.
24. Davies JP, Chesney PJ, Wand PJ, LaVenture M. Toxic-shock syndrome: epidemiologic features, recurrence, risk factors and prevention. N Engl J Med. 1980; 303:1429–35.
25. Chesney JP, Davis JP. Toxic shock syndrome. In: Feigin RD, Cherry JD, editors. Textbook of pediatric infectious diseases. 4th ed. Philadelphia: WB Saunders; 1998. pp. 830–52.
26. Chuang Y, Huang Y, Lin T. Toxic shock syndrome in children: epidemiology, pathogenesis, and management. Pediatr Drugs. 2005; 7:11–25.
27. Lowy FD. Staphylococcus aureus infections. 1998; 339:520–32.
28. Stevens DL. Invasive group A streptococcus infections. Clin Infect Dis. 1992; 14:2–11.
29. Stevens DL, Tanner MH, Winship J, et al. Severe group A streptococcal infections associated with a toxic shock–like syndrome and scarlet fever toxin A. N Engl J Med. 1989;321:1–7.
30. Bradley JS, Schlievert PM, Sample TG Jr. Streptococcal toxic shock–like syndrome as a complication of varicella. Pediatr Infect Dis J. 1991; 10:77–8.
31. Hribalova V. Streptococcus pyogenes and the toxic shock syndrome. Ann Intern Med. 1988; 108:772.
32. Luce JM. Pathogenesis and management of septic shock. Chest. 1987; 91:883–8.
33. Hotchkiss RS, Karl IE. The pathophysiology and treatment of sepsis. N Engl J Med. 2003; 348:138–50.
34. Remick DG. Pathophysiology of sepsis. Am J Pathol. 2007; 170:1435–44.
35. Arbour NC, Lorenz E, Schutte BC, et al. TLR4 mutations are associated with endotoxin hyporesponsiveness in humans. Nat Genet. 2005; 25:187–91.
36. Underhill DM, Ozinsky A. Toll-like receptors: key mediators of microbe infection. Curr Opin Immunol. 2002; 14:103–10.
37. Opal SM, Gluck T. Endotoxin as a drug target. Crit Care Med. 2003; 31:S57–S64.
38. Beutler B, Rietschel ET. Innate immune sensing and its roots: the story of endotoxin. Nat Rev Immunol. 2003; 3:169–76.

39. Akira S, Uematsu S, Takeuchi O. Pathogen recognition and innate immunity. Cell. 2006; 124:783–801.

40. Beutler B, Jiang Z, Georgel P, et al. Genetic analysis of host resistance: Toll-like receptor signaling and immunity at large. Annu Rev Immunol. 2006; 24:353–89.

41. Munoz C, Carlett J, Ritting C. Dysregulation of in vitro cytokine production by monocytes during sepsis. J Clin Invest. 1991; 88:1747–54.

42. Bohach GA, Fast DJ, Nelson RD, Schlievert PM. Staphylococcal and streptococcal pyrogenic toxins involved in toxic shock syndrome and related illnesses. Crit Rev Microbiol. 1990; 17:251–72.

43. Schmitt CK, Meysick KC, O'Brien AD. Bacterial toxins: friends or foes? Emerg Infect Dis. 1999; 5:224–34.

44. Proft T, Sriskandan S, Yang L, Fraser JD. Superantigens and streptococcal toxic shock syndrome. Emerg Infect Dis. 2003; 9:1211–18.

45. Sriskandan S, Ferguson M, Elliot V, et al. Human intravenous immunoglobulin for experimental streptococcal toxic shock: bacterial clearance and modulation of inflammation. J Antimicrob Chemother. 2006; 58:117–24.

46. King C. Evaluation and management of febrile infants in the emergency department. Emerg Med Clin N Am. 2003; 21:89–99.

47. Martin GS, Mannino DM, Moss M. The effect of age on the development and outcome of adult sepsis. Crit Care Med. 2006; 34:15–21.

48. Sprung CL, Peduzzi PN, Shatney CH, et al. The impact of encephalopathy on mortality and physiologic derangements in the sepsis syndrome. Crit Care Med. 1988; 16:398–405.

49. Kreger BE, Craven DE, Carling PC, McCabe WR. Gram-negative bacteremia. III. Reassessment of etiology, epidemiology and ecology in 612 patients. Am J Med. 1980; 68:332–43.

50. Vincent JL. Clinical sepsis and septic shock - definition, diagnosis and management principles. Langenbecks Arch Surg. 2008; 393:817–24.

51. Iberti TJ, Bone RC, Balk R, et al. Are the criteria used to determine sepsis applicable for patients 75 years of age? Crit Care Med. 1993; 21:S130.

52. Musher D. Cutaneous and soft-tissue manifestations of sepsis due to gram-negative enteric bacilli. Rev Infect Dis. 1980; 2:854–66.

53. El Baze P, Ortonne JP. Ecthyma gangrenosum. J Am Acad Dermatol. 1985; 13:299–300.

54. Huminer D, Siegman-Igra Y, Morduchowicz G, Pitlik SD. Ecthyma gangrenosum without bacteremia. Report of six cases and review of the literature. Arch Intern Med. 1987; 147:299–310.

55. Gucluer H, Ergun T, Demircay Z. Ecthyma gangrenosum. Int J Dermatol. 1999; 38:298–305.

56. Brogan PA, Raffles A. The management of fever and petechiae: making sense of rash decisions. Arch Dis Child. 2000; 83:506–7.

57. Crowson AN, Mihm MC Jr, Magro CM. Cutaneous vasculitis: a review. J Cutan Pathol. 2003; 30:161–73.

58. Macke SE, Jordon RE. Leukocytoclastic vasculitis. A cutaneous expression of immune complex disease. Arch Dermatol. 1982; 118:296.

59. Dagan R, Powell KR, Hall CB, Menegus MA. Identification of infants unlikely to have serious bacterial infection although hospitalized for suspected sepsis. J Pediatr. 1985; 107:855–60.

60. van Nguyen Q, Nguyen EA, Weiner LB. Incidence of invasive disease in children with fever and petechiae. Pediatrics. 1984; 74:77–80.

61. Van Deuren M, van Dijke BJ, Koopman RJ, et al. Rapid diagnosis of acute meningococcal infections by needle aspiration or biopsy of skin lesions. BMJ. 1993; 306:1229–32.

62. Robboy SJ, Mihm MC, Colman RW, Minna JD. The skin in disseminated intravascular coagulation. Prospective analysis of thirty-six cases. Br J Dermatol. 1973; 88:221–9.

63. Jackson RT, Luplow RE. Adult purpura fulminans and digital necrosis associated with sepsis and the factor V mutation. JAMA. 1998; 280:1829–30.

64. Bisharat N, Agmon V, Fenkelstein R. Clinical, epidemiological and microbiological features of Vibrio vulnificus biogroup 3 causing outbreaks of wound infection and bacteraemia in Israel. Lancet. 1999; 354:1421–4.

65. Fujisawa N, Yamada H, Kohda H, et al. Necrotizing fasciitis caused by Vibrio vulnificus differs from that caused by streptococcal infection. J Infect. 1998; 36:3113–16.

66. Swartz MN. Cellulitis and subcutaneous tissue infections. In: Mandell GL, editor. Principles and practice of infectious diseases. 5th ed. New York: Churchill Livingstone; 2000. pp. 1042–5.

67. Bisno AL, Stevens DL. Streptococcal infections of skin and soft tissues. N Engl J Med. 1996; 334:240–5.

68. Bolton CF, Young GB, Zochodne DW. The neurological complications of sepsis. Ann Neurol. 1993; 33:94–100.

69. Sprung CL, Peduzzi PN, Shatney CH, et al. Impact of encephalopathy on mortality in the sepsis syndrome. Crit Care Med. 1990; 18:801–5.

70. Gao F, Melody T, Daniels DF, et al. The impact of compliance with 6-hour and 24-hour sepsis bundles on hospital mortality in patients with severe sepsis: a prospective observational study. Crit Care. 2005; 9:R764–70.

CHAPTER 11

Staphylococcal Scalded Skin Syndrome

Eleonora Ruocco

Adone Baroni

Sonia Sangiuliano

Giovanna Donnarumma

Vincenzo Ruocco

STAPHYLOCOCCAL scalded skin syndrome (SSSS) is the term used to define a potentially life-threatening, blistering skin disease caused by exfoliative toxins (ETs) of certain strains of *Staphylococcus aureus*. The syndrome belongs to a wide spectrum of staphylococcal infections that range in severity from localized bullous impetigo to a generalized cutaneous involvement characterized by extensive blistering with superficial denudation and subsequent desquamation of the skin. SSSS is so-named because of its staphylococcal etiology and its remarkable resemblance to the clinical picture of scalding.

HISTORY

The original description of the syndrome dates back to 1878, when Ritter von Rittershain, director of an orphanage in Prague, reported approximately 300 cases of *dermatitis exfoliativa neonatorum*. A relationship between the disease and staphylococci was perceived at the beginning of the 20th century, but only in the early 1950s did the link between bullous impetigo and phage group 2 staphylococci become evident. Lyell's report on toxic epidermal necrolysis (TEN) in 1956 drew attention to the similarities between this drug-induced condition and the appearance of extensive scalding, but also led to a period of confusion between nonbacterial (immune-mediated) TEN and bacterial (staphylococcal) toxin-mediated scalded skin syndrome.[1] In the early 1970s, the development of a murine model of the staphylococcal disease clarified the situation.[2]

Nowadays, SSSS is clearly distinguished from other diseases of generalized epidermal necrolysis and the term *Ritter's disease* is still used to describe generalized SSSS in newborns.

EPIDEMIOLOGY

SSSS, which may be present in epidemic form as well as sporadically, is primarily a disease of infancy and early childhood with most cases occurring in children younger than 6 years. The median age of onset is 1 year 10 months. There has been one case report of congenital SSSS in a neonate with sepsis, born to a mother with staphylococcal chorioamnionitis.[3] Occasionally, adults with chronic renal insufficiency or who are immunosuppressed can be affected. Because the toxins responsible for the lesions are excreted renally, infants, who have naturally immature kidneys, and adults with renal failure are obviously the most common candidates for this disease.

Besides decreased toxin clearance, lack of immunity to the toxins may also play a role. Outbreaks of SSSS have often occurred in neonatal nurseries as a consequence of asymptomatic carriage of a toxigenic strain of *S. aureus* by health care workers or parents. In fact, standard infection control measures, such as the use of chlorhexidine hand washing, may not be always sufficient for prevention, because the presence of potentially pathogenic staphylococci in the nasal cavities of a healthy adult carrier can be a point source for infection.

Interestingly, a male-to-female predominance of SSSS has been documented (2:1 in sporadic cases; 4:1 in epidemics).[4]

ETIOLOGY

The cause of SSSS is related to bacteria belonging to the genus *Staphylococcus*. This genus encompasses spherical gram-positive bacteria, irregularly grouped in cluster-like formations. They are immobile and asporogenic microorganisms, and, from a metabolic perspective, are facultative aerobes–anaerobes (Figure 11.1, A and B). This genus includes bacteria that are pathogens for both humans and other mammals. Traditionally, staphylococci are subdivided into two groups according to their ability to coagulate plasma (Figure 11.1, C and D). *S. aureus*, which is pathogenic for humans, belongs to the coagulase-positive

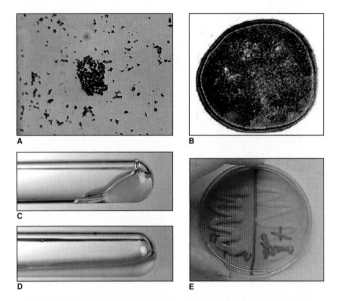

FIGURE 11.1: Etiology of staphylococcal scalded skin syndrome (SSSS). Panel A: Staphylococci grown in medium. Gram-positive cocci grouped in typical clusters. Panel B: Electron microscopy of a Staphylococcus species. Panels C and D: Coagulase test. A suspension of Staphylococcus aureus provokes coagulation of plasma contained in test tube (positive test, panel C). A suspension of Staphylococcus epidermidis does not provoke coagulation of plasma contained in test tube (negative test, panel D). Panel E: Isolation of S. aureus in Chapman's medium. The high NaCl content allows the growth of Staphylococcus species, but not other microorganisms. Only S. aureus causes the phenol red (indicator of pH) to change from red to yellow, through the fermenting of mannitol. (Photo courtesy of Maria Antonietta Tufano, Naples, Italy.)

group; the coagulase-negative group comprises 32 species that have been isolated in humans. The latter constitute the normal flora of the skin and mucosa, although some of them can cause infections in neonates, elderly persons, and immunodepressed subjects. *S. aureus* owes its name to the carotenoid pigment produced during multiplication that gives its colonies a yellow–orange color. To isolate *S. aureus* in samples contaminated by a mixed flora, a selective medium containing 7% NaCl is needed as this inhibits the multiplication of most microorganisms but not of *S. aureus*. If mannitol (Chapman's medium) is added to the NaCl medium, the sugar is fermented by *S. aureus* but not by the other staphylococci, thus allowing differentiation of the species (Figure 11.1E). *S. aureus* is a ubiquitous microorganism that permanently colonizes the epidermis around the nostrils in 20% of the population, is usually associated with transient flora, and can occasionally cause infections. *S. aureus* infections underlie several clinical patterns that differ considerably according to the site of infection and the means of transmission (direct extension or metastatic or hematogenous diffusion). *S. aureus*, in particular, is the most frequent etiological agent in common skin infections, such as folliculitis, furuncle, and carbuncle that arise in the sebaceous glands and hair follicles where

the microorganism produces lipolytic enzymes that allow both the degradation of the sebum (and as a result of the lipid components with antibacterial activity) and the use of the lipids themselves as a source of metabolic energy. The pathogenic action of *S. aureus* depends both on a series of factors that favor multiplication in vivo and on the production of numerous toxins and isoenzymes.

The strains of *S. aureus* responsible for the onset of SSSS are producers of epidermolytic or exfoliative toxin (ET) and are often penicillin resistant.[5] Although most toxigenic strains of *S. aureus* are identified by group 2 phage (types 71 and 55), toxin producers have also been identified among phage groups 1 and 3.[2] The frequency of isolation of strains of toxin-producing *S. aureus* varies from place to place, but is generally less than 10%. ET is produced by the microorganism in two antigenically distinct forms, both capable of causing the disease (ET-A and ET-B). ET-A, a thermostable protein, is encoded by a chromosomally located gene; ET-B, which is encoded by a gene located in the plasmids, is a thermolabile protein.[6,7]

PATHOGENESIS

More than 30 years ago it was shown that the blisters in SSSS are caused by an ET released by virulent strains of *S. aureus* dwelling in distant foci of infection, such as the pharynx, nose, ear, or conjunctiva. It was surmised that ET, produced by staphylococci, and released into circulation, reached the skin and caused blistering and shedding of the epidermis at sites that were distant from the infection. In fact, the formation of superficial epidermal blisters and extensive skin exfoliation, similar to those observed in patients with SSSS, were experimentally obtained in neonatal mice into which purified staphylococcal ET was injected. It was also noted that the presence of ET in the blood induced the production of protective neutralizing antibodies and, as a consequence, lasting immunity, which could account for the fact that adolescents and adults are rarely affected by SSSS. Subsequently, it was discovered that two major serotypes of this toxin, ET-A and ET-B, are responsible for the pathogenic changes of the syndrome.[8] ET-A is the predominant ET isoform in Europe and the United States, whereas ET-B is the most frequent isoform in Japan. ET-B–producing *S. aureus* is, however, the predominant strain isolated in generalized SSSS.

After the initial identification of the toxins, the mechanism by which ETs cause intraepidermal separation remained unknown for more than 3 decades. Early studies reported that ETs were mitogenic in human and murine lymphocytes, suggesting that the toxins act as superantigens and stimulate certain Vβ T lymphocyte clones nonspecifically via major histocompatibility complex class II molecules. Histopathological observations of the cutaneous lesions in SSSS patients, however, have generated controversy regarding the superantigen theory of ETs because the

SSSS skin lesions fail to show evidence of intense T-cell recruitment into the epidermis, where the blisters occur. In addition, patients exhibit only a loss of cell–cell adhesion, but no induced keratinocyte necrosis as would be expected with superantigen-stimulated T cells. Furthermore, because purified recombinant ET-A produced in a non–toxin-producing strain of *S. aureus* was unable to stimulate human and murine T cells, it was suggested that the superantigen activity of ETs was probably due to contamination by other mitogenic exotoxins.[7]

The potency of ETs as serine proteases also has been examined. Comparison of the deduced amino acid sequences of ET-A and ET-B (they comprise 242 and 246 amino acids, respectively, and share approximately 40% amino acid homology) showed that they share primary amino acid homology with staphylococcal V8 protease, which belongs to a family of trypsin-like serine proteases.

The crystal structure analyses of ET-A and ET-B revealed that their three-dimensional structures resemble those of known glutamate-specific serine proteases, including the presence of the catalytic triad, a putative active site comprising histidine, aspartic acid, and serine.[7]

Both ET isoforms cleave human and mouse desmoglein 1 (dsg 1), a desmosomal intercellular adhesion molecule, at one position after glutamic acid residue 381, between extracellular domain (EC) 3 and EC 4 This cleavage site is located in the putative calcium-binding site of dsg 1, and the removal of the calcium ions blocks the cleavage of dsg 1 by both ET-A and ET-B. The importance of this site was demonstrated by the replacement of the catalytic serine-195 of ET-A with a cysteine or glycine residue, which resulted in a loss of exfoliating activity after injection into neonatal mice.[6]

These findings suggest that the serine protease activities of ET-A and ET-B are involved in intraepidermal blister formation in patients with SSSS.[7] ET cleaves dsg 1 by the key-in-lock mechanism that is common to many proteolytic enzymes with limited substrate specificities. This remarkable mechanism efficiently targets one molecule, dsg 1, which allows *Staphylococcus* to grow below the epidermal barrier but superficially enough to be contagious through skin contact;[8] however, neither the enzymatic activities of ETs nor their specific substrates were recognized at the time. To determine whether ET-A cleaves dsg 1 directly, the toxin was incubated in vitro with baculovirus recombinant ECs of human dsg 1, human dsg 3, mouse dsg 1-α (one of three mouse dsg 1 isoforms), and mouse dsg 3. ET-A was shown to cleave human and mouse dsg 1-α in a dose-dependent fashion, but not dsg 3. ET-B also was found to cleave the ECs of human and mouse dsg 1-α specifically and directly.[9] A major breakthrough in understanding the mechanism of ET-mediated blistering came in 2000, when similarities were noted between SSSS and an autoimmune blistering skin disease, pemphigus foliaceus (PF).[10] In PF patients, immunoglobulin G (IgG) autoantibodies disrupt

TABLE 11.1: Similarities between Pemphigus Foliaceus (PF) and Staphylococcal Scalded Skin Syndrome

Clinical features: scaly and crusted superficial erosions

Skin (not mucous membranes) are involved

Site of cleavage: just below the stratum corneum

The crucial point where cleavage occurs is a Ca^{2+} binding domain in the extracellular region of desmoglein 1

Identical appearance of experimentally induced lesions in neonatal mice injected with either PF immunoglobulin G antibodies or staphylococcal exfoliative toxins

the intercellular adhesion of keratinocytes and cause epidermal blistering. The target molecule for IgG autoantibodies in PF is dsg 1. The extracellular region of dsg contains five cadherin repeats separated by putative calcium-binding domains. In humans, four dsg isoforms (dsg 1, 2, 3, 4) with tissue- and differentiation-specific distribution patterns have been identified. In all desmosome-bearing tissues dsg 2 is present, whereas dsg 1 and dsg 3 are found predominantly in stratified squamous epithelia. In humans, dsg 1 is expressed throughout the epidermis, but most intensely in superficial layers. The expression of dsg 3 is restricted to the basal and immediate suprabasal layers, although in human oral mucous membranes, dsg 1 and dsg 3 are expressed throughout the epithelia, with dsg 1 expression being much lower than that of dsg 3. The expression of dsg 2 and dsg 4 in the human epidermis is restricted to the basal layer and just below the cornified layer, respectively. In PF, blisters are observed exclusively in the superficial epidermis, where dsg 1 is predominantly expressed with no coexpression of other dsg isoforms.[7]

Five important clues from PF studies indicated that the substrate of the ETs might be dsg 1 (Table 11.1). These clues suggested that the ETs, such as PF IgG, might target dsg 1. If dsg 1 were cleaved specifically by the ETs, then, just as in PF, "desmoglein compensation" would account for the localization of the blisters in SSSS in the superficial epidermis and for the absence of the blisters in the mucous membrane. The dsg compensation theory rests on the following two observations: anti–dsg 1 or anti–dsg 3 autoantibodies inactivate only the corresponding dsg, and functional dsg 1 or dsg 3 alone is usually sufficient for cell–cell adhesion. Anti-dsg 1 IgG autoantibodies in serum from patients with PF cause superficial blisters in the skin; no blisters form in the lower epidermis or mucous membranes because dsg 3 maintains cell–cell adhesion in those areas. In SSSS, the ETs produced by *S. aureus* act as dsg 1–specific molecular scissors and cleave dsg 1 but not dsg 3, resulting in superficial epidermal blisters only, because, in the upper epidermal layers, the cohesive function of the impaired dsg 1 cannot be compensated by other dsgs isoforms, as occurs elsewhere. Therefore, although pemphigus and SSSS are unrelated diseases, the identical

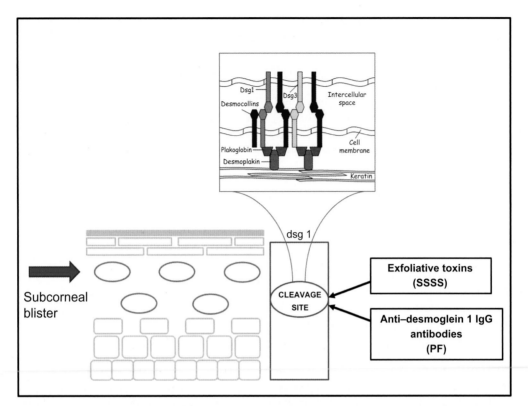

FIGURE 11.2: *Identical cleavage site in staphylococcal scalded skin syndrome (SSSS) and pemphigus foliaceus (PF). IgG, immunoglobulin G; dsg 1, desmoglein 1.*

histopathology of the superficial type of the IgG-mediated disorder (PF) and lesions in neonatal mice treated with staphylococcal ETs clearly indicates that staphylococcal ETs act on the same autoimmune target of PF (i.e., dsg 1), thus provoking identical specific cleavage within the superficial layer of the epidermis (Figure 11.2). Interestingly enough, about 2 centuries ago, astute clinicians realized that staphylococcal bullous diseases were clinically similar enough to pemphigus to name SSSS (along with its localized form, bullous impetigo) in infants "pemphigus neonatorum."[8]

CLINICAL FEATURES

The onset of SSSS may either be acute with fever and rash or be preceded by a prodrome of malaise, irritability, and cutaneous tenderness, often accompanied by purulent rhinorrhea, conjunctivitis, or otitis media. The typical rash presents as a faint, orange–red, macular exanthem, localized initially on the head (Figure 11.3A) and spreading within a few hours to the remainder of the body, with peculiar periorificial and flexural accentuation. Edema of the hands and feet may be observed. At this stage, cutaneous tenderness is a distinctive feature as proven by the easy disruption of skin after firm rubbing or pressure (Nikolsky sign) (Figure 11.3B). Within 24–48 hours, the macular exanthem gradually turns into a blistering eruption; in particular, a characteristic tissue-paper-like

wrinkling of the epidermis heralds the appearance of large, flaccid bullae. Blistering usually starts in the axillae and groins and on periorificial areas. Subsequently, the entire body is affected. One or two days later, the bullae rupture and their roofs are sloughed, leaving behind a moist, glistening, red surface along with varnish-like crusts. At this stage, the clinical appearance closely resembles that of extensive scalding (Figure 11.3C). The patient becomes irritable, sick, and feverish, with "sad man" facies, perioral crusting, lip fissuring, and mild facial edema. Mucous membranes are usually spared by bullae and erosions, but generalized mucous membrane erythema, especially intense in the conjunctiva (under which there may be hemorrhage), is often observed. Days later, due to generalized shedding of the epidermis, scaling and desquamation progressively occur. The skin returns to normal in 2–3 weeks. Scarring is not usually a feature.

An abortive form of SSSS, known as scarlatiniform variant (staphylococcal scarlet fever), also may be seen. The early erythrodermic picture evolves into a desquamative condition with the absence of a blistering stage. This clinical form is often associated with occult bone and joint infections or contaminated wounds.

PATHOLOGY

Under light microscopy SSSS is characterized by intraepidermal cleavage with clefts appearing in the granular layer

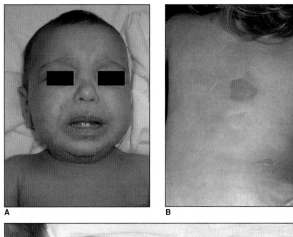

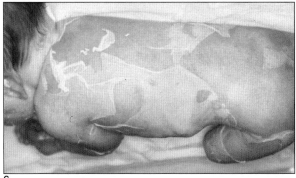

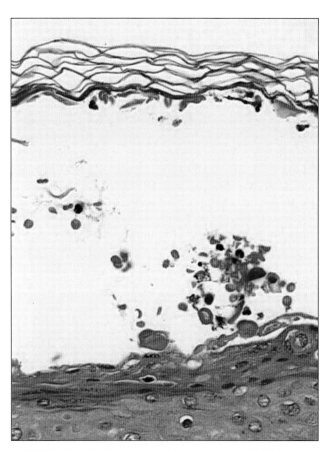

FIGURE 11.3: Clinical features of staphylococcal scalded skin syndrome. Panel A: Orange–red exanthema initially localized on the head. Panel B: Nikolsky sign: erosion following firm rubbing of the skin. (Photo courtesy of Carlo Gelmetti, Milan, Italy.) Panel C: Extensive sloughing of the skin closely resembling that of vast scalding. (Photo courtesy of Giovanni Angelini, Bari, Italy.)

FIGURE 11.4: Histology of staphylococcal scalded skin syndrome: subcorneal bullous cavity (hematoxylin and eosin, ×200). (Photo courtesy of Carlo Gelmetti, Milan, Italy.)

or just beneath the stratum corneum and leading to the formation of bullous cavities (Figure 11.4). Few or no inflammatory cells are present within the blister. A few acantholytic cells are often seen either adjoining the cleavage plane or free-floating in the bulla. A scanty lymphocytic infiltrate may surround superficial blood vessels in the dermis. In fresh lesions, no bacterial organisms can be seen on Gram stain of the biopsy specimens, whereas older lesions can become superinfected thus obscuring an SSSS diagnosis.

DIAGNOSIS

The diagnosis of SSSS is mainly clinical and should be taken into consideration in any child who develops a generalized, tender erythema, most prominent on periorificial (in particular perinostril and periocular) areas, associated with Nikolsky sign. Suspected SSSS is supported by the confirmation of staphylococcal infection in different sites (conjunctiva, nasopharynx, ear). Cultures taken from intact bullae are negative because fresh lesions do not harbor staphylococci. In the full-blown disease, shock is a typical feature, whereas postural dizziness may be an important diagnostic clue in the early stages or mild cases.

The main differential diagnosis is that of TEN, which usually affects adults and is uncommon in children. In this severe drug-induced reaction, the skin changes are widespread and severe mucosal involvement is common (erosive mucositis is part of the clinical presentation in TEN), whereas SSSS extends from the face and flexures and does not affect mucosae with erosions. Histologically, TEN shows subepidermal splitting, also in frozen sections, with full-thickness necrosis of the epidermis, whereas SSSS is characterized by subcorneal cleavage with a viable appearance of the epidermis. The two conditions can be rapidly differentiated by means of exfoliative cytology. A Tzanck smear taken from a fresh bulla shows necrotic keratinocytes with inflammatory cells in TEN and viable acantholytic or normal keratinocytes without inflammatory cells in SSSS, but accurate interpretation requires an experienced observer. Other differential diagnoses comprise Leiner and Kawasaki diseases. Leiner disease, the erythrodermic form of seborrhoeic dermatitis in newborns, lacks blisters or erosion, but yellowish scales are present all over the body. Prolonged fever, heart involvement, and generalized lymphadenopathy characterize Kawasaki disease. Slide latex agglutination, double immunodiffusion, and enzyme-linked immunosorbent assay tests – which can identify the staphylococcal toxins responsible for the intraepidermal splitting – are all useful in confirming a SSSS clinical diagnosis.

COURSE AND PROGNOSIS

The disease in newborns (Ritter's disease) is usually self-limiting, with rapid resolution of the skin blisters and complete recovery in a couple of weeks, but there is a mortality of 2%–3% due to progression of the staphylococcal infection (sepsis) or exfoliation complications (serious fluid and electrolyte disturbances). In children, with appropriate treatment, complications (cellulitis, pneumonia) are uncommon and the prognosis is usually good, with a low mortality risk (about 5%). In adults, SSSS carries a less favorable prognosis because of basic medical problems such as immunosuppression or kidney failure. Adults are much more likely than children to develop staphylococcal sepsis, which brings the mortality rate to more than 50%, despite appropriate antibiotic therapy.

MANAGEMENT

Patients with SSSS require hospitalization because, besides the appropriate systemic antibiotic therapy, intensive general supportive measures are needed. The mainstay of treatment is to eradicate staphylococci from the focus of infection, which in most cases requires intravenous (IV) antistaphylococcal antibiotics (e.g., methicillin, flucloxacillin). Subsequently, parenteral therapy may be replaced with 1-week oral treatment with a β-lactamase–resistant antibiotic (e.g., dicloxacillin, cloxacillin, cephalexin). Second-line therapies include IV macrolide (erythromycin or clarithromycin)[11] or vancomycin.[12] Due to the disrupted cutaneous barrier function, which may lead to dehydration and electrolyte imbalance, IV replacement of fluids and lacking electrolytes is recommended for prompt recovery. In each case, oral fluid intake and careful monitoring of urinary output should be encouraged. If required, analgesics should be used. The superficial nature of the erosions in SSSS paves the way to rapid reepithelialization following appropriate topical therapy. The therapy consists of nonirritant, nonsensitizing antiseptics (e.g., 1:1000 diluted aqueous potassium permanganate solution) on denuded, moist areas and bland, lubricating emollients on itching, tender, scaling areas. Newborns with SSSS should be kept in incubators to maintain body temperature. In neonatal care units, as well as in hospital-acquired cases of SSSS, it is of the utmost importance to identify health care workers who are possible carriers of toxigenic staphylococci. Useful prevention measures encompass strict enforcement of chlorhexidine hand washing, oral antibiotic treatment for infected workers, and the use of intranasal mupirocin ointment to eradicate persistent nasal carriage of toxigenic strains of *S. aureus*.[2]

FUTURE PERSPECTIVES

The increasing frequency of methicillin-resistant *S. aureus* (MRSA) strains raises the possibility that antibiotic-resistant, ET–producing staphylococci can become pathogens in future cases of SSSS. The development of innovative, alternative therapies may rapidly become an urgent necessity. Structural identification of the dsg 1 binding site of staphylococcal ETs and the generation of neutralizing antibodies that efficiently inhibit the reaction between enzyme and substrate will provide a novel therapeutic option for SSSS caused by MRSA.[7]

ACKNOWLEDGMENTS

We are greatly indebted to Prof. Maria Antonietta Tufano (Naples), Prof. Carlo Gelmetti (Milan), and Prof. Giovanni Angelini (Bari) for their courtesy in providing us with Figures 11.1 (MAT); 11.3A, 11.3B, and 11.4 (CG); and 11.3C (GA).

REFERENCES

1. Lyell A. Toxic epidermal necrolysis: an eruption resembling scalding of the skin. Br J Dermatol, 1956; 68:355–61.
2. Resnick SD, Elias PM. Staphylococcal scalded-skin syndrome. In: Freedberg IM, Eisen AZ, Wolff K, et al., editors. Fitzpatrick's dermatology in general medicine. 5th ed. Vol. 2. New York: McGraw-Hill: 1999. pp. 2207–13.
3. Loughead JL. Congenital staphylococcal scalded skin syndrome: report of a case. Pediatr Infect Dis J. 1992; 11:413–14.
4. Cribier B, Piemont Y, Grosshans E. Staphylococcal scalded skin syndrome in adults: a clinical review illustrated with a new case. J Am Acad Dermatol. 1994; 30:319–24.
5. Lowy FD. Staphylococcus aureus infections. N Engl J Med. 1998; 339:520–32.
6. Hanakawa Y, Schechter NM, Lin C, et al. Molecular mechanisms of blister formation in bullous impetigo and staphylococcal scalded skin syndrome. J Clin Invest. 2002; 110:53–60.
7. Nishifuji K, Sugai M, Amagai M. Staphylococcal exfoliative toxins: "Molecular scissors" of bacteria that attack the cutaneous defense barrier in mammals. J Dermatol Sci. 2008; 49:21–31.
8. Stanley JR, Amagai M. Pemphigus, bullous impetigo, and the staphylococcal scalded-skin syndrome. N Engl J Med. 2006; 355:1800–10.
9. Amagai M, Yamaguchi T, Hanakawa Y, et al. Staphylococcal exfoliative toxin B specifically cleaves desmoglein 1. J Invest Dermatol. 2002; 118:845–50.
10. Amagai M, Matsuyoshi N, Wang ZH, et al. Toxin in bullous impetigo and staphylococcal scalded-skin syndrome targets desmoglein 1. Nat Med. 2000; 6:1275–7.
11. Sturman SW, Malkinson FD. Staphylococcal scalded skin syndrome in an adult and a child. Arch Dermatol. 1976; 112:1275–9.
12. Strauss G, Mogensen AM, Rasmussen A, Kirkegaard P. Staphylococcal scalded skin syndrome in a liver transplant patient. Liver Transpl Surg. 1997; 3:435–6.

CHAPTER 12

Life-Threatening Cutaneous Viral Diseases

Aron J. Gewirtzman

Brandon Christianson

Anne Marie Tremaine

Brenda L. Pellicane

Stephen Tyring

VIRAL DISEASES frequently have cutaneous manifestations, most of which are self-limited and of little consequence; however, there are occasions when a viral cutaneous disease may be accompanied by systemic manifesttions that can be life threatening. In general, healthy children and adults are at little risk for these severe complications. Persons at highest risk for systemic involvement include patients who are immunosuppressed, as well as neonates, extremely elderly persons, and the undernourished population. Because many viruses have some form of cutaneous exanthem, almost any virus known to have systemic involvement can be considered a dermatological emergency. This chapter focuses mainly on those viruses in which the cutaneous findings would be likely to prompt dermatological investigation in an emergency situation.

HERPES SIMPLEX VIRUS

Presentation and Clinical Features

Herpes simplex virus (HSV) is not typically associated with life-threatening or emergency situations; rather, HSV is better known as an acute, self-limited infection that may recur in certain individuals. In rare instances, fatal and highly morbid complications can arise. Neonates and immunocompromised persons generally make up the vast majority of patients with these poor outcomes, but in extremely rare cases some immunocompetent patients suffer severe complications.

HSV can be divided into two subgroups (HSV-1 and HSV-2) based on molecular and immunologic characteristics. HSV-1 typically causes lesions in the oral mucosa and produces gingivostomatitis and pharyngitis in primary infections. Primary infections of HSV-2 most commonly cause genital lesions and produce acute vulvovaginitis and progenitalis. Infection with HSV-1 is generally acquired during childhood and is commonly asymptomatic, whereas HSV-2 infections are routinely found in postpubertal individuals who engage in sexual contact. Both HSV-1 and HSV-2 are associated with recurrent infections in patients with low immunologic status.

The classic HSV presentation is indurated erythema followed by grouped vesicles on an erythematous base. These vesicles eventually become pustules, which rupture and eventually crust. Sometimes the affected skin may become necrotic and result in a punched-out ulcerative appearance. Clinical manifestations, however, can vary and include acute gingivostomatitis, herpes labialis, ocular herpes, herpes genitalis, zosteriform herpes simplex, herpetic whitlow, eczema herpeticum, meningitis, encephalitis, visceral infections, and neonatal herpes. For mucocutaneous infections, the mainstay of therapy has been the synthetic purine nucleoside analogues acyclovir, valacyclovir, famciclovir, and penciclovir. In emergency situations intravenous (IV) acyclovir should be used.

Neonatal HSV. HSV in a neonate is considered a pediatric emergency, and antiviral therapy should be initiated as soon as there is clinical suspicion.[1] HSV is known to infect approximately 1 in 3200 deliveries.[2] Transmission to the neonate can occur by intrauterine (5%), intrapartum (85%), or postpartum (10%) infection.[3–7] The risk of neonatal herpes is greatest if a woman has a primary occurrence at delivery, lower if she has a recurrent episode, and lowest if there is a history of HSV but no lesions at delivery.[2] Although cesarean section has proven to be effective in decreasing the chances of HSV transmission to the neonate from a mother actively shedding virus from the genital tract, the majority of transmitted infections arise from mothers who do not have lesions at the time of delivery. Approximately 60%–80% of women who deliver

TABLE 12.1: Herpes Simplex Virus in Neonates

Type of neonatal HSV infection	Incidence[8]	Mortality without treatment[8,11]	Presentation[12]	Therapy[1]	Onset[1,13]
Skin, eye, and mouth infections	45%	0%	Discrete vesicles and keratoconjunctivitis to spastic quadriplegia, microcephaly, and blindness	IV acyclovir 20 mg/kg every 8 h for 14–21 days	10–11 days
Central nervous system	35%	50%	Seizures, lethargy, irritability, tremors, poor feeding, temperature instability, bulging fontanelle, or pyramidal tract signs	60 mg/kg/d in three divided doses for 21 days is advised	16–19 days
Disseminated multiorgan infection	20%	80%	Irritability, seizures, respiratory distress, jaundice, bleeding diatheses, shock, and vesicular exanthema	60 mg/kg/d in three divided doses for 21 days is advised	9–11 days

HSV, herpes simplex virus; IV, intravenous.

an HSV-infected infant have no evidence of genital HSV infection at the time of delivery, no past history of genital herpes, nor a sexual partner reporting a history of genital HSV.[2,8–10]

In neonates, HSV can manifest in three different types of infections (Table 12.1).

Neonatally disseminated HSV infection and central nervous system (CNS) HSV disease both have high mortality rates without treatment. In those individuals who do survive without treatment, significant neurologic impairment is common.[8,11] Although skin, eye, and mouth HSV neonatal infections typically do not cause mortality, without antiviral therapy, approximately 75% of infections will eventually develop into CNS or disseminated disease.[8]

HSV in Immunocompromised Patients. Immunocompromised individuals such as those with human immunodeficiency virus (HIV), recipients of organ transplantations, pregnant women, or patients with any other disease/state that affects T-cell function should also be monitored for dissemination and/or CNS involvement in HSV infections. These patients have been associated with higher mortality rates and worse recurrent episodes of HSV.

Herpes Simplex Encephalitis. Herpes simplex encephalitis (HSE) is the most commonly identified cause of acute, sporadic viral encephalitis in the United States, comprising 10%–20% of all cases.[14] It is estimated to have an incidence of approximately 1 case per 250,000 population per year.[15] Mortality in untreated patients is in excess of 70%, and only 2.5% of all patients recover full neurological function. The pathology of HSE varies and may occur in a primary or recurrent infection. Not all cases have skin lesions, and differentiation from other encephalitides can be very difficult. HSV DNA in the cerebrospinal fluid confirmed by

polymerase chain reaction is the most sensitive noninvasive test for early diagnosis.[16] HSE manifests as an acute onset of fever and focal (temporal) neurologic symptoms.[17] Patients typically complain of headache, nuchal rigidity, weakness, sensory abnormalities, aphasia, visual field defects, or cranial nerve palsies.[18]

Eczema Herpeticum. Eczema herpeticum is a potentially life-threatening dermatologic emergency that involves a herpetic superinfection of a preexisting skin disease. It is most commonly seen in individuals who have disruptive skin diseases (typically atopic dermatitis) or are immunocompromised (secondary to medication for the skin disease). It is commonly seen in children of all ages and all ethnic groups, with those in the first 2–3 years of life having the highest incidence.[19] Without rapid antiviral therapy, complete dissemination can occur, leading to fulminant hepatitis and possible death.[20,21]

Eczema herpeticum is similar to the classic skin lesions of HSV except that there are multiple clusters of vesicles in areas of previous skin disease involvement along with systemic symptoms (fever and malaise). Vesicles spread and result in punched-out erosions causing significant pain. Lesions may be discrete or confluent, and tend to occur in crops, resulting in many lesions at different stages.[22] Other signs and symptoms may include pruritus, vomiting, anorexia, diarrhea, lymphadenopathy, and/or secondary bacterial infection.[23,24]

Visceral Infections. The most common sites of visceral infections are the esophagus, lung, and liver; the infections usually result from viremia. Of these, lung and liver infections have the worse prognoses. Lung HSV infections frequently present as a focal necrotizing pneumonitis and are more common in severely immunocompromised patients. Mortality is considered to be greater than 80%.

HSV hepatitis also has a high association with mortality (near 80%) and can present with fever, abdominal or right upper quadrant pain, nausea and vomiting, abrupt elevations of bilirubin and serum aminotransferase levels, and leukopenia.[25] HSV hepatitis has been seen in immunocompetent and immunosuppressed persons.

Prevention and Treatment

IV acyclovir is highly recommended for all cases of neonatal HSV. Treatment of neonatal HSV with IV acyclovir is described in Table 12.1. For maximum benefit, antiviral therapy must be administered before widespread dissemination or significant replication of the virus in the CNS has occurred.[13] It is also recommended that dosing intervals for IV acyclovir be increased in premature infants due to their high creatinine clearance.[26] In rare cases, IV acyclovir has been associated with neutropenia and nephrotoxicity. Therefore, neutrophil counts and kidney function should be monitored in neonates when receiving IV acyclovir.[1] With acyclovir therapy the mortality of disseminated HSV and CNS HSV is reduced to 29% and 4%, respectively.[1] Preventing maternal primary infection is of the utmost importance because primary infection has the highest rate of transmission to the infant. To prevent maternal infection, condoms or suppressive oral acyclovir in late pregnancy has been beneficial for persons who are in sexual contact with partners who have genital herpes.

Immunocompromised patients should be treated with systemic antiviral therapy such as acyclovir. For patients who may have acyclovir-resistant HSV, foscarnet can be used, but it is generally reserved for patients with extensive mucocutaneous infections because of its high cost and toxicity.[27] Cidofovir has also been proven to work as a topical medication for HSV lesions and may also be used in acyclovir-resistant patients.

Prompt treatment is of the utmost importance to prevent the high mortality associated with HSE. It is recommended that HSE patients be treated with IV acyclovir at 30 mg/kg/d divided into 3 doses for 14–21 days.[28] Even in presumed HSE, IV acyclovir is recommended until an alternative diagnosis is made, and continued when the diagnosis of HSE is confirmed.[29]

For all visceral HSV infections, IV acyclovir is recommended. In some cases liver transplant plus high-dose acyclovir therapy has been used to treat fulminant HSV hepatic failure.[30,31]

VARICELLA ZOSTER VIRUS

Presentation and Clinical Features

Primary Varicella. Varicella zoster virus (VZV) presents as chickenpox (varicella) as a primary infection and shingles (herpes zoster) when the virus is reactivated. Varicella is generally a self-limited disease, usually of childhood, that causes outbreaks of vesicles and pustules classically described as "dewdrops on a rose petal." Lesions progress from a vesicle into a pustule that then produces an itchy scab. Classically, all of these stages are present simultaneously, as the lesions develop in successive crops. Varicella is common, as greater than 95% of adults in the United States have antibodies to the virus. In healthy children, the mortality rate is quite low, estimated at two deaths per 100,000 cases.[32] In immunocompromised patients and neonates, however, complications such as pneumonitis, thrombocytopenia, liver function impairment, and CNS involvement are more common and must be recognized and treated promptly.

Neonatal varicella is mostly caused by maternal chickenpox acquired during the last 3 weeks of pregnancy. Death may occur due to complications of generalized neonatal varicella in up to 20% of neonates if the mother develops a rash between days 4 and 5 antepartum to day 2 postpartum.[33] Whereas neonatal chickenpox occurring within the first 4 days after birth tends to be mild, a fatal outcome has been reported in 23% of cases occurring between 5 and 12 days of age.[33]

Primary varicella in adults is frequently more severe than in children. Fewer than 5% of cases of varicella occur in adults, yet 55% of varicella-related deaths occur in this age group, usually due to pneumonia and consequent respiratory failure.[32,34]

Herpes Zoster. Herpes zoster has a lifetime incidence between 10% and 25%, with the elderly population being at greater risk than the general population. Like varicella, herpes zoster is rarely life threatening in immunocompetent people. The disease is recognized by dermatomal pain and vesicular rash. Pain may be intense and can last for months after the rash heals (postherpetic neuralgia). Herpes zoster is generally limited to a single dermatome or a few adjacent dermatomes, but may disseminate, particularly in patients with immunosuppression due to HIV, hematological malignancy, organ transplantation, or chemotherapy. Disseminated zoster results from hematogenous spread of the virus resulting in involvement of multiple dermatomes, as well as potentially systemic involvement. Dissemination is life-threatening due to the potential to cause encephalitis, hepatitis, or pneumonitis.

Disseminated herpes zoster may present with visceral symptoms including hepatitis, pancreatitis, gastritis, or abdominal pain. Occasionally, these complaints are seen even without skin involvement at all, or can be the presenting feature before a rash develops.[35,36] CNS involvement may be seen in the form of cranial nerve palsies or encephalitis in up to one third of patients with disseminated zoster.[37]

Although the incidence of shingles among recipients of solid organ transplants is approximately 9%,[32] the complications of dissemination in these patients are particularly grave. A review of the literature of disseminated varicella infection in adult renal allograft recipients found a mortality rate of 34%.[38] Use of mycophenolate mofetil (a drug commonly used to prevent organ transplant rejection) has been associated with increased susceptibility to VZV infection.[39]

Of note, disseminated herpes zoster is not limited to immunocompromised persons. Although rare, there have been reported cases of disseminated cutaneous herpes zoster without any apparent immunosuppression. It has been proposed that significant age-related depression in cellular immunity can contribute to dissemination of herpes zoster; therefore, elderly patients should be recognized as a group in which dissemination risk is higher than the average immunocompetent host.[40]

Prevention and Treatment

A live, attenuated varicella zoster vaccination has been approved by the U.S. Food and Drug Administration (FDA) for prevention of varicella in children since 1995, and a similar vaccine to prevent herpes zoster outbreaks in adults received approval in 2006. Curtis and colleagues[41] reported a case of disseminated zoster in an elderly woman with a history of recurrent breast cancer undergoing chemotherapy that occurred 8 days following vaccination. This was the first known report of dissemination attributed to zoster vaccination with the Oka strain in a chemotherapy patient. Dissemination of varicella zoster following vaccination has been reported as the defining illness in a 16-month-old patient who was later diagnosed with acquired immune deficiency syndrome (AIDS).[42] Similarly, a novel deficiency in natural killer T cells was discovered following VZV dissemination after vaccination of an 11-year-old girl.[43] These multiple reports of disseminated infection resulting from the vaccine strain in immunocompromised patients point to the need for careful medical history-taking prior to vaccination to avoid vaccinating patients who are immunosuppressed. Disseminated zoster following vaccination in a patient with no known history of immunodeficiency should prompt a thorough workup. The most effective method to protect immunocompromised persons is to ensure that their potential susceptible contacts have been vaccinated.[34]

Treatment for classic herpes zoster may be given orally, either with acyclovir (800 mg 5 times a day for 7 days), valacyclovir (1 g 3 times a day for 7 days), or famciclovir (500 mg 3 times a day for 7 days). The treatment of choice for disseminated zoster is IV acyclovir 10 mg/kg every 8 hours for 7 days.[40] Likewise, IV acyclovir should be given for primary varicella in immunocompromised populations. To prevent severe neonatal chickenpox, passive immunization (i.e., with varicella immune globulin) is indicated.[33]

SMALLPOX (VARIOLA MAJOR) AND VACCINIA

Presentation and Clinical Features

Smallpox was, historically, one of the most lethal viruses known to man until it was eradicated in 1980 by a worldwide vaccination effort.[44] The last reported case of smallpox was in 1977; therefore, a significant percentage of the world's population is susceptible to smallpox infection.[32] Unfortunately, in the modern era, the potential use of smallpox as a weapon of bioterrorism makes this virus of continued interest to dermatologists.

Smallpox is spread by the respiratory route and has a prodromal phase of high fever, headache, and backache. Skin lesions are classically distributed in a centrifugal pattern with greater involvement of the face and extremities than of the trunk. Lesions begin as erythematous macules, which then evolve in synchrony (as opposed to chickenpox) into papules, pustules, and then crusts with the entirety of the rash lasting approximately 2 weeks. The mortality rate caused by smallpox averages approximately 30%.[45]

Prevention and Treatment

As just stated, smallpox was eradicated due to vaccination. The vaccinia virus is used to vaccinate against smallpox and produces a localized exanthem at the site of inoculation. The virus is inoculated through multiple punctures into the upper dermis. Persons with severe cell-mediated immunodeficiency should not receive the vaccination because of potential complications of encephalitis, generalized vaccinia (a self-limited eruption), progressive vaccinia, or accidental infection. Vaccinia necrosum is characterized by failure of the vaccination site to heal, followed by progressive necrosis and ulceration that may or may not spread to distant sites (skin, bones, and viscera).[46] Untreated progressive vaccinia can be fatal and should be treated with systemic vaccinia immune globulin and sometimes thiosemicarbazone.[47] Generalized and progressive vaccinia are uncommon complications in the absence of immunosuppression, and thus most cases occur in patients with undiagnosed immunodeficiency. Transmission of vaccinia following vaccination is possible, although the transfer rate is low if the vaccination site is kept covered until it heals. Vaccination against smallpox is no longer commonplace, although the possibility of reinstituting a vaccination program is being considered due to the high susceptibility of the world's population and potential use as biological warfare.

PARVOVIRUS B19

Presentation and Clinical Features

Parvovirus B19 (PVB 19), a small single-stranded DNA virus from the family Parvoviridae, is a virologic pathogen that often causes asymptomatic infection but may become life threatening in certain circumstances. The common dermatologic manifestations associated with PVB 19 infection include erythema infectiosum, papular purpuric "gloves-and-socks" syndrome, and nonspecific findings such as reticular erythema, petechiae, and/or purpura, and maculopapular eruptions.

Erythema infectiosum, otherwise known as fifth disease, is common in the pediatric population and is characterized by the classic "slapped-cheek" facial erythema and the fine reticulated (lacy) erythema involving the trunk and extremities. Papular purpuric "gloves-and-socks" syndrome is a disease seen in adulthood, and it presents with the hallmark symmetric, sharply demarcated erythema and edema of the hands and feet that evolves into petechiae and purpura over time.

Although PVB 19 infections are often mild and self-limited, patients who are immunosuppressed, have hematologic diseases, or are pregnant are at risk for serious complications. PVB 19 infects erythroid progenitor cells and temporarily halts red blood cell production, thereby causing a transient aplastic crisis. Individuals with hematologic conditions such as sickle cell anemia, thalassemia, autoimmune hemolytic anemia, and other similar conditions are at increased risk for developing an aplastic crisis. Often the crisis is transient and self-resolving, but the risk of a fatal complication increases in this subset of patients. Immunocompromised individuals lack the ability to mount an immune response to the virus and may have a course complicated by lingering cutaneous eruptions, persistent anemia, myocarditis, pericarditis, acute heart failure, acute liver failure, meningitis, and encephalitis.[48]

Maternal parvovirus infection during pregnancy can lead to vertical transmission of the virus to the unborn fetus. The incidence of maternal PVB 19 infection during pregnancy is 1%–2%, with vertical transmission occurring in 33%–51% of cases,[49–51] and fetal loss occurring in approximately 10% of all cases.[52,53] Fetal infection can result in miscarriage or nonimmune hydrops fetalis. The incidence of fetal morbidity and mortality is inversely related to gestational age, thus infection during the first trimester is the most dangerous.

Prevention and Treatment

The treatment for PVB 19 is mostly symptomatic, and immunocompetent patients do very well. Immunocompromised patients, pregnant women, and persons with hematologic disease must be closely monitored by their respective specialists. High-dose IV immunoglobulins have been shown to eliminate the virus from the bone marrow. Intrauterine transfusion can correct fetal anemia and reduce fetal death. Prevention is difficult because, when a patient presents with a rash, he or she is no longer contagious; thus no measures can be taken to avoid infecting others.[49,54]

CYTOMEGALOVIRUS

Presentation and Clinical Features

Cytomegalovirus (CMV, human CMV [HCMV], or human herpesvirus [HHV]-5) is a large double-stranded virus from the herpesvirus family. Most commonly, CMV mononucleosis is mild and asymptomatic, with no impact on the immune system. Immunocompromised individuals, such as those with HIV or a malignancy, or those who have had an organ transplant, may exhibit complications with CMV infection. Blood transfusion recipients and newborns are other patient populations that may have a lethal outcome from a CMV infection.

CMV infections are a frequent cause of morbidity and mortality among immunocompromised patients. The virus itself may not directly lead to the death of a patient, but it further lowers the patient's immune system, thus making him or her much more susceptible to other deadly diseases. For example, patients with HIV may die from a coinfection with CMV and *Pneumocystis carinii* (now renamed *Pneumocystis jiroveci*). Prognosis depends on the extent and interval of immunosuppression. CMV infection may increase the rate of organ rejection by inducing autoantibodies.[55] Patients with postperfusion syndrome (CMV mononucleosis acquired via blood transfusion) exhibit fever, malaise, hepatosplenomegaly, and jaundice; these patients carry a poor prognosis.[56]

Newborns can acquire CMV in utero (transplacentally), after exposure to genital secretions in the vaginal canal, or through breastfeeding.[57] Severe clinical manifestations of congenital CMV infection most often occur when the mother sustains a primary CMV infection rather than reactivation of a recurrent infection. The disease tends to be more severe if the infection is acquired earlier in gestation. The dermatologic manifestations of CMV infection include petechiae, purpura, jaundice, and "blueberry muffin" syndrome. Even if a newborn is born without overt symptoms, he or she is at risk for long-term complications such as hearing loss and/or mental retardation.

Prevention and Treatment

Immunocompromised patients should be treated concurrently with antiviral therapy (ganciclovir) and passive immunization with hyperimmune globulin (HIG). Little can be done in terms of prevention of CMV infection. Transplant centers use ganciclovir and HIG after organ transplant to prevent an infection. A live attenuated CMV vaccine (Towne strain) appears to be prophylactic against infection but it is not yet commercially available.

In pregnancy, prevention of CMV infection starts with hygienic behavior for seronegative women. Pregnant women with primary CMV infection can prevent transmission to the fetus by using CMV HIG. The effect of HIG on newborns is unknown, but there is evidence to suggest that it may also be effective. The efficacy of ganciclovir in pregnancy is unknown, and there is concern about possible teratogenic effects on the fetus. Ganciclovir, however, can be used safely and effectively in newborns. Pregnancy termination is an option if fetal infection is diagnosed via ultrasonography or amniocentesis.[58]

MEASLES (RUBEOLA)

Presentation and Clinical Features

The first sign of measles infection is usually high fever (approaching 40°C at its peak) beginning approximately 10–12 days after exposure and lasting 1–7 days. Other associated symptoms include coryza, conjunctivitis, and cough. Approximately 2–3 days later, a cutaneous exanthem appears, consisting of an erythematous rash composed of macules and papules (usually beginning on the face and upper neck) that coalesce and spread to the trunk and eventually to the extremities, hands, and feet. Often there is a diagnostic enanthem of bluish-gray areas on the tonsils (Herman spots) and punctate blue–white lesions surrounded by an erythematous ring on the buccal mucosa (Koplik spots).[59] The exanthem lasts for 5–6 days, then fades, whereas the enanthem occurs a few days prior to the exanthem and lasts 2–3 days.

For most persons, measles is an unpleasant mild or moderately severe illness. In poorly nourished young children, however, especially those who do not receive sufficient vitamin A, or whose immune systems have been weakened by HIV/AIDS or other diseases, severe complications including blindness, encephalitis, severe diarrhea (which can cause dehydration), pneumonia, and mortality from such complications can result.[60,61]

Encephalitis is estimated to occur in 1 of 800–1000 cases (although death and brain damage is limited to a small minority of cases), whereas pneumonia may occur in 5%–10% of cases. More uncommon is subacute sclerosing panencephalitis, which can develop in approximately 1 of 100,000 cases and cause mental and motor deterioration, seizures, coma, and death.[32]

Overall, the case fatality rate in developing countries is generally in the range of 1%–5%, but may be as high as 25% in populations with high levels of malnutrition and poor access to health care. In January 2007, the World Health Organization/United Nations Children's Fund (WHO/UNICEF) reported that implementation of measles mortality reduction strategies (including vaccinations and early treatment strategies) had reduced measles mortality by 60%, from an estimated 873,000 deaths worldwide in 1999 to 345,000 deaths in 2005.[62,63]

Prevention and Treatment

The best weapon we have against measles is vaccination to prevent disease. The measles vaccine is a live attenuated vaccine that first became available in 1963. In the United States, it is generally given as part of either the measles, mumps, rubella (German measles) (MMR) or MMR plus varicella (MMRV) vaccines. The vaccine is given in two shots, the first at 12–15 months and the second at 4–6 years of age.[64] After the second shot, approximately 99% of people become immune to the disease. Because it is a live vaccine (like the varicella vaccine), immunocompromised patients should not be vaccinated.

Severe complications of measles can usually be avoided. General nutritional support and the treatment of dehydration with oral rehydration solution are necessary. Should eye and ear infections or pneumonia result, antibiotics may be prescribed. In developing countries, persons diagnosed with measles should receive two doses of vitamin A supplements given 24 hours apart to help prevent eye damage and blindness. More important, vitamin A supplementation has been shown to reduce the number of deaths from measles by 50%.[65]

GERMAN MEASLES (RUBELLA)

Presentation and Clinical Features

Rubella tends to be milder than rubeola. Often called 3-day measles because of the duration of its classic rash, it is recognized by mild constitutional symptoms followed by an erythematous eruption that begins on the face and spreads from head to foot. Unlike measles, the rash of rubella is nonconfluent and tends to have a lesser degree of erythema. Additionally, petechiae of the palate may be present. In general, rubella is uncomplicated, but infection during pregnancy can lead to congenital rubella syndrome (CRS), an important cause of severe birth defects.[66] When a woman is infected with the rubella virus early in pregnancy, she has a greater than 50% chance of passing the virus on to her fetus, which may cause fetal demise or CRS, whereas infection later in pregnancy has a lower risk of CRS.[67] Common birth defects that may occur due to CRS are ocular defects, cardiovascular defects, CNS defects, deafness, microcephaly, mental retardation, and intrauterine growth retardation.

An uncommon but important systemic complication, particularly in adult women, is encephalitis. Rubella encephalitis occurs in approximately 1 in 6000 cases, and is fatal in approximately 20% of these cases.[68]

Prevention and Treatment

The currently used rubella vaccine is a live attenuated strain that was developed in 1979 and is given as part of the MMR or MMRV vaccine. The vaccine schedule includes a first shot at 12–15 months and a second at 4–6 years of age.[64] As it is a live virus vaccine, immunosuppressed patients should not be vaccinated. Treatment for rubella infection is supportive.

KAPOSI SARCOMA

Presentation and Clinical Features

Kaposi sarcoma (KS) is a vascular neoplasm with several distinct subtypes. Classic KS is an indolent disease in middle-aged to elderly men, generally of Southern and Eastern European origin. African cutaneous KS, which affects middle-aged Africans in tropical Africa, tends to be locally aggressive. African lymphadenopathic KS is an aggressive disease that affects young patients, usually younger than 10 years. KS is also seen in patients who are immunosuppressed, either by AIDS or by lymphoma or immunosuppressive therapy.[46]

Lesions of KS are reddish, violaceous, or bluish-black macules and patches that spread and coalesce to form nodules or plaques. They often appear on the toes or soles in the earliest stages. Regardless of the epidemiologic form, the prognosis of KS depends on the severity of visceral involvement. The gastrointestinal (GI) tract, particularly the small intestine, is the most frequent site of internal involvement in classic KS, although it may also affect the lungs, heart, liver, lymph nodes, and bone. Visceral involvement in classic KS occurs in approximately 10% of patients.[69] African cutaneous KS frequently has bone involvement as well as leg swelling caused by lymphedema. African lymphadenopathic KS, as the name suggests, involves the lymph nodes, which often precede the appearance of skin lesions. In AIDS-associated KS, 25% of patients have cutaneous involvement only, whereas 29% have visceral involvement only.[46] If AIDS is left untreated, more than 70% of patients with AIDS-associated KS will develop visceral involvement.

Due to its indolent course, patients with classic KS usually die of unrelated causes, often many years after initial diagnosis. In contrast, African cutaneous KS is aggressive and has early nodal involvement; this form of KS often results in death within 1–2 years. Despite often being widespread, AIDS-related KS tends not to be fatal, as most patients die of intercurrent infection.

Prevention and Treatment

KS lesions are radiosensitive, but they can also be locally excised and/or treated with cryotherapy, laser ablation, and intralesional injections (interferon, vincristine, vinblastine, and actinomycin D have all been reported). For disseminated, progressive, or symptomatic disease, systemic treatment options include interferon-α and chemotherapy including pegylated liposomal anthracyclines and paclitaxel.[70] Highly active antiretroviral therapy (HAART) in patients with AIDS has been shown both to decrease the incidence of KS as well as to treat existing lesions.[70,71] The fact that KS lesions tend to regress when a patient is on HAART leads to the assumption that improvement in immune function is responsible for the regression. Therefore, removal of the iatrogenic cause in patients with immunosuppression-related KS may result in KS resolution without therapy. There are no current preventative therapies for KS besides HAART in AIDS patients or removal of iatrogenic stresses on the immune system.

MOSQUITO-BORNE VIRUSES

Presentation and Clinical Features

Mosquitoes have been called the world's deadliest animals as diseases spread by these insects are responsible for more deaths than all mammals, amphibians, reptiles, birds, and fishes combined. Three such life-threatening viral diseases of concern to dermatologists include dengue, yellow fever, and West Nile virus.

Dengue causes fever as well as headache, retroorbital pain, myalgia, and arthralgia that may be followed by a skin eruption in up to 80% of patients during the remission of the fever. The rash classically consists of a mild macular eruption over the nape of the neck and face lasting up to 5 days. Petechiae or purpura as well as involvement of the palms and soles followed by desquamation and proximal spread to the arms, legs, and torso are also common.[32,66] This eruption is helpful diagnostically, as prior to the eruption the differential can include malaria, yellow fever, and influenza.[32] Dengue is associated with two life-threatening complications: hemorrhagic fever and shock syndrome. Hemorrhagic fever consists of a sudden temperature elevation lasting 2–7 days followed by bleeding from sites of trauma as well as the GI tract and urinary tract. The average case fatality is approximately 5%[32] but, in severe cases of dengue, hemorrhagic fever mortality may reach 50%.[66] Occasionally, shock syndrome may follow hemorrhagic fever. In these cases, circulatory and respiratory failure may occur, resulting in death in approximately 2% of cases.

Yellow fever has two disease phases. The first (acute phase) presents with fever, muscle pain (especially backache), headache, anorexia, and nausea and/or vomiting. Most patients improve after 3–4 days.[72] Approximately 15% of patients will enter a toxic phase consisting of fever reappearance, jaundice, and abdominal pain. Hemorrhage from the GI tract, mouth, nose, and eyes may occur. Liver and kidney failure may occur, and mortality can be as high as 40% in this toxic phase because of hepatorenal failure.[66] Dermatological findings in yellow fever include icteric skin (hence the name "yellow" fever) as well as hemorrhages or petechiae of the skin and mucous membranes.

West Nile virus can cause fever, headaches, GI symptoms, and (in up to 50% of cases) a skin eruption characterized by punctate, erythematous macules and papules most pronounced on the extremities.[32,66] Common serious complications include meningitis, encephalitis, and flaccid paralysis, although less than 1% of infections result in severe neurological illness. Persons at greatest risk for neurological disease are thoses older than 50 years.

Prevention and Treatment

Vaccination is available for yellow fever and is recommended every 10 years for persons visiting endemic countries.[66,73] There are no currently available vaccines for dengue or West Nile virus. The best form of prevention is to avoid mosquito bites. Using insect repellent; getting rid of mosquito breeding sites by emptying standing water from flower pots, buckets, or barrels; staying indoors between dusk and dawn (when mosquitoes are most active); and using screens on windows to keep mosquitoes out are all effective techniques. There are no antiviral treatments for the mosquito-borne viruses. Treatment for dengue and yellow fever is symptomatic, consisting of rehydration, rest, analgesia, and antiemetics, whereas therapy for West Nile virus is the same as for patients with meningoencephalitis.[66]

MARBURG AND EBOLA VIRUSES

Presentation and Clinical Features

The filoviridae viruses, Marburg and Ebola, cause severe hemorrhagic fever in human and nonhuman primates. The classic rash that may bring these infections to dermatological attention is a nonpruritic centripetal rash composed of macules and papules with varying degrees of erythema.[74] The rash occurs approximately 2 weeks after exposure and tends to desquamate by day 5 or 7 of the illness. Hemorrhagic manifestations include GI tract bleeding, bleeding into the oropharynx and lungs, petechiae, hemorrhage from puncture wounds, and massive gingival bleeding.[74] Mucosal bleeding and persistent vomiting are ominous symptoms in these diseases. Mortality due to Marburg and Ebola ranges between 30% and 90%, depending on the strain of the virus.[75,76]

Prevention and Treatment

There is no virus-specific treatment for either Marburg or Ebola virus; therefore, supportive therapy is the standard of care. Therapy should attempt to maintain effective blood volume and electrolyte balance that present due to hemorrhage.[74] Additionally, shock, cerebral edema, renal failure, coagulopathy, and secondary bacterial infection are commonplace and must be managed appropriately. Isolation is recommended to prevent spread of the disease to additional patients. When available, patients should be placed in a negative pressure room if experiencing symptoms of cough, vomiting, diarrhea, or hemorrhage.[77]

ONCOGENIC VIRUSES

Several viruses have the potential to be life threatening due to their oncogenic potential. Although these viruses are unlikely to require treatment on an emergent basis, recognizing some of the pathologies associated with these viruses is important.

Human papilloma viruses (HPV; there are >100 currently identified) are responsible for common warts and condyloma acuminata, and are encountered by dermatologists on a daily basis. Most warts are benign, but they can convert to malignant carcinomas, as is the case in patients with epidermodysplasia verruciformis.[78] Papilloma viruses are also found associated with human penile, uterine, and cervical carcinomas and are likely to be their cause. Of the multiple types of HPV, certain strains have been identified as having high oncogenic potential. Some of these strains, namely HPV 16 and 18 (along with nononcogenic types 6 and 11) have been targeted in a quadrivalent vaccine to prevent cervical cancer (Gardasil).[79]

Epstein–Barr virus (EBV) is a herpes virus that is strongly associated with cancer. It infects primarily lymphocytes and epithelial cells. EBV causes infectious mononucleosis, which itself is a benign self-limited disease characterized by fever, sore throat, swollen lymph glands, and occasionally hepatosplenomegaly. A pink, measles-like rash can occur and is more likely if the patient is given ampicillin or amoxicillin (approaching 70%–100% of patients who receive these medicines)[80] for a throat infection, which may prompt dermatological consultation. EBV is associated with multiple tumors, including Burkitt lymphoma (particularly in the tropics), nasopharyngeal cancer (particularly in China and Southeast Asia), B-cell lymphomas in immune suppressed individuals (such as in organ transplantation or HIV), and Hodgkin lymphoma (EBV has been detected in approximately 40% of affected patients).[81–83]

HHV-8 is widely known to be the viral cause of KS. It has also been associated with hematologic malignancies, including primary effusion lymphoma, Castleman disease, and various atypical lymphoproliferative disorders.[69,84]

Hepatitis B may come to dermatological attention if a patient develops Gianotti–Crosti syndrome, a cutaneous manifestation that is not specific to hepatitis B (it can also be associated with EBV among other diseases). This cutaneous eruption is characterized by monomorphous pale, pink-to flesh-colored or erythematous papules or papulovesicles distributed symmetrically and acrally over the extensor surfaces of the extremities, buttocks, and the face, with the trunk, knees, elbows, palms, and soles rarely involved.[46] Hepatitis B is thought to be associated with hepatocellular carcinoma (HCC), one of world's most common cancers. There is a strong correlation between HBsAg (hepatitis B virus surface antigen) chronic carriers and the incidence of HCC. In Taiwan, it has been shown that 72% of patients with HCC are carriers of HBsAg.[85] Fifty-one percent of deaths of HBsAg carriers are caused by liver cirrhosis or HCC compared to 2% of the general population.

SUMMARY

Most cutaneous viral diseases are self-limited in immunocompetent individuals. Due to the growing number of immunocompromised patients (whether because of HIV/AIDS or iatrogenic causes), life-threatening manifestations of these viral diseases are increasingly common. Although many of these diseases are classically seen in developing countries, air travel and the global economy have brought these infections to the attention of physicians and patients in developed nations as well. Doctors and health care workers must be careful not to overlook the potential for life-threatening complications of viral skin diseases. Vaccination when available is usually the best strategy for prevention of illness. On infection, prompt treatment is necessary to prevent avoidable morbidity and mortality.

REFERENCES

1. Kimberlin DW, Lin CY, Jacobs RF, et al. Safety and efficacy of high-dose intravenous acyclovir in the management of neonatal herpes simplex virus infections. Pediatrics. 2001; 108:230–8.
2. Brown ZA, Wald A, Morrow RA, et al. Effect of serologic status and cesarean delivery on transmission rates of herpes simplex virus from mother to infant. JAMA. 2003; 289:203–9.
3. Whitley RJ. Herpes simplex virus infections of women and their offspring: implications for a developed society. Proc Natl Acad Sci USA. 1994; 91:2441–7.
4. Hutto C, Arvin A, Jacobs R, et al. Intrauterine herpes simplex virus infections. J Pediatr. 1987; 110:97–101.
5. Baldwin S, Whitley RJ. Intrauterine herpes simplex virus infection. Teratology. 1989; 39:1–10.
6. Florman AL, Gershon AA, Blackett PR, Nahmias AJ. Intrauterine infection with herpes simplex virus. Resultant congenital malformations. JAMA. 1973; 225:129–32.
7. Stone KM, Brooks CA, Guinan ME, Alexander ER. National surveillance for neonatal herpes simplex virus infections. Sex Transm Dis. 1989; 16:152–6.
8. Whitley RJ, Corey L, Arvin A, et al. Changing presentation of herpes simplex virus infection in neonates. J Infect Dis. 1988; 158:109–16.

9. Whitley RJ, Nahmias AJ, Visintine AM, et al. The natural history of herpes simplex virus infection of mother and newborn. Pediatrics. 1980; 66:489–94.
10. Yeager AS, Arvin AM. Reasons for the absence of a history of recurrent genital infections in mothers of neonates infected with herpes simplex virus. Pediatrics. 1984; 73:188–93.
11. Kimberlin DW. Advances in the treatment of neonatal herpes simplex infections. Rev Med Virol. 2001; 11:157–63.
12. Whitley RJ, Kimberlin DW, Roizman B. Herpes simplex viruses. Clin Infect Dis. 1998; 26:541–53; quiz 54–5.
13. Kimberlin DW, Lin CY, Jacobs RF, et al. Natural history of neonatal herpes simplex virus infections in the acyclovir era. Pediatrics. 2001; 108:223–9.
14. Holland GN. Acquired immunodeficiency syndrome and ophthalmology: the first decade. Am J Ophthalmol. 1992; 114:86–95.
15. Whitley RJ, Roizman B. Herpes simplex virus infections. Lancet. 2001; 357:1513–18.
16. Lakeman FD, Whitley RJ. Diagnosis of herpes simplex encephalitis: application of polymerase chain reaction to cerebrospinal fluid from brain-biopsied patients and correlation with disease. National Institute of Allergy and Infectious Diseases Collaborative Antiviral Study Group. J Infect Dis. 1995; 171:857–63.
17. Whitley RJ, Soong SJ, Linneman C, Jr., et al. Herpes simplex encephalitis. Clinical Assessment. JAMA. 1982; 247:317–20.
18. Whitley RJ, Gnann JW. Viral encephalitis: familiar infections and emerging pathogens. Lancet. 2002; 359:507–13.
19. Novelli VM, Atherton DJ, Marshall WC. Eczema herpeticum. Clinical and laboratory features. Clin Pediatr (Phila). 1988; 27:231–3.
20. Sanderson IR, Brueton LA, Savage MO, Harper JI. Eczema herpeticum: a potentially fatal disease. Br Med J (Clin Res Ed). 1987; 294:693–4.
21. Wakkerman CT. A fatal case of Kaposi's varicelliform eruption. Dermatologica. 1967; 134:393–4.
22. Wheeler CE, Jr., Abele DC. Eczema herpeticum, primary and recurrent. Arch Dermatol. 1966; 93:162–73.
23. Ingrand D, Briquet I, Babinet JM, et al. Eczema herpeticum of the child. An unusual manifestation of herpes simplex virus infection. Clin Pediatrics (Phila). 1985; 24:660–3.
24. Monif GR, Brunell PA, Hsiung GD. Visceral involvement by herpes simplex virus in eczema herpeticum. Am J Dis Child. 1968; 116:324–7.
25. Kaufman B, Gandhi SA, Louie E, et al. Herpes simplex virus hepatitis: case report and review. Clin Infect Dis. 1997; 24:334–8.
26. Englund JA, Fletcher CV, Balfour HH, Jr. Acyclovir therapy in neonates. J Pediatr. 1991; 119:129–35.
27. Safrin S, Kemmerly S, Plotkin B, et al. Foscarnet-resistant herpes simplex virus infection in patients with AIDS. J Infect Dis. 1994; 169:193–6.
28. Whitley RJ, Alford CA, Hirsch MS, et al. Vidarabine versus acyclovir therapy in herpes simplex encephalitis. N Engl J Med. 1986; 314:144–9.
29. Whitley R, Lakeman AD, Nahmias A, Roizman B. DNA restriction-enzyme analysis of herpes simplex virus isolates obtained from patients with encephalitis. N Engl J Med. 1982; 307:1060–2.

30. Egawa H, Inomata Y, Nakayama S, et al. Fulminant hepatic failure secondary to herpes simplex virus infection in a neonate: a case report of successful treatment with liver transplantation and perioperative acyclovir. Liver Transpl Surg. 1998; 4:513–15.

31. Shanley CJ, Braun DK, Brown K, et al. Fulminant hepatic failure secondary to herpes simplex virus hepatitis. Successful outcome after orthotopic liver transplantation. Transplantation. 1995; 59:145–9.

32. Rebora A. Life-threatening cutaneous viral diseases. Clin Dermatol. 2005; 23:157–63.

33. Sauerbrei A, Wutzler P. Neonatal varicella. J Perinatol. 2001; 21:545–9.

34. Varicella-related deaths among adults–United States, 1997. Centers for Disease Control and Prevention (CDC). MMWR Morb Mortal Wkly Rep. 1997; 46(19):409–12.

35. Grant RM, Weitzman SS, Sherman CG, et al. Fulminant disseminated Varicella Zoster virus infection without skin involvement. J Clin Virol. 2002; 24:7–12.

36. Stratman E. Visceral zoster as the presenting feature of disseminated herpes zoster. J Am Acad Dermatol. 2002; 46:771–4.

37. Mehta J, Mahajan V, Khanna S. Disseminated zoster with polyneuritis cranialis and motor radiculopathy: letter to editor. Neurol India. 2002; 50:228–9.

38. Fehr T, Bossart W, Wahl C, Binswanger U. Disseminated varicella infection in adult renal allograft recipients: four cases and a review of the literature. Transplantation. 2002; 73:608–11.

39. Lauzurica R, Bayes B, Frias C, et al. Disseminated varicella infection in adult renal allograft recipients: role of mycophenolate mofetil. Transplant Proc. 2003; 35:1758–9.

40. Gupta S, Jain A, Gardiner C, Tyring SK. A rare case of disseminated cutaneous zoster in an immunocompetent patient. BMC Fam Pract. 2005; 6:50.

41. Curtis KK, Connolly MK, Northfelt DW. Live, attenuated varicella zoster vaccination of an immunocompromised patient. J Gen Intern Med. 2008; 23:648–9.

42. Kramer JM, LaRussa P, Tsai WC, et al. Disseminated vaccine strain varicella as the acquired immunodeficiency syndrome-defining illness in a previously undiagnosed child. Pediatrics. 2001; 108:E39.

43. Levy O, Orange JS, Hibberd P, et al. Disseminated varicella infection due to the vaccine strain of varicella-zoster virus, in a patient with a novel deficiency in natural killer T cells. J Infect Dis. 2003; 188:948–53.

44. Parrino J, Graham BS. Smallpox vaccines: past, present, and future. J Allerg Clin Immunol. 2006; 118:1320–6.

45. Nafziger SD. Smallpox. Crit Care Clin. 2005; 21:739–46, vii.

46. James WD, Berger TG, Elston DM, editors. Andrews' diseases of the skin: clinical dermatology. 10th ed. Philadelphia: WB Saunders: 2006.

47. Goldstein JA, Neff JM, Lane JM, Koplan JP. Smallpox vaccination reactions, prophylaxis, and therapy of complications. Pediatrics. 1975; 55:342–7.

48. Bultmann BD, Klingel K, Sotlar K, et al. Parvovirus B19: a pathogen responsible for more than hematologic disorders. Virchows Arch. 2003; 442:8–17.

49. de Jong EP, de Haan TR, Kroes AC, et al. Parvovirus B19 infection in pregnancy. J Clin Virol. 2006; 36:1–7.

50. Dembinski J, Eis-Hubinger AM, Maar J, et al. Long term follow up of serostatus after maternofetal parvovirus B19 infection. Arch Dis Child. 2003; 88:219–21.

51. Trotta M, Azzi A, Meli M, et al. Intrauterine parvovirus B19 infection: early prenatal diagnosis is possible. Int J Infect Dis. 2004; 8:130–1.

52. Miller E, Fairley CK, Cohen BJ, Seng C. Immediate and long term outcome of human parvovirus B19 infection in pregnancy. Br J Obstet Gynaecol. 1998; 105:174–8.

53. Norbeck O, Papadogiannakis N, Petersson K, et al. Revised clinical presentation of parvovirus B19-associated intrauterine fetal death. Clin Infect Dis. 2002; 35:1032–8.

54. Katta R. Parvovirus B19: a review. Dermatol Clin. 2002; 20:333–42.

55. Adler SP, Marshall B. Cytomegalovirus infections. Pediatr Rev. 2007; 28:92–100.

56. Prince SE, Cunha BA. Postpericardiotomy syndrome. Heart Lung. 1997; 26:165–8.

57. Griffiths PD, Walter S. Cytomegalovirus. Curr Opin Infect Dis. 2005; 18:241–5.

58. Adler SP, Nigro G, Pereira L. Recent advances in the prevention and treatment of congenital cytomegalovirus infections. Semin Perinatol. 2007; 31:10–18.

59. Cunha BA. Smallpox and measles: historical aspects and clinical differentiation. Infect Dis Clin North Am. 2004; 18:79–100.

60. Caulfield LE, de Onis M, Blossner M, Black RE. Undernutrition as an underlying cause of child deaths associated with diarrhea, pneumonia, malaria, and measles. Am J Clin Nutr. 2004; 80:193–8.

61. Moss WJ, Fisher C, Scott S, et al. HIV type 1 infection is a risk factor for mortality in hospitalized Zambian children with measles. Clin Infect Dis. 2008; 46:523–7.

62. Progress in global measles control and mortality reduction, 2000–2006. Centers for Disease Control and Prevention (CDC). MMWR Morb Mortal Wkly Rep. 2007; 56(47):1237–41.

63. Wolfson LJ, Strebel PM, Gacic-Dobo M, et al. Has the 2005 measles mortality reduction goal been achieved? A natural history modelling study. Lancet. 2007; 369:191–200.

64. Update: recommendations from the Advisory Committee on Immunization Practices (ACIP) regarding administration of combination MMRV vaccine. MMWR Morb Mortal Wkly Rep. 2008; 57:258–60.

65. Hussey GD, Klein M. A randomized, controlled trial of vitamin A in children with severe measles. N Engl J Med. 1990; 323:160–4.

66. Carneiro SC, Cestari T, Allen SH, Ramos e-Silva M. Viral exanthems in the tropics. Clin Dermatol. 2007; 25:212–20.

67. De Santis M, Cavaliere AF, Straface G, Caruso A. Rubella infection in pregnancy. Reprod Toxicol. 2006; 21:390–8.

68. Gulen F, Cagliyan E, Aydinok Y, et al. A patient with rubella encephalitis and status epilepticus. Minerva Pediatr. 2008; 60:141–4.

69. Martinelli PT, Tyring SK. Human herpesvirus 8. Dermatol Clin. 2002; 20:307–14, vii–viii.

70. Aldenhoven M, Barlo NP, Sanders CJ. Therapeutic strategies for epidemic Kaposi's sarcoma. Int J STD AIDS. 2006; 17:571–8.

71. Noy A. Update in Kaposi sarcoma. Curr Opin Oncol. 2003; 15:379–81.

72. Lupi O, Tyring SK. Tropical dermatology: viral tropical diseases. J Am Acad Dermatol. 2003; 49:979–1000; quiz, 2.

73. Monath TP. Yellow fever: an update. Lancet Infect Dis. 200; 1:11–20.

74. Rowe AK, Bertolli J, Khan AS, et al. Clinical, virologic, and immunologic follow-up of convalescent Ebola hemorrhagic fever patients and their household contacts, Kikwit, Democratic Republic of the Congo. Commission de Lutte contre les Epidemies a Kikwit. J Infect Dis. 1999; 179 Suppl 1:S28–35.

75. Freed EO. Virology. Rafting with Ebola. Science. 2002; 296:279.

76. Portela Camara F. Epidemiology of the Ebola virus: facts and hypotheses. Braz J Infect Dis. 1998; 2:265–8.

77. Update: management of patients with suspected viral hemorrhagic fever–United States. Centers for Disease Control and Prevention (CDC). MMWR Morb Mortal Wkly Rep. 1995; 44(25):475–9.

78. Gewirtzman A, Bartlett B, Tyring S. Epidermodysplasia verruciformis and human papilloma virus. Curr Opin Infect Dis. 2008; 21:141–6.

79. Krogstad P, Cherry JD. Quadrivalent human vaccine – a call to action and for additional research. Pediatr Res. 2007; 62:527.

80. Jappe U. Amoxicillin-induced exanthema in patients with infectious mononucleosis: allergy or transient immunostimulation? Allergy. 2007; 62:1474–5.

81. Brady G, MacArthur GJ, Farrell PJ. Epstein-Barr virus and Burkitt lymphoma. J Clin Pathol. 2007; 60:1397–402.

82. Kapatai G, Murray P. Contribution of the Epstein Barr virus to the molecular pathogenesis of Hodgkin lymphoma. J Clin Pathol. 2007; 60:1342–9.

83. Lin X, Gudgeon NH, Hui EP, et al. CD4 and CD8 T cell responses to tumour-associated Epstein-Barr virus antigens in nasopharyngeal carcinoma patients. Cancer Immunol Immunother. 2008; 57:963–75.

84. Cathomas G. Kaposi's sarcoma-associated herpesvirus (KSHV)/human herpesvirus 8 (HHV-8) as a tumour virus. Herpes. 2003; 10:72–7.

85. Merican I, Guan R, Amarapuka D, et al. Chronic hepatitis B virus infection in Asian countries. J Gastroenterol Hepatol. 2000; 15:1356–61.

CHAPTER 13

Life-Threatening Cutaneous Fungal and Parasitic Diseases

Marcia Ramos-e-Silva

Carlos Gustavo Costanza

Sueli Coelho Carneiro

CUTANEOUS FUNGAL and parasitic diseases are frequent and usually do not threaten the physical integrity of the patient. There are, however, some that may acquire a severe clinical picture and may even cause death. Some of the most important and/or dangerous of these life-threatening cutaneous fungal (as systemic candidosis, paracoccidioidomycosis, sporotrichosis, zygomycosis, and histoplasmosis) and parasitic diseases (Chagas disease, schistosomiasis amebiasis, and leishmaniasis) are discussed in this chapter.

FUNGAL INFECTIONS

Systemic Candidosis

First observed by Langenbeck in 1839, the genus *Candida* suffered several taxonomic modifications until its present classification. It presents about 200 species of fungi and shelters the most important yeasts that infect mankind. Many species are opportunistic pathogens; however, the majority do not infect humans.[1]

Although the last decade has observed an increase of infections by the non-albicans *Candida* species (such as *C. tropicalis, C. glabra, C. krusei, C. dubliniensis,* and *C. parapsilosis*), *C. albicans* remains the dimorphic yeast responsible for 70%–90% of all infections of this type.[2,3] It is frequently found as a saprophyte of humans colonizing the mucosa of the digestive system, and by contiguity, the vaginal mucosa of the majority of mammals.

The term "candidiasis" or "candidosis" (more frequent in Canadian and UK literature) has a generic connotation and encompasses a wide spectrum of clinical manifestations.

Factors related to the host's immunity, mainly the cell immunity, and characteristics of the microorganism's virulence will determine the spectrum of the disease, which varies from superficial infection of the mucous membranes and skin, to visceral and systemic infections.[1,2]

Neutropenia, hematological neoplasias, cancers in solid organs, transplants, and other situations of immunosupression are the main substrata for installation of systemic candidosis. Additional aggravating factors to those scenarios are extensive hospital internments, prolonged use of broad-spectrum antibiotics, hemodialysis, multiple gastrointestinal (GI) procedures, parenteral feeding, and medium- to long-term intravascular catheters.[3–5]

Systemic candidosis is a severe infection, associated with great mortality (approximately 40%–60%)[1,3,5,6] caused mainly by difficulties in its diagnosis, leading to a delay in its recognition. The clinical manifestations are unspecific, and tools for diagnosis are not sensitive enough.

The most relevant clinical finding is persistent fever, despite the use of appropriate antibiotics for the supposed bacterial picture. The remaining manifestations are inherent to the organs affected and to septic syndrome.

Dermatological lesions affect approximately 10%–13% of patients. Despite *C. albicans* ruling absolute as the cause of systemic disease, *C. tropicalis* is isolated with greater frequency in cases of systemic candidosis with dermatological manifestations. It is speculated that a greater tropism by cutaneous tissue occurs in the latter.[7,8]

Newborns present more frequent dermatological alterations when compared to adults with systemic candidosis.

A 35.8% rate of cutaneous manifestations associated with systemic candidosis has been observed.[7] In the present study, 52.6% of the patients with dermatological manifestations had onset of dermatitis concurrently with fever and, of these, four patients (40%) presented a triad of fever, cutaneous eruption, and myalgia.

The cutaneous lesions are varied and multiple: macules, nodules, and erythematous plaques, some purple, with a central lighter hue, affecting especially the trunk and extremities. In some cases, numerous vesicles can mimic herpes zoster. Also worthy of mention are reports of cellulite lesions and gangrenous ecthyma-like lesions. Some

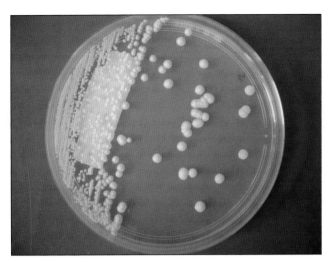

FIGURE 13.1: Candida albicans – *culture. (Photo courtesy of Mycology Laboratory – HUCFF/UFRJ.)*

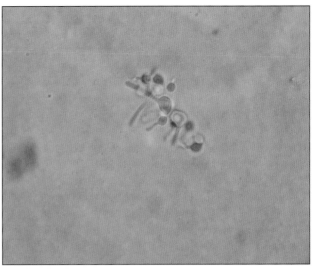

FIGURE 13.2: Candida albicans – *germ tubes. (Photo courtesy of Mycology Laboratory – HUCFF/UFRJ.)*

authors blame the purple lesions on the frequent thrombocytopenia found in those patients.[7,9,10]

Systemic candidosis is a disease of difficult diagnosis. Within some clinical coherence, biopsies of suspect cutaneous lesions and affected organs may suggest the diagnosis; however, the usual stains and immunofluorescence methods fail in identifying the species.

The dermatopathological findings can identify spores and/or hypha, mainly in the upper dermis, surrounding small vessels with varied degrees of vascular damage from dilations, thrombus, red cell extravasation, and even vasculitis.[7]

The gold standard is hemoculture, but cultures from other suspect sites can help in the diagnosis (Figures 13.1 and 13.2). The lack of sensitivity (only 50% of the affected patients) and a delay in identifying the agent (approximately 1 week) make the method unacceptable for a basis to begin therapy. Furthermore, the method has little capacity to identify the species of *Candida*, crucial for an appropriate treatment, because some species are naturally less sensitive

or resistant to commonly employed systemic antifungals (Table 13.1).[11]

Serological tests, using several resources (radioimmunoassay, enzyme-linked immunosorbent assay [ELISA], latex agglutination (LA), and reversed passive latex agglutination [RPLA] assay) aimed at identifying fungus antigens and metabolites, as well as detecting serum antibodies, are difficult to interpret and have low sensitivity.

New methods for biomolecular identification with amplification of deoxyribonucleic acid (DNA) by polymerase chain reaction (PCR) are promising. Recent publications praise the systems called "real-time" PCRs (TaqMan system® and LightCycler system®), promising immediate results, with optimal sensitivity and specificity. Those tools still present prohibitive costs, require standardization, and are not available in the majority of clinical laboratories.[6,12,13]

The fast and adequate institution of antifungal therapy is primordial for the reduction of mortality rates.

TABLE 13.1: Susceptibility of *Candida* Species

Candida spp.	Amphotericin B	Fluconazole	Itraconazole	Voriconazole	Caspofungin
C. albicans	S	S	S	S	S
C. tropicalis	S	S	S	S	S
C. parapsilosis	S	S	S	S	S[a]
C. glabrata	S to I	S-DD to R	S-DD to R	S to I	S
C. kruzei	S to I	R	S-DD to R	S	S
C. lusitaniae	S to R	S	S	S	S

Note: Interpretation based on the use of the National Committee for Clinical Laboratory Standards (CLSI) M27-A methodology.

S, susceptible; S-DD, susceptible-dose dependent; I, intermediate; R, resistant.

[a] MIC90 (the minimum inhibitory concentration required to inhibit the growth of 90% of organisms) is higher than in other *Candida* species, but clinical significance is unknown (breakpoints not yet defined).

Data adapted from (3).

TABLE 13.2: Empirical Therapy for *Candida* Bloodstream Infections

Setting	First choice	Alternatives
Non-neutropenic patient and no previous exposure to azoles	Fluconazole 800 mg IV (1st dose), then 400 mg/d IV	Amphotericin B deoxycholate 1 mg/kg/d IV Or Caspofungin 70 mg IV (1st dose), then 50 mg/d IV Or Voriconazol 6 mg/kg IV q12h on day 1, then 4 mg/kg q12h IV
Non-neutropenic patient and previous exposure to azoles	Amphotericin B deoxycholate 1 mg/kg/d IV Or Caspofungin 70 mg IV (1st dose) then 50 mg/d IV	Liposomal Amphotericin B (AmBisome®) 3 mg/kg/d IV
Neutropenic patient	Amphotericin B deoxycholate 1 mg/kg/d IV	Caspofungin 70 mg IV (1st dose) then 50 mg/d IV[a] Or Liposomal Amphotericin B (AmBisome®) 3 mg/kg/d IV
Severe sepsis or septic shock	Caspofungin 70 mg IV (1st dose) then 50 mg/d IV[a,b]	Liposomal Amphotericin B (AmBisome®) 3 mg/kg/d IV Or Voriconazole 6 mg/kg IV q12h on day 1, then 4 mg/kg q12h IV[a,b] If no previous azole exposure

[a] Few clinical data are available on the use of azoles and echinocandins in neutropenic patients with documented invasive candidosis. In vitro, azoles are fungistatic; echinocandins are fungicidal. In some experimental models (e.g., *Candida* endocarditis, disseminated candidosis in neutropenic animals), azoles are less efficacious than amphotericin B or echinocandins.

[b] Amphotericin B deoxycholate is not recommended in critically ill patients with severe sepsis/septic shock: risk of acute nephrotoxicity or of underdosing due to infusion-related toxicity. Caspofungin (Cancidas®) is first choice or alternative, respectively, in this setting.

[c] According to susceptibility testing. Some experts would add voriconazole to the list of first choice agents for the treatment of *C. glabrata* infections.

Data adapted from (3).

It is worthwhile to treat, when possible, the predisposing underlying factors, such as the removal of deep vein accesses.

The choice of the employed agent will depend on factors such as 1) the patient's state (hemodynamically stable, sepsis/shock, predisposing factors to renal inadequacy, etc.); 2) use of previous antifungal medication before the current picture; 3) isolation of specific microorganisms with known resistance to certain agents (Table 13.2).

For decades, amphotericin B deoxycholate, a polyenic antibiotic of broad-spectrum fungicide action, was used as a treatment of choice for invasive candidosis. Unfortunately, that drug is ill-tolerated, presenting immediate adverse reactions (related to the speed of its infusion; fever, shivers, hypoxemia, and hypotension) and late effects (nephrotoxicity; reduction of glomerular filtration rate and depletion of potassium, magnesium, and bicarbonate).

Lipid-based formulations were created to minimize undesired effects from amphotericin B deoxycholate, mainly nephrotoxicity. The high cost and scarcity of effective results in comparative studies led the lipid-based formulations to be used for second-line treatment of systemic candidosis.[3,14–16]

With the emergence of triazolic compounds (fluconazole and itraconazole), fluconazole became the most employed medication in the treatment of non-neutropenic and hemodynamically stable patients. It presents a wide action spectrum and good bioavailability; however,

C. krusei and *C. glabrata* present respectively resistance and low sensitivity to fluconazole. The azolic compounds, acting on enzymes of the cytochrome P450 system, interact with several drugs.[3,14–16]

Already available in intravenous (IV) formulations, itraconazole has variable bioavailability and low serum concentration when compared to other tissues (liver, lungs, and bones) and has a higher interaction with other medications.[14,15,17]

The second generation of triazolic compounds (voriconazole, posaconazole, and ravuconazole) is in advanced study phases. These compounds present an expanded spectrum with smaller risks of interactions with several drugs. Voriconazole and posaconazole are already available in venous and oral formulations, and initial comparative studies showed promising results.[3,14–16,18]

The echinocandins (caspofungin, micafungin, and anidulafungin), a recent class of antifungals with parenteral action, have fungicide action on different species of *Candida*, including samples resistant to fluconazole and amphotericin B. Different from the remaining antifungals, the echinocandins act on the fungal cell wall. Caspofungin and, later, micafungin were approved by the U.S. Food and Drug Administration with good action spectrum and minimal collateral effects being reserved for patients with severe sepsis or systemic shock and averting risks of renal damage from amphotericin B deoxycholate.[14,15,17]

Investigations encompassing combinations of antifungal agents are scarce and, in certain cases, disappointing. In vivo studies showed antagonism between the simultaneous use of amphotericin B and azoles. The classic association between amphotericin B deoxycholate and 5-fluorocitosin did not show a clear advantage as in the cases of cryptococcosis in immunodepressed patients. In contrast, the combination of caspofungin and meropenem, an ultra–broad-spectrum antibiotic in hospital use, showed a significant superiority to monotherapy.[3,19]

Paracoccidioidomycosis

Paracoccidioidomycosis was first described in Brazil by Adolfo Lutz, in 1908, and, later, investigated by Afonso Splendore and Floriano Almeida, in 1912 and 1930, respectively, both with relevant contributions. Lutz–Splendore–Almeida disease and South American blastomycosis are less common names for paracoccidioidomycosis, a term acknowledged by the United Nations since 1971.[20–22]

Paracoccidioidomycosis is a deep mycosis, the isolated agent of which is the dimorph fungus *Paracoccidioides brasiliensis*, the causative agent of the granulomatous process, predominantly chronic, and implicated on rare occasions in acute and subacute diseases. It is characterized by polymorphism of the lesions and can affect virtually any organ, especially the lymph nodes, lungs, nasal mucosa, and GI tract, besides suprarenal glands and the central nervous system (CNS).[21]

The geographic distribution of the fungus is directly related to the climate, being found predominantly in tropical and subtropical regions with acid soils. It is an endemic disease in Latin America, with great incidence in South American countries, mainly Brazil, Venezuela, Colombia, Ecuador, and Argentina, without reports of autochthonous cases either in Chile or in the Antilles. There are few cases of the disease in Central America, with predominance in Mexico.

The infection happens in general in the first two decades of life; however, it can remain latent for many years until generating the disease.

Incidence before age 12 is similar in both sexes, with greater risk for the acute and subacute forms of paracoccidioidomycosis. After age 12, there is greater predominance in men (young or middle-aged men, and men who work in rural areas [who are at greater risk of developing the disease in the chronic form]).

The extremely low percentage of women affected during childbearing age can be explained by the assumed inhibition of β-estradiol by the transformation of the mycelia into hyphae, infecting forms of *P. brasiliensis*, after finding receivers of that hormone in the cytoplasm of the fungus.

The greatest risk factor for infection is represented by activities involving handling of polluted soil. Tabagism and alcoholism are frequently associated with the disease.

TABLE 13.3: Classification of the Clinical Forms of Paracoccidioidomycosis

Paracoccidioidomycosis disease
    Acute/subacute form (juvenile type)
    Chronic form (adult type)
    Unifocal
    Multifocal
    Residual form or sequel

Data adapted from (23).

Different than other systemic mycoses, paracoccidioidomycosis is rarely related to immunodepressive diseases. There have been reports of this mycosis in patients with acquired immune deficiency syndrome (AIDS), neoplasias, and (more rarely) transplants.

The most important infection modality is through the respiratory tract, by inhalation of the spores of the fungus, although there is a report of the disease by direct cutaneous and mucosal inoculation. Starting from the penetration site, the fungus can multiply and disperse into neighboring tissues, reaching the regional lymph nodes or disseminating hematogenically.

Varied clinical forms can be observed in paracoccidioidomycosis, from located benign to disseminated and progressive disease, often with a fatal outcome. Genetic, hormonal, nutritional, and immunologic factors are involved in the development of the infection and its clinical manifestations.[21]

The classification proposed by the consensus on paracoccidioidomycosis of 2006, developed by the Brazilian Society of Tropical Medicine and adapted at the International Colloquium on Paracoccidioidomycosis (held in February 1986) is shown in Table 13.3.[23]

After penetration of *P. brasiliensis* into the host, a paracoccidioidomycosis infection results that may resolve spontaneously, progress to a disease, or remain latent, according to the patient's immunity. The main types of paracoccidioidomycosis disease are the acute/subacute forms (juvenile type) and the chronic type. The acute/subacute form is responsible for approximately 5% of the cases of paracoccidioidomycosis, prevailing in children and teenagers of both sexes, presenting rapid evolution. We highlight occurrence of lymph-node involvement, hepatosplenomegaly, intraabdominal masses, jaundice, ascites, osteoarticular and cutaneous lesions (approximately 50% of the cases), in addition to rare lung involvement (<5% of the cases).

The chronic form prevails in 90% of the cases of the disease, affecting adults older than 20 years, and can be divided into unifocal or multifocal, according to the number of organs or systems affected, in direct relation to the degree of cellular and humoral immunity.

The oral cavity involvement (Figure 13.3) is predominantly caused by contamination from lung secretions, although a direct inoculation of the fungus can also occur.

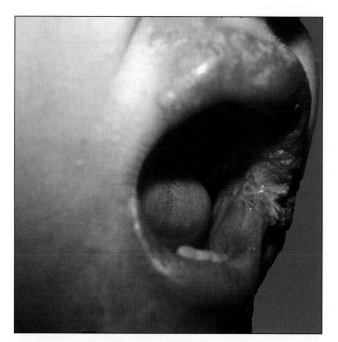

FIGURE 13.3: Paracoccidioidomycosis – oral lesion.

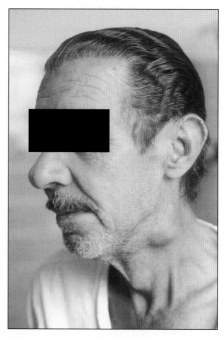

FIGURE 13.5: Paracoccidioidomycosis – lymph-node enlargement.

The most affected sites are lower lip, mucous membrane, and sublingual area. The lesions can extend to the pharynx, tonsils, and larynx. The typical presentation is erythematous ulcerated lesions, with granulomatous bases, intermixed with hemorrhagic spots, called moriform stomatitis of Aguiar-Pupo (Figure 13.4).

The characteristic cutaneous lesions are ulcers or vegetations, but crusted papules, erythematous plates, and nodules may be present. They are located more frequently in the central face area, limbs, and trunk. Cervical lymph-node involvement (Figure 13.5) tends to suppurate, resembling scrofuloderma.

Visceral commitment is varied and always present. Lungs (Figure 13.6), adrenals, liver, spleen, GI tract, genitourinary tract, CNS, and bones can also be affected.

The residual form or sequel is observed in advanced stages of the disease, where the chronic inflammatory process generates fibrosis and functional restrictions of the affected organs, with lung fibrosis being the preferred one.

In view of a clinical and epidemiologic suspicion of paracoccidioidomycosis, methods for isolation and identification of the fungus are required, in addition to serological techniques that help in the diagnosis and follow-up.[22]

The direct mycological examination of fresh or Giemsa-stained material shows rounded cells, of double contour, well refringent, varying from 5 to 25 μm in diameter (Figure 13.7). Simple or multiple gemulations can be observed, both by direct examination as in histopathology.

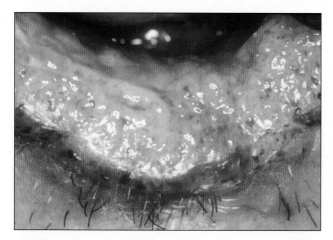

FIGURE 13.4: Paracoccidioidomycosis – stomatitis of Aguiar Pupo.

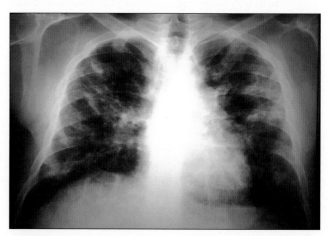

FIGURE 13.6: Paracoccidioidomycosis – x-ray showing lung involvement.

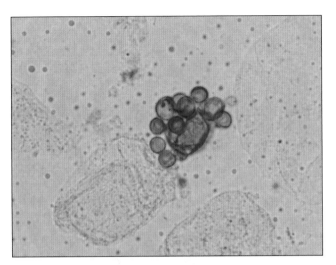

FIGURE 13.7: Paracoccidioides brasiliensis – *direct examination of cutaneous biopsy in potassium hydroxide (KOH) and Parker ink. (Photo courtesy Mycology Laboratory – HUCFF/UFRJ.)*

A typical finding is multiple gemulation in the form of a rudder wheel, with multiple gemulation around the fungus.[21,24]

Cultures are made in Sabouraud or blood agar, with an approximate 20-day duration,[24] and they are different if the culture is maintain at 37°C or 25°C (Figure 13.8).

At histopathology, we observe a granulomatous pattern, rich in giant and epithelioid cells, some containing different amounts of fungi. The finding of a parasitic element with double walls with simple or multiple gemulation is a positive diagnosis. *P. brasiliensis* can be visualized by hematoxylin and eosin (H&E) stain, but special colorations are required for fungi; periodic acid–Schiff (PAS) and Gomori methenamine–silver (GMS) stains are required when the amount of parasites is low.

Currently, several serological techniques for identification of antigens of *P. brasiliensis*, mainly gp43 and gp70,

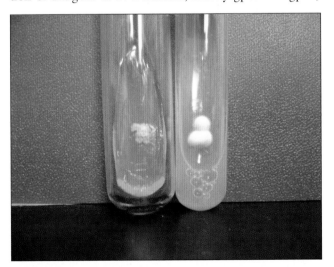

FIGURE 13.8: Paracoccidioides brasiliensis – *cultures at 37°C and 25°C showing dimorphism. (Photo courtesy of Mycology Laboratory – HUCFF/UFRJ.)*

are available from reference services. Double immunodiffusion, counterimmunoelectrophoresis, indirect immunofluorescence, ELISA, and immunoblot are examples that, besides aiding in the diagnosis, present relevant roles in the segment, with important information on the prognosis and activity of the disease.

The titer of specific anti-*P. brasiliensis* antibody is correlated to the severity in the clinical forms, being higher in the acute/subacute forms of the disease. Cases of false-negative serologies can be justified for located forms of the disease, immunodepressed hosts, or AIDS patients. False-positive results are found in patients with histoplasmosis and aspergillosis.[23]

For its simplicity, acceptable cost, and good sensitivity and specificity, double immunodiffusion was considered the main technique for diagnosis of paracoccidioidomycosis by consensus of the Brazilian Society of Tropical Medicine.

Other more complex tests are subject to clinical suspicion or initial alterations that predict the involvement of CNS, lung, GI, osteoarticular, or adrenal dysfunction.

The treatment of paracoccidioidomycosis should obligatorily encompass support measures for clinical complications associated with local and systemic involvement of the mycosis, in addition to specific antifungal therapeutics.

Most of the systemic antifungal drugs available present action against *P. brasiliensis*, such as amphotericin B, sulfamides (sulfadiazine and sulfamethoxazole/trimethoprim), terbinafine, and azolic antifungals, (ketoconazole, fluconazole, itraconazole, and voriconazole).

In mild-to-moderate cases, itraconazole is the option of choice. For its low cost and availability at the public health services, the association of sulfamethoxazole/trimethoprim is widely used in Brazil. Terbinafine has in vitro activity, against *P. brasiliensis*, similar to itraconazole, and was used successfully in the treatment of the disseminated disease, in a dosage of 500 mg/day, with a 2-year follow-up.[22,25] In patients with severe forms of the disease, amphotericin B or IV sulfamethoxazole/trimethoprim is used.

IV fluconazole can be considered in an attack dosage (400–800 mg/day for 1 month) for cases of neuroparacoccidioidomycosis because of its good penetration into the CNS.[21] Voriconazole, a second-generation triazolic compound available in oral and IV formulations, is an alternative therapeutic option of great potential.

Treatment is long, related to the severity of the disease as well as to the type of drug employed, and should be maintained until reaching cure criteria based on clinical, mycological, radiological, and serological parameters. Clinical cure means resolution of the signs and symptoms referring to the disease, healing of the tegumentary lesions, and regression of adenopathy and recovery of body weight. The demonstration of the agent's elimination or its nonviability represents the mycological cure. The stabilization of the radiological findings and regression, characteristically slow of the lung images, predict radiological cure.[26] Serological cure occurs when double immunodiffusion shows negative titers or stabilization of the values less than or equal to 1:2 observed in two samples collected in a 6-month interval after the period of specific treatment.[23]

Every patient presents a potential risk of a late reactivation; for that reason, after observing the criteria for cure, and after treatment interruption, patients should be followed half-yearly in the first year with clinical and serological tests, if necessary.[21,23]

Vaccines containing antigen gp43 DNA demonstrated capability to generate protective immunity against *P. brasiliensis* and to be a potential weapon in the prevention of future cases.[27,28]

Visceral and Disseminated Sporotrichosis

The first case of sporotrichosis was reported in 1896 by Benjamin Schenck, who was at that time a medical student. He isolated the suspect organism and forwarded it to Erwin Smith, a mycology teacher, who concluded that it belonged to the *Sporotrichum* genus. Later, in 1900, Hekton and Perkins classified the pathogenic fungus as *Sporothrix schenckii*.[29,30]

Although it is found worldwide, *S. schenckii* is more prevalent in the tropics and in hot areas of temperate regions. This dimorph fungus is present in decaying vegetation, sphagnum moss, and soil. Commonly, contamination occurs by cutaneous inoculation of the organism, preceded by local trauma.

Another less common contamination modality, but related to more severe forms of the disease, is through inhalation of fungal conidia, generating primary lung lesions (diffuse fibrosis, abscesses, and lymph-node enlargement) with posterior hematogenic dissemination.[31]

Farmers, gardeners, horticulturists, and forest workers are most susceptible to the infection. Sporotrichosis can be transmitted by scratches and bites from digging animals that carry the microorganism in their paws and teeth.[32] Recently, an epidemic of sporotrichosis in cats occurred with a consequent increase of reports of infections transmitted by those sick animals.[33,34]

Classified among the subcutaneous mycoses, most reports of sporotrichosis are restricted to the skin and subcutaneous tissue. Osteoarticular, visceral, and disseminated lesions are uncommon and present greater morbidity. Osteoarticular manifestations are the most frequent among the cases of extracutaneous disease. The immune conditions of the host and the contamination route are the factors of greater relevance for the severity of the disease.

Kong and colleagues[35] demonstrated the possibility of virulence factors associated with different genotypes of *S. schenckii* being contributors to the distinct forms of presentation of sporotrichosis.

Patients with AIDS, chronic alcoholics, and malnourished, transplanted, or immunodepressed patients in

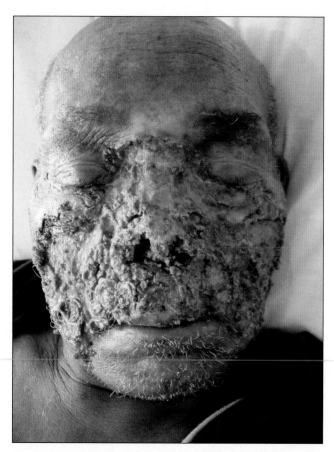

FIGURE 13.9: *Sporotrichosis – cutaneous lesion patient with lymphoma. (Photo courtesy of Nurimar Fernandes, MD, PhD, and Hugo Alves, MD, Rio de Janeiro, RJ, Brazil.)*

general are most susceptible to the disseminated forms (Figures 13.9 and 13.10). Patients with AIDS present a special risk for developing more severe forms. The diagnosis of cutaneous or lymphocutaneous sporotrichosis in an AIDS patient justifies the search for disseminated lesions

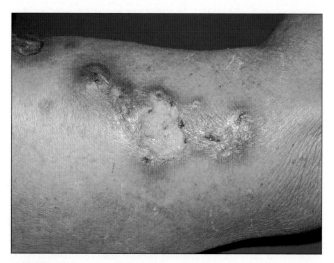

FIGURE 13.10: *Sporotrichosis – cutaneous lesion with multiple myeloma.*

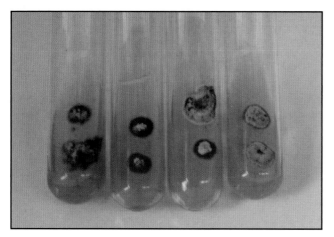

FIGURE 13.11: Sporothrix schenckii – *cultures at 25° C. (Photo courtesy of Mycology Laboratory – HUCFF/UFRJ.)*

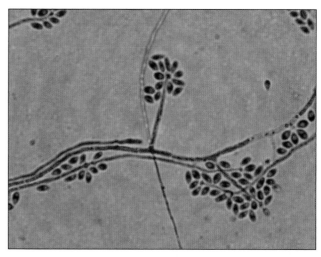

FIGURE 13.12: Sporothrix schenckii – *culture microscopy microculture in potato-dextrose agar (PDA) stained in blue. (Photo courtesy of Mycology Laboratory – HUCFF/UFRJ).*

in other organs, including the CNS. Disseminated lesions may result in arthritis, mastitis, meningitis or multiple cerebral abscesses, orchitis, pyelonephritis, and bone infections.

Cutaneous manifestations can arise in the process of disease dissemination and are characterized by painful nodules that evolve into ulcers. Papules, pustules, and other elementary lesions are occasionally observed.[30]

Due to the few reported cases and similarity of their clinical manifestations to other more common diseases such as tuberculosis, paracoccidioidomycosis, cryptococcosis, and sarcoidosis, the diagnosis of visceral sporotrichosis is frequently delayed.

Culture is the gold standard for diagnosis. Aspirates, scrapings, and biopsies of suspect lesions, cutaneous or not, can serve as substrata. Cultures of synovial liquid and/or liquor can be adequately accomplished. The culture is initially white, acquiring a darker color later (Figure 13.11). In 89% of cases, isolation of *S. schenckii* is obtained in approximately 8 days. The growth of the fungus can occur later, sometimes taking up to 4 weeks. Microscopy of the culture shows conidia in a flower head arrangement (Figure 13.12). Direct examination does not help due to the very small amount of fungal cells, commonly present in the examined materials.

A histopathologic study can disclose an unspecific granulomatous reaction with pseudoepitheliomatous hyperplasia and intraepidermal abscesses. Rarely, in PAS or silver stain, oval and cigar-shaped organisms are observed, with diameters of 3–5 mm inside the granuloma. The asteroid bodies are observed in 40% of the rare cases in which these microorganisms are found. They can be seen in other granulomatous reactions, however, extracellular structures made of spiculae of eosinophilic material involved by a center containing yeasts (Splendore-Hoeppli phenomenon) are specific of the asteroid bodies in sporotrichosis.[30,31,36]

The test of late reaction with sporotrichin is of little use in cases of visceral infections or in dealing with patients with inadequate immune response, in addition to the incapacity of differentiating previous exposure. Serological examinations did not prove useful in the diagnosis of sporotrichosis and are not widely available.

The cutaneous and cutaneolymphatic lesions are responsive to the therapy using a saturated solution of potassium iodide (SSKI), triazoles (especially itraconazole), terbinafine, and even local heat application.[37]

With the exception of osteoarticular lesions, with reasonable response to itraconazole, the remaining extracutaneous infections (visceral and disseminated) fail to respond to commonly used medications. Present guidelines for management of sporotrichosis are summarized in Table 13.4.[31]

In cases of disseminated or visceral disease, administration of amphotericin B is mandatory, preferably in lipidic formulations. After a favorable response, the parenteral medication can be replaced with itraconazole for a minimum of 12 months. In patients with AIDS, itraconazole can be used indefinitely, as collateral prevention, in a dosage of 200 mg/dia. Surgical treatment combined with amphotericin B can be recommended in localized visceral cases, mainly in pulmonary sporotrichosis.

Among the second-generation triazoles, voriconazole showed less antifungal activity against *S. schenckii* than did itraconazole and without indications in cases of sporotrichosis. Posaconazole presents activity against isolated *S. schenckii* samples, but no comparative study has been published so far.

In a published Mexican study[38] the production of melanin by *Sporothrix* was demonstrated. This fact might positively influence the discovery of effective therapeutic interventions. Herbicides directed to melanin biosynthesis, such as tricyclazole, are available for agricultural use.[31]

TABLE 13.4: Summary of Recommendations

Lymphocutaneous/ Cutaneous	Itr 200 mg/d	Itr 200 mg b.i.d.; or terbinafine 500 mg b.i.d.; or SSKI with increasing doses; or fluconazole 400–800 mg/d; or local hyperthermia[a]
Osteoarticular	Itr 200 mg b.i.d.	Lipid AmB 3–5 mg/kg/d; or deoxycholate AmB 0.7–1 mg/kg/d[b]
Pulmonary	Lipid AmB 3–5 mg/kg/d, then Itr 200 mg b.i.d.; or Itr 200 mg b.i.d	Deoxycholate AmB 0.7–1 mg/kg/d, then Itr 200 mg b.i.d.; surgical removal[c]
Meningitis	Lipid AmB 5 mg/kg/d, then Itr 200 mg b.i.d.	Deoxycholate AmB 0.7–1 mg/kg/d, then 200 mg b.i.d.[d]
Disseminated	Lipid AmB 3–5 mg/kg/d, then Itr 200 mg b.i.d.	Deoxycholate AmB 0.7–1 mg/kg/d, then 200 mg/ b.i.d.[e]
Pregnant women	Lipid AmB 3–5 mg/kg/d or deoxycholate AmB 0.7–1 mg/kg/d for severe disease; local hyperthermia for cutaneous disease	_____[f]
Children	Itr 6–10 mg/kg/d (400 mg/d maximum) for mild disease; deoxycholate AmB 0.7–1 mg/kg/d for severe disease	SSKI with increasing doses for mild disease.[g]

AmB, amphotericin B; b.i.d., twice per day; Itr, itraconazole; SSKI, saturated solution of potassium iodide.

[a] Treat for 2–4 weeks after lesions resolve.
[b] Switch to Itr after favorable response if AmB used. Treat for a total of at least 12 months.
[c] Treat severe disease with an AmB formulation followed by Itr. Treat less severe disease with Itr. Treat for a total of at least 12 months.
[d] Length of therapy with AmB is not established, but therapy for at least 4–5 weeks is recommended. Treat for a total of at least 12 months. May require long-term suppression with Itr.
[e] Therapy with AmB should be continued until the patient shows objective evidence of improvement. Treat for a total of at least 12 months; may require long-term suppression with Itr.
[f] It is preferable to wait until after delivery to treat non–life-threatening forms of sporotrichosis.
[g] Treat severe disease with an AmB formulation followed by Itr.

Data adapted from (31).

Zygomycoses

The term "zygomycosis" characterizes any disease caused by fungi of the *Zygomycetes* class, and includes two groups of pathogenic microorganisms of medical importance: the order of the *Mucorales* and that of the *Entomophthorales*.[39] Several species of genera *Rhizopus* (Figures 13.13 and 13.14), *Mucor*, and *Absidia* may cause the disease.

Mucorales cause an aggressive disease called mucormycosis, which is angioinvasive, rapidly destructive, and in most cases fatal.

Although *Entomophthorales*, responsible for entomophthoromycoses, are known for causing mucocutaneous and subcutaneous, painless, and chronic infections, recently a change in the profile of virulence and geographic distribution of those fungi was found that can cause clinical syndromes that are indistinguishable from those caused by the *Mucorales*, making a differentiation between the two orders impossible, based solely on epidemiologic observation or even at histopathologic examination.[40]

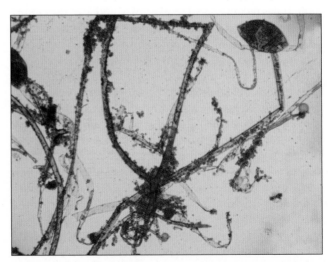

FIGURE 13.14: Rhizopus sp. – culture microscopy. (Photo courtesy of Mycology Laboratory – HUCFF/UFRJ.)

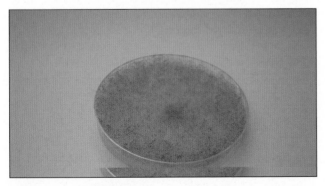

FIGURE 13.13: **Rhizopus** *sp. – culture. (Photo courtesy of Mycology Laboratory – HUCFF/UFRJ.)*

TABLE 13.5: Factors Predisposing Patients to Zygomycosis

Diabetes mellitus
Diabetic ketoacidosis
Poorly controlled diabetes mellitus
Chronic metabolic acidosis
Renal failure
Chronic salicylate poisoning
Deferoxamine therapy
Iron overload
Immunosuppression
Neutropenia (due to malignances or chemotherapy)
Corticosteroid therapy
Organ or hematopoietic cell transplantation
Human immunodeficiency virus infection
Skin or soft tissue breakdown
Burn
Trauma
Surgical wound
Miscellaneous
Intravenous illicit drug use
Neonatal prematurity
Malnourishment
Prolonged use of broad-spectrum antimicrobial agents

Data adapted from (39).

Despite the majority of zygomycosis cases being caused by *Mucorales*, the term zygomycosis is preferable to mucormycosis, for being more encompassing and designating disease even when the cultures are not available and identification of the fungus is not made.

Recent studies show that zygomycosis is an emerging non-*Aspergillus* mycosis of relevant significance, in part due to the constant increase of cases of diabetes and growing use of immunosuppressive drugs available from the progress of modern medicine.

Inhalation, ingestion, and cutaneous exposure to microorganisms are the main infection sources, and the predisposing factors are listed in Table 13.5.[39]

Diabetes mellitus with metabolic acidosis is implicated in the most cases (36%–88%), although zygomycosis has been observed in metabolically controlled diabetes patients.

The average survival rate in diabetic patients with zygomycosis is approximately 60%. The relative treatment facility of acute complications, compared with the remaining immunocompromising conditions, helps to explain the lower mortality rate in cases of zygomycosis associated with diabetes mellitus.

The excess of iron (by transfusion or by dyserythropoiesis) in addition to therapy with deferoxamine for treatment of excessive albumin and/or iron in patients in dialysis is an important risk factor for angioinvasive zygomycoses.

Some recent studies show, that 78% of patients in dialytic regime and with zygomycosis were treated with deferoxamine.[41] The more common presentation of the disease was the disseminated (44%), followed by the rhinocerebral form (31%).

Zygomycosis associated with deferoxamine therapy presents great mortality, approximately 80%,[39] and in immunosuppressed patients it is frequently fatal (68%–100%). A prolonged neutropenia represents the greatest risk factor of this group, approximately 15% of all cases of zygomycosis.

Pulmonary disease is the most common presentation in neutropenic patients, with the disseminated form more common in individuals with greater immunosuppression. Systemic steroids are another factor favoring zygomycosis, whether by action of macrophages and neutrophils or by steroid-induced diabetes. Patients with AIDS are known to be at risk; however, the majority of cases of zygomycosis in human immunodeficiency virus (HIV)-infected persons are also associated with IV drug abuse.[42]

Temporary local trauma and burns can also lead to accidental inoculation of fungus spores, generating cutaneous disease even in immunocompetent hosts. The use of broad-spectrum antibiotics and topical preparations with antibacterial effect in burned patients seems to increase the risk of cutaneous fungal infection significantly, including cutaneous zygomycosis.[43]

Other predisposing factors include abuse of illicit IV drugs, premature neonatality, malnutrition, sites of IV catheter insertion, and extensive therapy with broad-spectrum antimicrobials.

Recent reports of prolonged use of voriconazole for prophylaxis and treatment of invasive fungal infections revealed great risk for several forms of zygomycosis.[39,44]

Based on the clinical presentations and involvement sites, zygomycoses can be classified as rhinocerebral, pulmonary, cutaneous, GI, disseminated, and miscellaneous, as involvement of CNS without alteration of the paranasal sinuses, endocarditis, and pyelonephritis.

Primary cutaneous commitment varies among edemas, pustules, plates, bullae, nodules, ulcerations, gangrene-like ecthyma lesions, necrotizing fasciitis, osteomyelitis, and dissemination of the infection.[39] Cutaneous manifestations of hematogenic dissemination frequently result in painful erythematous lesions, cellulite-like, with central necrosis and eschar, resulting from the angioinvasive action of the fungus.[39]

There is a certain correlation between the predisposing factor and the clinical site or form of the disease, as can be seen in Table 13.6.

In case of a clinical suspicion, the diagnosis of zygomycosis can be made thru histopathologic examination of the supposedly committed tissues, in which characteristic broad, hyaline, ribbon-like, wide-angled branching, pauciseptate irregular fungal hyphae accompanying tissue necrosis and angioinvasion of the fungi are found. The tissue invasion by hyphae is essential for the diagnosis. The samples can be stained routinely by H&E, but the fungal elements are better observed by special stains such as the GMS, PAS, or calcofluor white stain. Perineural invasion

TABLE 13.6: Relationship between Predisposing Condition and Site of Infection

Predisposing condition	Predominant site of infection (in decreasing order of frequency)
Diabetic ketoacidosis	Rhinocerebral and pulmonary
Iron overload and deferoxamine	Disseminated and rhinocerebral
Neutropenia	Pulmonary and disseminated
Corticosteroids and immunosuppression	Pulmonary, disseminated, or rhinocerebral
Trauma, catheter/injection sites	Cutaneous/subcutaneous
Malnourishment	GI
Prolonged broad-spectrum azole use	Pulmonary, disseminated, GI, or rhinocerebral

GI, gastrointestinal.
Data adapted from (44).

is seen in 90% of tissues containing such elements for sampling. The inflammatory response can be absent, or there may be neutrophils or granulomas.[39]

Large hyaline, nonseptated or irregularly septated, thick-walled hyphae (coenocytic hyphae) can be observed directly in samples from a bronchoalveolar wash and also from other materials prepared with potassium hydroxide (Figure 13.15). Direct immunofluorescence can be employed with samples prepared for maceration by potassium hydroxide and use of calcofluor white, blank fluor, or UVITEX.

The differentiation between zygomycoses (mucormycosis/entomophthoromycosis) can be made by some histopathologic peculiarities: broad fungal hyphae with sparsely found septum surrounded by eosinophilic granular material (Splendore–Hoeppli phenomenon) and peripheral eosinophilia, which are not usually seen in *Mucorales*, favoring the suspicion of *Entomophthorales*.[39]

Hemocultures in all forms of zygomycoses are frequently negative, even when fungal hyphae are observed at histopathologic examination, but it is important that the physician endeavors to exhaustively try to identify the agent, aiming at better guiding his or her therapy, because the differentiation of *Mucorales/Entomophthorales* with other filamentous fungi at histopathologic examination is difficult.

Contamination of clinical samples by *Zygomycetes* is common due to the small size of the sporangiospores, facilitating their airborne dissemination. In any case, isolation of *Mucorales/Entomophthorales* from sterile sites or repeatedly positive nonsterile cultures in patients with significant risk factors should be considered highly suspect.

Different techniques of molecular serological examinations are appearing, but are not being recommended as routine procedures because of lack of studies and few satisfactory results.

Despite the growing clinical suspicion of the cases of zygomycoses, based on the best knowledge of the predisposing factors, more than half of the mucormycosis diagnoses are obtained postmortem.

The treatment of patients with zygomycosis by *Mucorales* is frustrating; therefore, an early diagnosis should be the objective in patients with high risk, and treatment should be initiated as soon as possible. A multifactor approach should be initiated as early as possible. They are appropriate antifungal therapy, surgical debridement, and correction or resolution of the predisposing factors, such as control of comorbidities and adjuvant therapies for improving the host's immune response.

Despite frequent use of amphotericin B deoxycholate (1–1.5 mg/kg/d), lipidic amphotericin B formulations represent the first line of treatment because it is potentially the least toxic and it has better clinical response than do high doses. Those compounds should be used in initial doses of 5 mg/kg/d, increasing to significant doses and for an extended time, not less than 6–8 weeks.[44]

Among the azolic compounds, itraconazole has action in some strains of *Mucorales*; however, it has been implicated as a risk factor for zygomycosis in prolonged use. Of the second-generation imidazoles, voriconazole is not effective in vitro. It has also been frequently implicated in cases of zygomycosis with long-term use after prophylaxis for other systemic fungal infections. Posaconazole and

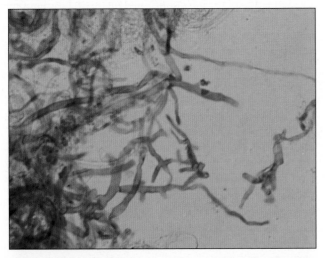

FIGURE 13.15: *Zygomycosis – direct examination – kenocytic hyphae in KOH and Parker ink. (Photo courtesy of Mycology Laboratory – HUCFF/UFRJ.)*

ravuconazole have in vitro action against agents of mucormycosis. There are promising reports regarding the use of posaconazole as monotherapy or in combination with lipidic formulations of amphotericin B.[44]

Caspofungin and micafungin seem to be ineffective as monotherapy, but present a synergic effect when used with amphotericin B.[44]

Zygomycosis (mucormycosis) is rapidly progressive, and an antifungal therapy alone is inadequate to control the infection. The numerous agents of zygomycosis have a wide spectrum of susceptibility to drugs used, and some can be highly resistant to amphotericin B. Additionally, thrombosis and tissue necrosis resulting from angioinvasion generate an environment with poor penetration by systemic agents into the sites affected by the infection.[39] Even if the causative agent is susceptible and the drug does penetrate the affected site appropriately, tissue necrosis is not prevented with the death of the microorganism.[39] Surgical debridement is crucial and highly recommended, and should be initiated quickly and repeated several times, which may cause deformities.

Correction of the metabolic disturbances and reversal of the immunosuppression are essential for the treatment of zygomycosis. In patients with diabetic ketoacidosis, the hyperglycemia and the acidosis should be corrected as soon as possible. Immunosuppressors, especially systemic steroids, should be discontinued, if possible, or at least have their doses significantly reduced.

The main role of iron metabolism in the pathogenesis of zygomycosis suggests the possibility of using iron chelate as therapeutic adjuvant. In contrast to deferoxamine, other oral iron chelates did not allow an iron offer to the microorganism and did not favor the growth of the same in vitro.[44]

Ibrahim and colleagues[45] demonstrated the protecting action of deferasirox in mice.

Despite cytokines not being recommended as routine, granulocyte-macrophage colony-stimulating factor and granulocyte colony-stimulating factor as adjuvant therapy have been considered in cases of conventional therapy failure.

The use of hyperbaric oxygen therapy finds support in the hypothesis that the high oxygen pressure might improve the capacity of the macrophages to fight the infection.[44]

HISTOPLASMOSIS

Histoplasma capsulatum var. capsulatum infection is a common infection in areas of the United States and Latin America where it is endemic, but some cases have also been reported from Europe. In the United States, most cases have occurred within the Ohio and Mississippi River valleys (moderate climate, humidity, and soil characteristics). Bird and bat excrement enhances the growth of the organism in soil by accelerating sporulation. Air currents carry the conidia for miles, exposing individuals who were unaware of contact with the contaminated site. Histoplasmosis causes

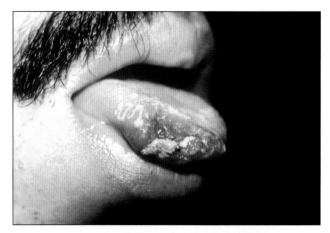

FIGURE 13.16: *Histoplasmosis – lesion on the tongue in a patient with AIDS.*

progressive infection in immunocompromised individuals and in persons with underlying chronic lung disease. Certain forms of histoplasmosis cause life-threatening illnesses and result in considerable morbidity, whereas other manifestations cause either no symptoms or minor self-limited illnesses.[46]

In some cases of immune depression (Figures 13.16 and 13.17), disseminated histoplasmosis appears in the eyes, oral cavity, larynx, CNS, GI tract, and, more rarely, the nasosinusal region.[47]

Laboratory diagnosis is made by direct examination in which, with special staining, small round intracellular fungal structures may be observed (Figure 13.18). The small round forms, similar to *Leishmania*, can also be seen in histopathological preparations. At 25°C, the colonies have a cotton aspect and are a white to beige color, whereas at 37°C they are leveduriform (Figures 13.19 and 13.20). In microscopy, hyaline, septated, and branched hyphae; thick and spiculated walled, round macroconidia; and oval microconidia are observed (Figure 13.21).

The treatment is indicated only in patients with chronic pulmonary disease and in those with severe forms of acute pulmonary illnesses or in those with the disseminated form of infection with mild to moderately severe manifestations. In patients with AIDS, the treatment may fail because the absorption is variable, resulting in the inability to achieve therapeutic concentrations in blood.[48,49]

PARASITIC DISEASES

American Trypanosomiasis or Chagas Disease

Trypanosomiasis is a tropical and mainly rural parasitic disease of blood and various organs. There are two different entities: African, caused by trypanosomes of the *Trypanosoma brucei* group (*T. gambiense* and *T. rhodesiense*), transmitted by tsetse flies, also called sleeping sickness; and Chagas disease, also known as American trypanosomiasis.[50]

Chagas disease, described in 1909 by Carlos Chagas, occurs in rural areas, in wattle and daub houses in

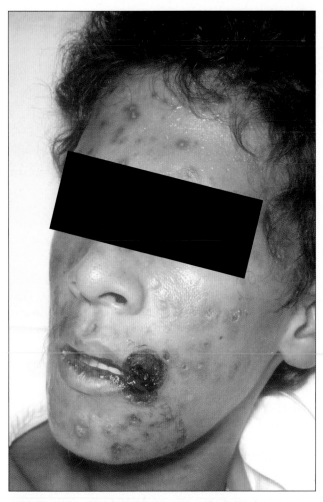

FIGURE 13.17: *Histoplasmosis – disseminated lesions and herpes infection on the left side of the lip in a patient with AIDS.*

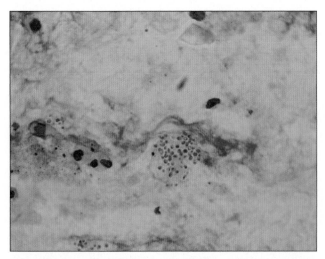

FIGURE 13.18: Histoplasma capsulatum – *direct examination – Giemsa stain. (Photo courtesy of Mycology Laboratory – HUCFF/UFRJ.)*

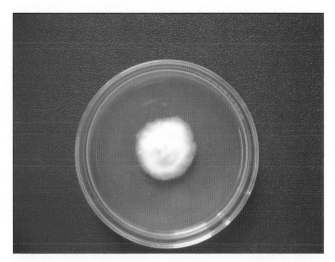

FIGURE 13.19: Histoplasma capsulatum – *culture at 25°C. (Photo courtesy of Mycology Laboratory – HUCFF/UFRJ.)*

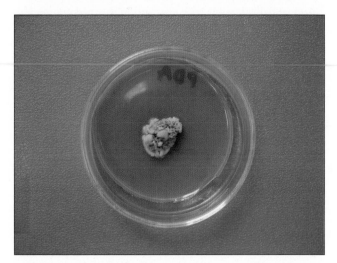

FIGURE 13.20: Histoplasma capsulatum – *culture at 37°C. (Photo courtesy of Mycology Laboratory – HUCFF/UFRJ.)*

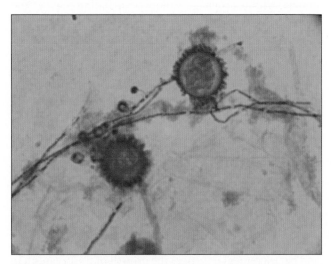

FIGURE 13.21: Histoplasma capsulatum – *culture microscopy. (Photo courtesy of Mycology Laboratory – HUCFF/UFRJ.)*

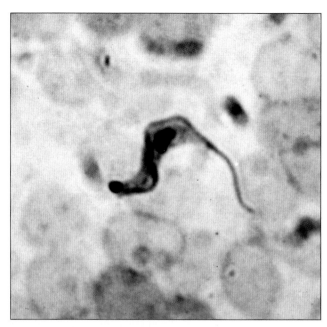

FIGURE 13.22: *Trypanosoma cruzi. (Photo courtesy of Luis Rey, MD, Rio de Janeiro, RJ, Brazil.)*

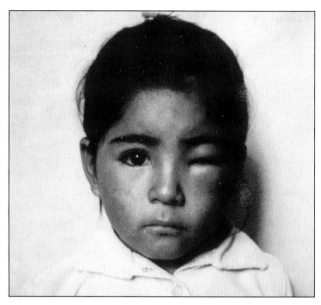

FIGURE 13.24: *Chagas disease – Romaña sign. (Photo courtesy of João Dias, MD, and Luis Rey, MD, Rio de Janeiro, RJ, Brazil.)*

tropical zones of the Americas. It is also called Trypanosomiasis americana and is caused by *Trypanosoma cruzi*, a parasite of humans and domestic or wild animals. The transmission is through a sting by the vector animal, the triatominae ("*barbeiro*"). Age, sex, and race do not influence the incidence of the disease, despite the acute phase being more frequent in children.[51]

Chagas disease is produced by a hemoflagellated protozoan, *Trypanosoma cruzi* (Chagas, 1909) (Figure 13.22), affecting humans and various domestic or wild mammals that act as reservoirs. It is transmitted by bloodsucking invertebrates of the order Hemiptera, genera *Triatoma*, *Panstrongylus*, and *Rhodnius*, called reduviid, assassin, or kissing bugs and "barbeiro" in Brazil (Figure 13.23). Transfusional and congenital infections are also possible, although rare.[50]

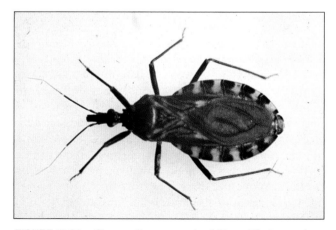

FIGURE 13.23: *Chagas disease – reduviid bug. (Photo courtesy of Luis Rey, MD, Rio de Janeiro, RJ, Brazil.)*

Two cycles of circulation of the parasite are known in nature: the wild and the domestic. The wild cycle occurs among marsupials, rodents, monkeys, mice, rabbits, and the triatomid. The domestic cycle results from contamination of animals that live in the vicinity of human dwellings. The trypomastigote form circulates in the peripheral blood of vertebrates; undergoes transformation in the organism of the vector to the epimastigote form; and multiplies, becoming metacyclic trypomastigotes in the digestive system of the triatomine.[51] The main species of this arthropod is *Triatoma infestans* (Argentina, Bolivia, Brazil, Chile, Paraguay, Peru, and Uruguay), *Rhodnius prolixus* (Colombia, Guyana, Venezuela, and Central America), and *Panstrongylus megistus* (Brazil). Transmission occurs through the feces of triatominae, which habitually defecate while feeding.[52–54]

Acute Chagas disease is more frequently seen in children and begins with inflammatory lesions at the inoculation site of the parasite in the skin or conjunctiva, called Romaña sign (Figure 13.24). The inoculation chagoma is a macular or papulonodular lesion, erythematous-violet, hard and painless, that can ulcerate, but tends to regress in 3 weeks. Other signs of disease are satellite lymphadenitis, fever, indisposition, cephalea, myalgia, hepatosplenomegaly, and maculopapular, morbilliform, or urticariform cutaneous rashes (schizotrypanis).

The following phases may present megaesophagus megacolon and affection of the heart, with myocarditis, arrhythmias, and complete blocking.[50,53,55]

During the acute phase, direct examination of Giemsa-stained blood smears, imprints of skin, or lymph-node biopsy can easily show the parasite.[50] The search for anti-*T. cruzi* immunoglobulin M antibodies by indirect immunofluorescence and PCR and (in the chronic phase) serological tests with indirect hemagglutination, indirect immunofluorescence, and ELISA are useful.[56] They can also be demonstrated by blood culture in NNN medium or by animal inoculation.[50]

Xenodiagnosis of Brumpt is also helpful. For this an uninfected reduviid bug is allowed to bite and feed on the forearm of the suspect patient; 30–60 days later, the insect's feces are examined for the infective form. During the chronic phase, the Machado–Guerreiro complement fixation test using antigens of cultured T. cruzi is most useful. ELISA, hemagglutination, indirect immunofluorescence, and PCR can also diagnose the disease.[50]

The therapeutics are unsatisfactory, and treatment does not change the serological reactions or degradation of cardiac function in chronic phases, despite possibly curing the patient in the acute phase. The two main drugs, benznidazole and nifurtimox, are active against circulating and tissue forms and should be administered for 30–90 days.[51,55,57]

For patients with stable chronic disease, the treatment includes antiarrhythmics and control of the affected systems. Prevention of the disease requires sanitary education and use of insecticides.[51,57]

Schistosomiasis

Schistosomiasis is one of the most important helminthic infections because of its wide geographical distribution and extensive pathological effect. It is a systemic disease, and its causative agents are human trematodes or flukes. These trematodes affect approximately 200 million people worldwide, mainly in the tropical and subtropical latitudes; sometimes entire communities are affected. Most infected persons experience few, if any, signs and symptoms, and only a small minority develop significant disease.[58,59]

Schistosomiasis or bilharziasis is an infection caused by five types of blood flukes of the genus *Schistosoma*. Humans are infected by the cercarial stage of the parasites released from freshwater snails in ponds, canals, lake edges, and streams. Penetration of intact skin occurs rapidly, and the schistosomes migrate into the portal system to mate and then to a part of the venous system to lay eggs. High infection rates persist among both the rural and urban poor. Rural living, poor housing and water supplies, and low educational level are major factors in schistosomiasis occurrence among agricultural populations.[60]

In Brazilian urban areas, prevailing living conditions in shantytowns and labor migrations from and periodic return movements to rural areas were predictive of schistosomiasis. The risk of the establishment of new transmission foci exists in both rural and urban areas, conferred by and affecting poorer people.[61–63]

In sub-Saharan Africa there is high prevalence of parasitic worm infections, such as schistosomiasis. The hypothesis of whether a helminth infection increases the susceptibility of the host to acquire de novo infection with

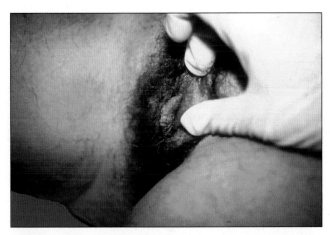

FIGURE 13.25: *Schistosomiasis – vulval granuloma.* Reproduced from Parish et al. (2001).[60]

an immunodeficiency virus after mucosal exposure, which is the predominant route of HIV transmission in humans, has been tested by Chenine and colleagues.[64] They quantified the amount of a clade C simian–human immunodeficiency virus needed to infect rhesus macaques that had acute *Schistosoma mansoni* infections compared with control animals exposed to virus alone. The schistosome-infected monkeys also had significantly higher levels of initial virus replication and loss of a certain subset of memory T cells, both predictors of a more rapid progression to immune dysfunction. Research suggested that worm infections may increase the risk of individuals with viral exposures becoming infected with HIV-1 and also suggested that control programs for schistosomiasis and perhaps other parasitic worm infections may also be useful in helping to reduce the spread of HIV/AIDS in developing countries where helminths are endemic.

Contrary to previous reports that indicated no transmission of schistosomiasis at altitudes higher than >1400 m, John and colleagues[65] found that schistosomiasis transmission can take place at an altitude range of 1487–1682 m above sea level in western Uganda.

Eggs laid in bladder and pelvic and rectal venous plexuses return to the local water supply to complete the cycle through the snail population. Cercarial penetration of the skin may produce an itch eruption, which may be followed by myalgia, headache, and abdominal pain.

Abdominal pain, diarrhea, malabsorption, and (occasionally) intestinal obstruction and rectal prolapse; cirrhosis of the liver associated with portal hypertension, splenomegaly, and esophageal varices; recurrent hematuria and eventually bladder calcification; and obstructive uropathy and renal failure are late manifestations of the disease. Periovular or schistosomotic granuloma may rarely occur on the skin or vulva (Figure 13.25). Migration of eggs to the lungs may cause massive chronic fibrosis.

Detection of the characteristic ova in the stools, in urine, or on biopsy (Figure 13.26) or with an ELISA make the

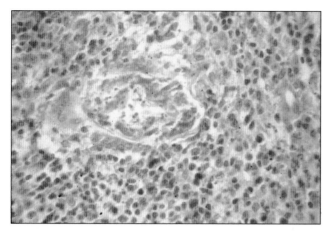

FIGURE 13.26: *Schistosomiasis – biopsy of vulval granuloma showing egg and inflammatory infiltrate. Reproduced from Parish et al. (2001).[60]*

diagnosis. Treatment of patients is made with praziquantel given as a single dose.[61–63]

Amebiasis

Amebiasis is an intestinal parasitic disease that may sometimes affect the skin, especially perianal and genital. It is caused by a common and worldwide intestinal unicellular parasite, *Entamoeba histolytica*, the only human pathogenic species of this genus. The invasive form found in the tissues is a 20- to 40-μm elongated cell, with pseudopods on its surface.[50,66]

E. histolytica is the pathogenic ameba that can cause invasive intestinal and extraintestinal disease. The most frequent manifestations of invasive amebiasis are colitis and liver abscesses. *E. histolytica* invades the colonic mucosa, and the patient suffers from bloody diarrhea. It is one of the most common parasitic infections worldwide, and the possibility of amebiasis must always be considered in a patient who complains of bloody diarrhea and has recently returned from a developing country. In industrialized counties where the *E. histolytica* endemicity is generally low, invasive disease may occur in men who have sex with men.[67]

In tissues, the trophozoites – with a basophilic and elongated cytoplasm, single eccentric nucleus, and central spherical karyosome – are difficult to observe. In cutaneous and mucosal lesions, they are more easily seen in biopsies of the borders rather than the center of the ulcer.[50]

E. histolytica is a pathogenic ameba that recent studies indicate is an increased risk for invasive amebiasis among persons with HIV.[68] The infestation by this species is a public health concern because it has the potential to become endemic and to cause severe disease, such as acute dysenteric symptoms (malaise, fever, abdominal pain, and frequent loose stools containing blood and mucus); granulomatous masses in the bowel wall (amoeboma); liver abscess; and pleura, lung, and pericardium involvement.[56]

Vegetative forms of amebae should be sought in fresh stools or in scrapings from bowel ulcers at sigmoidoscopy. Ultrasound, computed tomography, or aspiration diagnoses suspected liver abscess. The effective treatment is made with metronidazole.[56]

Patients can be rapidly cured in 7–20 days with metronidazole, 20–40 mg/kg/day, divided in three daily doses, for up to 8 days. Tinidazole, in a single daily dosage, 2 g for adults and 50–60 mg/kg for children, for 3–5 days, also shows good and fast results. IV or intramuscular dehydroemetine hydrochloride, the drug of choice in the past, is cardiotoxic. Diiodohydroxyquinoline, paromomycin, and diloxanide furoate can also be used. Severe dysentery associated with mucosal or cutaneous involvement requires support measures.[50,66]

Mucocutaneous Leishmaniasis

Leishmaniasis is an anthropozoonosis of worldwide distribution, being considered a public health problem in 88 countries, distributed in four continents, in the Americas, Europe, Africa, and Asia. On the American continent there are records of cases from the extreme southern part of the United States to north of Argentina, with the exception of Chile and Uruguay.[20,56,57,66,69]

Leishmania belongs to the Trypanosomatidae family of protozoa. It is a mandatory intracellular parasite of the mononuclear phagocyte system, with two main forms: a flagellated or promastigote, observed in the digestive tube of the vector insect, and another aflagellated or amastigote, found in the tissues of vertebrate hosts. Currently in the Americas, there are 11 known dermotropic species of *Leishmania* causative of disease in humans and eight species described only in animals, all belonging to the subgenera *Viannia* and *Leishmania*. The three main species are: *L.(V.) braziliensis*, *L.(V.) guyanensis*, and *L.(L.) amazonensis*.[57,69]

The vectors are insects called Phlebotominae, belonging to the order Diptera, family *Psychodidae*, subfamily *Phlebotominae*, genus *Lutzomyia*, also known popularly as sandflies, and, depending on the geographical location in Brazil, as *mosquito palha*, *tatuquira*, and *birigui*, among others. The reservoirs can be forest animals (such as rodents and marsupials), synanthropic and domestic (canidae, felidae, and equidae, considered accidental hosts of the disease).[57]

The transmission occurs through a sting by the infected transmitter insects without distinction regarding sex, race, or age, without person-to-person transmission. The majority of cases occur in men between 20 and 40 years old. The disease incubation period in humans may vary from 2 weeks to 2 years, with an average of 2–3 months.[57,66] Epidemiological analyses have suggested changes in the transmission pattern of the disease passing from a sylvestral animal zoonosis to a disease of rural zones, in practically barren and periurban areas. There are three epidemiological profiles: sylvestral, in which the transmission occurs in areas of primary vegetation (zoonosis of sylvestral animals);

occupational, associated with irregular forest exploration and forest slashing (anthropozoonosis); and rural or peri-urban, in areas around cities or colonized regions, where the vector undergoes an adaptation to the peridomicile (zoonosis of residual woods and/or anthropozoonosis).[57]

The transmission cycles differ according to the geographic variations, involving several types of parasites, vectors, reservoirs, and hosts. *L. (L.) amazonensis* is present in primary and secondary forests of the "Legal Amazonia" (Amazonas, Pará, Rondônia, Tocantins, and Maranhão), and also in the states of the Northeast Region (Bahia), Southwest (Minas Gerais and São Paulo), Midwest (Goiás), and South (Paraná) of Brazil. It causes localized cutaneous ulcers and, occasionally, some individuals can develop a classical diffuse cutaneous leishmaniasis. *L. (V.) guyanensis* is found in onshore forests and is apparently restricted to the North Region of Brazil (Acre, Amapá, Roraima, Amazonas, and Pará) and Guyana, Suriname, and French Guiana. It causes single or multiple cutaneous ulcers, with the latter resulting from simultaneous stings of several infected phlebotoma or secondary lymphatic metastases. Mucous involvement is rare. In endemic areas, besides young males, a great number of children can be affected. *L. (V.) braziliensis* is a widespread species, occurring from Central America and all over Brazil to the North of Argentina. In the areas of modified environments, transmission occurs in the surroundings of the dwellings, affecting individuals of both genders and all age groups, with a tendency to concentrate the cases in a single focus. The lesions that are characterized by cutaneous ulcer (single or multiple) or the main complication, which is the hematogenic metastasis to the mucous membranes of the nasopharynx, with tissue destruction, can occur in the eyelids or in areas usually covered by clothes, suggesting that the transmission with great frequency occurs inside human dwellings.[57,69]

When introduced into the skin, promastigotes meet the immune system cells, as T and B lymphocytes, macrophages, Langerhans cells, and mastocytes. Through a not entirely clarified mechanism, the parasite adheres to the surface of the macrophages and Langerhans cells, passing into the intracellular media and changing into the amastigote form, characteristic of parasitism in mammals. The leishmania develop defense mechanisms capable of subverting the microbicidal capacity of the macrophages, surviving and multiplying until cell rupture occurs, when they are freed to infect other macrophages and propagate the infection. The location of the amastigote in the interior of macrophages makes the control of the infection become dependent on the immune response mediated by the cells. The main effecting cell is the macrophage itself, after its activation by T-helper lymphocyte cells. Even with the diversity of *Leishmania* species, the spectrum of clinical manifestations of the disease depends not only on the species involved, but also on the infected individual's immunologic state. With cutaneous leishmaniasis, the cutaneous test with leishmanin, the intradermal

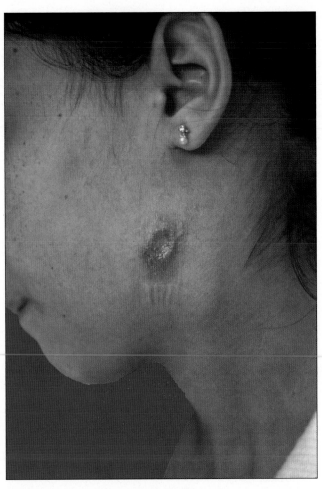

FIGURE 13.27: *Leishmaniasis – ulcer on the side of the neck with a visible lymph-node enlargement.*

reaction of Montenegro (IDRM), and other in vitro tests are positive. Cutaneous leishmaniasis can be caused by all dermotropic species of *Leishmania*. There are clinical differences, however, such as those observed in lesions caused by *L. (L.) amazonensis* that present more infiltrated borders, with great amounts of parasites, whereas in those caused by the subgenus *Viannia*, few macrophages and parasites are present.[57,66,69]

An infection is called unapparent when characterized by positive serological and IDRM tests in apparently healthy individuals, living in areas of mucocutaneous leishmaniasis without previous clinical history. Lymph-node leishmaniasis is characterized by localized lymph adenopathy without tegumentary lesion. Cutaneous leishmaniasis presents as a rounded or oval painless ulcer, of few or several millimeters, located in exposed sites of the skin, with an erythematous and infiltrated base, with well-delimited and raised borders, reddish background, and coarse granulations (Figure 13.27). Vegetating lesions also occur, either papillomatous or verrucous, as well as lesions with associated bacterial infection (Figure 13.28). The lesions tend to cure spontaneously with atrophic, depressed scars, with hypo- or hyperpigmentation and fibrosis in variable periods, but

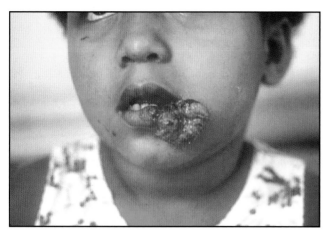

FIGURE 13.28: *Leishmaniasis – vegetating lesion on the lip. Reproduced from Ramos-e-Silva et al. (2002).*[69]

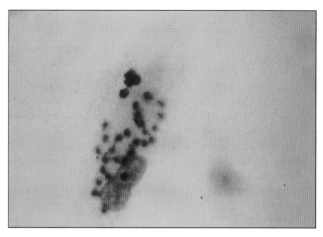

FIGURE 13.29: *Leishmaniasis – amastigote inside a macrophage.*

may remain active for several years and coexist with later emergence of mucous lesions. The disseminated mucocutaneous leishmaniasis form is relatively rare, being observed in up to 2% of the cases. The two species recognized as causes of this syndrome are *L. (V.) braziliensis and L. (L.) amazonensis*. There is emergence of multiple papular lesions with an acneiform aspect, on several segments of the body, mainly in face and trunk, followed by hematic or lymphatic dissemination of the parasite, sometimes within 24 hours, causing distant lesions from the site of the sting. Concurrent mucous affection has been observed in up to 30% of the patients, and systemic manifestations can also appear, as fever, general indisposition, muscle pains, weight loss, and anorexia, among others. Finding the parasite in the disseminated form is uncommon when compared to the diffuse form. The titers of serous anti-Leishmania antibodies are high, and the response to the IDRM is variable. In individuals co-infected by HIV, ulcerated lesions prevail. The diffuse cutaneous form is severe, albeit rare, and occurs in patients with lack of energy and specific deficiency in the cellular immune response to Leishmania antigens. In Brazil, it is caused by *L. (L.) amazonensis*. The response to the therapeutics is poor or absent, and IDRM is usually negative. It is estimated that 3%–5% of cutaneous cases develop a painless mucous lesion, destructive of the upper respiratory tract due to hematic or lymphatic dissemination. Patients with multiple cutaneous, extensive lesions with more than 1 year of evolution and located above the waist are the group with greater risk of developing metastases in the mucous membrane. The etiologic agent causative of mucosal lesions, in Brazil, is mainly *L. (V.) braziliensis*. IDRM is strongly positive; however, it has difficult parasitological confirmation due to the scarceness of parasites, presents difficult therapeutic response, has a higher complication frequency, is mainly infectious, and may result in death in 1% of the cases.[66]

The clinical–epidemilogical diagnosis is complemented by positive IDRM. Direct demonstration of the parasite is the procedure of first choice because it is faster, less expensive, and easy to execute (Figure 13.29). The probability of finding the parasite is inversely proportional to the time of evolution of the cutaneous lesion, being rare after a year. The isolation in cultivation in vitro is a method that allows the subsequent identification of the species of Leishmania involved. The intradermal test, IDRM, or leishmanin test is based in the response of retarded cellular hypersensibility. Patients with mucous disease usually present an exacerbated IDRM, with several centimeters of hardening, vesiculation in the center of the reaction, possibly with ulceration and local necrosis. In diffuse cutaneous forms, IDRMs are usually negative. Other methods, such as detection of circulating antibodies and PCR, can also be used.[56,69]

The drugs of first choice in the treatment of leishmaniasis are the pentavalent antimonials, considered as leishmanicide drugs, because they interfere in the bioenergetic processes of the amastigote forms of Leishmania. In the case of unsatisfactory response with pentavalent antimonials, the second choice of drugs are amphotericin B and pentamidines. The cure criterion is clinical, being recommended a regular follow-up for 12 months. Cure is defined by epithelization of the ulcerated lesions and total regression of the infiltration and erythema, up to 3 months after the end of treatment. Recurrence is defined as reappearance of the lesion in any part of the body in the period of up to 1 year after clinical cure, discarding the possibility of reinfection. The prophylactic measures are use of insect repellents; use of fine-mesh mosquito nets, as well as the screening of doors and windows; and environmental handling through cleaning of backyards and land areas.[56,57,66]

REFERENCES

1. Segal E. Candida, still number one – what do we know and where are we going from there? Mycoses. 2005; 48 Suppl 1:3–11.
2. Fidel PL Jr. Immunity to Candida. Oral Dis. 2002; 8 Suppl 2:69–75.

3. Flückiger U, Marchetti O, Bille J, et al. Fungal Infection Network of Switzerland (FUNGINOS). Treatment options of invasive fungal infections in adults. Swiss Med Wkly. 2006; 136:447–63.

4. Ferretti G, Mandala M, Di Cosimo S, et al. Catheter-related bloodstream infections, part II: specific pathogens and prevention. Cancer Control. 2003; 10:79–91.

5. Raad I, Hanna H, Maki D. Intravascular catheter-related infections: advances in diagnosis, prevention, and management. Lancet Infect Dis. 2007; 7:645–57.

6. Ellepola AN, Morrison CJ. Laboratory diagnosis of invasive candidiasis. J Microbiol. 2005; 43:65–84.

7. Bae GY, Lee HW, Chang SE, et al. Clinicopathologic review of 19 patients with systemic candidiasis with skin lesions. Int J Dermatol. 2005; 44:550–5.

8. Grossman ME, Silvers DN, Walther RR. Cutaneous manifestations of disseminated candidiasis. J Am Acad Dermatol. 1980; 2:111–16.

9. Fine JD, Miller JA, Harrist TJ, Haynes HA. Cutaneous lesions in disseminated candidiasis mimicking ecthyma gangrenosum. Am J Med. 1981; 70:1133–5.

10. Bodey GP, Luna M. Skin lesions associated with disseminated candidiasis. JAMA. 1974; 229:1466–8.

11. Ruhnke M. Epidemiology of Candida albicans infections and role of non-Candida-albicans yeasts. Curr Drug Targets. 2006; 7:495–504.

12. Anane S, Khalfallah F. [Biological diagnosis of systemic candidiasis: difficulties and future prospects] Pathol Biol (Paris). 2007; 55:262–72.

13. Dunyach C, Bertout S, Phelipeau C, et al.Detection and identification of Candida spp. in human serum by LightCycler real-time polymerase chain reaction. Diagn Microbiol Infect Dis. 2008; 60:263–71.

14. DiNubile MJ, Lupinacci RJ, Strohmaier KM, et al. Invasive candidiasis treated in the intensive care unit: observations from a randomized clinical trial. J Crit Care. 2007; 22:237–44.

15. Martinez R. An update on the use of antifungal agents. J Bras Pneumol. 2006; 32:449–60.

16. Spellberg BJ, Filler SG, Edwards JE Jr. Current treatment strategies for disseminated candidiasis. Clin Infect Dis. 2006; 42:244–51.

17. Maertens J, Boogaerts M. The place for itraconazole in treatment. J Antimicrob Chemother. 2005; 56 Suppl 1:i33–i38.

18. Scott LJ, Simpson D. Voriconazole: a review of its use in the management of invasive fungal infections. Drugs. 2007; 67:269–98.

19. Ozcan SK, Budak F, Willke A, et al. Efficacies of caspofungin and a combination of caspofungin and meropenem in the treatment of murine disseminated candidiasis. APMIS. 2006; 114:829–36.

20. Ramos-e-Silva M. Facial and oral aspects of some venereal and tropical diseases. Acta Dermatovenerol Croat. 2004; 12:173–180.

21. Ramos-e-Silva M, Saraiva Ldo E. Paracoccidioidomycosis. Dermatol Clin. 2008; 26:257–69.

22. Costa RO. Micoses subcutâneas e sistêmicas. In: Ramos-e-Silva M, Castro MCR, editors. Fundamentos de dermatologia. Rio de Janeiro: Atheneu; 2009. pp. 861–73.

23. Shikanai-Yasuda MA, Telles Filho Fde Q, Mendes RP, et al. Guidelines in paracoccidioidomycosis. Rev Soc Bras Med Trop. 2006; 39:297–310.

24. Franco M, Sano A, Kera K, et al. Chlamydospore formation by Paracoccidioides brasiliensis mycelial form. Rev Inst Med Trop Sao Paulo. 1989; 31:151–7.

25. Marques, S. Paracoccidioidomicose: atualização epidemiológica, clínica e terapêutica. An Bras Dermatol. 2003; 78:135–46.

26. Valle ACF, Guimarães RR, Lopes DJ, et al. Aspectos radiológicos torácicos na paracoccidioidomicose. Rev Inst Med Trop S Paulo. 1992; 34:107–15.

27. Felipe MS, Torres FA, Maranhão AQ, et al. Functional genome of the human pathogenic fungus Paracoccidioides brasiliensis. FEMS Immunol Med Microbiol. 2005; 45:369–81.

28. Pinto AR, Puccia R, Diniz SN, et al. DNA-based vaccination against murine paracoccidioidomycosis using the gp43 gene from paracoccidioides brasiliensis. Vaccine. 2000; 18: 3050–8.

29. Morris-Jones R. Sporotrichosis. Clin Exp Dermatol. 2002; 27:427–31.

30. Ramos-e-Silva M, Vasconcelos C, Carneiro S, Cestari T. Sporotrichosis. Clin Dermatol. 2007; 25:181–7.

31. Kauffman CA, Bustamante B, Chapman SW, Pappas PG; Infectious Diseases Society of America. Clinical practice guidelines for the management of sporotrichosis: 2007 update by the Infectious Diseases Society of America. Clin Infect Dis. 2007; 45:1255–65.

32. Conti Diaz IA. Epidemiology of sporotrichosis in Latin America. Mycopathologia. 1989; 108:113–16.

33. Schuback TMP, Melo M, Valle A, et al. Clinical evolution of feline and canine sporotrichosis in Rio de Janeiro. Braz J Vet Sci. 2000; 7 Suppl:38.

34. Barros MB, Schubach Ade O, do Valle AC, et al. Cat-transmitted sporotrichosis epidemic in Rio de Janeiro, Brazil: description of a series of cases. Clin Infect Dis. 2004; 38:529–35.

35. Kong X, Xiao T, Lin J, et al. Relationships among genotypes, virulence and clinical forms of Sporothrix schenckii infection. Clin Microbiol Infect. 2006; 12:1077–81.

36. Wu JJ, Pang KR, Huang DB, Tyring SK. Therapy of systemic fungal infections. Dermatol Ther. 2004; 17:523–31.

37. Kauffman CA. Old and new therapies for sporotrichosis. Clin Infect Dis. 1995; 21:981–5.

38. Romero-Martinez R, Wheeler M, Guerrero-Plata A, et al. Biosynthesis and functions of melanin in Sporothrix schenckii. Infect Immun. 2000; 68:3696–703.

39. Chayakulkeeree M, Ghannoum MA, Perfect JR. Zygomycosis: the re-emerging fungal infection. Eur J Clin Microbiol Infect Dis. 2006; 25:215–29.

40. Gonzalez CE, Rinaldi MG, Sugar AM. Zygomycosis. Infect Dis Clin North Am. 2002; 16:895–914.

41. Boelaert JR, Fenves AZ, Coburn JW. Deferoxamine therapy and mucormycosis in dialysis patients: report of an international registry. Am J Kidney Dis. 1991; 18:660–7.

42. Van Den Saffele JK, Boelaert JR. Zygomycosis in HIV-positive patients: a review of the literature. Mycoses. 1996; 39:77–84.

43. Nash G, Foley FD, Goodwin MN Jr., et al. Fungal burn wound infection. JAMA. 1971; 215:1664–6.

44. Spellberg B, Edwards J Jr., Ibrahim A. Novel perspectives on mucormycosis: pathophysiology, presentation, and management. Clin Microbiol Rev. 2005; 18:556–69.

45. Ibrahim AS, Gebermariam T, Fu Y, et al. The iron chelator deferasirox protects mice from mucormycosis through iron starvation. J Clin Invest. 2007; 117:2649–57.

46. Kauffman CA. Histoplasmosis: a clinical and laboratory update. Clin Microbiol Rev. 2007; 20:115–32.

47. Ceccato F, Gongora V, Zunino A, et al. Unusual manifestation of histoplasmosis in connective tissue diseases. Clin Rheumatol. 2007; 26:1717–19.

48. Mora DJ, dos Santos CT, Silva-Vergara ML. Disseminated histoplasmosis in acquired immunodeficiency syndrome patients in Uberaba, MG, Brazil. Mycoses. 2008; 51:136–40.

49. Wheat LJ, Freifeld AG, Kleiman MB, et al. Clinical Practice Guidelines for the Management of Patients with Histoplasmosis: 2007 Update by the Infectious Diseases Society of America. Clin Infect Dis. 2007; 45:807–25.

50. Ramos-e-Silva M. Diseases of the oral cavity caused by protozoa. In: Lotti TM, Parish LC, Rogers III RS, editors. Oral diseases. Textbook and Atlas. Berlin: Springer-Verlag; 1999. pp. 122–5.

51. Gurtler RE, Diotaiuti L, Kitron U. Chagas disease: 100 years since discovery and lessons for the future. Int J Epidemiol. 2008; 37:698–701.

52. Gurtler RE, Segura EL, Cohen JE. Congenital transmisión of Trypanosoma cruzi infection in Argentina. Emerg Infect Dis. 2003; 9:29–32.

53. Rassi A Jr., Rassi A, Little WC, et al. Development and validation of a risk score for predicting death in Chagas' heart disease. N Engl J Med. 2006; 355:799–808.

54. Dias JP, Bastos C, Araújo E, et al. Acute Chagas disease outbreak associated with oral transmission. Rev Soc Bras Med Trop. 2008; 41:296–300.

55. Kroll-Palhares K, Silvério JC, Silva AA, et al. TNF/TNFR1 signaling up-regulates CCR5 expression by CD8+ T lymphocytes and promotes heart tissue damage during Trypanosoma cruzi infection: beneficial effects of TNF-a blockade. Mem Inst Oswaldo Cruz. 2008; 103:375–85.

56. Forbes CD, Jackson WF. Infections. In: Forbes CD, Jackson WF, editors. Color atlas and text of clinical medicine. London: Mosby; 2003. pp. 1–64.

57. Sangüeza OP, Lu D, Sangüeza M, Pereira CP. Protozoa and worms. In: Bolognia JL, Jorizzo JL, Rapini RP, editors. Dermatology. 2nd ed. London: Mosby: 2008. pp. 1295–319.

58. McKee PH, Wright E, Hutt SR. Vulval schistosomiasis. Clin Exp Dermatol. 1983; 8:189–94.

59. Gonzalez E. Schistosomiasis, cercarial dermatitis and marine dermatitis. Dermatol Clin. 1989; 7:291–300.

60. Ramos-e-Silva M, Fernandes NC. Parasitic diseases including tropical. In: Parish LC, Brenner S, Ramos-e-Silva M, editors. Women's dermatology: from infancy to maturity. Lancaster (UK): Parthenon; 2001. pp. 291–302.

61. Souza MA, Barbosa VS, Wanderlei TN, Barbosa CS. [Temporary and permanent breeding sites for Biomphalaria in Jaboatão dos Guararapes, PE.] Rev Soc Bras Med Trop. 2008; 41:252–6.

62. Grant AV, Araujo MI, Ponte EV, et al. High heritability but uncertain mode of inheritance for total serum IgE level and Schistosoma mansoni infection intensity in a schistosomiasis-endemic Brazilian population. J Infect Dis. 2008; 198:1227–36.

63. Kloos H, Correa-Oliveira R, Quites HF, et al. Socioeconomic studies of schistosomiasis in Brazil: a review. Acta Trop. 2008; 108:194–201.

64. Chenine AL, Shai-Kobiler E, Steele LN, et al. Acute Schistosoma mansoni infection increases susceptibility to systemic SHIV clade C infection in rhesus macaques after mucosal virus exposure. PLoS Negl Trop Dis. 2008; 2: e265.

65. John R, Ezekiel M, Philbert C, Andrew A. Schistosomiasis transmission at high altitude crater lakes in Western Uganda. BMC Infect Dis. 2008; 8:110.

66. Machado-Pinto J, Pimenta-Gonçalves MP. Dermatoses por protozoários. In: Ramos-e-Silva M, Castro MCR, editors. Fundamentos de dermatologia. Rio de Janeiro: Atheneu; 2009. pp. 1029–41.

67. Stark D, van Hal SJ, Matthews G, et al. Invasive amebiasis in men who have sex with men, Australia. Emerg Infect Dis. 2008; 14:1141–3.

68. Stark D, Fotedar R, van Hal S, et al. Prevalence of enteric protozoa in human immunodeficiency virus (HIV)–positive and HIV-negative men who have sex with men from Sydney, Australia. Am J Trop Med Hyg. 2007; 76:549–52.

69. Ramos-e-Silva M, De Moura Castro Jacques C. Leishmaniasis and other dermatozoonoses in Brazil. Clin Dermatol. 2002; 20:122–34.

CHAPTER 14

Life-Threatening Stings, Bites, and Marine Envenomations

Dirk M. Elston

BITES AND STINGS

Major causes of death related to arthropod bites and stings include anaphylaxis, reactions to venom, and vector-borne disease. This chapter addresses each of these causes.

ANAPHYLAXIS

Background

Anaphylaxis related to insect stings is estimated to occur in 3 of every 100 adults.

Clinical and Laboratory

Skin tests can be used to verify a history of sting allergy. Radioallergosorbent testing (RAST) is less sensitive, but does not carry a risk of anaphylaxis during the testing. It is important to note that neither the size of a skin test reaction nor the RAST level is a reliable predictor of the severity of subsequent sting reactions.[1] In vitro methods of testing also include western blot and in vitro basophil activation tests that measure histamine and sulphidoleukotrien released (Cellular Antigen Stimulation Test [CAST]) or activation markers on the cell surface detected by means of flow cytometric analysis (Flow CAST).[2] Basophil activation tests using either CD63 or CD203c show promise in the in vitro diagnosis of patients with bee or wasp venom allergy.[3]

Patients with mastocytosis who develop severe hypotension after wasp or bee stings typically do not demonstrate specific immunoglobulin E (IgE). Similar patients have been described with no skin lesions to suggest mastocytosis. In some patients, serum tryptase elevations suggest subclinical mastocytosis, and bone-marrow biopsy may reveal systemic mastocytosis.[4]

Cardiac medications such as beta-blockers and angiotensin-converting enzyme inhibitors may increase the severity of anaphylactic reactions, placing the patient at greater risk for a bad outcome.[5] In contrast, previous large local reactions to insect stings does not increase the risk of subsequent anaphylaxis.[6] In a study of 115 patients with a history of an anaphylactic reaction to a wasp sting and specific IgE to Vespula and/or Polistes, the mean age was higher in patients with no cutaneous symptoms and cardiovascular involvement was more frequent in males, but the clinical pattern was not predicted by a history of atopy.[7] Vespids remain the major cause of insect-related anaphylaxis. In a retrospective review of 98 adult patients with anaphylactic reactions to vespids, 18 patients (18%) suffered a reaction to wasp venom while at work. The rest of the reactions occurred during leisure time. Most (94%) of the patients with work-related anaphylaxis had a personal history of atopy, whereas only 22% of those with sting-induced anaphylaxis outside of the workplace had an atopic diathesis. Previous systemic reactions had occurred in 17% of the patients. Gardening was the occupation most closely associated with a risk of vespid-induced anaphylaxis. Vespula IgE was detected in all patients, and Polistes IgE was detected in 78%.[8]

Among patients with bumblebee allergy, two groups have been identified, patients with IgE that is highly cross-reactive with honeybee venom and patients, frequently stung only by bumblebees, who require immunotherapy with purified bumblebee venom.[9]

Children with insect-induced anaphylaxis have a higher incidence of honeybee allergy than adults have, but severe systemic reactions are less common than in adults. Those patients with moderate to severe systemic reactions have a 30% chance of a similar reaction years later. Fortunately, the long-term immune tolerance induced by immunotherapy is greater in children than adults.[10]

Membranous winged insects other than wasps and bees can also cause anaphylaxis – most notably, the fire ants *Solenopsis invicta* and *Solenopsis richteri*. A diverse array of other ant species belonging to six different subfamilies (Formicinae, Myrmeciinae, Ponerinae, Ectatomminae, Myrmicinae, and Pseudomyrmecinae) have also been associated with anaphylactic reactions.[11] Although hymenopterids remain the major cause of arthropod-induced anaphylaxis, other arthropods, such as the European pigeon tick (*Argas reflexus*) have also been implicated. This tick has demonstrated the potential for both IgE-mediated sensitizations and anaphylactic reactions.[12]

Therapy

Although intramuscular injections of epinephrine remain the standard type of epinephrine therapy for vespid-related anaphylaxis, rapidly disintegrating sublingual epinephrine tablets show promise for oral treatment of anaphylaxis.[13] Biphasic reactions are common, and patients need extended observation after their initial response to therapy.[14] Desensitization improves quality of life and is preferred by patients.[15] All patients with sting-related anaphylaxis should be referred to an allergist to discuss the option of desensitization. Venom immunotherapy is thought to be 75%–98% effective in preventing future episodes of anaphylaxis. Rush regimens of hymenoptera venom immunotherapy have been shown to be safe and effective.[16]

Course and Prognosis

Risk factors for fatal anaphylactic reactions include preexisting cardiovascular disease and a high mast-cell load as evidenced by clinical evidence of mastocytosis or an elevated baseline serum tryptase level.[17] Patients with vespid allergy who also have mastocytosis are at greater risk for life-threatening sting reactions, but most tolerate venom immunotherapy well with few systemic symptoms.[18]

REACTIONS TO VENOM

Background

A wide variety of reactions to arthropods relate directly to the venom. Manifestations vary from disseminated intravascular coagulation (DIC) to rhabdomyolysis.

Clinical and Laboratory

Rhabdomyolysis with acute renal failure has been described after fire ant bites.[19] Life-threatening facial edema has been reported after exposure to pine caterpillars.[20] Neurologic symptoms are common after centipede bites, but are usually self-limited. Acute myocardial infarction in a previously healthy young man has been reported after a centipede bite.[21]

Death from scorpion envenomation relates to the potency of the toxin, the age of the patient, and preexisting conditions such as heart disease. In some studies, all fatalities involved children younger than 10 years.[22] In Bangkok, a strip of Teflon tape is wrapped around each piling supporting a house to prevent scorpions from climbing the pilings and entering the house. It has reduced infant mortality related to scorpionism.

Tityus zulianus is a major cause of scorpionism in Latin America. *Mesobuthus tamulus* (the Indian red scorpion) is often associated with fatal envenomation. The toxin produces an autonomic storm and has been associated with

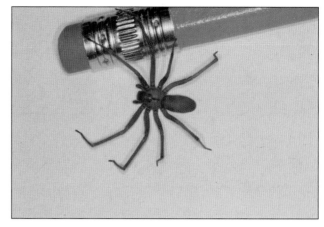

FIGURE 14.1: *Brown recluse spider.*

bilateral cerebellar infarction.[23] Prazosin reverses the autonomic storm characteristic of Indian red scorpion envenomation and is superior to antivenin.[24]

Brown spiders of the genus *Loxosceles* include *Loxosceles reclusa*, the brown recluse spider (Figure 14.1). All spiders in this genus are capable of producing dermonecrotic reactions and may also produce DIC. A generalized vasculitic exanthem has also been described following *Loxosceles reclusa* envenomation.[25]

Brown recluse spiders have three sets of eyes (rather than the usual four) and a characteristic violin-shaped marking on the dorsum of the cephalothorax. Sphingomyelinase D is the primary dermonecrotic factor. The toxin depletes clotting factors VIII, IX, XI, and XII and prolongs the activated partial thromboplastin time in a dose-dependent manner.[26] The venom induces rapid coagulation and occlusion of small capillaries, causing subsequent tissue necrosis. Enzyme-linked immunosorbent assay methods can be used for the diagnosis of loxoscelism with noninvasive tissue sampling.[27] Both tissue swabbing and hair pluck techniques have been used.

Immunologic studies have demonstrated cross-reactivity between *L. boneti* and *L. reclusa* venoms, and between anti-*L. gaucho* and anti-*L. laeta* venoms. In contrast, the venom of the South American *L. laeta* shows little cross-reactivity with North American *Loxosceles* antivenoms. The lack of cross reaction limits the worldwide distribution of spider antivenin.[28]

Widow spiders are widely distributed throughout the world. Genetically, widow spiders can be divided into two large groups. The *geometricus* clade includes *Latrodectus rhodesiensis* from Africa, and the more widespread *L. geometricus*. The *mactans* clade contains all other *Latrodectus* species in Africa, the Middle East, the Iberian Peninsula, Australia, New Zealand, and North and South America.[29]

The venom of black widow spiders (Figure 14.2) is more toxic than that of brown widow spiders, and black widow spiders are found throughout the continental United

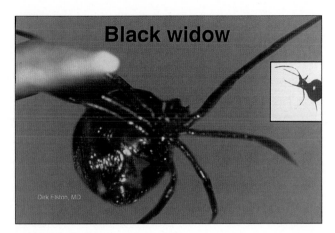

FIGURE 14.2: Black widow spider.

States and southern Canada. The venom contains latrotoxins that act by depolarizing neurons, resulting in increasing intracellular calcium and release of neurotransmitters. Female black widow spiders can be as much as 20 times larger than the males and have much more potent venom. The female can be identified by the red hourglass pattern on the ventral aspect of her large, shiny, roughly spherical abdomen. Alpha-latrotoxin induces release of acetylcholine, norepinephrine, dopamine, and enkephalin. The result is abdominal rigidity that may mimic an acute surgical abdomen.

Widow spiders are named for their cannibalistic behavior. The female mates, then kills. Some female spiders do not even wait until mating is complete before taking the first bite from their mates. Some male *Latrodectus* spiders have developed strategies to prolong their survival long enough to maximize their chance of passing on their genes. Female redback spiders (*Latrodectus hasselti*) have paired sperm-storage organs that are inseminated during two separate copulations. If a male can survive to copulate twice, he ensures the transmission of his genes. Males have developed a reflexive abdominal constriction during courtship that increases their chance of survival from cannibalistic injury inflicted during the first copulation.[30] It is hardly romantic, but effective nonetheless. In a study of redback spider envenomation, the median duration of symptoms was 48 hours, with severe pain lasting more than 24 hours occurring in more than half of the patients. Systemic signs and symptoms occurred in more than one third of the patients. Local diaphoresis and pain are characteristic features. The Australian funnel web spider (*Atrax* and *Hadronyche* spp.) pose a significant risk in Australia. They are not related to the funnel web spiders (*Tegenaria agrestis*) of the Pacific Northwest. In a prospective Australian study of 750 spider bites with expert identification of the spider, clinically significant effects occurred in 44 bites (6%), including 37 of 56 redback spider bites. The major symptom was pain lasting more than 24 hours. One severe neurotoxic envenomation

by an Australian funnel web spider required antivenin therapy.[31] Brazilian *Phoneutria* "armed spiders" have a limited range, but are an important cause of life-threatening bites in Brazil. Antivenins are available for both the neurotoxic Australian funnel web spider and the Brazilian armed spider, but relatively few data exist regarding efficacy.

Lonomia caterpillars in South America cause a hemorrhagic diathesis. No antivenin exists. Tick paralysis in North America is typically associated with *Dermacentor* ticks. Tick paralysis typically occurs in children who present with rapidly progressive ascending paralysis. Symptoms resolve rapidly when the tick is removed, but *Dermacentor* ticks (Figure 14.3) tend to attach to the scalp where they are hidden by the hair. As a result, tick paralysis carries a death rate of approximately 10%. *Ixodes* tick paralysis is a common cause of death in Australian dogs, but is less likely to affect humans.

Therapy

Although in vitro data and rabbit studies suggest that dapsone and tetracyclines[32] could be of benefit in the treatment of brown recluse spider bites, a "real life" delay in the onset of therapy negates any beneficial effect of dapsone therapy. In a rabbit model, the only therapy that showed a trend toward less thrombosis was intralesional triamcinolone.[33]

The primary treatment for black widow spider envenomation is the administration of antivenin, although antispasmodics such as valium and calcium gluconate play some role. The antivenin is horse serum, and serum sickness can result from subsequent use.

Redback spider antivenin is effective at controlling local symptoms, but did not demonstrate a conclusive effect against systemic toxicity.[34] It should be noted that redback antivenin is routinely given intramuscularly, which may not be as effective as the intravenous route.[35]

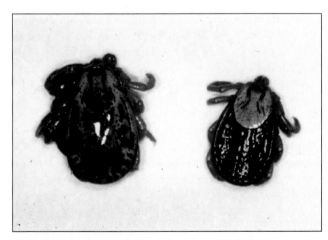

FIGURE 14.3: Male (left) and female (right) Dermacentor andersoni.

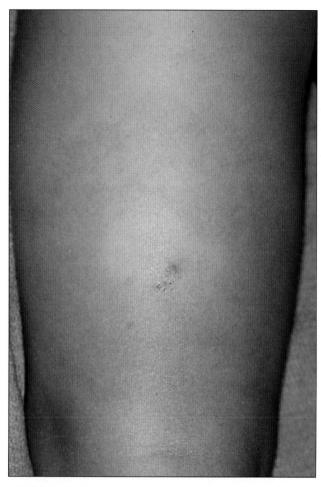

FIGURE 14.4: *Erythema migrans of Lyme disease.*

VECTOR-BORNE DISEASE

Background

Arthropod-borne diseases remain a serious threat throughout most of the world. Malaria remains the single most important vector-borne disease and kills thousands every year. Other important vector-borne diseases worldwide include viral encephalitis, viral hemorrhagic fevers, African and New World types of trypanosomiasis, and leishmaniasis. In the United States, mosquitoes are more likely to carry West Nile virus, St. Louis encephalitis, equine encephalitis, or dengue. North American ticks are important vectors of Lyme disease (Figure 14.4), Rocky Mountain spotted fever (RMSF), ehrlichiosis, Colorado tick fever, relapsing fever, tularemia, and babesiosis.

Clinical and Laboratory

Persons in the developing world are at particular risk for transmission of arthropod-borne diseases, partly because of sophisticated vector-control programs in developed countries and partly because of the indoor, air-conditioned lifestyle common to subtropical areas of the developed world. An outbreak of dengue along the United States–Mexican border demonstrated this effect. Disease transmission was greater on the Mexican side of the border, even though the vector was more abundant on the U.S. (Texas) side.[36]

Whereas mosquito-borne illness predominates in much of the world, tick-borne illness is more common in North America, Northern Europe, and even parts of Africa. *Amblyomma* ticks carry *Ehrlichia chaffeensis*, the agent of human monocytic ehrlichiosis, as well as RMSF and southern tick–associated rash illness (southern Lyme disease), as well as African tick bite fever. *Dermacentor variabilis* is the major North American vector for RMSF. *Dermacentor andersoni* also carries RMSF and serves as a vector for Colorado tick fever, Q fever, and tularemia. RMSF carries a high mortality rate if antibiotic therapy is delayed. In endemic areas, it is best to "treat now and ask questions later" for any patient with fever and a headache, regardless of a history of tick bite. Spotless fever is particularly prone to misdiagnosis, and treatment should never be delayed because of the absence of dermatitis.

Rhipicephalus ticks are common brown dog ticks in both North America and Europe. They are important vectors for RMSF as well as canine ehrlichiosis, Boutonneuse fever, babesiosis, and Congo–Crimean hemorrhagic fever virus. *Ixodes* ticks carry Lyme disease, babesiosis, anaplasmosis (human granulocytic ehrlichiosis), and viral encephalitis.

Trombiculid mites are important vectors of scrub typhus in East Asia, and rickettsial pox is transmitted by *Liponyssoides sanguineus* (the house mouse mite). Body lice are important vectors for Bartonella endocarditis among homeless persons in urban areas.[37–39] Fleas are important vectors of plague, bacillary angiomatosis, and endemic typhus.

Therapy

Most tick-borne diseases respond readily to tetracycline, with viral fevers and babesiosis being notable exceptions. Antibiotic prophylaxis after tick bites is controversial. Although it is not indicated after most tick attachments, an argument can be made for prophylaxis in highly endemic areas with ticks that are heavily engorged, evidence that they have been attached long enough to transmit disease.

Primary prevention of vector-borne disease requires a multifaceted approach including infrastructure measure for control of important vectors, use of screens and mosquito netting, and personal protection with repellents. Prompt tick removal also plays an important role in disease prevention. Secondary prevention of disease and morbidity can be accomplished with malaria chemoprophylaxis, prophylactic antibiotics after a tick bite, or early treatment of illness. Although malaria chemoprophylaxis may be reasonable for visitors to an area, it is not feasible for the entire indigenous population. Malaria-carrying anopheline mosquitoes feed mostly at night, emphasizing the importance of screens and mosquito netting. Screening can be impregnated with pyrethroids to improve their effectiveness. Because the mosquitoes that carry dengue typically bite during the day, vector control, repellents, and protective clothing play important roles in disease prevention.[40,41]

Infrastructure changes to control mosquito vectors include draining stagnant water, stocking water with fish or turtles to eat larvae, spraying with insecticide, and using gas or electric mosquito traps. Most mosquito traps generate carbon dioxide. Although some use chemical attractants such as octenol and butanone in areas with *Aedes* mosquitoes, it should be noted that some *Culex* mosquitoes are repelled by octenol.[42–44]

N,N-diethyl-3-methylbenzamide (DEET) remains the most commonly used repellent, although picaridin is gaining market share. Although DEET has a long safety record, rare cases of bullous dermatitis, anaphylaxis, and toxic encephalopathy have been reported.[45–48] For children, the American Academy of Pediatrics recommends slow-release products that require less frequent application. The Academy notes that such products plateau in efficacy at concentrations of 30% and that there is no published evidence to support the use of higher concentrations in children. It should be noted that many extended duration products formulated for children have concentrations of 10% or less and that these appear to be perfectly adequate in most instances.

Whereas DEET products can generally be applied to both exposed skin and clothing, permethrin products are to be applied to fabric. The combination of DEET repellent and permethrin-treated clothing is effective against a wide range of biting arthropods.[49,50]

Picaridin has been used in Europe and Australia and is now available in North America. In tests, it has shown good efficacy against a range of mosquitoes. A soybean oil–based product (marketed as Bite Blocker for Kids in the United States) shows reasonable efficacy against some mosquitoes and may be a good choice for persons who wish to avoid chemical repellents. Neem oil products perform reasonably well against various mosquitoes, whereas citronella has limited efficacy.[51,52]

Permethrin-treated clothing offers significant protection against ticks and chiggers, with good substantivity through a number of wash cycles.[53–55] In southwest Asia and North Africa, some ticks are attracted by permethrin, but this has not been reported in other areas.[56]

Deer fencing, border beds, insecticidal sprays, and even fire ants help keep residential and recreational areas free of ticks.[57,58] Area sprays of insecticides are more effective if leaf debris is removed. Removal of leaf debris also reduces tick numbers by means of dehydration.[59,60] Various other methods have been employed, including deer-feeding stations outfitted to deliver topical acaricides to the deer. This approach is more cost effective than adding a systemic acaricide to the deer corn.[61–63]

MARINE ENVENOMATIONS

Background

Marine animals contain some of the most potent toxins known. Most minor envenomations result in severe pain. As the toxins tend to be heat labile, immersion in hot, but not scalding, water is the preferred form of therapy. This section focuses on the more severe life-threatening envenomations.

Clinical Features

Chironex fleckeri, the Pacific box jellyfish or sea wasp, is responsible for many deaths as a result of shock and drowning. Confirmation of envenomation can be made by identification of the jelly or by means of tape stripping nematocysts from the skin.[64] Other jellies cause painful eruptions but are much less likely to result in serious reactions. Important jellies around the world include *Physalia physalis* (the Portuguese Man o' War, endemic to the southern waters of the Atlantic), *Physalia utriculus* (the Pacific bluebottle jellyfish), as well as *Cyanea* and *Chrysaora* sea nettles. These may cause severe allergic reactions in some individuals, but generally lack the severe toxicity associated with *Chironex fleckeri*. All jellyfish produce serpiginous patterns of stings that follow the course of the tentacles attached to skin.

Sponge dermatitis is related to calcium and silica spicules that become embedded in the skin and is rarely life threatening. In contrast, sponge diver's disease is not caused by the sponge at all, but rather by sea anemones attached to the base of the sponge. In addition to local symptoms similar to jellyfish stings, systemic symptoms may occur, such as nausea, vomiting, and headache. More severe reactions are possible in predisposed individuals.

Life-threatening envenomation by mollusks may occur with the blue-ringed octopus and with some cone shells. The blue-ringed octopus is a small cephalopod (about 10 cm long) found in waters off the coast of Australia. The distinctive blue rings may cause some foolish divers to get too close to the mollusk, but most envenomations occur completely by accident. Cone shells are marine gastropods with pretty shells and highly potent venom. The mortality rate from cone shell envenomation may approach 20%. The shells are approximately 10 cm in length and tend to be found in shallow water, mostly in tropical and subtropical waters.

Death has been reported after penetrating chest injury from stingrays. The death may occur as a direct result of the injury or by means of venom-induced myocardial necrosis.[65] Envenomation by stonefish and lionfish is becoming more common as these fish move from tropical waters to a much more cosmopolitan distribution. Stings commonly result in pain, erythema, bulla formation, and tissue necrosis. Systemic symptoms may be life threatening, but death is more likely a result of drowning related to disorientation following the sting. Catfish spine injuries may be associated with local pain, severe bleeding, and systemic symptoms, but are rarely fatal.

Treatment

As with other bites and stings, knowledge and avoidance are the best means of preventing injury. Drowning is the most common cause of death from marine envenomation, and the swimmer should be removed from the water immediately. Supportive treatment for shock may be necessary in severe envenomations. Initial treatment for most marine envenomations includes soaking the site in hot, but not scalding, water to denature as much of the venom as possible. Sea wasp antivenin is available, but data on other systemic agents (such as calcium channel blockers) are mixed. Physicians in coastal areas should consult current recommendations for treatment of local venomous species.

Course and Prognosis

The prognosis depends on the potency of the toxicity, comorbidities such as cardiac disease or hypertension, and prompt removal from the water to prevent drowning.

ACKNOWLEDGMENTS

Images were produced while the author was a full-time federal employee. They are in the public domain.

REFERENCES

1. Golden DB. Insect sting anaphylaxis. Immunol Allergy Clin North Am. 2007; 27:261–72, vii.
2. Tavares B. Hymenoptera venom allergy–new diagnostic methods. Acta Med Port. 2005; 18:445–51.
3. Eberlein-König B, Varga R, Mempel M, et al. Comparison of basophil activation tests using CD63 or CD203c expression in patients with insect venom allergy. Allergy. 2006; 61:1084–5.
4. Sonneck K, Florian S, Müllauer L, et al. Diagnostic and subdiagnostic accumulation of mast cells in the bone marrow of patients with anaphylaxis: monoclonal mast cell activation syndrome. Int Arch Allergy Immunol. 2007; 142:158–64.
5. Stumpf JL, Shehab N, Patel AC. Safety of angiotensin-converting enzyme inhibitors in patients with insect venom allergies. Ann Pharmacother. 2006; 40:699–703.
6. Brand PL. Anaphylaxis: facts and fallacies. Ned Tijdschr Geneeskd. 2007; 151:574–7.
7. Pérez Pimiento AJ, Prieto Lastra L, Rodríguez Cabreros MI, et al. Systemic reactions to wasp sting: is the clinical pattern related to age, sex and atopy? Allergol Immunopathol (Madr). 2007; 35:10–14.
8. Pérez Pimiento A, Prieto-Lastra L, Rodríguez-Cabreros M, et al. Work-related anaphylaxis to wasp sting. Occup Med (Lond). 2007; 57:602–4.
9. de Groot H. Allergy to bumblebees. Curr Opin Allergy Clin Immunol. 2006; 6:294–7.
10. Golden DB. Insect allergy in children. Curr Opin Allergy Clin Immunol. 2006; 6:289–93.
11. Klotz JH, deShazo RD, Pinnas JL, et al. Adverse reactions to ants other than imported fire ants. Ann Allergy Asthma Immunol. 2005; 95:418–25.
12. Kleine-Tebbe J, Heinatz A, Gräser I, et al. Bites of the European pigeon tick (Argas reflexus): risk of IgE-mediated sensitizations and anaphylactic reactions. J Allergy Clin Immunol. 2006; 117:190–5.
13. Sicherer SH, Leung DY. Advances in allergic skin disease, anaphylaxis, and hypersensitivity reactions to foods, drugs, and insects. J Allergy Clin Immunol. 2007; 119:1462–9.
14. Cortellini G, Corvetta A, Campi P, et al. A case of fatal biphasic anaphylaxis secondary to multiple stings: adrenalin and/or a longer observation time could have saved the patient? Allerg Immunol (Paris). 2005; 37:343–4.
15. Oude Elberink JN, Van Der Heide S, Guyatt GH, Dubois AE. Analysis of the burden of treatment in patients receiving an EpiPen for yellow jacket anaphylaxis. J Allergy Clin Immunol. 2006; 118:699–704.
16. Pasaoglu G, Sin BA, Misirligil Z. Rush hymenoptera venom immunotherapy is efficacious and safe. J Investig Allergol Clin Immunol. 2006; 16:232–8.
17. Mueller UR. Cardiovascular disease and anaphylaxis. Curr Opin Allergy Clin Immunol. 2007; 7:337–41.
18. Ruëff F, Placzek M, Przybilla B. Mastocytosis and Hymenoptera venom allergy. Curr Opin Allergy Clin Immunol. 2006; 6:284–8.
19. Koya S, Crenshaw D, Agarwal A. Rhabdomyolysis and acute renal failure after fire ant bites. J Gen Intern Med. 2007; 22:145–7.
20. Inal A, Altintas DU, Güvenmez HK, et al. Life-threatening facial edema due to pine caterpillar mimicking an allergic event. Allergol Immunopathol (Madr). 2006; 34:171–3.
21. Yildiz A, Biçeroglu S, Yakut N, et al. Acute myocardial infarction in a young man caused by centipede sting. Emerg Med J. 2006; 23:e30.
22. Mejías RJ, Yánez CA, Arias R, et al. [Occurrence of scorpionism in sanitary districts of Mérida State, Venezuela.] Invest Clin. 2007; 48:147–53.
23. Gadwalkar SR, Bushan S, Pramod K, et al. Bilateral cerebellar infarction: a rare complication of scorpion sting. J Assoc Physicians India. 2006; 54:581–3.
24. Bawaskar HS, Bawaskar PH. Utility of scorpion antivenin vs prazosin in the management of severe Mesobuthus tamulus (Indian red scorpion) envenoming at rural setting. J Assoc Physicians India. 2007; 55:14–21.
25. Robb CW, Hayes BB, Boyd AS. Generalized vasculitic exanthem following Loxosceles reclusa envenomation. J Cutan Pathol. 2007; 34:513–14.
26. McGlasson DL, Harroff HH, Sutton J, et al. Cutaneous and systemic effects of varying doses of brown recluse spider venom in a rabbit model. Clin Lab Sci. 2007; 20:99–105.

27. Stoecker WV, Green JA, Gomez HF. Diagnosis of lox-oscelism in a child confirmed with an enzyme-linked immunosorbent assay and noninvasive tissue sampling. J Am Acad Dermatol. 2006; 55:888–90.

28. de Roodt AR, Estevez-Ramírez J, Litwin S, et al. Toxicity of two North American Loxosceles (brown recluse spiders) venoms and their neutralization by antivenoms. Clin Toxicol (Phila). 2007; 45:678–87.

29. Garb JE, González A, Gillespie RG. The black widow spider genus Latrodectus (Araneae: Theridiidae): phylogeny, biogeography, and invasion history. Mol Phylogenet Evol. 2004; 31:1127–42.

30. Andrade MC, Gu L, Stoltz JA. Novel male trait prolongs survival in suicidal mating. Biol Lett. 2005; 1:276–9.

31. Isbister GK, Gray MR. A prospective study of 750 definite spider bites, with expert spider identification. QJM. 2002; 95:723–31.

32. Paixão-Cavalcante D, Van Den Berg CW, Gonçalves-de-Andrade RM, et al. Tetracycline protects against dermonecrosis induced by Loxosceles spider venom. J Invest Dermatol. 2007; 127:1410–18.

33. Elston DM, Miller SD, Young RJ, et al. Comparison of colchicine, dapsone, triamcinolone, and diphenhydramine therapy for the treatment of brown recluse spider envenomation. A double blind, controlled study in a rabbit model. Arch Dermatol. 2005; 141:595–7.

34. Isbister GK, Gray MR. Latrodectism: a prospective cohort study of bites by formally identified redback spiders. Med J Aust. 2003; 179:88–91.

35. Isbister GK, Graudins A, White J, Warrell D. Antivenom treatment in arachnidism. J Toxicol Clin Toxicol. 2003; 41:291–300.

36. Reiter P, Lathrop S, Bunning M, et al. Texas lifestyle limits transmission of dengue virus. Emerg Infect Dis. 2003; 9:86–9.

37. Guibal F, de La Salmoniere P, Rybojad M, et al. High seroprevalence to Bartonella quintana in homeless patients with cutaneous parasitic infestations in downtown Paris. J Am Acad Dermatol. 2001; 44:219–23.

38. Foucault C, Barrau K, Brouqui P, Raoult D. Bartonella quintana bacteremia among homeless people. Clin Infect Dis. 2002; 35:684–9.

39. Raoult D, Foucault C, Brouqui P. Infections in the homeless. Lancet Infect Dis. 2001; 1:77–84.

40. Coosemans M, Van Gompel A. The principal arthropod vectors of disease. What are the risks of travellers' to be bitten? To be infected? Bull Soc Pathol Exot. 1998; 91:467–73.

41. Carnevale P. Protection of travelers against biting arthropod vectors. Bull Soc Pathol Exot. 1998; 91:474–85.

42. Rueda LM, Harrison BA, Brown JS, et al. Evaluation of 1-octen-3-ol, carbon dioxide, and light as attractants for mosquitoes associated with two distinct habitats in North Carolina. J Am Mosq Control Assoc. 2001; 17:61–6.

43. Kline DL. Comparison of two American biophysics mosquito traps: the professional and a new counterflow geometry trap. J Am Mosq Control Assoc. 1999; 15:276–82.

44. Kline DL, Mann MO. Evaluation of butanone, carbon dioxide, and 1-octen-3-OL as attractants for mosquitoes associated with north central Florida bay and cypress swamps. J Am Mosq Control Assoc. 1998; 14:289–97.

45. Brown M, Hebert AA. Insect repellents: an overview. J Am Acad Dermatol. 1997; 36:243–9.

46. Fradin MS. Mosquitoes and mosquito repellents: a clinician's guide. Ann Intern Med. 1998; 128:931–40.

47. McKinlay JR, Ross V, Barrett TL. Vesiculobullous reaction to diethyltoluamide revisited. Cutis. 1998; 62:44.

48. Miller JD. Anaphylaxis associated with insect repellent. N Engl J Med. 1982; 307:1341–2.

49. Young GD, Evans S. Safety and efficacy of DEET and permethrin in the prevention of arthropod attack. Mil Med. 1998; 163:324–30.

50. Gupta RK, Sweeny AW, Rutledge LC. Effectiveness of controlled-release personal use arthropod repellent and permethrin-treated clothing in the field. J Mosq Control Assoc. 1987; 3:556–60.

51. Lindsay LR, Surgeoner GA, Heal JD, Gallivan GJ. Evaluation of the efficacy of 3% citronella candles and 5% citronella incense for protection against field populations of Aedes mosquitoes. J Am Mosq Control Assoc. 1996; 12:293–4.

52. Caraballo AJ. Mosquito repellent action of Neemos. J Am Mosq Control Assoc. 2000; 16:45–6.

53. Young GD, Evans S. Safety and efficacy of DEET and permethrin in the prevention of arthropod attack. Mil Med. 1998; 163:324–30.

54. Gupta RK, Sweeny AW, Rutledge LC. Effectiveness of controlled-release personal use arthropod repellent and permethrin-treated clothing in the field. J Mosq Control Assoc. 1987; 3:556–60.

55. Schreck CE, Mount GA, Carlson DA. Wear and wash persistence of permethrin used as a clothing treatment for personal protection against the lone star tick (Acari: Ixodidae). J Med Entomol. 1982; 19:143–6.

56. Fryauff DJ, Shoukry MA, Schreck CE. Stimulation of attachment in the camel tick, Hyalomma dromedarii (Acari: Ixodidae): the unintended result of sublethal exposure to permethrin-impregnated fabric. J Med Entomol. 1994; 31:23–9.

57. Stafford KC 3rd. Reduced abundance of Ixodes scapularis (Acari: Ixodidae) with exclusion of deer by electric fencing. J Med Entomol. 1993; 30:986–96.

58. Daniels TJ, Fish D, Schwartz I. Reduced abundance of Ixodes scapularis (Acari: Ixodidae) and Lyme disease risk by deer exclusion. J Med Entomol. 1993; 30:1043–9.

59. Strey OF, Teel PD, Longnecker MT, Needham GR. Survival and water-balance characteristics of unfed Amblyomma cajennense (Acari: Ixodidae). J Med Entomol. 1996; 33:63–73.

60. Slowik TJ, Lane RS. Nymphs of the western black-legged tick (Ixodes pacificus) collected from tree trunks in woodland-grass habitat. J Vector Ecol. 2001; 26:165–71.

61. Mount GA, Haile DG, Daniels E. Simulation of management strategies for the blacklegged tick (Acari: Ixodidae) and the Lyme disease spirochete, Borrelia burgdorferi. J Med Entomol. 1997; 34:672–83.

62. Pound JM, Miller JA, George JE. Efficacy of amitraz applied to white-tailed deer by the '4-poster' topical treatment device in controlling free-living lone star ticks (Acari: Ixodidae). J Med Entomol. 2000; 37:878–84.

63. Solberg VB, Miller JA, Hadfield T, et al. Control of Ixodes scapularis (Acari: Ixodidae) with topical self-application of permethrin by white-tailed deer inhabiting NASA, Beltsville, Maryland. J Vector Ecol. 2003; 28:117–34.

64. Currie BJ, Wood YK. Identification of Chironex fleckeri envenomation by nematocyst recovery from skin. Med J Aust. 1995; 162:478–80.

65. Fenner PJ, Williamson JA, Skinner RA. Fatal and non-fatal stingray envenomation. Med J Aust. 1989; 151:621–5.

CHAPTER 15

Severe, Acute Adverse Cutaneous Drug Reactions I: Stevens–Johnson Syndrome and Toxic Epidermal Necrolysis

Ronni Wolf

Batya B. Davidovici

ADVERSE CUTANEOUS drug reactions (ADRs) are frequent, affecting 2%–3% of all hospitalized patients. Fortunately, only approximately 2% of ADRs are severe, and few are fatal.

Stevens–Johnson syndrome (SJS) and toxic epidermal necrolysis (TEN) are acute, severe, life-threatening diseases with a mortality rate reaching 30%. Only prompt recognition, diagnosis, and referral to an intensive care unit or burn care unit might improve the prognosis and save the patient's life.

HISTORICAL BACKGROUND

In his classic 1866 treatise "On Disease of the Skin," Ferdinand von Hebra precisely described and gave the name to erythema multiforme (EM).[1] In 1922, two American physicians, Stevens and Johnson, described two patients, boys 7 and 8 years old, who had "an extraordinary, generalized eruption with continued fever, inflamed buccal mucosa, and severe purulent conjunctivitis"[2] that was later given the name "Stevens–Johnson syndrome." In 1950, Thomas divided EM into two categories: erythema multiforme minor (von Hebra) and erythema multiforme major, also known as SJS.[3] In 1956, Alan Lyell wrote the most highly cited article ever to appear in *The British Journal of Dermatology*: He described four patients with a scalding disease, which was later given the name toxic epidermal necrolysis (TEN), or the Lyell syndrome or Lyell disease.[4,5] These severe, acute, life-threatening ADRs were not classified and defined according to their clinical appearance and/or linked to their etiology and prognosis until around 1993.[6]

DEFINITION AND CLASSIFICATION

EM was initially described as an acute self-limited skin disease, symmetrically distributed on the extremities with typical concentric "target" lesions and often recurrent.[1] The terminology "EM minor" was later proposed to separate the mild cutaneous syndrome from more severe forms with involvement of several mucous membranes ("EM major"). SJS for years had been considered an extreme variant of EM, and TEN as being a different entity. In 1993,[6] a group of experts proposed a new classification in which they separated SJS from the EM spectrum and added it to TEN, thereby creating a new spectrum of drug-related severe diseases, for example, SJS/TEN. Two disease spectra were created: 1) EM consisting of EM minor and EM major, and 2) SJS/TEN. The former are often recurrent, postinfectious disorders (especially herpes and mycoplasma) with low morbidity and almost no mortality. The latter are usually severe drug-induced reactions with high morbidity and poor prognosis.

According to the new "consensus definition and classification,"[6] categorization of these diseases is determined essentially by the percentage of skin detachment and by the characteristic appearance of the typical individual "EM-like" or "target" lesions.

The clinical pattern of the individual skin lesion was classified into the following four types:

1. *Typical targets* – individual lesions less than 3 cm in diameter with a regular round shape, well-defined border, and at least three different zones (i.e., two concentric rings around a central disk). One ring consists of palpable edema, paler than the center disk.

2. *Raised atypical targets* – round, edematous, palpable lesions, similar to EM but with only two zones and/or a poorly defined border.

3. *Flat atypical targets* – round lesions characteristic of EM but with only two zones and/or a poorly defined border and nonpalpable with the exception of a potential central blister.

TABLE 15.1: Original Classification

EM	SJS/Overlap/TEN
Typical targets	Flat atypical targets
Raised atypical targets	Macules with/without blisters

EM, erythema multiforme; SJS, Stevens–Johnson syndrome; TEN, toxic epidermal necrolysis.

TABLE 15.2: Proposed New Classification

EM	SJS/Overlap/TEN
Raised typical targets	Flat typical targets
Raised atypical targets	Flat atypical targets
	Macules with/without blisters

EM, erythema multiforme; SJS, Stevens–Johnson syndrome; TEN, toxic epidermal necrolysis.

4. *Macules with or without blisters* – nonpalpable, erythematous, or purpuric macules with an irregular shape and size and often confluent. Blisters often occur on all or part of the macule.

The involved body surface area (BSA) should measure the extent of detached and detachable epidermis (which is often much less than the area of erythema) at the worst stage of the disease.

These authors then proposed the following consensus classification (five categories):

1. *EM* – detachment <10% of BSA, localized typical targets or raised atypical targets.
2. *SJS* – detachment <10% of BSA, widespread erythematous or purpuric macules or flat atypical targets.
3. *Overlap SJS/TEN* – detachment between 10% and 30% of BSA, widespread purpuric macules or flat atypical targets.
4. *TEN with spots* – detachment >30% of BSA, widespread purpuric macules or flat atypical targets.
5. *TEN without spots* – detachment >10% of BSA, large epidermal sheets and no purpuric macules.

They went on to suggest a practical algorithm in the definition and categorization of these diseases based on their classification. The first question that the clinician needs to ask is: "What is the percentage of detachment?" The second question is: "What is the nature of the discrete lesions?" They also suggested that their purely descriptive clinical classification might indicate a causative agent, namely, that SJS, TEN, and overlap are drug induced, whereas the diseases in the EM group are caused by infectious agents.

Because the involved area of detachment is defined as such at the worst stage of the disease, it cannot always be delineated when the clinician first sees the patient. Consequently, the most – and often the only – reliable means of classifying the cases is through observing the pattern of the individual lesions.

We recently proposed a small modification of the current classification to enable the clinician to pinpoint quickly and precisely the type of lesion to implement the appropriate treatment without delay.[7]

We have noticed that patients of the SJS/TEN group occasionally have typical targets that are flat and are missing the palpable ring around the center. We therefore suggested adding an additional type of lesion to the nomenclature, namely, a flat typical target, and calling the original typical target a raised typical target. The new classification will thus contain five types of lesions, instead of four (Tables 15.1 and 15.2).

As to the questions "Why a new classification?" and "Why an additional type of lesion that, at first glance, seems only to complicate the existing classification and make it more cumbersome?" we contend that our proposed modification gives the classification better leeway, incorporating all the variations characteristic of these lesions. We also believe that the new addition makes the classification more compact, easier to understand, and (not less important) easier to remember. How can extending a classification make it more compact? In our proposed modified classification, all the lesions that are found in the EM group are raised, whereas all lesions that characterize the SJS/TEN group are flat, which makes the classification easy to remember and to use. Accordingly, if a patient is found to have raised lesions (raised typical or raised atypical targets), we are directed toward a diagnosis of postinfectious EM. In contrast, if a patient has flat lesions (flat typical targets, flat atypical targets, or macules with or without blisters), we should immediately consider the diagnosis of drug-induced SJS/TEN.

CLINICAL PATTERN

The initial symptoms of TEN (i.e., before the appearance of frank mucocutaneous sloughing) include fever (all cases) as well as conjunctivitis (32% of cases), pharyngitis (25% of cases), and pruritus (28% of cases). These signs usually last 2–3 days and can resemble an upper respiratory infection. There is speculation that the fever is caused by drugs, release of pyrogens from epidermal necrosis, or both, but that it is not due to infection. Mucous membranes (in increasing order of frequency: oropharynx, eyes, genitalia, anus) are commonly affected 1–3 days before the skin lesions appear.[8] The cutaneous lesions begin with a burning and painful eruption initially not typical. This

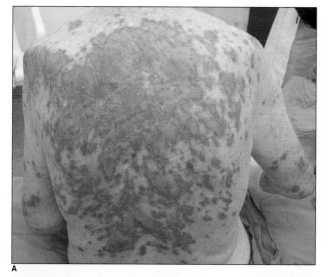

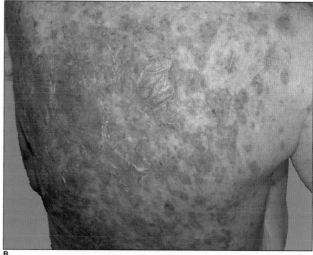

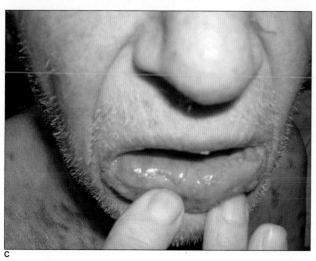

FIGURE 15.1: A, B, and C. 78-year-old man with toxic epidermal necrolysis (TEN) that appeared 5 days after he had been treated with cefuroxime for an upper respiratory infection. (Photos courtesy of S. Halevy, MD, Soroka University Medical Center, Ben Gurion and University of the Negev, Beer-Sheva, Israel.)

eruption extends symmetrically from the face and upper part of the body to the entire body, predominantly on the trunk and proximal limbs. The initial lesions are poorly defined macules with darker centers. Maximal extension of lesions usually occurs in 2 or 3 days, but can be manifest in a few hours. There is a sheet-like loss of epidermis and the appearance of flaccid blisters that spread with pressure. The Nikolsky sign is positive over large areas involved by confluent erythema. Traumatized sites leave a dark red oozing dermis. The entire skin surface may be involved, with up to 100% of epidermal sloughing. Widespread painful mucosal erosions result in impaired alimentation, photophobia, and painful micturition. (See Figures 15.1A–15.1C.) Keratitis and corneal erosions are less frequent, but they are known to occur. Asthenia, skin pain, and anxiety are extreme. Gastrointestinal or tracheobronchial epithelium can be involved via a process of necrosis resulting in profuse diarrhea or respiratory dis-

tress, respectively, and causing high morbidity.[9,10] Prerenal azotemia is common. Fluid losses are massive and accompanied by electrolyte imbalance. During the first days, skin lesions are usually colonized by *Staphylococcus aureus*; they are later invaded by gram-negative rods. Thermoregulation is impaired, and energy expenditure is increased.[11,12] Alteration of immunologic functions increases the risk of sepsis.

Reepidermization begins after a few days, and most of the skin surface is reepithelialized in 3 weeks. Pressure areas and mucosal lesions often remain eroded and crusted for an additional 2 weeks. Scarring may occur in areas of pressure or infection. Disturbances in pigmentation are characteristically present and lead to a patchwork of pigmented and hypopigmented areas. Ocular sequelae are frequent and severe, affecting approximately 40% of survivors.[13,14] Abnormal nail regrowth, phimosis, and vaginal synechiae may be present as well.[14]

DIFFERENTIAL DIAGNOSIS

The preceding classification is intended to help physicians to differentiate EM from SJS/TEN; however, there are several other dermatoses that must be differentiated from these diseases.

Although the clinical presentation and patient history make the diagnosis of the classical form of SJS (with its target lesions and mucosal involvement) and of TEN obvious, other conditions should be considered in the differential diagnosis, particularly in the early stages of disease when the full-blown picture may not be fully apparent. These simulators include staphylococcal scalded skin syndrome (SSSS); linear immunoglobulin A (IgA) bullous dermatosis; paraneoplastic pemphigus and acute graft versus host disease (GVHD); drug-induced pemphigus and pemphigoid, urticarial vasculitis, or lupus erythematosus; Sweet syndrome, particularly the recently described variant of neutrophilic dermatosis of the dorsal hands. Linear IgA bullous dermatosis, SSSS, and drug-induced pemphigus usually do not show mucosal membrane involvement. All other diseases – except SSSS, Sweet syndrome, and acute GVHD – are not accompanied by fever.

In any event, two biopsy specimens are recommended: one for routine, formalin-fixed hematoxylin and eosin processing, and the other for immediate frozen sections. Epidermis must be present to make the diagnosis, as epidermal necrosis is the pathognomonic finding in this entity.

LABORATORY CHANGES

Blood abnormalities are also almost always present. Anemia and lymphopenia are found in virtually all patients, neutropenia in 30% of patients (indicating a poor prognosis), and thrombocytopenia in 15% of patients.[15] The peculiarity of the anemia lies in its regenerative character, with concomitant medullary erythroblastopenia and blood reticulocytopenia. It does not appear to be secondary to the inflammatory process, because the regenerative capacity returns before the peak of the inflammatory phase. Lymphopenia is also commonly present (90% of patients) due to depletion of CD4+ helper T lymphocytes.[16,17] Disseminated intravascular coagulation (DIC) has been reported, and some authors advocate prophylactic treatment with heparin.[18]

Approximately 30% of patients have elevated transaminase enzymes[19] and elevated levels of amylase and lipase without other evidence of pancreatic involvement.[20]

Proteinuria is present in more than one half of patients, but usually at a level less than 1 g per 24 hours. Renal tubular enzyme secretion and microalbuminuria are increased in all patients, but the glomerular filtration rate remains normal. This profile is suggestive of both proximal tubule involvement and secondary effects of glomerular structure.[21]

CAUSATIVE DRUGS

Drugs are clearly the leading causative factor and are associated with nearly 90% of TEN cases and more than 50% of SJS cases.[22]

Recent studies suggested a strong association between human leukocyte antigen (HLA) alleles and susceptibility to drug hypersensitivity.[23] The genetic associations can be drug specific, such as HLA-B*1502 being associated with carbamazepine-induced SJS/TEN, HLA-B*5701 with abacavir hypersensitivity, and HLA-B*5801 with allopurinol-induced severe cutaneous adverse reactions. A genetic association can also be phenotype specific (e.g., B*1502 is associated solely with carbamazepine–SJS/TEN, and not with either maculopapular eruption of hypersensitivity syndrome).[24] Furthermore, a genetic association can also be ethnicity specific; carbamazepine–SJS/TEN associated with B*1502 is seen in Southeast Asians, but not in whites, which may be explained by the different allele frequencies.[25]

More than 100 drugs have been associated with the development of SJS/TEN in single case reports or retrospective studies. In 1995, results of the first prospective case–control study to assess the relative risk for different drugs for being associated with SJS/TEN were published.[26] In this study, sulfonamides were the most strongly associated with TEN (crude relative risk, 172; 95% confidence interval, 75 to 396) followed by antibiotic drugs (in descending order of frequency: cephalosporins, quinolones, aminopenicillins, tetracyclines, macrolides), imidazole antifungals, anticonvulsants (phenobarbital, phenytoin, valproic acid, carbamazepine, and lamotrigine), then nonsteroidal antiinflammatory drugs (especially oxicam), allopurinol, and others.

TREATMENT

Both SJS and TEN are life-threatening diseases, so the management of patients must be prompt. Early diagnosis with the early recognition and withdrawal of all potential causative drugs is essential to a favorable outcome. Morbidity and mortality decrease if the culprit drug is withdrawn no later than the day when blisters or erosions first occurred.[27]

The patient must be transferred to an intensive care unit or a burn center. Prompt referral reduces risk of infection, mortality rate, and length of hospitalization.[28–30]

The main types of symptomatic treatment are the same as for burns, and the experience of burn units is helpful for the treatment of TEN: environmental temperature control, careful and aseptic handling, sterile field creation, avoidance of any adhesive material, and maintenance of venous peripheral access distant from affected areas.

Intravenous (IV) fluid replacement must be initiated immediately on admission and use macromolecules or saline solutions. The rate and amount of fluid and electrolyte administration must be adjusted daily. The early fluid requirement of TEN patients is two thirds to three fourths of that of patients with burns covering the same area.[31]

Like most other authors, we do not advocate the use of prophylactic antibiotics. Catheters should be changed and cultured regularly, and bacterial sampling of the skin lesions must be performed at least every 48 hours.

Early initiation of massive oral nutrition by nasogastric tube to minimize protein losses promotes healing and decreases the risk of stress ulcer. The environmental temperature should be increased to 30°C, and heat shields, infrared lamps, and an air-fluidized bed should be provided.

Thromboembolism and DIC are important causes of morbidity and death: Effective anticoagulation with heparin is recommended for the duration of hospitalization.[27]

Like patients with major burns, TEN patients suffer severe pain as well as emotional instability and extreme anxiety, which should be treated appropriately.[32]

Pulmonary care includes aerosols, bronchial aspiration, and physical therapy. Intubation and mechanical ventilation are nearly always necessary if the trachea and bronchi are involved.

The SJS/TEN disease spectrum remains an important cause of severe visual loss in a significant number of patients. Therefore, daily examination by an ophthalmologist and vigorous treatment are mandatory. Antiseptic or antibiotic eyedrops and eye ointments, with or without corticosteroids, should be instilled every 2 hours. Lid–globe adhesions should be cautiously removed with a glass rod twice daily to avoid occlusion of the fornices, taking care not to strip pseudomembranes which may lead to bleeding and increased conjunctival scarring.[33]

There is no consensus about topical care. Topical antiseptics (0.5% silver nitrate or 0.05% chlorhexidine) are usually used to paint, bathe, or dress the patients. Silver sulfadiazine, which is popular in burn units, should be avoided because sulfonamides are frequently implicated in the etiology of TEN and can cause hemolysis in glucose-6-phosphate dehydrogenase–deficient patients. Although most surgeons in burn units advocate large operative debridement of nonviable epidermis followed by immediate wound cover with biologic dressings such as Biobrane® or xenograft,[34] dermatologists are more conservative, leaving in place the epidermis that has not yet peeled off. Dressings may be gauzes with petrolatum, silver nitrate, or polyvidone iodine; hydrogels; Hydrone; Vigilon (semipermeable dressings); SoftSorb; and others, which can also be impregnated with silver nitrate.

CORTICOSTEROIDS AND OTHER "DISEASE-MODIFYING" DRUGS

For years, corticosteroids have been the mainstay therapy for TEN and SJS in most[32,35–42] (although not all[43,44]) dermatological centers, including ours, in the belief that they suppress the intensity of reaction, control the extension of the necrolytic process, decrease the involved area, reduce fever and discomfort, and prevent damage to internal organs when given at an early stage and in a sufficiently high dosage. There are no randomized clinical trials on the use of corticosteroids in the treatment of these life-threatening diseases.

The early approach to treatment was followed by a complete turnabout at the beginning of the 1980s when the management of SJS/TEN shifted to specialized burn centers and was taken over by nondermatologists, mostly surgeons, who rejected the use of steroids almost out of hand. They regarded them as being hazardous and a potential iatrogenic source of decreased host resistance, increased morbidity and complications (e.g., sepsis, leukopenia, thromboembolism, gastrointestinal ulcerations), prolonged recovery, worse and deteriorated prognosis, reduced survival and, for all intents and purposes, a contraindicated mode of therapy.[45–50]

In the absence of well-controlled trials, many dermatology departments adopted the concept of large burn units to avoid the use of steroids, in our opinion more as a matter of practicing "defensive medicine" and being on the safe (rather than on the effective) side.

The simple fact is that burns and TEN are two separate disease entities, and, although there is an "acute skin failure" in both conditions, they differ in terms of etiology and pathomechanism. Specifically, burns are a one-time, acute event that affects the skin from the outside, whereas TEN is a more complex, probably immune (T lymphocyte)-mediated process that reaches the skin from within. Above all, unlike thermal burns, in TEN, the disease continues to progress and becomes more intensified over a period of several days after its first appearance; therefore, it would make good sense to turn to aggressive disease-modifying drugs that are capable of halting disease progression, reduce the extent of skin detachment, decrease the inflammatory cytokines and, consequently, the symptoms, discomfort, organ damage (less relevant for burns), and perhaps mortality. The important role of burn units in the treatment of these patients notwithstanding, we think it has been a mistake to ignore our collective clinical experience and own good judgment and be swayed by the stand taken by plastic surgeons who view TEN and thermal burns as similar entities.

It is our hope that, with the introduction of new immunomodulating drugs, the pendulum will swing again in the opposite direction (i.e., toward advocating disease-modifying agents). The first step in this long journey has already been taken with the introduction in 1998 of IV immunoglobulins (IVIG) in the treatment of TEN patients.

Following the observation that antibodies present in IVIG block Fas-mediated keratinocyte apoptosis in vitro, and in light of the fact that the Fas–Fas ligand pathway of apoptosis is considered the first or pivotal step in the pathogenesis of TEN,[51] Viard and colleagues[52] tried this treatment in their patients. In their initial article, all 10 patients benefited from this therapy, an observation that was confirmed in several additional studies,[53–59] but contradicted by at least one prospective noncomparative study based on 34 patients from a single referral center.[60]

In a recent study from a plastic surgery and burn center from Italy,[61] the experience using IVIG together with the local conservative approach (the change to conservative approach by plastic surgeons is noteworthy) was related to previous treatments, which consisted of an aggressive approach with a wide debridement. The group treated with IVIG and conservative local approach showed a reduction in mortality rate from 75% to 26%.

The recommended approach today is early treatment at a total dose of 3 g/kg over 3 consecutive days (1 g/kg/d for 3 days).[61,62] It is of note that there are significant batch-to-batch variations concerning Fas-inhibitory activity of IVIG, which might also explain some of the variability in the response-rate of TEN patients to this therapy.

We hope that, with the meteoric advances being made in biologic therapy and the continuing development of target monoclonal antibodies against cytokines and receptors, new therapies will emerge that will more selectively and specifically target the underlying processes, thus avoiding treatment-related side effects. Until these new therapies are available for clinical use, we advocate treating TEN patients with what we have here and now, namely, IVIG and corticosteroids.

PROGNOSIS

In 2000, a mathematical tool called SCORTEN (Severity-of-Illness Score for Toxic Epidermal Necrolysis) was developed to asses severity of illness and predict mortality.[63]. SCORTEN should be computed within the first 24 hours after admission and again on Day 3.[64] The score is the sum of 7 easily measured clinical variables: 1) age (>40); 2) tachycardia (>120 bpm) ; 3) the presence of malignancy; 4) initial surface of epidermal detachment (>10%); 5) serum urea (>10 mmol/L); 6) serum glucose (>14 mmol/L; >252 mg/dL); and 7) bicarbonate (<20 mmol/L [mEq/L]). One point is given for each variable if positive and zero if negative. Computing the sum of the scores for each parameter results in a SCORTEN ranging from 0 to 7, with the mortality increasing sharply with each additional point (Table 15.3).

TABLE 15.3: Mortality and Severity-of-Illness Score for Toxic Epidermal Necrolysis)

SCORTEN	Mortality
0–1	3.2%
2	12.1%
3	35.3%
4	58.3%
≥5	90.0%

SCORTEN, Severity-of-Illness Score for Toxic Epidermal Necrolysis.

The scoring system that was developed with a French patient cohort has been validated in a U.S.-based patient cohort[65] and is proving to be a valuable tool for predicting patient outcome.

CONCLUDING REMARKS

"Any substance that is capable of producing a therapeutic effect can also produce unwanted or adverse effects."[66] ADR had occurred since the beginning of ancient medicine. To our great fortune, the most severe ADRs described here in SJS/TEN are rare. Despite their low incidence they are still frequent enough that primary care physicians and dermatologists will probably be involved with the management of at least one affected individual during their practice, but they are too infrequent to acquire any real degree of familiarity with them.

Because there is no specific and definitely effective treatment for SJS/TEN, prompt recognition and diagnosis and early identification and withdrawal of all potential causative drugs and prompt referral to a burn unit are generally agreed-upon steps and, for the time being, the best we can do for our patients to most significantly influence outcome and prognosis. Beyond that, however, considerable controversy exists. Evidence both pro and con exists for the use of IVIG, systemic corticosteroids, and other measures.

In this chapter, we present practical and comprehensive information on the two most severe acute cutaneous drug eruptions – SJS and TEN – concentrating on their definition, classification, clinical appearance, management, and prognosis. It is intentionally clinically oriented and covers what is most relevant to the clinicians in their practice, omitting the theoretical aspects of the pathogenesis of the diseases, unless they are relevant to diagnosis or treatment.

REFERENCES

1. Fabbri P, Panconesi E. Erythema multiforme ("minus" and "maius") and drug intake. Clin Dermatol. 1993; 11:479–89.
2. Stevens A, Johnson F. A new eruptive fever associated with stomatitis and ophthalmia. Am J Dis Child. 1922; 24:526.

3. Thomas B. The so-called Stevens-Johnson syndrome. Br Med J. 1950; 1:1393–7.

4. Lyell A. Toxic epidermal necrolysis: an eruption resembling scalding of the skin. Br J Dermatol. 1956; 68:355–61.

5. Lyell A. Drug-induced toxic epidermal necrolysis. I. An overview. Clin Dermatol. 1993; 11:491–2.

6. Bastuji-Garin S, Rzany B, Stern RS, et al. Clinical classification of cases of toxic epidermal necrolysis, Stevens-Johnson syndrome, and erythema multiforme. Arch Dermatol. 1993; 129:92–6.

7. Wolf R, Wolf D, Davidovici B. In the pursuit of classifying severe cutaneous adverse reactions. Clin Dermatol. 2007; 25:348–9.

8. Rasmussen J. Toxic epidermal necrolysis. Med Clin North Am. 1980; 64:901–20.

9. Chosidow O, Delchier JC, Chaumette MT, et al. Intestinal involvement in drug-induced toxic epidermal necrolysis. Lancet. 1991; 337:928.

10. Timsit JF, Mion G, Rouyer N, et al. Bronchopulmonary distress associated with toxic epidermal necrolysis. Intensive Care Med. 1992; 18:42–4.

11. Timsit JF, Mion G, Le Gulluche Y, et al. Severe hypothermia occurring during the course of toxic epidermal necrolysis in patients treated with air-fluidized beds. Arch Dermatol. 1991; 127:739–40.

12. Timsit JF, Mion G, Le Gulluche Y, Carsin H. Hypothermia and air-fluidized beds during toxic epidermal necrolysis management. Intensive Care Med. 1991; 17:506.

13. Forman R, Koren G, Shear NH. Erythema multiforme, Stevens-Johnson syndrome and toxic epidermal necrolysis in children: a review of 10 years' experience. Drug Saf. 2002; 25:965–72.

14. Magina S, Lisboa C, Leal V, et al. Dermatological and ophthalmological sequels in toxic epidermal necrolysis. Dermatology. 2003; 207:33–6.

15. Bombal C, Roujeau JC, Kuentz M, et al. [Hematologic anomalies in Lyell's syndrome. Study of 26 cases]. Ann Dermatol Venereol. 1983; 110:113–19.

16. Roujeau JC, Moritz S, Guillaume JC, et al. Lymphopenia and abnormal balance of T-lymphocyte subpopulations in toxic epidermal necrolysis. Arch Dermatol Res. 1985; 277:24–7.

17. Goens J, Song M, Fondu P, et al. Haematological disturbances and immune mechanisms in toxic epidermal necrolysis. Br J Dermatol. 1986; 114:255–9.

18. Kvasnicka J, Rezac J, Svejda J, et al. Disseminated intravascular coagulation associated with toxic epidermal necrolysis (Lyell's syndrome). Br J Dermatol. 1979; 100:551–8.

19. Kamaliah MD, Zainal D, Mokhtar N, Nazmi N. Erythema multiforme, Stevens-Johnson syndrome and toxic epidermal necrolysis in northeastern Malaysia. Int J Dermatol. 1998; 37:520–3.

20. Chosidow O, el Wady Z, Devanlay M, et al. Hyperamylasemia in toxic epidermal necrolysis. Arch Dermatol. 1993; 129:792–3.

21. Blum L, Chosidow O, Rostoker G, et al. Renal involvement in toxic epidermal necrolysis. J Am Acad Dermatol. 1996; 34:1088–90.

22. Schopf E, Stuhmer A, Rzany B, et al. Toxic epidermal necrolysis and Stevens-Johnson syndrome. An epidemiologic study from West Germany. Arch Dermatol. 1991; 127:839–42.

23. Chung WH, Hung SI, Chen YT. Human leukocyte antigens and drug hypersensitivity. Curr Opin Allergy Clin Immunol. 2007; 7:317–23.

24. Man CB, Kwan P, Baum L, et al. Association between HLA-B*1502 allele and antiepileptic drug-induced cutaneous reactions in Han Chinese. Epilepsia. 2007; 48:1015–18.

25. Lonjou C, Thomas L, Borot N, et al. A marker for Stevens-Johnson syndrome . . . : ethnicity matters. Pharmacogenomics J. 2006; 6:265–8.

26. Roujeau JC, Kelly JP, Naldi L, et al. Medication use and the risk of Stevens-Johnson syndrome or toxic epidermal necrolysis. N Engl J Med. 1995; 333:1600–7.

27. Garcia-Doval I, LeCleach L, Bocquet H, et al. Toxic epidermal necrolysis and Stevens-Johnson syndrome: does early withdrawal of causative drugs decrease the risk of death? Arch Dermatol. 2000; 136:323–7.

28. George Sm, Harrison DA, Welch CA, et al. Dermatological conditions in intensive care: a secondary analysis of the Intensive Care National Audit & Research Centre (INCNARC) Case Mix Programme Database. Crit Care 2008;Euppl1:S1–S10.

29. McGee T, Munster A. Toxic epidermal necrolysis syndrome: mortality rate reduced with early referral to regional burn center. Plast Reconstr Surg. 1998; 102:1018–22.

30. Demling RH, Ellerbe S, Lowe NJ. Burn unit management of toxic epidermal necrolysis. Arch Surg. 1978; 113; 758–9.

31. Roujeau JC, Revuz J. Intensive care in dermatology. In: Champion R, Pye R, editors. Recent advances in dermatology. Edinburgh: Churchill Livingstone; 1990. pp. 85–99.

32. Anhalt G, Snelling CF. Toxic epidermal necrolysis. Case report. Plast Reconstr Surg. 1978; 61:905–10.

33. Power WJ, Ghoraishi M, Merayo-Lloves J, et al. Analysis of the acute ophthalmic manifestations of the erythema multiforme/Stevens-Johnson syndrome/toxic epidermal necrolysis disease spectrum. Ophthalmology. 1995; 102: 1669–76.

34. Palmieri TL, Greenhalgh DG, Saffle JR, et al. A multicenter review of toxic epidermal necrolysis treated in U.S. burn centers at the end of the twentieth century. J Burn Care Rehabil. 2002; 23:87–96.

35. Bjornberg A. Fifteen cases of toxic epidermal necrolysis (Lyell). Acta Derm Venereol. 1973; 53:149–52.

36. Ohlenschlaeger K. Toxic epidermal necrolysis and Stevens-Johnson's disease. Acta Derm Venereol. 1966; 46: 204–9.

37. Sherertz EF, Jegasothy BV, Lazarus GS. Phenytoin hypersensitivity reaction presenting with toxic epidermal necrolysis and severe hepatitis. Report of a patient treated with corticosteroid "pulse therapy." J Am Acad Dermatol. 1985; 12:178–81.

38. Patterson R, Dykewicz MS, Gonzales A, et al. Erythema multiforme and Stevens-Johnson syndrome. Descriptive and therapeutic controversy. Chest. 1990; 98:331–6.

39. Prendiville JS, Hebert AA, Greenwald MJ, Esterly NB. Management of Stevens-Johnson syndrome and toxic epidermal necrolysis in children. J Pediatr. 1989; 115:881–7.

40. Tegelberg-Stassen MJ, van Vloten WA, Baart de la Faille H. Management of nonstaphylococcal toxic epidermal

necrolysis: follow-up study of 16 case histories. Dermatologica. 1990; 180:124–9.

41. Patterson R, Grammer LC, Greenberger PA, et al. Stevens-Johnson syndrome (SJS): effectiveness of corticosteroids in management and recurrent SJS. Allergy Proc. 1992; 13:89–95.

42. Cheriyan S, Patterson R, Greenberger PA, et al. The outcome of Stevens-Johnson syndrome treated with corticosteroids. Allergy Proc. 1995; 16:151–5.

43. Rasmussen JE. Erythema multiforme in children. Response to treatment with systemic corticosteroids. Br J Dermatol. 1976; 95:181–6.

44. Rasmussen JE. Toxic epidermal necrolysis. A review of 75 cases in children. Arch Dermatol. 1975; 111:1135–9.

45. Halebian P, Corder VJ, Herndon D, Shires GT. A burn center experience with toxic epidermal necrolysis. J Burn Care Rehabil. 1983; 4:176–83.

46. Halebian PH, Corder VJ, Madden MR, et al. Improved burn center survival of patients with toxic epidermal necrolysis managed without corticosteroids. Ann Surg. 1986; 204:503–12.

47. Jones WG, Halebian P, Madden M, et al. Drug-induced toxic epidermal necrolysis in children. J Pediatr Surg. 1989; 24:167–70.

48. Halebian PH, Shires GT. Burn unit treatment of acute, severe exfoliating disorders. Annu Rev Med. 1989; 40:137–47.

49. Kelemen JJ III, Cioffi WG, McManus WF, et al. Burn center care for patients with toxic epidermal necrolysis. J Am Coll Surg. 1995; 180:273–8.

50. Sheridan RL, Weber JM, Schulz JT, et al. Management of severe toxic epidermal necrolysis in children. J Burn Care Rehabil. 1999; 20:497–500.

51. Abe R, Shimizu T, Shibaki A, et al. Toxic epidermal necrolysis and Stevens-Johnson syndrome are induced by soluble Fas ligand. Am J Pathol. 2003; 162:1515–20.

52. Viard I, Wehrli P, Bullani R, et al. Inhibition of toxic epidermal necrolysis by blockade of CD95 with human intravenous immunoglobulin. Science. 1998; 282:490–3.

53. Stella M, Cassano P, Bollero D, et al. Toxic epidermal necrolysis treated with intravenous high-dose immunoglobulins: our experience. Dermatology. 2001; 203:45–9.

54. Tristani-Firouzi P, Petersen MJ, Saffle JR, et al. Treatment of toxic epidermal necrolysis with intravenous immunoglobulin in children. J Am Acad Dermatol. 2002; 47:548–52.

55. Tan A, Tan HH, Lee CC, Ng SK. Treatment of toxic epidermal necrolysis in AIDS with intravenous immunoglobulins. Clin Exp Dermatol. 2003; 28:269–71.

56. Prins C, Vittorio C, Padilla RS, et al. Effect of high-dose intravenous immunoglobulin therapy in Stevens-Johnson syndrome: a retrospective, multicenter study. Dermatology. 2003; 207:96–9.

57. Prins C, Kerdel FA, Padilla RS, et al. Treatment of toxic epidermal necrolysis with high-dose intravenous immunoglobulins: multicenter retrospective analysis of 48 consecutive cases. Arch Dermatol. 2003; 139:26–32.

58. Trent JT, Kirsner RS, Romanelli P, Kerdel FA. Analysis of intravenous immunoglobulin for the treatment of toxic epidermal necrolysis using SCORTEN: The University of Miami Experience. Arch Dermatol. 2003; 139:39–43.

59. Sidwell RU, Swift S, Yan CL, et al. Treatment of toxic epidermal necrolysis with intravenous immunoglobulin. Int J Clin Pract. 2003; 57:643–5.

60. Bachot N, Revuz J, Roujeau JC. Intravenous immunoglobulin treatment for Stevens-Johnson syndrome and toxic epidermal necrolysis: a prospective noncomparative study showing no benefit on mortality or progression. Arch Dermatol. 2003; 139:33–6.

61. Stella M, Clemente A, Bollero D, et al. Toxic epidermal necrolysis (TEN) and Stevens-Johnson syndrome (SJS): experience with high-dose intravenous immunoglobulins and topical conservative approach. A retrospective analysis. Burns. 2007; 33:452–9.

62. Teo L, Tay YK, Liu TT, Kwok C. Stevens-Johnson syndrome and toxic epidermal necrolysis: efficacy of intravenous immunoglobulin and a review of treatment options. Singapore Med J 2009; 50:29–33.

63. Bastuji-Garin S, Fouchard N, Bertocchi M, et al. SCORTEN: a severity-of-illness score for toxic epidermal necrolysis. J Invest Dermatol. 2000; 115:149–53.

64. Guegan S, Bastuji-Garin S, Poszepczynska-Guigne E, et al. Performance of the SCORTEN during the first five days of hospitalization to predict the prognosis of epidermal necrolysis. J Invest Dermatol. 2006; 126:272–6.

65. Trent JT, Kirsner RS, Romanelli P, Kerdel FA. Use of SCORTEN to accurately predict mortality in patients with toxic epidermal necrolysis in the United States. Arch Dermatol. 2004; 140:890–2.

66. Edwards IR, Aronson JK. Adverse drug reactions: definitions, diagnosis, and management. Lancet. 2000; 356:1255–9.

CHAPTER 16

Severe, Acute Adverse Cutaneous Drug Reactions II: DRESS Syndrome and Serum Sickness-Like Reaction

Ronni Wolf

Batya B. Davidovici

DRUG RASH WITH EOSINOPHILIA AND SYSTEMIC SYMPTOMS

Background

Drug rash with eosinophilia and systemic symptoms (DRESS) syndrome, formerly termed "drug hypersensitivity syndrome" (HSS), is a severe, potentially fatal adverse drug reaction characterized by skin rash, fever, lymph-node enlargement, and single- or multiple-organ involvement, characteristically occurring in a delayed fashion between 3 and 8 weeks after starting treatment with the culpable drug for the first time.

Phenytoin HSS was first described in 1939,[1] 1 year after phenytoin had been introduced in the treatment of convulsive disorders. Similar reactions were reported during the following years, initially to various anticonvulsant drugs[2,3] and later to many other drugs.[4–6] Consequently, the name of this reaction was changed to the more widely inclusive HSS, instead of anticonvulsant-, sulfone-, or dapsone-hypersensitivity syndrome. The word "hypersensitivity" itself, however, is ambiguous and uninformative insofar as it may apply to any idiosyncratic reaction that fits one phase of the classic Gell and Coombs classification. Therefore, a more informative, precise, and clinically relevant term was proposed, "drug rash with eosinophilia and systemic symptoms" or DRESS.[7] The suitability of the term DRESS has recently been questioned because eosinophilia need not necessarily be present in this syndrome, and a return to "drug-induced HSS" has been suggested.[8]

DRESS is characteristically defined by a triad of symptoms consisting of fever, skin eruption, and internal organ involvement. In this context, it should be mentioned that serum sickness (SS) or serum sickness-like reaction (SSLR), which have many features in common with DRESS syndrome, are distinct diseases that have another pathogenesis and, as such, should be distinguished from DRESS syndrome (Table 16.1).

Epidemiology and Causative Drugs

The true incidence of DRESS syndrome is unknown because its variable presentation confounds uniform diagnosis. It is estimated to occur in between 1 in 1000 and 1 in 10,000 exposures with drugs such as anticonvulsants and sulfonamides.[9] In a record linkage study, the risk for developing DRESS syndrome within 60 days of the first or second prescription in new adult users of phenytoin or carbamazepine was estimated to be 2.3–4.5 per 10,000 exposures, respectively.[10]

The aromatic anticonvulsants (phenylhydantoin, phenobarbital, carbamazepine)[9,11–14] and sulfonamides[15] are the most common causes of DRESS syndrome, but a large variety of other drugs have been associated with it, notably among them lamotrigine[16,17] (see Figure 16.1), allopurinol,[18,19] nonsteroidal antiinflammatory drugs, captopril, antibiotics, tuberculostatic drugs, calcium channel blockers, mood stabilizers, neuroleptics, dapsone, terbinafine, methyldopa, minocycline, and antiretroviral drugs.[20,21]

TABLE 16.1: Comparison between DRESS Syndrome and SS/SSLR

Symptom	DRESS syndrome	SS/SSLR
Rash	Exanthematous (mostly)	Urticarial (mostly)
Onset of symptoms	1–8 weeks	>2 weeks
Fever	Present	Present
Internal organ involvement	Present	Absent
Arthralgia	Absent	Present
Lymphadenopathy	Present	Present

DRESS, drug rash with eosinophilia and systemic symptoms; SS/SSLR, serum sickness/serum sickness-like reaction.

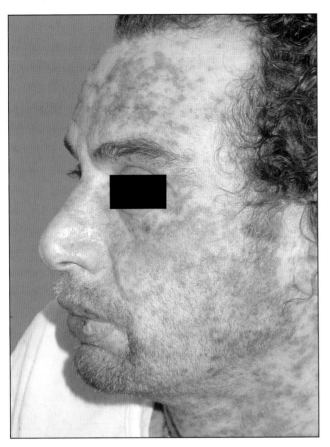

FIGURE 16.1: *A 43-year-old man with lamotrigine-induced drug rash with eosinophilia and systemic symptoms (DRESS). Note the typical periorbital edema.*

Clinical and Laboratory Aids Required for Diagnosis

DRESS syndrome occurs most frequently on first exposure to the drug, with initial symptoms starting between 1 and 8 weeks afterward.[22] The syndrome may occur within 1 day upon rechallenge in previously sensitized individuals.

The syndrome commonly begins with a fever shortly followed by a maculopapular rash and varying degrees of lymphadenopathy. Body temperature ranges from 38°C to 40°C, with spikes that usually generate the concern of an underlying infection. The spiking fever often persists for as long as weeks despite discontinuation of the offending drug.[23]

An eruption occurs in approximately 70%–100% of patients.[8] In most cases, the cutaneous eruption starts as a macular erythema that often evolves into a red, symmetrical, pruritic, confluent, and papular rash. Pustules, either follicular or nonfollicular, may also be present. The upper trunk and face are initially affected, with later involvement of the lower extremities. Facial and periorbital edema is a frequent occurrence, and can lead to such gross distortion of the patients' features that they can become unrecognizable. Notably, there is usually no mucosal involvement, a feature that helps to distinguish DRESS from other forms of severe drug eruptions, such as Stevens–Johnson syndrome (SJS) or toxic epidermal necrolysis (TEN).

As for internal organ involvement, again there is a large degree of variability among patients with regard to both the target organs involved and the severity of the involvement. It is important to emphasize, however, that the severity of cutaneous changes does not necessarily reflect the severity of internal organ involvement. Therefore, meticulous assessment is necessary for patients suspected of DRESS syndrome and internal organ involvement. It is also important to bear in mind that internal organ involvement may not develop for 1–2 weeks into the reaction, and even not until 1 month later.

The liver is the most frequently involved internal organ, with tender hepatomegaly and sometimes with splenomegaly. Liver involvement can range from mild elevations in serum transaminase levels[24] to granulomatous hepatitis or fulminant hepatic necrosis.[25–28] The degree of hepatitis is related to the interval between the onset of the syndrome and the discontinuation of the drug.[29] Prompt recognition of the syndrome and withdrawal of the drug are therefore of utmost importance to the prognosis.

The kidney is another organ frequently involved, and the nephrotic condition can range from mild hematuria, to nephritis, to acute renal failure, usually following acute granulomatous interstitial nephritis, even despite discontinuation of the offending drug.[30,31]

Rarer manifestations of DRESS syndrome are colitis, pneumonitis, pancreatitis, myocarditis, encephalitis, arthritis, and myositis.[8,32] Thyroiditis with autoantibodies has also been reported. Its acute hyperthyroid phase may be missed by the clinician because of fever, tachycardia, and malaise, which are part of DRESS syndrome, and may thus be identified only several months later when hypothyroidism develops.[33]

Lymphadenopathy is perhaps the most frequent finding associated with DRESS syndrome. In the early stages of the disease, lymph-node histology shows benign hyperplasia, but histological changes may progress to reveal atypical lymphoid cells. In rare cases, pseudolymphoma or lymphoma may develop if the drug is not discontinued.[34]

Notably, no single symptom, including fever or peripheral eosinophilia, is necessarily present in all cases of DRESS, and cutaneous lesions apparently are, in fact, the most often reported signs. The clinical pattern of skin changes is, however, quite variable, ranging, according to the present definition, from a faint generalized exanthematous eruption to SJS or TEN. The same is true for the other associated symptoms, organ dysfunction, and laboratory abnormalities.[8,32,35]

In 2006, a Japanese consensus group proposed a set of criteria for diagnosis of DRESS (or, as suggested by them, drug-induced hypersensitivity syndrome, DIHS).[21] That group established 6 diagnostic criteria for DIHS/DRESS to which they subsequently added a 7th:[36] 1) maculopapular rash developing more than 3 weeks after starting therapy; 2) prolonged clinical symptoms 2 weeks after discontinuation of the causative drug; 3) fever higher than 38°C; 4) at least one leukocyte abnormality (i.e., leukocytosis >11 × 10^8/L), atypical lymphocytosis >5%, or eosinophilia >1.5 × 10^8/L); 5) liver abnormalities (alanine aminotransferase >100U/L), which can be replaced with other organ involvement, such as the kidney; 6) lymphadenopathy; and 7) human herpesvirus 6 (HHV-6) reactivation. The diagnosis is confirmed by the presence of all seven of these criteria (typical DIHS) or of the first five (atypical DIHS). The most novel and innovative of the proposed criteria is undoubtedly HHV-6 reactivation. The authors state that their series of more than 60 patients diagnosed by clinical findings had consistently shown that HHV-6 reactivation can be detected in the vast majority of patients who satisfy the other six criteria and show clinical manifestations consistent with the classical triad, but not in patients with other types of drug eruption, such as papulomacular rash, SJS, and TEN. Moreover, HHV-6 was rarely detected in patients with a tendency toward milder disease. Without entering into any debate about the appropriateness of this criterion, the fact that it usually appears 2–3 weeks after the onset of rash means that it can be used for studies and late analyses, but not when we first see our patient and have to make urgent decisions. The same holds true, of course, for their second criterion.

We especially espouse two features of this newly suggested classification: 1) it narrows the wide definition of cutaneous rash, in particular by excluding cases with cutaneous manifestations of SJS and TEN, a characteristic that we had emphasized long ago,[20,35] and 2) it provides cutoff points for delineating hematological and other laboratory abnormalities.

Although most authors agree that the existence of DRESS as a clinically distinctive and unique entity is unarguable,[8,37] its diagnosis is complicated because, in addition to its highly variable presentation, it is a diagnosis by exclusion. Its main features, such as rash, fever, and organ involvement, can also be attributed to a wide range of other causes, most notably infections (with which it is also often associated). The similarity between DRESS and infection diseases is of particular importance considering our efforts to avoid prescribing for patients with DRESS additional drugs because they can cross-react with other drugs or initiate drug neosensitization[38] during DRESS, whereas we usually use drugs such as analgesics/antipyretics and antibiotics in the case of infections.

Treatment

DRESS is potentially life threatening. The mortality rate is estimated at nearly 10%, although complete recovery can be achieved.[39] DRESS syndrome must be promptly recognized and all potential culprit drugs withdrawn.

Skin care may include the use of topical steroids to alleviate symptoms. The main principles of therapy for extensive rash or erythroderma are the same as those for major burns: warming of the environment, correction of electrolyte disturbances, high caloric intake, and prevention of sepsis.

As for the controversy about the use of systemic corticosteroids, unlike their position on the administration of these medications to patients with SJS/TEN, most authors do not regard them as either hazardous or contraindicated and suggest their use "when internal organ involvement exists."[40,41] Because internal organ involvement is a prerequisite for this syndrome (remember, the requisite triad of fever, rash, and internal organ involvement!), however, systemic steroids should be considered in most cases of DRESS syndrome, particularly in patients with severe organ damage. Furthermore, corticosteroids are known for their beneficial effects in diseases with blood eosinophilia (e.g., hypereosinophilic syndrome), where eosinophils are responsible for organ damage, and thus might be expected to be of benefit in DRESS, insofar as eosinophil accumulation is also thought to account for the internal organ involvement in this disease.

SERUM SICKNESS AND SERUM SICKNESS-LIKE REACTION

Background

SS, first described in humans by von Pirquet and Schick in 1905, is a type III hypersensitivity reaction (of the classic Gell and Coombs classification) resulting from the administration of foreign protein or of heterologous serum, usually equine, serving as an antitoxin.[42]

The syndrome includes fever, cutaneous eruptions (mostly urticaria), edema, arthralgias, and lymphadenopathy. Although fatalities from this reaction are rare, it has been traditionally included in the group of severe adverse cutaneous reactions to drugs[43] because it requires hospitalization (and, often, intensive care) and might cause extensive organ damage.

During the first 4 decades of the 19th century, it was not uncommon for up to 50% of patients to develop this reaction after treatment with horse serum as an antiserum to diphtheria, tetanus, rabies, or other organisms. It has almost disappeared in these settings with the advent of effective immunization procedures, antimicrobial therapy, and the development of specific human immune serum globulins. More recently, SS has made a comeback with the introduction of targeted immune modulators – commonly referred to as biological response modifiers or simply "biologics." It is also commonly seen with the use of antivenom therapy used to treat envenomations by snakes, spiders, scorpions, and so forth. The SSLR that is similar to classic SS may result from the administration of a number of nonprotein drugs, such as antibiotics (particularly cefaclor and minocycline), psychiatric drugs, analgesic/

antiinflammatory drugs, antineoplastic drugs, and many others.

Clinical and Laboratory Aids Required for Diagnosis

Early recognition and accurate diagnosis are the keys to the management of SS because treatment is highly effective in reversing all symptoms. Recognition and diagnosis, however, are made more difficult by a lack of diagnostic and laboratory criteria and by the protean manifestations of this reaction.

An attempt was recently made to gather signs and symptoms and produce diagnostic criteria for SS.[44] Four major criteria were established: 1) more than 7 days since initial drug (thymoglobulin) administration, 2) persistent high fevers (>101°F), 3) persistent arthritis/arthralgias, and 4) positive heterologous antibodies on enzyme-linked immunosorbent assay. Rash was considered a minor criterion. These criteria are, however, in disagreement with earlier studies, in which cutaneous rash appeared in more than 90% of patients.[45–48] The clinical manifestations of SS begin at 4–21 days (usual range 7–10 days) after initial exposure to the causative antigen. Symptoms usually include fever, a cutaneous eruption (morbilliform, urticaria, or the combination of these two reaction patterns) in more than 90% of patients, arthralgias in up to 50%, lymphadenopathy, and myalgias. Headache and gastrointestinal complaints may occasionally occur as well. Less common manifestations include arthritis, nephritis, neuropathy, and other organ involvement.

The diagnosis is made on the basis of clinical findings because there are no pathognomonic laboratory tests specific for the diagnosis of SS or SSLRs in the acute setting. The erythrocyte sedimentation rate is noncontributory because it may be elevated, normal, or low. Leukopenia or leukocytosis may be present, and SS is one of the few illnesses in which plasmocytosis may be detected in the peripheral blood smear. The urine analysis may show proteinuria, hematuria, or hemoglobinuria. Serum creatinine and transaminases may be transiently elevated. Circulating immune complexes may rise and fall before symptoms and signs appear. Serum concentrations of C3, C4, and total complement are depressed because of the formation of immune complexes, but they tend to rapidly return to normal.[49] Direct immunofluorescence microscopy of lesional skin from patients with SS had demonstrated immunoreactants in seven of nine subjects, with immunoreactants being confined to the walls of dermal blood vessels and consisting of immunoglobulin M, C3, immunoglobulin E, and immunoglobulin A. Immunoglobulin G was not identified in any of the specimens.[46]

Therapy

We, like others,[44] recommend the administration of high-dose steroids for 3–5 days, followed by a prednisone taper,

depending on the severity of the disease and its activity. Typically, there is a noticeable improvement in the fevers and arthralgias within the first 48 hours of treatment, and resolution of symptoms is seen over approximately 8–10 days.[50] Some groups consider plasmapheresis the first-line therapy for SS.[51,52] Like others,[44] however, we think that plasmapheresis should be reserved for steroid-resistant cases.

Vasculitis

Vasculitis is inflammation of vessel walls. It has many causes, although they result in only a few histologic patterns of vascular inflammation. Vessels of any type in any organ can be affected; this fact results in a wide variety of signs and symptoms. These manifold clinical manifestations, combined with the etiologic nonspecificity of the histologic lesions, complicate the diagnosis of specific forms of vasculitis. The difficulty in diagnosis is problematic because different vasculitides with indistinguishable clinical presentations have different etiologies, associations with specific diseases, involvement in certain organs, prognoses, and treatments. To make things even more complicated, there are many classifications and no agreed-upon diagnostic criteria for the various categories of vasculitis, particularly the small-vessel vasculitides.

Drugs cause approximately 10% of vasculitic skin lesions and should be considered in any patient with small-vessel vasculitis.[53–55] Withdrawal of the offending agent alone is often sufficient to induce prompt resolution of clinical manifestations, obviating the need for systemic corticosteroids or more powerful forms of immunosuppression.

For more details on this topic, readers are directed to Chapter 23 in this book, which is devoted entirely to purpura and vasculitis of any kind.

REFERENCES

1. Merrit H, Putnam T. Sodium diphenylhydantoinate in treatment of convulsive disorders: toxic symptoms and their prevention. Arch Neurol Psych. 1939; 42:1053–8.
2. Shear NH, Spielberg SP. Anticonvulsant hypersensitivity syndrome. In vitro assessment of risk. J Clin Invest. 1988; 82:1826–32.
3. Haruda F. Phenytoin hypersensitivity: 38 cases. Neurology. 1979; 29:1480–5.
4. Tomecki KJ, Catalano CJ. Dapsone hypersensitivity. The sulfone syndrome revisited. Arch Dermatol. 1981; 117: 38–9.
5. Wolf R, Tamir A, Werbin N, Brenner S. Methyldopa hypersensitivity syndrome. Ann Allergy. 1993; 71:166–8.
6. Knowles SR, Shapiro L, Shear NH. Serious adverse reactions induced by minocycline. Report of 13 patients and review of the literature. Arch Dermatol. 1996; 132:934–9.
7. Bocquet H, Bagot M, Roujeau JC. Drug-induced pseudolymphoma and drug hypersensitivity syndrome (Drug Rash with Eosinophilia and Systemic Symptoms: DRESS). Semin Cutan Med Surg. 1996; 15:250–7.

8. Peyriere H, Dereure O, Breton H, et al. Variability in the clinical pattern of cutaneous side-effects of drugs with systemic symptoms: does a DRESS syndrome really exist? Br J Dermatol. 2006; 155:422–8.

9. Schlienger RG, Shear NH. Antiepileptic drug hypersensitivity syndrome. Epilepsia. 1998; 39 Suppl 7:S3–S7.

10. Tennis P, Stern RS. Risk of serious cutaneous disorders after initiation of use of phenytoin, carbamazepine, or sodium valproate: a record linkage study. Neurology. 1997; 49:542–6.

11. Shear NH, Spielberg SP. Anticonvulsant hypersensitivity syndrome. In vitro assessment of risk. J Clin Invest. 1988; 82:1826–32.

12. Knowles SR, Shapiro LE, Shear NH. Anticonvulsant hypersensitivity syndrome: incidence, prevention and management. Drug Saf. 1999; 21:489–501.

13. Bessmertny O, Pham T. Antiepileptic hypersensitivity syndrome: clinicians beware and be aware. Curr Allergy Asthma Rep. 2002; 2:34–9.

14. De Vriese AS, Philippe J, Van Renterghem DM, et al. Carbamazepine hypersensitivity syndrome: report of 4 cases and review of the literature. Medicine (Baltimore). 1995; 74: 144–51.

15. Cribb AE, Lee BL, Trepanier LA, Spielberg SP. Adverse reactions to sulphonamide and sulphonamide-trimethoprim antimicrobials: clinical syndromes and pathogenesis. Adverse Drug React Toxicol Rev. 1996; 15:9–50.

16. Bessmertny O, Pham T. Antiepileptic hypersensitivity syndrome: clinicians beware and be aware. Curr Allergy Asthma Rep. 2002; 2:34–9.

17. Knowles SR, Shapiro LE, Shear NH. Anticonvulsant hypersensitivity syndrome: incidence, prevention and management. Drug Saf. 1999; 21:489–501.

18. Hamanaka H, Mizutani H, Nouchi N, et al. Allopurinol hypersensitivity syndrome: hypersensitivity to oxypurinol but not allopurinol. Clin Exp Dermatol. 1998; 23:32–4.

19. Sommers LM, Schoene RB. Allopurinol hypersensitivity syndrome associated with pancreatic exocrine abnormalities and new-onset diabetes mellitus. Arch Intern Med. 2002; 162:1190–2.

20. Wolf R, Orion E, Marcos B, Matz H. Life-threatening acute adverse cutaneous drug reactions. Clin Dermatol. 2005; 23:171–81.

21. Shiohara T, Inaoka M, Kano Y. Drug-induced hypersensitivity syndrome (DIHS): a reaction induced by a complex interplay among herpesviruses and antiviral and antidrug immune responses. Allergol Int. 2006; 55:1–8.

22. Shear NH, Spielberg SP. Anticonvulsant hypersensitivity syndrome. In vitro assessment of risk. J Clin Invest. 1988; 82:1826–32.

23. Kennebeck GA. Anticonvulsant hypersensitivity syndrome. J Am Board Fam Pract. 2000; 13:364–70.

24. Baba M, Karakas M, Aksungur VL, et al. The anticonvulsant hypersensitivity syndrome. J Eur Acad Dermatol Venereol. 2003; 17:399–401.

25. Crantock L, Prentice R, Powell L. Cholestatic jaundice associated with captopril therapy. J Gastroenterol Hepatol. 1991; 6:528–30.

26. Parker WA, Shearer CA. Phenytoin hepatotoxicity: a case report and review. Neurology. 1979; 29:175–8.

27. Morkunas AR, Miller MB. Anticonvulsant hypersensitivity syndrome. Crit Care Clin. 1997; 13:727–39.

28. Mahadeva U, Al Mrayat M, Steer K, Leen E. Fatal phenytoin hypersensitivity syndrome. Postgrad Med J. 1999; 75: 734–6.

29. Vittorio CC, Muglia JJ. Anticonvulsant hypersensitivity syndrome. Arch Intern Med. 1995; 155:2285–90.

30. Fervenza FC, Kanakiriya S, Kunau RT, et al. Acute granulomatous interstitial nephritis and colitis in anticonvulsant hypersensitivity syndrome associated with lamotrigine treatment. Am J Kidney Dis. 2000; 36:1034–40.

31. Hegarty J, Picton M, Agarwal G, et al. Carbamazepine-induced acute granulomatous interstitial nephritis. Clin Nephrol. 2002; 57:310–13.

32. Kosseifi SG, Guha B, Nassour DN, et al. The dapsone hypersensitivity syndrome revisited: a potentially fatal multisystem disorder with prominent hepatopulmonary manifestations. J Occup Med Toxicol. 2006; 1:9.

33. Gupta A, Eggo MC, Uetrecht JP, et al. Drug-induced hypothyroidism: the thyroid as a target organ in hypersensitivity reactions to anticonvulsants and sulfonamides. Clin Pharmacol Ther. 1992; 51:56–67.

34. Vittorio CC, Muglia JJ. Anticonvulsant hypersensitivity syndrome. Arch Intern Med. 1995; 155:2285–90.

35. Wolf R, Davidovici B, Matz H, et al. Drug rash with eosinophilia and systemic symptoms versus Stevens-Johnson Syndrome–a case that indicates a stumbling block in the current classification. Int Arch Allergy Immunol. 2006; 141:308–10.

36. Shiohara T, Iijima M, Ikezawa Z, Hashimoto K. The diagnosis of a DRESS syndrome has been sufficiently established on the basis of typical clinical features and viral reactivations. Br J Dermatol. 2007; 156:1083–4.

37. Kardaun SH, Sidoroff A, Valeyrie-Allanore L, et al. Variability in the clinical pattern of cutaneous side-effects of drugs with systemic symptoms: does a DRESS syndrome really exist? Br J Dermatol. 2007; 156:609–11.

38. Gaig P, Garcia-Ortega P, Baltasar M, Bartra J. Drug neosensitization during anticonvulsant hypersensitivity syndrome. J Investig Allergol Clin Immunol. 2006; 16:321–6.

39. Ghislain PD, Roujeau JC. Treatment of severe drug reactions: Stevens-Johnson syndrome, toxic epidermal necrolysis and hypersensitivity syndrome. Dermatol Online J. 2002; 8:5.

40. Tas S, Simonart T. Management of drug rash with eosinophilia and systemic symptoms (DRESS syndrome): an update. Dermatology. 2003; 206:353–6.

41. Auret-Leca E, Norbert K, Bensouda-Grimaldi L, et al. DRESS syndrome, a drug reaction which remains bad known from paediatricians. Arch Pediatr. 2007; 14:1439–41.

42. von Pirquet C, Schick B. Die Serumkrankheit. Leipzig: Deuticke; 1905.

43. Roujeau JC, Stern RS. Severe adverse cutaneous reactions to drugs. N Engl J Med. 1994; 331:1272–85.

44. Lundquist AL, Chari RS, Wood JH, et al. Serum sickness following rabbit antithymocyte-globulin induction in a liver transplant recipient: case report and literature review. Liver Transpl. 2007; 13:647–50.

45. Bielory L, Gascon P, Lawley TJ, et al. Human serum sickness: a prospective analysis of 35 patients treated with equine

anti-thymocyte globulin for bone marrow failure. Medicine (Baltimore). 1988; 67:40–57.

46. Bielory L, Yancey KB, Young NS, et al. Cutaneous manifestations of serum sickness in patients receiving antithymocyte globulin. J Am Acad Dermatol. 1985; 13:411–17.

47. LoVecchio F, Welch S, Klemens J, et al. Incidence of immediate and delayed hypersensitivity to Centruroides antivenom. Ann Emerg Med. 1999; 34:615–19.

48. Chao YK, Shyur SD, Wu CY, Wang CY. Childhood serum sickness: a case report. J Microbiol Immunol Infect. 2001; 34:220–3.

49. Gamarra RM, McGraw SD, Drelichman VS, Maas LC. Serum sickness-like reactions in patients receiving intravenous infliximab. J Emerg Med. 2006; 30:41–4.

50. Bielory L, Gascon P, Lawley TJ, et al. Human serum sickness: a prospective analysis of 35 patients treated with equine anti-thymocyte globulin for bone marrow failure. Medicine (Baltimore). 1988; 67:40–57.

51. Christiaans MH, van Hooff JP. Plasmapheresis and RATG-induced serum sickness. Transplantation. 2006; 81:296.

52. Pham PT, Pham PM, Miller JM, Pham PC. Polyclonal antibody-induced serum sickness presenting as rapidly progressive descending paralysis. Transplantation. 2007; 83: 1657.

53. Ekenstam E, Callen JP. Cutaneous leukocytoclastic vasculitis. Clinical and laboratory features of 82 patients seen in private practice. Arch Dermatol. 1984; 120:484–9.

54. Sanchez NP, Van Hale HM, Su WP. Clinical and histopathologic spectrum of necrotizing vasculitis. Report of findings in 101 cases. Arch Dermatol. 1985; 121:220–4.

55. Jennette JC, Falk RJ. Small-vessel vasculitis. N Engl J Med. 1997; 337:1512–23.

CHAPTER 17

Severe, Acute Complications of Dermatologic Therapies

Ronni Wolf

Jasna Lipozenčić

Batya B. Davidovici

ALTHOUGH PHYSICIANS from other specialties, like the population at large, still consider cutaneous maladies as being mainly aesthetic, skin deep, and insignificant, they are generally aware that treating these diseases often requires a variety of potent systemic drugs and not only topical treatments. These powerful medications may cause many adverse reactions, some of them severe, acute, or even life threatening.

"There are no really 'safe' biologically active drugs. There are only 'safe' physicians."[1] A "safe" physician must, first and foremost, be well informed about adverse reactions at the time of prescribing a drug, during the follow-up period, and especially when one of these rare catastrophes suddenly occurs. Because the diversity of severe adverse reactions to dermatologic therapies is almost endless, we focus on new drugs and the less known adverse effects.

TARGETED IMMUNE MODULATORS/BIOLOGICS

Targeted immune modulators (TIMs) – commonly referred to as biological response modifiers or simply "biologics" – are a relatively new category of medications used in the treatment of certain types of immunologic and inflammatory diseases, including dermatologic diseases, most notably psoriasis.

Overall, TIMs appear to have a good tolerability profile, although some rare but acute serious adverse events, such as infections, hematologic events, neurologic events, infusion reactions, congestive heart failure, nephrotic syndrome, and others, are of concern. The following sections describe adverse events associated with TIMs.

Infusion Reactions

As is the case with any foreign protein–derived agent, infusion with chimeric antibodies that contain murine antibodies, such as infliximab (containing 25% murine proteins), can lead to either acute or delayed infusion reactions. Overall, these reactions occur in up to 10%–20% of patients and usually during or within 2 hours after infusion.[2] They can, in most cases, be easily managed.

Clinical manifestations of acute infusion reaction include fever, chest pain and/or discomfort (e.g., tightening pressure), hypotension or hypertension, palpitations, urticaria, and hyperemia. Although such a reaction might very well be a harrowing experience to the uninformed, most of the symptoms improve substantially or resolve completely after stopping the infusion or slowing its rate. The Division of Clinical Immunology Infusion Center at Mount Sinai Medical Center has developed a protocol for the treatment of initial severe acute reactions[3,4] that recommends stopping the infusion and starting an infusion of normal saline. The airway must be maintained, and oxygen is given. Epinephrine (0.1–0.5 mL, 1:1000) is administered subcutaneously and can be repeated every 5 minutes for three doses. Intravenous (IV) hydrocortisone (100 mg) or IV methylprednisolone (20–24 mg) is also given, followed by IV diphenhydramine (25–50 mg) and oral acetaminophen (650 mg). It should be noted that epinephrine and diphenhydramine have a rapid onset of action and, in cases of severe reactions, should be given before steroids, which have a slower onset of action.

Although those authors[3,4] recommend restarting TIM infusion at a slower rate after resolution of the symptoms, and that a "prophylaxis protocol" be followed for retreatment of patients who experienced severe reactions, we believe that there is no logical justification to do so, especially in view of the facts that we are treating a benign disease and that there are many other alternative medications from which to choose.

Infections

Following U.S. Food and Drug Administration (FDA) approval and the more widespread use of TIMs (particularly, anti–tumor necrosis factor-α [TNF-α] for rheumatic disease and inflammatory bowel disease [IBD]), postmarketing surveillance data from the FDA MedWatch database revealed a disturbing number of reports of serious infections in patients treated with these agents.[5] The FDA has issued black box warnings about an increased risk of infections for all TNF-α inhibitors, stating that "Serious infections, including sepsis and pneumonia, have been reported in patients receiving TNF-α–blocking agents. Some of these infections have been fatal."

The true incidence of infections and the effect of TNF-α–blocking agents on these numbers cannot be ascertained with accuracy, particularly in view of the fact that rheumatologic patients have a higher risk for infection than do nonrheumatologic patients, and that they are also usually receiving other disease-modifying drugs that are associated with considerable risk of infections. We will discuss several of the most significant infections reported so far, without entering into the issue of the quantitative effect of anti-TNFs to their incidence.

Tuberculosis. At the forefront of interest concerning serious infections and the use of TNF-α inhibitors are mycobacterial infections, particularly *Mycobacterium tuberculosis.*

An estimated one third of the world's population (outside the United States, where the disease is uncommon) has latent tuberculosis infection (LTBI), which can potentially progress to disease and further spread of the epidemic. In LTBI, the person has a small number of "latent" *M. tuberculosis* bacilli that are contained in granulomas in their bodies. These organisms are viable and are possibly in a slow state of replication. These bacilli will never cause disease in most infected persons, but the ones who do reactivate disease suffer considerable morbidity and mortality and are also the major source of transmission of the disease, fueling the continued epidemic. Even though TB is usually not rapidly fatal, the disease may show a fulminant course in immunocompromised patients, and may also have an atypical pattern and presentation. In a review of 70 TB cases associated with infliximab therapy reported to the FDA,[6] more than half of the patients had extrapulmonary TB (lymph-node disease, peritoneal disease, pleural disease, meningeal disease, etc.), and approximately one quarter had disseminated TB. In contrast, among cases of TB in immunocompetent patients, approximately 18% were manifested as extrapulmonary disease, and disseminated disease accounted for less than 2%. TNFs have a central role in the host defense against *M. tuberculosis*. The human immune response is highly effective in controlling primary infection resulting from exposure to *M. tuberculosis*. TNF-α is involved in the killing of mycobacteria by activating macrophages and preventing the dissemination of infection by stimulating granuloma formation. Physicians should be aware of the increased risk of reactivation of TB among patients who are receiving anti-TNFs and, in particular,

of the unusual clinical manifestations of the disease, of the high mortality rates in this group (12%),[7] and its sometimes fulminant course. Both infliximab and adalimumab have black box warnings on their product labels citing this risk, and discussion with the FDA is ongoing regarding an update to the package labeling for etanercept.[8] The Centers for Disease Control and Prevention (CDC) recommends TB screening with tuberculin skin test for all patients being treated with any TNF-α inhibitor. Although other biologic medications that are not anti-TNFs (such as alefacept or efalizumab) have not been reported to cause reactivation of LTBI, they are immunosuppressive, and the majority of advisors from the medical board of the National Psoriasis Foundation perform baseline TB testing before initiating therapy with either agent.[8] Physicians should also bear in mind that a negative skin purified protein derivative (PPD) skin test and negative chest x-ray are not always reliable in patients with concomitant immunosuppression.[9] Indeed, anergy to PPD testing has been reported to be as high as 50% in rheumatic arthritis patients, compared with 7% in controls.[10] When active TB is suspected, treatment with TIMs should be immediately stopped until the diagnosis has been ruled out or the infection has been treated with anti-TB agents. In contrast, TB following therapy with anti-TNFs may be initially refractory to treatment because of lingering TNF-α blockers in the system.[11]

Other Bacterial Infections. There are no reliable post-licensure data on the rates of serious bacterial infections in patients treated with TNF-α inhibitors because infections with commonly acquired organisms are less likely to be reported to the authorities. Nonetheless, the clinician is certain to encounter serious bacterial infections, including those requiring a critical care setting, in individuals exposed to TNF-α antagonists. There are no specific guidelines for the recognition or treatment of suspected infections in these patients, but a heightened awareness and suspicion on the part of the clinician for these infections and rapid evaluation and treatment cannot be emphasized enough.

Histoplasmosis and Other Fungal Infections

Host responses to pulmonary inoculation with the fungus *Histoplasma capsulatum* are similar to pulmonary mycobacterial infection. Histoplasmosis is the most prevalent endemic mycosis in the United States, and approximately 250,000 individuals are infected per year. As with TB, 90%–95% of exposed immunocompetent hosts will develop latent asymptomatic disease, but reactivation and dissemination, which can be severe and fatal, may occur in the context of therapy with immunosuppressants.[12]

There were no cases of histoplasmosis in clinical trials with etanercept and infliximab, but two cases were documented in phase I trials with adalimumab. By May 2002, 22 cases of histoplasmosis were reported to the FDA

MedWatch database. Of these 22, 19 were associated with infliximab and three with etanercept. Five of the 22 resulted in death. All 22 cases occurred in the United States, and most resided in the Ohio and Mississippi River valleys. The majority of the cases presented with disseminated disease. Typical presenting symptoms included fever, dyspnea, malaise, weight loss, and intestinal pneumonitis.[12] Cases of histoplasmosis are uncommon outside the United States. Currently no reliable serologic or skin testing is available for screening for latent histoplasmosis infection. Due to this lack of a diagnostic tool, and because manifestations of infection can mimic any other infection, a high index of suspicion, particularly of physicians in endemic areas, is crucial for early diagnosis.

Pneumocystis carinii pneumonia (PCP; now renamed Pneumocystis *jiroveci*) is a common opportunistic infection in immunocompromised persons. As of June 2002, there have been 44 cases of PCP in the United States following the use of infliximab, and five cases of PCP following etanercept, with six fatal cases among them.[13]

Case reports and case series of other severe fungal infections have also been reported in association with the use of TNF-α inhibitors. These include disseminated cryptococcal infections, disseminated sporotrichosis, invasive pulmonary aspergillosis, systemic candidiosis, and others.[12,14]

In summary, disseminated fungal infections should be carefully considered in the differential diagnosis of patients who present to the emergency room or intensive care setting with a serious febrile illness in the setting of anti-TNF therapy, especially in areas of high disease prevalence.

Congestive Heart Failure

Worsening or exacerbation of congestive heart failure (CHF) is inarguably a serious, life-threatening, and frightening adverse effect. The question is, to what extent, if at all, are TNF-α antagonists involved in this event?

It is known that worsening CHF has been associated with elevated serum levels of TNF-α. Indeed, initial data from animal models and from preclinical and pilot studies were encouraging, showing some anecdotal efficacy of TNF-α antagonist therapy in the treatment of CHF.[15,16] Two larger, multicenter, randomized, placebo-controlled clinical trials (i.e., RECOVER [Research into Etanercept Cytokine Antagonism in Ventricular Dysfunction] and RENAISSANCE [Randomized Etanercept North American Strategy to Study Antagonism of Cytokines]) failed to show any significant difference in composite clinical function score for anti–TNF-α therapy versus placebo. Both studies were terminated early because interim analysis did not show any benefit of etanercept on morbidity or mortality. For the RENAISSANCE study, the key finding was a trend toward higher mortality in etanercept-treated subjects, a concern heightened by the apparent dose–response relationship.[15,16] A phase II trial with infliximab

indicated a strong trend toward an increase in the percentage of patients with worsening clinical status with increasing infliximab dose, largely due to an increase in deaths or hospitalization for CHF at weeks 14 (primary endpoint) and 28.[17]

In an examination of case reports[18] of all patients who developed new or worsening CHF while receiving TNF-α antagonist therapy, investigators obtained a total of 47 reported cases from the FDA's MedWatch system. After receiving TNF-α antagonist therapy, 38 patients developed new-onset CHF and 9 patients experienced CHF exacerbation. Of the 38 patients with new-onset CHF, 19 (50%) had no identifiable risk factor, and 10 patients were younger than 50 years. After TNF-α antagonist therapy was discontinued and heart failure therapy was started in these 10 patients, 3 had complete resolution of heart failure, 6 improved, and 1 died, an outcome that supports a causal relationship between TNF-α therapy and CHF.

There are currently no concrete guidelines for the evaluation and treatment of patients with suspected CHF. It is generally agreed upon that infliximab (>5 mg/kg) is contraindicated in patients with severe CHF. Likewise, patients who develop new-onset CHF while on anti-TNF therapy should immediately stop medication, undergo a prompt evaluation, and receive appropriate treatment. We currently advise against the reinstitution of anti-TNF therapy in such patients with dermatological diseases. As for patients with well-compensated mild CHF, each patient's risk versus benefit should be considered before therapy is begun.

Serious Neurological Events

Seizure Disorder. Seizure disorder following anti-TNF therapy is rare, having been reported in 29/170,000 patients who had been exposed to infliximab, in 26/104,000 exposed to etanercept, and in none exposed to adalimumab.[13,19] In view of these data, it was suggested that preexisting seizure disorder does not seem to be a contraindication to anti-TNF therapy for rheumatic patients.[13,19] We, however, think that dermatologic patients should nevertheless have an alternative therapy.

Demyelination

As is the case for TNF-α antagonists and CHF, the fact that patients with multiple sclerosis (MS) show elevated TNF-α levels in serum and cerebrospinal fluid (CSF) prompted researchers to try this form of therapy for patients with MS. To this end, a TNF-α blocker named lenercept, which was developed and studied specifically for patients with MS, resulted in an increase in MS exacerbations and a shortened time to flare.[20] An open-label, phase I safety study of infliximab carried out on two patients with MS showed a worsening of the disease.[21]

Demyelinating disorders have been described in postmarketing surveillance and in published case reports for all three TNF-α blockers.[13,14,19] The incidence of demyelinating disease, however, does not appear to be increased in patients on anti-TNF therapy compared with the background rate in the general population.[13,14,19] Nonetheless, it has been recommended that, for the sake of safety, these agents should be avoided in patients with preexisting demyelinating conditions until more data are available on the relationship between TNF-α blocker and demyelination.[13,14,19] In this context, it is important that physicians are aware of the signs and symptoms of demyelinating diseases, such as weakness, paresthesias, visual disturbances, confusion, and gait disturbances. Obviously, therapy with TNF-α inhibitors should be immediately stopped if a patient develops any suspicious neurological signs, and the patient should be sent for evaluation.

Serious Hematological Events

Although extremely rare, serious and acute hematological dyscrasias, such as aplastic anemia and pancytopenia, have been described in association with the use of TNF-α inhibitors. There are no current recommendations for regular monitoring of blood counts, but physicians should be aware of the possibility of hematological adverse events. If one occurs, TNF blockers should be stopped and the patient should be checked for evidence of other underlying disease or other causative medications before ascribing the event as potentially related to the TNF blockade.[13,19,22]

Efalizumab, an immunosuppressive recombinant humanized immunoglobulin G1 (IgG1) κ isotype monoclonal antibody that binds to human CD11a, is another biological therapy utilized in the treatment of psoriasis.

Four cases of hemolytic anemia have been reported with efalizumab. Two cases that were reported during clinical trials required discontinuation of therapy and blood transfusions. There is no descriptive information about the other two cases. A precaution regarding immune-mediated hemolytic anemia was added to the package insert for efalizumab.[23,24] Eight cases of thrombocytopenia (0.3%) were reported in a combined safety database of 2762 patients who received it, all eight being consistent with an immune-mediated process. Three individuals were asymptomatic and three required hospitalization, including one with heavy uterine bleeding. Five of the eight patients were treated with systemic steroids. Postmarketing cases of thrombocytopenia have also been reported. Prescribing information for efalizumab advocates monitoring for signs and symptoms of thrombocytopenia along with baseline and periodic assessments of platelet counts.[23,24] The reporting of one case of efalizumab-induced autoimmune pancytopenia resulted in the recommendation of close monitoring of all blood cell counts.[23]

Miscellaneous

Vasculitis. Rare cases of vasculitis associated with anti-TNF therapy have been reported, some of them severe. The causal relationship between the drug and the vasculitis remains uncertain, however, because the possibility of rheumatoid vasculitis cannot be excluded.[25,26]

Hepatotoxicity. Although TNF-α inhibitors have no confirmed liver toxicity, rare cases of serious liver disease suspected of having been induced by these drugs have been reported.[27,28]

Autoantibodies and Drug-Induced Lupus. TNF-α inhibitors can lead to the formation and increased titers of autoantibodies and antinuclear antibodies. The formation of these antibodies is not associated with any specific clinical syndrome. In contrast, a clinical syndrome of systemic *lupus erythematosus* (SLE) occurs rarely (approximately 0.2%) and seems to be associated with TNF-α inhibitors. The outcome of the disease has been favorable, with the disease being reversible on cessation of the drug. No patient thus far has reportedly developed neurological or renal disease.[13,14]

Recently, the manufacturer of efalizumab (Raptiva) has voluntarily withdrawn the drug from the market because of the association of efalizumab with an increased risk of progressive multifocal leukoencephalopathy (PML).

Since the approval of Raptiva (efalizumab) in October 2003, the FDA has received reports of three confirmed cases and one possible case of PML in patients 47 to 73 years of age who were using Raptiva for the treatment of moderate to severe plaque psoriasis. Two of the patients with confirmed PML and one patient with possible PML died. All four patients were treated with Raptiva continuously for more than three years. None of the patients were receiving other treatments that suppress the immune system while taking Raptiva.

METHOTREXATE

Since the mid-1950s, methotrexate (MTX) has become the gold standard by which other systemic psoriasis medications are measured.[29] MTX has been safely prescribed to thousands of patients with psoriatic and rheumatoid conditions with great therapeutic benefit. Indeed, the fact that 58% of surveyed dermatologists used MTX to treat patients with severe psoriasis in 1987[30] indicates that dermatologists feel comfortable with this form of therapy. A significant number of dermatologists are, however, still unwilling to treat psoriasis with MTX, reflecting a persistent bias against it. The good benefit/toxicity ratio, low cost, extensive experience over decades, and relatively good tolerability of MTX notwithstanding, it is, like the majority of cancer medications, a toxin and an antimetabolite and, as such, it can cause acute toxicity. In this section we focus on some acute, serious adverse reactions of MTX.

Pancytopenia

Bone-marrow toxicity (specifically, pancytopenia) is certainly the most serious, acute, and, therefore, frightening side effect of MTX, with an estimated incidence of 1.4%.[31] MTX-induced bone-marrow suppression develops suddenly, rapidly, and without warning signs. It seems unlikely, therefore, that a more frequent monitoring schedule would substantially avoid its occurrence. Although it usually occurs late into treatment,[32] there are several reports on early occurrence, even after one or two doses of MTX.[31,33] The outcome is grave, with a reported mortality rate ranging from 17%[31] to as high as 44%,[33] most commonly resulting from infections and bleeding disorders.

Physicians need to be alerted to this potentially life-threatening complication, if not to avoid it, then at least to recognize it as early as possible and promptly take the appropriate measures.

Pulmonary Complications

Although the major safety concern of MTX is its hepatotoxicity, it is less known that pulmonary toxicity is only slightly less common and not less serious: It is the reason for withdrawal of MTX in 1 in 108 patient-years compared with 1 in 35 patient-years for hepatotoxicity. The prevalence of MTX-induced pneumonitis is reported to be 0.3%–7.5%,[34] and more than 120 cases have been reported in the English language literature since its first description in 1969.[34] Pneumonitis following MTX is a serious, potentially fatal hypersensitivity reaction and is far less predictable than hepatic and hematological toxicity. A review of 123 published cases of MTX-induced pneumonitis showed a mortality rate of 13%.[34] Although most patients with MTX pneumonitis have the subacute type with progression over several weeks, a life-threatening, acute type with rapid progression over only a few days has also been reported.[34,35] Differentiation between MTX pneumonitis and acute respiratory infection is not always easy, despite the accepted diagnostic criteria.[36] A suggested management approach[34,35] for a patient with suspected MTX-related lung pathology consists of MTX discontinuation, supportive therapy, and (most important) a comprehensive diagnostic procedure to exclude infection. It should consist of extensive cultures of sputum, blood, and bronchoalveolar lavage (BAL) fluid and serological testing for common respiratory viruses, *Mycoplasma*, *Rickettsia*, and *Legionella*. Microscopic examination of BAL fluid is recommended to exclude *P. jiroveci*, fungi, and mycobacteria. Because excluding infection might sometimes be difficult and time consuming in cases where rapid treatment might

be needed, it is suggested to start empirical antimicrobial treatment and, in some cases, IV corticosteroids until there is evidence of clinical and radiological improvement.

CYCLOSPORINE A

Cyclosporine A (CsA) has a range of side effects that is the subject of much concern. It may seem surprising that this drug is generally well tolerated and, ironically, the good tolerability itself can represent a hazard, because patients are not likely to be aware of any signs of its chronic toxicity.

Nephrotoxicity and Hypertension

The major safety concerns of CsA are nephrotoxicity, hypertension, and the potential risk of malignancy. There are three different forms of CsA nephrotoxicity: 1) reversible acute renal dysfunction, 2) hemolytic-uremic–like syndrome, and 3) irreversible chronic nephrotoxicity.

CsA-induced acute nephrotoxicity is a hemodynamically mediated phenomenon characterized by the absence of permanent structural changes and by reversibility with decrease or discontinuation of the drug. It is a dose-related, clinically asymptomatic increase in serum creatinine, which can occur even when drug blood levels are in the therapeutic range. In these patients, renal histology is usually normal or shows only nonspecific changes, such as vacuolization or the presence of giant mitochondria in tubular cells.[37]

Recurrent or de novo hemolytic-uremic syndrome is rare, generally multifactorial, and seldom related exclusively to CsA.[37,38] It occurs mainly in bone-marrow and solid-organ–transplanted patients and has not been reported in patients on CsA therapy for dermatological diseases.[39]

Chronic CsA nephrotoxicity is an insidious condition associated with an irreversible and progressive renal interstitial fibrosis, followed by decrease in renal function.[37] It is a clinicopathologic entity related to long-term exposure to CsA, and is never acute.

Neurotoxicity

Observations of acute neurotoxicity in conjunction with high concentrations of CsA in blood were reported soon after CsA's introduction into clinical practice in 1979.[40] Subsequently, severe neurotoxicity resulting from CsA treatment was frequently reported in bone-marrow and solid organ recipients, but also in patients with dermatological[41] or autoimmune diseases.[42] Neurotoxicity had been less well known, but with growing experience, central nervous system side effects are now reported in up to 40% of patients treated with CsA.[43–45] The most commonly noted neurologic finding is tremor, appearing in 20%–40% of patients treated with the drug.[43,44] This side effect is not particularly distressing for most patients and tends to diminish with time. Visual hallucinations are less frequently reported, and cortical blindness is extremely rare and reversible in most (although not all) patients.[44] A mild encephalopathy due to CsA was reported in up to 30% of patients, and cessation or reduction in dose is usually followed by relief of symptoms.[43,44] Severe encephalopathy, altered level of consciousness, psychosis, and coma have all been reported as well.[43,44]

Seizures were reported to occur in 1.5%–6% of CsA-treated patients. Most patients suffer a single seizure, without recurrence after dose reduction, although rare cases with status epilepticus have been reported.[43]

In summary, CsA induces neurological side effects in up to 40% of patients. The symptoms can be mild (e.g., tremor, headache, and neuralgia), moderate (e.g., visual disturbances and cortical blindness), or severe (affecting up to 5% of patients; e.g., altered level of consciousness, confusion, seizures, and coma). These side effects are almost always reversible on reduction or cessation of treatment; however, permanent changes have also been reported. Physicians should be aware of these acute side effects of the drug.

RETINOIDS (ISOTRETINOIN)

Isotretinoin (13-*cis*-retinoic acid) is a synthetic oral retinoid that has high efficacy against severe, recalcitrant, and nodulocystic acne.

Isotretinoin, a vitamin A derivative, interacts with many of the biologic systems of the body and, as such, has a diverse pattern of adverse effects, not unlike that seen in hypervitaminosis A. The side effects involve the mucocutaneous, musculoskeletal, metabolic, gastrointestinal, hepatobiliary, ophthalmic, and central nervous systems, as well as headaches. Most of the adverse effects are mild and temporary and resolve after the drug is discontinued: Some rare complications persist; these will be discussed here.

In a recent retrospective analysis of 1193 suspected pediatric adverse drug reactions (ADRs) reported to Health Canada (1998–2002),[46] 41 reports included a fatal outcome of which isotretinoin was responsible for two, making it second (together with six other drugs) to olanzapine, with 3 fatal cases. Of 14 cases that were defined as "recovered with sequelae," isotretinoin with three cases was alone in first place.

Psychiatric Disorders

Grave side effects attributed to isotretinoin are depression, psychosis, suicide, and suicide attempts. On February 25, 1998, the FDA mandated a change in the label warning to include, "Psychiatric disorders: Accutane may cause depression, psychosis and rarely, suicide ideation, suicide attempt and suicide. Discontinuation of Accutane therapy may be insufficient; further evaluation may be

necessary."[47] This warning notwithstanding, the issue is still not entirely clear. Although studies (mostly sponsored) conclude that the existing reports do not meet the required criteria for establishing causality between the ingestion of isotretinoin and suicide or major depression, and furthermore claim that the risk of depressed mood is no greater during isotretinoin therapy than during other therapy of an age-matched acne group, the link between psychiatric disorders and isotretinoin remains a controversial issue.[47–50]

Intracranial Hypertension

Severe headache is the most frequently reported adverse effect of isotretinoin.[51,52] About one fourth of the cases are caused by pseudotumor cerebri. Although this side effect is almost always reversible and leaves no sequelae, it can have a devastating outcome (there are cases of irreversible blindness), if not recognized early enough and treated appropriately.

Ocular Side Effects

These are common although rarely serious. Fraunfelder and colleagues[53] described a number of cases of optic neuritis, cortical blindness, corneal ulcers, and glaucoma that were possibly associated with isotretinoin.

Gastrointestinal and Hepatobiliary Side Effects

Gastrointestinal together with hepatobiliary side effects are the second most commonly reported adverse reactions after psychiatric disorders.[46]

Although IBD is described as a possible ADR in the product information of isotretinoin, this association has been given little attention in the literature. There are many cases of IBD reported to the FDA and World Health Organization (101 reports on isotretinoin and ulcerative colitis, and 35 reports on isotretinoin and Crohn disease), and cases of IBD are significantly more often reported in association with isotretinoin than with other drugs, thus supporting an association between the drug and the condition.[54]

Derangements of lipid metabolism leading to increased triglyceride and cholesterol levels are well-known side effects of retinoid therapy and are usually harmless, although the rare cases of marked hyperlipidemia associated with pancreatitis are always serious and of major concern.[50,55,56]

IV IMMUNOGLOBULIN

IV immunoglobulin (IVIG) is a blood product consisting primarily of intact IgG molecules, which are derived from pooled normal human plasma of between 1000 and 15,000 donors per batch. Its dermatological uses are Kawasaki disease, therapy-resistant dermatomyositis, toxic epidermal necrolysis, and the blistering diseases, particularly pemphigus. Examples of conditions for which the evidence consists mainly of case series or reports include atopic dermatitis, chronic immune urticaria, scleromyxedema, erythema multiforme, and others.

Several serious, acute, and potentially fatal adverse effects are known to be associated with IVIG therapy. Fortunately, these side effects are rare.

Acute Renal Failure

One of the most significant concerns of IVIG therapy is its association with acute renal failure. Interestingly, it is not the immunoglobulins that mostly cause renal insufficiency, but the sugar that is added to some of the products to stabilize the solution and minimize aggregate formation. Up to 90% of the IVIG-associated renal adverse events have been linked to sucrose-containing preparations.[57,58] The pathomechanism is osmotic nephrosis. Sucrose is a disaccharide that is enzymatically cleaved into glucose and fructose when it is ingested orally; however, the cleaving enzyme is not present in the blood or kidney, so, when given IV, the sucrose molecule remains intact and is excreted through the kidney. During this process, the sucrose is taken up (pinocytosed) into the proximal tubular cells, causing an osmotic gradient and leading to the entrance of fluid into the cells and to cell damage ("osmotic nephrosis").

An extensive review of the literature[58] comparing a group of patients with IVIG nephrotoxic effects published as case reports (Group A) with patients whose data were collected by the FDA (Group B) provides a useful picture of the demographic and clinical data of this side effect. In Group A, 45% of the patients had preexisting renal disease. Most (90%) of the patients in Group B and 72% of the patients in Group A received sucrose-containing IVIG products (a difference that might stem from the tendency to report unusual cases). Acute renal failure onset was between 1 and 10 days following IVIG administration. A high percentage of patients required hemodialysis (i.e., 31% in the published cases and 40% in the FDA report). The duration of the renal failure ranged from 3 to 45 days and was reversible in about 85% of the cases, with return of serum creatinine levels to baseline. Death occurred in 10%–15% of all patients in both groups despite treatment. All deaths involved patients with severe underlying medical conditions (pneumonia, cardiac disease, and SLE): The extent to which renal failure contributed to their deaths was undetermined.

General guidelines have been established to minimize the incidence of acute renal failure from IVIG.[59,60] Patients should be adequately hydrated prior to any infusion. If their clinical condition permits, they can skip the morning dose of a diuretic on the days of infusion. The recommended dose of IVIG should not be exceeded, and recommended infusion rates should be strictly followed. Urine output should be monitored during the infusion. Periodic monitoring of the serum creatinine level is indicated in high-risk patients. The infusion should be discontinued if deterioration in renal function is detected. The need for dialysis therapy is determined on an individual basis.

Stroke

Stroke is a rare but potentially fatal side effect of IVIG therapy. One review of a series of 16 cases[61] and an additional 13 case reports[59] provided the clinical features of this unusual occurrence. Most patients had received an IVIG dose of 2 g/kg/cycle. All of them had received IVIG at the recommended infusion rate or slower. Most patients developed stroke within 24 hours of completing an infusion, indicating a direct temporal relationship to the administration of IVIG. Slightly more than one half of the patients were receiving their first cycle of IVIG, suggesting that factors intrinsic to certain patients may have put them at higher risk for stroke than others. Common risk factors for stroke were present in most of the patients.

Currently, there is no clear understanding of the pertinent pathophysiology of this serious and sometimes fatal side effect, so there are no recommendations for prophylaxis and treatment. The only suggestion we can offer is that all patients who are being evaluated for potential IVIG therapy need to be questioned about known risk factors for stroke. The risk-to-benefit ratio of using IVIG in these patients needs to be discussed with patients and family members.[59]

Arterial and Venous Thrombotic Complications Including Myocardial Infarction

One series and review of literature analyzing this complication was recently published in a dermatologic journal.[62] This series demonstrates that IVIG-related thrombotic arteriovenous complications are not uncommon in patients with autoimmune disorders (6 [13%] of 46 patients developed IVIG-related thrombotic complications). Thrombotic complications frequently occurred during IVIG infusion (50%), although they were also observed within 1–8 days following IVIG infusion in other patients. Three of six patients developed deep venous thrombosis or pulmonary embolism, two developed myocardial infarction, and one suffered a stroke. Although the outcome of the thrombotic complications was favorable in all their patients, the authors' literature review indicates a serious outcome with a mortality rate of 20%–30%,[62] with 15% of the patients dying of IVIG-associated thrombosis.

In another large series of 279 IVIG-treated patients,[63] 5 (1.8%) developed acute myocardial infarction during or shortly after (3–5 hours) infusion. These cases occurred with the use of only one brand (Polygam).

As with other complications of this therapy, there are no specific recommendations except for reweighing the risk-to-benefit ratio, close monitoring, infusion at a slow rate, and (if possible) administering not-too-high doses after good hydration in patients with underlying predisposing factors. No consensus has been reached on the use of prophylactic antiplatelets or anticoagulants.

Aseptic Meningitis

Aseptic meningitis is an inflammation of the meninges that clinically presents with headache, nausea, vomiting, fever, photophobia, painful eye movements, and nuchal rigidity. Drug-induced aseptic meningitis (DIAS) is usually benign, the clinical course is short lived, and there is spontaneous resolution of the symptoms without sequelae within hours to days after discontinuation of therapy. No deaths were reported in association with this syndrome.[64,65]

The main challenge for the clinician is, however, the diagnosis. The differential diagnosis of DIAS is broad and includes infectious causes. Bacterial meningitis has symptoms that are similar, if not identical, to those of DIAS, and these two entities cannot be distinguished on clinical grounds. Bacterial culture of the CSF may help in the diagnosis. Treatment with third-generation cephalosporins has been suggested in cases where the presence of bacterial meningitis is a possibility.[64] Viral aseptic meningitis is another important consideration in terms of frequency, although less critical in terms of prognosis and management. Finally, other noninfectious causes of aseptic meningitis should be considered, such as SLE aseptic meningitis, as well as other drugs that can cause the syndrome. Intracranial bleeding, especially in patients with idiopathic thrombocytopenic purpura and bleeding disorders, must also be considered. Computed tomographic scans can be used to rule out hemorrhage.

CONCLUSIONS

Dermatologists have the good fortune to work on the most accessible organ of the body. This gives them numerous advantages and greatly facilitates not only the diagnosis but also the treatment of the skin disease, because many inflammatory and neoplastic conditions can be effectively managed using a wide range of externally applied modalities. All this notwithstanding, many serious, widespread, and life-threatening dermatoses often need to be treated with potent systemic therapies. Because systemic drugs are increasingly available, and are often essential and indispensable for the treatment of dermatological diseases, drug toxicity and adverse events are a significant problem. In view of the continuing development of new and effective therapies, it is expected that their incidence will not decrease. Whereas this book is mostly devoted to the treatment of serious dermatological diseases, this chapter deals with the other side of the coin – namely, the adverse effects, consequences, and risks of our treatments.

This chapter identified five major drugs or drug groups (biologics, MTX, CSA, retinoids, and IVIG) used in dermatology that are associated with an element of risk in causing serious and sometimes fatal adverse reactions. Basic principles of diagnosing, monitoring, and treating these adverse effects were presented.

REFERENCES

1. Kaminetzky HA. A drug on the market. Obstet Gynecol. 1963; 21:512–13.
2. Kapetanovic MC, Larsson L, Truedsson L, et al. Predictors of infusion reactions during infliximab treatment in patients with arthritis. Arthritis Res Ther. 2006; 8:R131.
3. Cheifetz A, Smedley M, Martin S, et al. The incidence and management of infusion reactions to infliximab: a large center experience. Am J Gastroenterol. 2003; 98:1315–24.
4. Cheifetz A, Mayer L. Monoclonal antibodies, immunogenicity, and associated infusion reactions. Mt Sinai J Med. 2005; 72:250–6.
5. US Food and Drug Administration Arthritis Advisory Committee. Briefing information from the March 4, 2003 meeting of Arthritis Advisory Committee. 3 April 2007. Available from: http://www.fda.gov/ohrms/dockets/ac/03/briefing/3930b1.htm.
6. Keane J, Gershon S, Wise RP, et al. Tuberculosis associated with infliximab, a tumor necrosis factor alpha-neutralizing agent. N Engl J Med. 2001; 345:1098–104.
7. Gomez-Reino JJ, Carmona L, Valverde VR, et al. Treatment of rheumatoid arthritis with tumor necrosis factor inhibitors may predispose to significant increase in tuberculosis risk: a multicenter active-surveillance report. Arthritis Rheum. 2003; 48:2122–7.
8. Doherty SD, Van VA, Lebwohl MG, et al. National Psoriasis Foundation consensus statement on screening for latent tuberculosis infection in patients with psoriasis treated with systemic and biologic agents. J Am Acad Dermatol. 2008; 59:209–17.
9. Stas P, D'Hoore A, Van AG, et al. Miliary tuberculosis following infliximab therapy for Crohn disease: a case report and review of the literature. Acta Gastroenterol Belg. 2006; 69:217–20.
10. Paimela L, Johansson-Stephansson EA, Koskimies S, Leirisalo-Repo M. Depressed cutaneous cell-mediated immunity in early rheumatoid arthritis. Clin Exp Rheumatol. 1990; 8:433–7.
11. Taylor JC, Orkin R, Lanham J. Tuberculosis following therapy with infliximab may be refractory to antibiotic therapy. Rheumatology (Oxford). 2003; 42:901–2.
12. Giles JT, Bathon JM. Serious infections associated with anticytokine therapies in the rheumatic diseases. J Intensive Care Med. 2004; 19:320–34.
13. Khanna D, McMahon M, Furst DE. Safety of tumour necrosis factor-alpha antagonists. Drug Saf. 2004; 27:307–24.

14. Scheinfeld N. A comprehensive review and evaluation of the side effects of the tumor necrosis factor alpha blockers etanercept, infliximab and adalimumab. J Dermatolog Treat. 2004; 15:280–94.

15. Behnam SM, Behnam SE, Koo JY. TNF-alpha inhibitors and congestive heart failure. Skinmed. 2005; 4:363–8.

16. Mousa SA, Goncharuk O, Miller D. Recent advances of TNF-alpha antagonists in rheumatoid arthritis and chronic heart failure. Expert Opin Biol Ther. 2007; 7:617–25.

17. Chung ES, Packer M, Lo KH, et al. Randomized, double-blind, placebo-controlled, pilot trial of infliximab, a chimeric monoclonal antibody to tumor necrosis factor-alpha, in patients with moderate-to-severe heart failure: results of the anti-TNF Therapy Against Congestive Heart Failure (ATTACH) trial. Circulation. 2003; 107:3133–40.

18. Kwon HJ, Cote TR, Cuffe MS, et al. Case reports of heart failure after therapy with a tumor necrosis factor antagonist. Ann Intern Med. 2003; 138:807–11.

19. Desai SB, Furst. DE Problems encountered during anti-tumour necrosis factor therapy. Best Pract Res Clin Rheumatol. 2006; 20:757–90.

20. TNF neutralization in MS: results of a randomized, placebo-controlled multicenter study. The Lenercept Multiple Sclerosis Study Group and The University of British Columbia MS/MRI Analysis Group. Neurology. 1999; 53:457–65.

21. van Oosten BW, Barkhof F, Truyen L, et al. Increased MRI activity and immune activation in two multiple sclerosis patients treated with the monoclonal anti-tumor necrosis factor antibody cA2. Neurology. 1996; 47:1531–4.

22. Furst DE, Breedveld FC, Kalden JR, et al. Updated consensus statement on biological agents, specifically tumour necrosis factor {alpha} (TNF{alpha}) blocking agents and interleukin-1 receptor antagonist (IL-1ra), for the treatment of rheumatic diseases, 2005. Ann Rheum Dis. 2005; 64 Suppl 4:iv2–14.

23. Tom WL, Miller MD, Hurley MY, et al. Efalizumab-induced autoimmune pancytopenia. Br J Dermatol. 2006; 155:1045–7.

24. Scheinfeld N. Efalizumab: a review of events reported during clinical trials and side effects. Expert Opin Drug Saf. 2006; 5:197–209.

25. Mohan N, Edwards ET, Cupps TR, et al. Leukocytoclastic vasculitis associated with tumor necrosis factor-alpha blocking agents. J Rheumatol. 2004; 31:1955–8.

26. Saint MB, De Bandt M. Vasculitides induced by TNF-alpha antagonists: a study in 39 patients in France. Joint Bone Spine. 2006; 73:710–3.

27. Tobon GJ, Canas C, Jaller JJ, et al. Serious liver disease induced by infliximab. Clin Rheumatol. 2007; 26:578–81.

28. Wahie S, Alexandroff A, Reynolds NJ. Hepatitis: a rare, but important, complication of infliximab therapy for psoriasis. Clin Exp Dermatol. 2006; 31:460–1.

29. Roenigk HH, Jr., Auerbach R, Maibach H, et al. Methotrexate in psoriasis: consensus conference. J Am Acad Dermatol. 1998; 38:478–85.

30. Peckham PE, Weinstein GD, McCullough JL. The treatment of severe psoriasis. A national survey. Arch Dermatol. 1987; 123:1303–7.

31. Gutierrez-Urena S, Molina JF, Garcia CO, et al. Pancytopenia secondary to methotrexate therapy in rheumatoid arthritis. Arthritis Rheum. 1996; 39:272–6.

32. Lim AY, Gaffney K, Scott DG. Methotrexate-induced pancytopenia: serious and under-reported? Our experience of 25 cases in 5 years. Rheumatology (Oxford). 2005; 44:1051–5.

33. Kuitunen T, Malmstrom J, Palva E, Pettersson T. Pancytopenia induced by low-dose methotrexate. A study of the cases reported to the Finnish Adverse Drug Reaction Register from 1991 to 1999. Scand J Rheumatol. 2005; 34:238–41.

34. Imokawa S, Colby TV, Leslie KO, Helmers RA. Methotrexate pneumonitis: review of the literature and histopathological findings in nine patients. Eur Respir J. 2000; 15:373–81.

35. Barrera P, Laan RF, van Riel PL, et al. Methotrexate-related pulmonary complications in rheumatoid arthritis. Ann Rheum Dis. 1994; 53:434–9.

36. Searles G, McKendry RJ. Methotrexate pneumonitis in rheumatoid arthritis: potential risk factors. Four case reports and a review of the literature. J Rheumatol. 1987; 14:1164–71.

37. Cattaneo D, Perico N, Gaspari F, Remuzzi G. Nephrotoxic aspects of cyclosporine. Transplant Proc. 2004; 36:234S–239S.

38. Jumani A, Hala K, Tahir S, et al. Causes of acute thrombotic microangiopathy in patients receiving kidney transplantation. Exp Clin Transplant. 2004; 2:268–72.

39. Vercauteren SB, Bosmans JL, Elseviers MM, et al. A meta-analysis and morphological review of cyclosporine-induced nephrotoxicity in auto-immune diseases. Kidney Int. 1998; 54:536–45.

40. Calne RY, Rolles K, White DJ, et al. Cyclosporin A initially as the only immunosuppressant in 34 recipients of cadaveric organs: 32 kidneys, 2 pancreases, and 2 livers. Lancet. 1979; 2:1033–6.

41. Humphreys TR, Leyden JJ. Acute reversible central nervous system toxicity associated with low-dose oral cyclosporine therapy. J Am Acad Dermatol. 1993; 29:490–2.

42. Porges Y, Blumen S, Fireman Z, et al. Cyclosporine-induced optic neuropathy, ophthalmoplegia, and nystagmus in a patient with Crohn disease. Am J Ophthalmol. 1998; 126:607–9.

43. Gijtenbeek JM, Van Den Bent MJ, Vecht CJ. Cyclosporine neurotoxicity: a review. J Neurol. 1999; 246:339–46.

44. Bechstein WO. Neurotoxicity of calcineurin inhibitors: impact and clinical management. Transpl Int. 2000; 13:313–26.

45. Serkova NJ, Christians U, Benet LZ. Biochemical mechanisms of cyclosporine neurotoxicity. Mol Interv. 2004; 4:97–107.

46. Carleton BC, Smith MA, Gelin MN, Heathcote SC. Paediatric adverse drug reaction reporting: understanding and future directions. Can J Clin Pharmacol. 2007; 14:e45–e57.

47. Strahan JE, Raimer S. Isotretinoin and the controversy of psychiatric adverse effects. Int J Dermatol. 2006; 45:789–99.

48. Strauss JS, Krowchuk DP, Leyden JJ, et al. Guidelines of care for acne vulgaris management. J Am Acad Dermatol. 2007; 56:651–63.

49. Goldsmith LA, Bolognia JL, Callen JP, et al. American Academy of Dermatology Consensus Conference on the safe and optimal use of isotretinoin: summary and recommendations. J Am Acad Dermatol. 2004; 50:900–6.

50. Orion E, Matz H, Wolf R. The life-threatening complications of dermatologic therapies. Clin Dermatol. 2005; 23:182–92.

51. Friedman DI. Medication-induced intracranial hypertension in dermatology. Am J Clin Dermatol. 2005; 6:29–37.

52. Bigby M, Stern RS. Adverse reactions to isotretinoin. A report from the Adverse Drug Reaction Reporting System. J Am Acad Dermatol. 1988; 18:543–52.

53. Fraunfelder FT, Fraunfelder FW, Edwards R. Ocular side effects possibly associated with isotretinoin usage. Am J Ophthalmol. 2001; 132:299–305.

54. Passier JL, Srivastava N, van Puijenbroek EP. Isotretinoin-induced inflammatory bowel disease. Neth J Med. 2006; 64:52–4.

55. Greene JP. An adolescent with abdominal pain taking isotretinoin for severe acne. South Med J. 2006; 99:992–4.

56. Jamshidi M, Obermeyer RJ, Govindaraj S, et al. Acute pancreatitis secondary to isotretinoin-induced hyperlipidemia. J Okla State Med Assoc. 2002; 95:79–80.

57. Gelfand EW. Differences between IGIV products: impact on clinical outcome. Int Immunopharmacol. 2006; 6: 592–9.

58. Orbach H, Tishler M, Shoenfeld Y. Intravenous immunoglobulin and the kidney – a two-edged sword. Semin Arthritis Rheum. 2004; 34:593–601.

59. Hamrock DJ. Adverse events associated with intravenous immunoglobulin therapy. Int Immunopharmacol. 2006; 6:535–42.

60. Epstein JS, Zoon KC. Important drug warning: immune globulin intravenous (human) (IGIV) products. Neonatal Netw. 2000; 19:60–2.

61. Caress JB, Cartwright MS, Donofrio PD, Peacock JE, Jr. The clinical features of 16 cases of stroke associated with administration of IVIg. Neurology. 2003; 60:1822–4.

62. Marie I, Maurey G, Herve F, Hellot MF, Levesque H. Intravenous immunoglobulin-associated arterial and venous thrombosis; report of a series and review of the literature. Br J Dermatol. 2006; 155:714–21.

63. Vo AA, Cam V, Toyoda M, et al. Safety and adverse events profiles of intravenous gammaglobulin products used for immunomodulation: a single-center experience. Clin J Am Soc Nephrol. 2006; 1:844–52.

64. Moris G, Garcia-Monco JC. The challenge of drug-induced aseptic meningitis. Arch Intern Med. 1999; 159:1185–94.

65. Sekul EA, Cupler EJ, Dalakas MC. Aseptic meningitis associated with high-dose intravenous immunoglobulin therapy: frequency and risk factors. Ann Intern Med. 1994; 121:259–62.

CHAPTER 18

Severe, Acute Allergic and Immunological Reactions I: Urticaria, Angioedema, Mastocytosis, and Anaphylaxis

Samuel H. Allen

BACKGROUND

Local wheals (synonyms: "nettle rash," hives) and erythema that resemble the effect of the common stinging nettle (*Urtica dioica*) on the skin is known as urticaria. The edema involves superficial skin to the mid-dermis. Pruritus is common.

Angioedema (synonyms: angioneurotic edema, Quinke's edema) produces a similar eruption but with larger edematous areas that affect both the dermal and subcutaneous and/or submucosal tissues. Angioedema is usually painful rather than itchy and is less well defined or normal in color. Both types of reaction can be triggered by drug allergies, insect stings or bites, desensitisation injections, cold temperature, other physical stimuli, or ingestion of certain foods, particularly eggs, shellfish, nuts, or fruits.

Mastocytosis is caused by an abnormal conglomeration of mast cells at a particular site. Degranulation, through rubbing or contact, triggers release of excessive histamine, resulting in localized swelling.

Anaphylaxis represents an extreme form of acute allergic reactions that is mediated by immunoglobulin E (IgE). Anaphylaxis is an example of a type I hypersensitivity reaction (see Chapter 19). Although erythema, urticaria, and angioedema may all occur, it is the systemic hypotension and shock that determine the outcome. It is a clinical emergency characterized by profound shock that may rapidly lead to cardiorespiratory arrest. A similar picture from nonallergic causes is called an "anaphylactoid reaction."

URTICARIA

Urticaria (see Figure 18.1) may result from different stimuli on an immunologic or nonimmunologic basis. The most common immunologic mechanisms are hypersensitivity mediated by IgE and activation of the complement cascade.

The physical urticarias, which account for approximately 25% of cases, include dermatographism and the pressure, cold, heat, solar, cholinergic, and aquagenic urticarias (Table 18.1). The trigger may not always be identified, even when such reactions are recurrent. This can be a frustration to the patient and the dermatologist alike. Urticaria may accompany, or even be the first symptom of, severe viral infection including hepatitis, infectious mononucleosis, and rubella. Similar lesions may precede, or be associated with, vasculitis (urticarial vasculitis), pemphigoid, or dermatitis herpetiformis.

Dermatographism is a wheal-and-flare reaction seen after scratching or stroking the skin firmly with a hard object, and is caused by an exaggerated release of histamine. Pressure urticaria is caused by sustained pressure from tight clothing, hard seats, and stiff footwear and may present as an immediate or late (4–6 hours, occasionally 24 hours) reaction to the pressure stimulus. Cold urticaria varies in severity and is induced by cold wind or bathing in cold water. Bronchospasm and histamine-mediated shock occur in extreme cases and may result in drowning. In its rare familial form it appears in infancy. Abnormal serum proteins may be found.

Warm environments often exacerbate the physical urticarias, but pure heat urticaria is rare. Solar urticaria is likewise a rare condition in which ultraviolet rays from sunlight cause an urticarial eruption. Aquagenic urticaria is independent of temperature and occurs on skin contact with water. Cholinergic urticaria appears to be caused by an unusual sensitivity to acetylcholine and is characterized by small, highly pruritic, discrete wheals surrounded by a large penumbra of erythema that occur after exertion, stress, or heat exposure. A skin challenge test using methacholine 1:5000 may reproduce the lesions in about one third

TABLE 18.1: Physical Urticarias

Pressure	e.g., dermatographism
Cold	
Heat	
Solar	
Cholinergic	
Aquagenic	

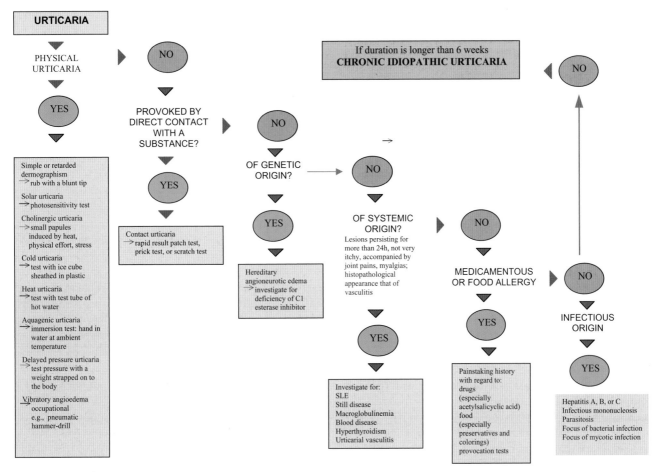

FIGURE 18.1: *Algorithmic approach to urticaria. Adapted from Lachapelle JM, Tennstedt D, Marot L. In Atlas of Dermatology. SLE, systemic lupus erythematosus.*

of cases. A more reliable diagnostic method is to induce the urticarial reaction through exercising the subject with occlusive dressing to promote sweating.

Chronic urticaria and angioedema with symptoms lasting more than 6 weeks are more difficult to explain; only rarely can a specific cause be found.[1] Some patients with chronic urticaria demonstrate autoantibodies directed against mast-cell epitopes with histamine-releasing activity, but these are the exception. Occasionally, chronic ingestion of an unsuspected drug or chemical is responsible (e.g., from antibiotics used in animal husbandry that may be present in small quantities in meat for human consumption, from the use of nonprescription drugs, or from preservatives, dyes, or other food additives) (Table 18.2).

Despite anecdotal reports of urticaria occurring with lymphoma and systemic malignancy, no association was found in a large epidemiological study by Lindelöf and colleagues.[2] In contrast, a higher frequency of autoimmune disease is found among patients with ordinary urticaria.[3]

TABLE 18.2: Nonphysical Urticarias

Food allergens	Fish, shellfish (lobster, shrimp, crab), eggs, dairy products, chocolate, nuts (especially peanuts), strawberries, pork, tomatoes, apples, oranges, bananas, celery, beans
Food additives	Tartazine, food dyes, sodium benzoate, MSG
Salicylates	Aspirin, mesalazine, sulfsalazine, NSAIDs
Other drugs	Penicillins, cephalosporins, blood products, vaccines, insulin
Infection	Bacterial, viral, protozoal, helminthic
Systemic disorders	Autoimmune and collagen-vascular diseases, reticuloses, SLE
Contact urticaria	Meat, fish, vegetables, plants (common stinging nettle, poison ivy, giant hogweed, sumac), animals, insects, caterpillars
Papular urticaria	Site of insect bites, bee sting
Inhalants	House dust mite, animal dander, feathers, grass, pollen

MSG, monosodium glutamate; NSAIDs, nonsteroidal antiinflammatory drugs; SLE, systemic lupus erythematosus.

ANGIOEDEMA

A familial form of urticaria was described by Milton and termed hereditary angioedema in 1876.[4] It is transmitted as an autosomal dominant trait and thus affects successive generations. The term of angioneurotic edema was introduced a few years later, as it was believed that mental stress could precipitate attacks.[5] Hereditary angioedema is now known to be associated with a deficiency in serum inhibitor of the activated first component of complement.[6]

The genetic defect has been mapped to chromosome 11. More than 100 different mutations of the C1-inhibitor gene have been described. In 85% of cases, the deficiency is due to lack of C1 esterase inhibitor; in the remainder, a malfunction to C1 inhibitor is the cause. A spontaneous mutation is found in up to 25% of cases.[7]

Worldwide, the incidence of hereditary angioedema varies between 1:10,000 and 1:150,000. Seventy-five percent of patients present before the age of 15 years.

In contrast to urticaria, angioedema affects both the reticular dermis and subcutaneous tissues. Recent data suggest that histamine-releasing immunoglobulin G (IgG) antibody directed against ε region of the constant fragment (F_c), or anti-F_cε antibodies are the cause of the disease, removal or suppression by immunomodulation being followed by remission.[8]

Most patients with hereditary angioedema have a personal or family history of recurrent attacks of angioedema or abdominal pain. An important exception to this is where a spontaneous mutation has occurred. Attacks are often precipitated by trauma including surgical procedures, pregnancy, viral illness, emotional stress, and drugs such as estrogen and angiotensin-converting enzyme (ACE) inhibitors. The combination of ACE inhibitors and estrogens is contraindicated.

Cutaneous angioedema of the extremities is the first presenting sign in 75% of patients. The edema tends to be recurrent, is nonpitting in nature, and demonstrates a rapidly expanding unifocal, indurated swelling that is painful rather than pruritic. Urticaria is not part of the syndrome. The areas usually affected are the extremities, genitalia, and face. Twenty-five percent of patients also suffer from gastrointestinal (GI) symptoms including abdominal cramps, nausea, vomiting, colic, and (occasionally) signs of obstruction.

Cutaneous signs of angioedema usually develop gradually over 12–36 hours and may last up to 5 days whereas the GI symptoms usually subside with 24 hours. Conversely, upper airway obstruction may develop rapidly within 20 minutes of onset resulting in an acute respiratory syndrome that may prove fatal. Up to 40% of all undiagnosed patients die as a result of upper airway obstruction.

MASTOCYTOSIS

Mastocytosis is a condition of unknown etiology characterized by an excessive accumulation of mast cells in various body organs and tissues. Mastocytosis occurs in three forms: 1) mastocytoma (a benign cutaneous tumor), 2) urticaria pigmentosa that is characterized by multiple colored or brown macules or papules that urticate when stroked and may become vesicular or even bullous, and 3) systemic mastocytosis in which there are mast-cell infiltrates in the skin, lymph nodes, liver, spleen, GI tract, and bones.

Patients with mastocytosis suffer from arthralgias, bone pain, and anaphylactoid reactions. Other symptoms result from overstimulation of H_2 histamine receptors, leading to peptic ulcer disease and chronic diarrhea.

ANAPHYLAXIS

Anaphylaxis is an acute systemic reaction that occurs in a previously sensitized person who is reexposed to the sensitizing antigen. The most common antigens are foreign serum, parenteral enzymes, blood products, β-lactam antibiotics, other drugs, and wasp and bee stings. Anaphylaxis may be aggravated or even induced by exercise. It is an IgE-mediated reaction that occurs when antigen (foreign protein, polysaccharide or hapten coupled with a carrier protein) reaches the circulation. Leukotrienes, histamine, and other mediators are generated or released when the antigen reacts with IgE on sensitized mast cells and basophils. These mediators cause smooth muscle contraction responsible for wheeze and GI symptoms as well as vascular dilatation that leads to circulatory collapse. Capillary leakage into the tissues causes urticaria and angioedema and results in a further decrease in the plasma volume leading to shock. Fluid may leak into the alveoli and produce pulmonary edema. Obstructive angioedema of the upper airway may also occur. Finally, profound hypotension may result in arrhythmia and cardiogenic shock.

Typically the patient feels uneasy for approximately 1–15 minutes after exposure to the allergen. The patient then becomes more agitated and flushed. He or she may experience palpitations, paresthesias, pruritus, throbbing in the ears, coughing, sneezing, and difficulty in breathing due to laryngeal edema or bronchospasm. Urticaria and angioedema may be evident. Nausea, vomiting, and abdominal pain and diarrhea are less common. Shock develops within another 1–2 minutes, and the patient may become incontinent, convulse, and lose consciousness.

CLINICAL AND LABORATORY AIDS REQUIRED FOR DIAGNOSIS

Urticaria

Urticaria is a clinical diagnosis. In urticaria, pruritus (generally the first symptom) is followed shortly by the appearance of wheals that may remain small (1–5 mm) or may enlarge. The larger ones tend to clear in the center and may be noticed first as large rings (>20 cm across) of erythema and edema. Ordinarily, crops of hives come and go; a lesion may appear in one site for several hours, then disappear only to reemerge at another site later. The changing morphology of lesions that may evolve over minutes to hours may lead to geographic or bizarre patterns.

The cause of acute urticaria is usually self-evident. Even when it is not so obvious, a diagnostic investigation is seldom required because of the self-limiting nature of the eruption.

In cases of chronic urticaria, a careful history, examination, and screening tests should be carried out to eliminate possible underlying systemic lupus erythematosus, polycythemia rubra vera, vasculitis syndrome, or infection. A few patients with intractable urticaria are hyperthyroid. A serum-sickness–like prodrome with urticaria may be associated with acute hepatitis B. Quantitative immunoglobulins, cryoglobulins, cryofibrinogens, and antinuclear antibodies are often sought in cold urticaria but rarely found. Although often suspected, controllable psychogenic factors are rarely identified.

The histological changes may be very slight but usually there is edema, vascular and lymphatic dilatation, and a variable perivascular cellular infiltrate of lymphocytes, monocytes, polymorphs, and histiocytes. On electron-microscopy, dermal mast cells show signs of degranulation. Various vasoactive substances are thought to be involved including histamine, kinins, leukotrienes, prostaglandins, and complement.

Urticarial lesions lasting more than 24 hours raise the possibility of this being a vasculitic disorder. Urticarial lesions of vasculitic etiology are more fixed than in classical urticaria. They last for 2–3 days and are frequently accompanied by joint pains and fever. Reduced serum complement levels with raised inflammatory markers are observed. A skin biopsy is most useful in these circumstances as urticarial vasculitis is an uncommon entity.

Angioedema

Angioedema represents a more diffuse swelling affecting the loose subcutaneous and/or submucosal tissues. The dorsum of the hands or feet, eyelids, lips, and genitalia are the usual sites affected. Involvement of the mucous membranes may present as wheeze or stridor that may be mistaken for asthma. Edema of the upper airway is potentially life-threatening.

The diagnosis of hereditary angioedema is made by measuring complement C4 levels, which remain low, even between attacks. This test carries 100% sensitivity and 100% negative predictive value in an untreated patient. A low C1 inhibitor level will confirm the diagnosis. If the C1 inhibitor is unexpectedly normal, a C1 functional assay can be performed.

Mastocytosis

In localized mastocytosis, the histamine content in tissue is usually high, commensurate with the elevated mast cell concentration. In systemic mastocytosis, urinary excretion of histamine and its metabolites are high. Plasma histamine and prostaglandin D_2 may also be elevated.

Anaphylaxis

The diagnosis of anaphylaxis is usually self-evident when there has been exposure to a known allergen. In the case of unknown exposure, increased IgE and serum tryptase levels will strongly support the diagnosis. It is worth remembering, however, that anaphylaxis may be immediate or delayed. Even in the case of a bee sting, anaphylaxis may be delayed for up to 20 minutes due to the rate of absorption of the toxin from the embedded sting sac. Acute life-threatening edema of the airway can occur more immediately when there is local swelling following a bee or wasp sting to the pharynx, which may occur when the insect has inadvertently fallen into a beer can or glass and is unknowingly drunk by the unsuspecting partygoer.

DIFFERENTIAL DIAGNOSIS

Differential diagnosis for urticaria and angioedema includes persistent papular eruptions from insect bites such as flea or gnat bites. These eruptions can usually be distinguished from the urticarias by their central punctum.

Contact urticaria may be caused by a host of substances varying from chemicals to foods to medications, but it is usually limited to areas exposed to the contactant. Streaked urticarial lesions may be seen in acute allergic plant dermatitis (e.g., poison ivy, oak, or sumac). Phytophotodermatitis is caused by the exposure of skin to plant extracts and sun and is common in hot climates (e.g., where lime juice is used in cocktails). The possibility of protoporphyria should be considered in any sun-related pruritic reaction.

The differential diagnosis for anaphylaxis includes all causes of shock (e.g., acute internal hemorrhage, sepsis syndrome, cardiogenic shock) and the Waterhouse–Friderichsen syndrome.

THERAPY

Urticaria

Acute urticaria is a self-limited condition that generally subsides in 1–7 days. Treatment is chiefly palliative. If the etiological trigger is known, it should be avoided. A specific exclusion diet (e.g., salicylate and tartrazine-free diet) may be helpful. If the cause is not apparent, all nonessential drugs should be discontinued until the reaction has subsided.

If treatment is indicated, the initial management will include H_1 antihistamines. Doses should be increased weekly to tolerance. Antihistamines from different classes may be systematically tried if initial choice is ineffective or intolerable. Combinations of different antihistamines are often effective.

Most symptoms can usually be relieved with diphenhydramine 50–100 mg every 4 hours, hydroxyzine 25–100 twice a day, or cyproheptadine 4–8 mg every 4 hours. Hydroxyzine is the preferred drug for cholinergic urticaria; anticholinergic drugs are ineffective at tolerable doses.

Terfenadine (60 mg b.i.d.) is a nonsedating antihistamine that has been reported to be effective in chronic idiopathic urticaria. Concomitant use with erythromycin (and related macrolide antibiotics) or ketoconazole (and related imidazole) leads to increases in the plasma levels that may cause cardiac arrhythmias. It is not recommended in lactating or pregnant women. Another nonsedating antihistamine, astemizole, has been reported to be effective in the majority of patients with seasonal allergic rhinitis and chronic idiopathic urticaria.[9,10] The long half-life of astemizole is a major disadvantage if skin-prick testing is needed or if the patient becomes pregnant while on therapy. Another less sedating antihistamine approved for use is loratadine in a dosage of 10 mg daily. It has a shorter half-life than astemizole and is similar to the other antihistamines in its effectiveness. It appears not to interact with imidazole antifungals or macrolide antibiotics.

Oral antihistamines with tranquilizing properties are usually beneficial (e.g., hydroxyzine 25–50 mg b.i.d. or cyproheptadine 4–8 mg q 4–8 h for adults; for children, hydroxyzine 2 mg/kg/day divided q 6 h, and cyproheptadine 0.25–0.5 mg/kg/day divided q 6–8 h).

Doxepin (a tricyclic antidepressant) 25–50 mg twice daily, or more commonly 25–75 mg at bedtime, may be the most effective agent for some adult patients. It should be used with caution because of its anticholinergic side effects and promotion of cardiac arrhythmias.

Prednisone in a dose of 40 mg daily may be necessary in more severe cases of urticaria and in cases of angioedema.[11] It will usually suppress both acute and chronic forms of urticaria; however, the use of systemic glucocorticoids is rarely indicated because properly selected combinations of agents with less toxicity are usually effective. Furthermore, after steroids are withdrawn, the urticaria virtually always returns if it had been chronic.

Other agents with some promise as adjuvant therapy include calcium channel blockers (used for at least 4 weeks), terbutaline 1.25–2.5 mg three times a day, and colchicine 0.6 mg twice a day.

Local treatment is rarely of benefit. Starch baths twice daily or Aveeno baths, prepared by adding one cupful of finely refined cornstarch or a packet of Aveeno to a comfortably warm bath, may alleviate symptoms in some patients. Alternatively, one may use a lotion containing 0.5% camphor, 0.5% menthol, and 0.5% phenol topically or in addition to the bathing. Topical glucocorticoids should not be used.

Hereditary Angioedema

Hereditary angioedema may present as a medical emergency that requires rapid therapeutic intervention. The edema progresses until the complement components have been consumed. Iatrogenic cases are not uncommon.

Acute attacks that threaten to produce airway obstruction should be treated promptly by establishing an airway. Aminocaproic acid 8 g every 4 hours may succeed in terminating the attack. Epinephrine, an antihistamine, and a glucocorticoid should be administered even though the evidence base is unproven. Parenteral pain relief, antiemetics, and intravenous fluid replacement are recommended for abdominal attacks.

Replacement therapy using C1 inhibitor is the only therapy that has been successfully used in a prospective double-blind, placebo-controlled trial.[12] Although not available in the United States, it has been the treatment of choice in Europe for more than 20 years.

A partially purified C1 inhibitor fraction of pooled plasma has been shown to be safe and effective for prophylaxis (e.g., prior to a dental procedure or endoscopy).[13] Alternatively, 2 units of fresh frozen plasma can be given. Although a complement substrate in the plasma might provoke an attack, this has not been observed in symptom-free patients.

Long-term management will have to take into account both the frequency and severity of attacks as well as special circumstances such as pregnancy, surgical procedures, and children. For long-term prophylaxis of hereditary angioedema, androgens are effective. One of the impeded androgens should be used. Treatment is commenced with stanozolol 2 mg times a day or danazol 200 mg three times a day. When control is achieved, the dosage should be reduced as much as possible to minimize masculinizing side effects in women and reduce the cost. These drugs are not only effective but also have been shown to raise the low C1 inhibitor and C4 toward normal.

Mastocytosis

Cutaneous mastocytosis usually develops in childhood. The solitary mastocytoma will usually involute spontaneously. Urticaria pigmentosa either clears completely or is substantially improved by adolescence. These conditions rarely, if ever, progress to systemic mastocytosis. Treatment with an H_1 antihistamine is usually all that is needed.

If systemic mastocytosis ensues, the symptoms should be treated with an H_1 or H_2 antihistamine. Aspirin therapy may be tried, but with caution as this may enhance production of leukotrienes. For GI symptom control, oral cromolyn sodium 200 mg four times a day (100 mg four times a day for children 2–12 years old) should be given. There is no effective treatment available to reduce the number of tissue mast cells.

Anaphylaxis

Severe reactions with generalized swelling, urticaria, angioedema, dizziness, sweating, pounding headache, stomach cramps, chest tightness, and a sensation of choking or impending doom may signify an impending anaphylaxis.

In cases of acute pharyngeal or laryngeal angioedema, epinephrine 1:1000, 0.5 mL by subcutaneous injection should be given immediately. Nebulized epinephrine 1:100 dilution and intravenous antihistamine (e.g., diphenhydramine 50–100 mg) will usually prevent airway obstruction. Urgent intubation or emergency tracheostomy may be required, followed by 100% O_2 therapy and resuscitation. (See Chapter 19. Allergy to bee sting as an example of a type I allergic hypersensitivity [anaphylaxis] reaction.)

Confirmation that an allergic reaction has taken place can be made by measuring the serum tryptase. Most deaths will occur because of delays in accessing emergency treatment.

COURSE AND PROGNOSIS

Most episodes of acute urticaria and angioedema are acute and self-limited and resolve spontaneously over a period of 1–2 weeks. In about half the cases of chronic urticaria, spontaneous remissions occur within 2 years. Control of stress often helps to reduce the frequency and severity of episodes. Alcohol, coffee, and tobacco should be avoided as these may aggravate the symptoms. Certain drugs, such as aspirin, may also exacerbate symptoms. When urticaria is produced by aspirin, sensitivity to other nonsteroidal anti-inflammatory drugs and to foods or drugs containing the additive tartazine should be investigated.

Patients with chronic mastocytosis generally have a good prognosis. The course of an anaphylactic reaction is unpredictable and is largely determined by the speed with which the patient can access appropriate emergency services.

All patients with a history of anaphylaxis should carry a preloaded epinephrine syringe (EpiPen; 300 μg) for emergencies. Any person with a history of allergy should wear a MedicAlert bracelet at all times bearing the details of this allergy.

REFERENCES

1. Greaves MW. Chronic urticaria. N Engl J Med. 1995; 332:1767.
2. Lindelöf B, Sigurgeirsson B, Wahlgren CF, Eklund G. Chronic urticaria and cancer: an epidemiological study of 1155 patients. Br J Dermatol. 1990; 123:453–6.
3. O'Donnell BF, Swana GT, Kobza Black A. Organ and non-organ specific autoimmunity in chronic urticaria. Br J Dermatol. 1995; 153 Suppl 45:42A.
4. Milton JL. On giant urticaria. Edinb Med J. 1876; 22:513–26.
5. Quinke H. Uber akutes umschriebenes Hautodem. Monatshefte Prakt Dermatol. 1882; 1:129–31.
6. Donaldson VH, Evans RR. A biochemical abnormality in hereditary angioneurotic edema; absence of serum inhibitor of C'1-esterase. Am J Med. 1963; 35:37–44.
7. Tosi M. Molecular genetics of C-inhibitor. Immunobiology. 1998; 199:358–65.
8. Kaplan AP, Greaves MW. Angioedema. J Am Acad Dermatol. 2005; 53:373–88.
9. Breneman D, Bronsky EA, Bruce S, Kalivas JT, et al. Cetirizine and astemizole therapy for chronic idiopathic urticaria: a double-blind, placebo-controlled, comparative trial. J Acad Dermatol. 1995; 33:192–8.
10. Krausse HF. Therapeutic advances in the management of allergic rhinitis and urticaria. Otolaryngol Head Neck Surg. 1994; 111:364.
11. Pollack CV Jr., Romano TJ. Outpatient management of acute urticaria: the role of prednisone. Ann Emerg Med. 1995; 26:547.
12. Longhurst HJ. Emergency treatment of acute attacks in hereditary angioedema due to C1 inhibitor deficiency: what is the evidence? Int J Clin Pract. 2005; 59:594–9.
13. Gompels MM, Lock RJ, Abinun M, Bethune CA, et al. C1 inhibitor deficiency: consensus document. Clin Exp Immunol. 2005; 139:379–94.

CHAPTER 19

Severe, Acute Allergic and Immunological Reactions II: Other Hypersensitivities and Immune Defects, Including HIV

Samuel H. Allen

HYPERSENSITIVITY REACTIONS

A hypersensitivity reaction (HSR) is an uncommon, usually immune-mediated response to a drug or other substance. It is estimated that HSRs account for approximately 5%–10% of all drug-related adverse events. Although severe drug hypersensitivity is rare, it is of concern because it can cause serious illness or death. There are four basic types of immune-mediated hypersensitivity (Table 19.1).

Type I – Immediate (Atopic or Anaphylactic)

Type I hypersensitivity is an allergic reaction provoked by exposure to a specific type of antigen known as an allergen. Exposure may be by ingestion, inhalation, injection, or direct contact. Type I reactions are characterized by an exaggerated release of immunoglobulin E (IgE), which binds to mast cells and basophils. Later exposure to the same allergen results in cross-linking of bound IgE on the sensitized cells. This cross-linking causes degranulation and secretion of pharmacological mediators (such as histamine, leukotriene, and prostaglandin) that act on the surrounding tissues, causing vasodilatation and smooth muscle contraction. The reaction may be local or systemic, and symptoms may vary from mild irritation to anaphylactic shock, which is the result of an acute systemic reaction and can be fatal.

Examples of type I reactions and their triggers include allergic asthma (house dust mite), hay fever (grass pollen), allergic rhinitis (animal dander), and nut and drug allergies. Because it takes some time to produce IgE antibodies, type I HSRs usually begin at least several days after starting a new drug. If a person stops the drug and restarts it later, the reaction can be immediate, because the immune system is already primed to respond to it. Occasionally, HSRs can occur for the first time several months (and sometime years) after starting a drug.

Skin eruptions occur in approximately 90% of type I HSRs. The most common manifestation is an itchy red measles-like eruption that typically develops 1–4 weeks after starting a new drug. A rash often appears first on the trunk and then spreads outward. The mucous membranes may be involved.

In Stevens–Johnson syndrome (SJS) and erythema multiforme major, patients develop blisters on the skin and mucous membranes. Other manifestations may include fever, aphthous ulcers, and injection of the eyes. Extensive skin loss may occur in toxic epidermal necrolysis. Sections of the skin may die and peel off, leaving raw areas

TABLE 19.1: Types of Hypersensitivity Reaction

Type	Alternative name	Associated disorders	Mediator(s)
I	Allergic	Atopy, anaphylaxis, asthma	IgE
II	Cytotoxic, antibody dependant	Erythroblastosis fetalis, Goodpasture syndrome, autoimmune hemolytic anemia	IgM or IgG (complement)
III	Immune complex disease	Serum sickness, Arthus reaction, SLE	IgG (complement)
IV	Cell mediated	Contact dermatitis, tuberculosis, chronic transplant rejection	Cell mediated

ALLERGY TO BEE STING AS AN EXAMPLE OF A TYPE I ALLERGIC HYPERSENSITIVITY (ANAPHYLAXIS) REACTION

Insects of the order *Hymenoptera* include wasps and bees. Stinging is a defense mechanism designed to incapacitate other insects. Bees differ from wasps in that their stinging apparatus is inserted into the victim on stinging. Sting venom comprises proteolytic enzymes, phospholipases, metalloproteinases, and toxins. Antigen 5 (or Ves g V) from yellow jacket wasps (*Vespula germanica*) and phospholipase (Api m II) from honeybees (*Apis millifera*) are the major allergy-provoking venom components. Sensitization to insect venom can occur after a single sting. Although cross-reaction allergy can occur, most people remain allergic to either wasp or bee, but not both.

Pain, redness, and swelling normally occur at the site of a sting. This is not an allergy, but rather a local toxic reaction to the venom. This reaction evolves over a period of a few hours and settles within 1–2 days without any adverse consequences. A more immediate and severe reaction can occur, however, in an individual who has been sensitized by a previous wasp or bee sting. If allergic, he or she may develop a reaction that can vary from mild localized swelling to life-threatening anaphylaxis. Typically there is localized redness and swelling spanning two joints, intense itching, and pain. More severe reactions cause generalized swelling, urticaria, angioedema, dizziness, sweating, pounding headache, stomach cramps, chest tightness, and a sensation of choking and/or impending doom. Symptoms may develop up to 20 minutes after the sting. This represents the time between the release of the sting and the effect of the venom components on the victim following the insect attack.

If stung by a bee, the sting sac will continue to actively pump venom if left in situ. Therefore, if the stinging apparatus is visible, it should be carefully extricated from the flesh of the victim to prevent further toxin release. The sac should be removed without squeezing. The honeybee (*Apis* spp.) is unique in that it possesses a barbed stinging organ. The female honeybee, however, carries the stinger and dies shortly after discharging a sting.

TREATMENT OF WASP OR BEE STING ALLERGIC REACTION

A double dose of oral antihistamine such as chlorpheniramine 8 mg should be administered in adults and older children. In the case of a generalized reaction, one should administer immediate intramuscular chlorpheniramine 10 mg, oral corticosteroid (prednisone 30 mg) and give a β-agonist inhaler or nebulizer.

In the case of shock or respiratory difficulties, 0.5 mL of intramuscular epinephrine (1:1000) plus intramuscular chlorpheniramine 10 mg and hydrocortisone 200 μg should be administered and arrangements made to transport the patient to a suitable treatment facility.

All patients with a history of allergy should carry a preloaded epinephrine syringe (EpiPen 300 μg) for emergencies. Repeat injections should be administered every 5 minutes until a satisfactory response is achieved. For children younger than 5 years, 0.1–0.3 mL of epinephrine (1:1000) should be administered according to size and age, and arrangements made to transport the child to an emergency department for further monitoring. Confirmation that an allergic reaction has taken place can be made by measuring the serum tryptase.

A person known to be wasp or bee allergic should have a MedicAlert bracelet carrying details of this allergy.

DESENSITIZATION

Venom desensitization immunotherapy is a useful means of treatment for patients with severe generalized venom allergy and is particularly useful for beekeepers, horticulturists, and gardeners. Weekly injections are given during the initial treatment phase and then monthly for another 3 years. At the end of the therapy the patient should be able to tolerate 100 μg of venom – equivalent to two bee stings – with no adverse reaction. This therapy should be carried out only in specialist clinics where resuscitation facilities are available because there is a small risk of inducing an allergic reaction. Anti-wasp and anti-bee venom vaccines are available, but these are wasp and bee species-specific.

that resemble burns. These reactions are not true allergic reactions but appear to involve the release of inflammatory cytokines in response to a superantigen such as in toxic shock syndrome (toxic shock syndrome toxin 1 and/or exfoliatin A or B).

Fever is a common feature of drug-induced hypersensitivity. Other manifestations include soft-tissue swelling, enlarged lymph nodes, sore throat, cough, difficulty breathing, gastrointestinal (GI) symptoms, dizziness, muscle and joint pain, blood cell abnormalities, blood vessel inflammation, and liver or kidney dysfunction.

The most severe type of drug-induced allergic reaction is anaphylaxis, which can occur within seconds or minutes after restarting a drug to which the person has previously been exposed. Symptoms include hives, swelling, constriction of the upper airway, falling blood pressure, rapid heartbeat, shock, and cardiovascular collapse.

Treatment depends on the severity of the reaction. Antihistamines and corticosteroids are usually indicated. In the case of anaphylaxis, immediate epinephrine to maintain blood pressure should be administered. In all situations, the provocative agent should be avoided.

Type II – Antibody-Dependent

In type II hypersensitivity, the antibodies produced by the immune response bind to antigens on the patient's own cell surfaces. The antigens recognized in this way may be either intrinsic (self) or extrinsic (foreign) antigens. These cells are recognized by macrophages and dendritic cells that act as antigen-presenting cells, causing B cells to respond by producing antibodies against the foreign protein. Examples of this type of reaction include autoimmune hemolytic anemia, transfusion reactions, transplant rejection, Goodpasture syndrome, pemphigus, Graves' disease, myasthenia gravis, and rheumatic fever. Because the reaction is antibody mediated, the reaction will evolve over a period of 1–3 days.

Type III – Immune Complex

Type II hypersensitivity occurs when antigens and antibodies are present in roughly equal measure, causing extensive cross-linking. Large immune complexes that cannot be cleared are deposited in tissue to induce an inflammatory response. The reaction develops over days to weeks. Examples of this type of reaction include rheumatoid arthritis, serum sickness, systemic lupus erythematosus (SLE), Arthus reaction, farmer's lung, and polyarteritis nodosa.

Type IV – Cell-Mediated (Delayed-Type Hypersensitivity)

Type IV hypersensitivity is often called delayed type as the reaction takes 2–3 days to develop. Unlike other types, it is not antibody mediated but rather represents a type of cell-mediated response.

Cytotoxic (CD8+) and helper (CD4+) T cells recognize antigens in a complex with the major histocompatibility complex molecules class I or II, respectively. The antigen-presenting cells are macrophages or dendritic cells that secrete interleukin-12 (IL-12). This secretion stimulates further CD4+ T-cell proliferation. These T cells secrete IL-2 and interferon-γ, inducing type I cytokines. Activated CD8+ cells destroy target cells, and activated macrophages transform into multinucleated giant cells. This type of reaction is seen in contact dermatitis (e.g., poison ivy), atopic dermatitis, leprosy, and tuberculosis. The Mantoux reaction is an example of a delayed-type HSR.

IMMUNE DEFECTS

Deficiencies of the immune system may result in recurrent infections, autoimmunity, and susceptibility to malignancy. Although intrinsic congenital immunodeficiencies are rare, the widespread use of corticosteroid and immunosuppressive therapies (as well as the spread of the human immunodeficiency virus [HIV] pandemic) means that the dermatologist is increasingly being called to assess problems relating to immunosuppression. In the context of an immune defect, the patient is often systemically unwell and the dermopathy may constitute an emergency.

Immunodeficiency may be congenital or acquired (Table 19.2). Dysfunction may occur in either the quantitative (number of cells) or the qualitative (function of cells) aspect. These aspects include deficiencies of

- neutrophils (and monocytes/macrophages),
- complement pathway,
- B-cell defects (causing antibody deficiency),
- T-cell defects (causing impaired cell-mediated immunity), or
- combinations of any of the preceding aspects.

More than 100 different congenital immunodeficiencies due to specific genetic defects have been described; most

TABLE 19.2: Congenital and Acquired Immunodeficiencies

Congenital	Acquired
Neutophil deficiency	
Congenital neutropenia	Drug-induced myelosuppression
Cyclical neutropenia	Hypersplenism
Leukocyte adhesion defects	Autoimmune neutropenia
Hyper IgE syndrome	Corticosteroid therapy
Shwachman syndrome	Diabetes mellitus
Chronic granulomatous disease	Hypophosphatemia
Storage diseases	Myeloid leukaemia
Chediak–Higashi syndrome	Influenza
Complement deficiency	
C3, C1q, I, H deficiency	
C5, 6, 7, 8, 9 deficiencies	
Mannan-binding lectin deficiency	
Antibody deficiency (B-cell defects)	
X-linked hypogammaglobulinemia	Myeloma
Common variable immunodeficiency	Lymphoma
Specific IgA deficiency	Splenectomy
Specific antibody deficiency	Congenital rubella
T-cell deficiencies	
DiGeorge anomaly	Measles
IL-2 deficiency	Corticosteroids
Signal transduction defect	Calcineurin inhibitors (e.g., cyclosporine)
Combined T- and B-cell deficiencies	
Severe combined immunodeficiency	Protein–calorie malnutrition
Wiskott–Aldrich syndrome	Immunodeficiency of prematurity
Ataxia telangiectasia	HIV/AIDS
Hyper IgM syndrome	
Duncan syndrome	

TABLE 19.3: Immune Defects and Associated Opportunistic Infections

---

Neutrophil deficiency

Staphylococcus aureus	Coagulase-negative staphylococcus
Escherichia coli	*Klebsiella pneumoniae*
Pseudomonas aeruginosa	*Serratia marcescens*
Bacteroides spp.	*Aspergillus fumigatus*
Candida spp. (systemic)	*Mucor* spp.
Absidia spp.	

B-cell (antibody) deficiency

Campylobacter spp.	*Echovirus*
Mycoplasma spp.	*Ureaplasma* spp.

Complement deficiency (lytic pathway C5–C9)

Meningococcus	Gonococcus (disseminated)

T-cell–mediated immunodeficiency

Listeria monocytogenes	*Legionella pneumophila*
Salmonella spp. (nontyphi)	*Nocardia* spp.
Mycobacterium tuberculosis	*Atypical mycobacteria* spp.
Candida spp. (mucocutaneous)	*Toxoplasma gondii*
Cryptococcus neoformans	*Histoplasma capsulatum*
Pneumocystis jiroveci	Herpes simplex
Herpes zoster	Measles virus
Cytomegalovirus	Epstein–Barr virus

---

are rare. They usually present in childhood, but some types and the less severe forms may not become apparent until adulthood. Much more common are acquired immunodeficiencies, which can result from malnutrition, splenectomy, immunosuppressive therapy, drug side effects, and/or infection. The most common infective cause is HIV, which leads to acquired immune deficiency syndrome (AIDS).

Opportunistic infections occur when there is weakness of host defense mechanisms regardless of the cause. The nature of the infection may sometimes indicate the specific type of immune defect (Table 19.3). Opportunistic infections usually present insidiously. An underlying immune defect should be suspected in patients presenting with recurrent infections, particularly with unusual organisms or at unusual sites (Table 19.4).

TABLE 19.4: Warning Signs of Immune Deficiency

- 8 respiratory tract infections/year in a child, or
- >4 respiratory tract infections/year in an adult
- >1 infection requiring hospital admission or intravenous antibiotics
- Infections with unusual organisms
- Infections at unusual sites
- Chronic infection unresponsive to usual treatment
- Early end-organ damage (e.g., bronchiectasis)
- Positive family history

Defects in Neutrophils

Defects of neutrophils result in a predisposition to bacterial infections that results in extracellular infection. The risk of infection rises steeply once the neutrophil count falls below 0.5×10^9/L. The gut is normally colonized with potentially pathogenic bacteria that can readily lead to septicemia following immunosuppression from whatever cause. The duration of neutropenia can be reduced by use of granulocyte colony-stimulating factor or granulocyte–macrophage colony-stimulating factor. Prompt antiinfective therapy for febrile episodes during neutropenia is essential. Often, preemptive prophylaxis is prescribed to commence approximately 1 week after chemotherapy – the time to clinically significant neutropenia following immunosuppressive therapy. A particular and typically benign variant of neutropenia is cyclical neutropenia, which produces cycles of neutropenia every 3–5 weeks.

Defects of neutrophil function include autosomal recessive congenital leukocyte adhesion defect, hyper-IgE syndrome, and Shwachman syndrome that may resemble cystic fibrosis. Hyper-IgE syndrome produces recurrent frequent staphylococcal boils and furuncles – hence its synonym, Job syndrome – and is associated with elevated levels of IgE. Unusual eczema-like skin eruptions and severe lung infections resulting in pneumatoceles may occur. Many patients with autosomal dominant hyper-IgE syndrome fail to lose their baby teeth and have two sets simultaneously.

Chronic granulomatous disease usually presents in early or late childhood. Patients present with chronic suppurative granulomas or abscesses affecting the skin, lymph nodes, and sometimes the lung and liver, as well as osteomyelitis. Because macrophages are also affected, cell-mediated opportunistic infections may also be seen, such as atypical mycobacteria, *Nocardia*, and salmonellae. Diagnosis is established by the nitroblue tetrazolium test.

Complement Deficiency

Complement deficiencies are rare. They can be associated with increased susceptibility to infection with *Haemophilus* and pneumococcal infection, especially in early childhood prior to development of a sufficiently wide specific antibody repertoire.

There are two major patterns of infection associated with complement deficiency: Deficiency of C3, C1q, or factors I or H give rise to an increased susceptibility to capsulated bacteria, such as *Haemophilus influenza*, pneumococcus, meningococcus, and Group B streptococcus. These patients may also develop SLE-like immune complex disorders. Conversely, deficiency of the lytic complement pathway, C5–9, causes susceptibility to disseminated neisserial infections, meningococcemia, and gonococcemia. C1 esterase inhibitor deficiency is not associated with infection but with hereditary angioedema (see Chapter 18).

B-Cell Defects (Antibody Deficiency)

In X-linked hypogammaglobulinemia, B cells and plasma cells are reduced resulting in a profound reduction in all the immunoglobulin classes. T cells are normal. The specific gene defect is found on the X chromosome. X-linked hypogammaglobulinemia typically presents with infections such as meningitis and mycoplasmal infection after the first 3–6 months of life, when passively transferred maternal antibody has largely been lost. Intravenous immunoglobulin (IVIg) replacement therapy is successful, and most patients are able to treat themselves at home.

Common variable immunodeficiency is a late-onset antibody deficiency that may present in childhood or adult life. Immunoglobulin G (IgG) levels are especially low. It is similar to X-linked hypogammaglobulinemia, but a particular feature is lymph-node hyperplasia that may express itself as nodular lymphadenopathy and lymphoreticular malignancy. The findings of reduced immunoglobulin levels with normal B-cell numbers indicate the diagnosis. Regular immunoglobulin replacement therapy (IVIg) with antimicrobials for opportunistic infection is the mainstay of management.

Specific immunoglobulin A (IgA) deficiency is extremely common, affecting 1 in 600 of the UK population. Most cases are asymptomatic, but some patients have an associated celiac disease or other autoimmune disorder.

Hypogammaglobulinemia is seen in the immune paresis of patients with myeloma and chronic leukemia or lymphoma. Splenectomy causes impaired defense against capsulated bacteria, particularly pneumococcus. Hyposplenism associated with severe sickle cell disease is responsible for the increased risk of infection in such patients. Pneumococcal, meningococcal, and *Haemophilus influenzae* type B (Hib) vaccination before elective splenectomy and the use of penicillin prophylaxis can largely eliminate the risk of serious infection. Hypogammaglobulinemia can also occur in congenital rubella.

T-Cell Defects

DiGeorge syndrome (22q11 deletion syndrome) occurs in 1 in 4000 live births. It is a defect of branchial arch development leading to abnormal thymic growth. Associated features include dysmorphic facies, hypoparathyroidism, and cardiac defects. Patients present with features of impaired T cells including mucocutaneous candidosis and *Pneumocystis carinii* pneumonia (now renamed *Pneumocystis jiroveci*) (PcP), often with chronic diarrhea due to a variety of pathogens. The absent thymus can be documented radiologically. CD3+ and CD4+ T-cell subsets are reduced, and T-cell–proliferative responses are impaired. Immunoglobulin production is usually normal. Management entails prompt treatment of opportunistic infections. Thymic transplant and bone-marrow transplant have had some success.

Combined B- and T-Cell Defects

The most severe immunodeficiencies are those that affect both B- and T-cell responses. These immunodeficiencies can stem from a variety of defective mechanisms but tend to have rather similar clinical features, combining the opportunistic infections of cell-mediated immunodeficiency with those of antibody deficiency.

Severe combined immunodeficiency (SCID) syndrome usually presents in the first weeks of life. Failure to thrive, absent lymphoid tissue, lymphopenia, and hypogammaglobulinemia with multiple severe infections are typical. Immunoglobulin therapy is effective for the antibody deficiency, but the cell-mediated opportunistic infections are the main determinants of outcome. Bone-marrow transplantation is the definitive approach and has had significant success, especially if carried out early in the disease course. More recently, gene therapy and attempts to correct adenosine deaminase deficiency associated with SCID have had some success.

Failure of class switching from immunoglobulin M (IgM) to other classes of antibody leads to normal or high levels of IgM associated with low IgG and IgA. T-cell function is impaired, leading to opportunistic infection with *P. jirovecii*, *Cryptosporidium* (including sclerosing cholangitis), herpes virus infections, candidosis, and cryptococcosis.

Wiskott–Aldrich syndrome is an X-linked, mainly cell-mediated defect associated with falling immunoglobulins. Clinical features may include eczema, thrombocytopenia, autoimmune defects, and lymphoreticular malignancies.

Epstein–Barr virus (EBV)-associated immunodeficiency (Duncan syndrome) results in polyclonal EBV-driven lymphoproliferation, combined immunodeficiency, aplastic anemia, and lymphoid malignancy.

HIV AND AIDS

AIDS was first recognized in 1981.[1] It is caused by human immunodeficiency virus-1 (HIV-1). HIV-2 causes a similar illness to HIV-1 but is less aggressive and restricted mainly to western Africa.

In 2007, the World Health Organization estimated that there were 33.2 million people living with HIV/AIDS.[2] The cumulative death toll since the pandemic began is more than 20 million. The vast majority of deaths have been in sub-Saharan Africa, but Asia, which currently bears about one fifth of the burden of disease, could surpass this.

Combination therapy, composed of three active drugs ("triple cocktail") from two or more different drug classes, constitutes highly active antiretroviral therapy (HAART). As of 2008, there were more than 25 different antiretroviral drugs from 7 different drug classes (Table 19.5), offering the HIV-infected patient the potential for lifelong suppression of viral replication, even if the prospect of achieving eradication of the virus, either through a vaccine or potent combination therapy, remains illusive. Although HAART

TABLE 19.5: Antiretroviral Drug Classes

Drug class	Drug (abbreviation)
Nucleoside reverse transcriptase inhibitors (NRTI)	Zalcitabine (ddC) Didanosine (ddI) Lamivudine (3TC) Zidovudine (AZT) Stavudine (d4T) Abacavir Darunavir Emitricitabine (FTC)
Nucleotide reverse transcriptase inhibitor (NtRTI)	Tenofovir (TDF)
Non-nucleoside reverse transcriptase inhibitors (NNRTI)	Nevirapine Delaviridine[a] Efavirenz Etravirine (TMC-125)
Protease inhibitors (PI)	Indinavir[b] Ritonavir Nelfinavir Lopinavir[c] Atazanavir[b] Fosamprenavir[b] Saquinavir[b] Amprenavir[a,b] Tipranavir[a,b]
Fusion inhibitors	Enfuvirtide (T-20)
Integrase inhibitors	Raltegravir
CCR5 co-receptor inhibitors	Maraviroc

[a] Restricted use.
[b] Coformulated with low-dose ritonavir.
[c] Usually given with boosting low-dose ritonavir.

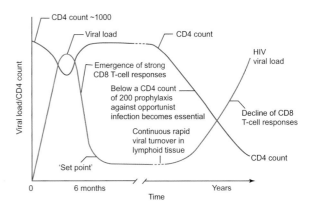

FIGURE 19.1: Natural history of human immunodeficiency virus (HIV) and acquired immune deficiency syndrome (AIDS).

reaction in the presence of a negative or equivocal HIV antibody test following recent exposure to HIV.

The principal dermatological manifestation, occurring in up to 75% of cases of acute seroconversion, is a non-specific rash. This usually appears as a maculopapular erythematous exanthem, notably of the face, palms, and soles (Figure 19.2). Painful oral ulceration, genital ulceration, has resulted in great benefit to patients, novel side effects to these drugs have emerged, many of which affect the skin.

Natural History of HIV and AIDS

Without treatment, a person with HIV may develop one or more opportunistic infections and/or cancers. Death results from these illnesses, which the HIV has made the body more vulnerable to, and not directly from the HIV virus itself (Figure 19.1).

HIV Seroconversion

HIV seroconversion illness develops in approximately 75% of persons following acute infection with HIV. It occurs 2–6 weeks after exposure and lasts a few days to several months but usually less than a fortnight. The symptoms are nonspecific but may mimic a flu-like illness with headache. It can be mistaken for infectious mononucleosis with lassitude, fever, arthralgia, myalgia, and lymphadenopathy. Weight loss, nausea, and diarrhea are common. Rarely, presentation may be neurological (aseptic meningitis, Bell palsy, encephalitis, myelitis, polyneuritis, or Guillain–Barré syndrome).[3] Diagnosis is confirmed by a positive HIV polymerase chain

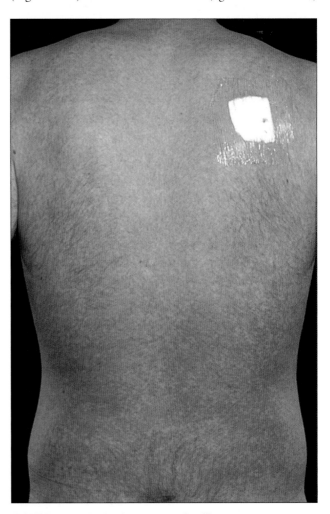

FIGURE 19.2: Rash of seroconversion illness.

TABLE 19.6: Cutaneous Manifestations of HIV Infection

Neoplasia	Kaposi sarcoma	B-cell lymphoma
	Non-Hodgkin lymphoma	Squamous cell carcinoma
	Anal carcinoma	
Infections	Herpes simplex (genital/oral/labial)	
	Herpes zoster (multidermatomal and disseminated)	
	Candidiasis (oral/vulvovaginal)	
	Tinea cruris/pedis	Scabies
	Tinea versicolor/rosea	Bacillary angiomatosis
	Chancroid	Molluscum contagiosum
	Lymphogranuloma venereum	Oral hairy leukoplakia
	Syphilis	Pyomyositis
	Cryptococcosis	Histoplasmosis
	Warts (oral/genital)	Mycobacterial infections
Other eruptions	Dry skin and scalp	Onychomycosis
	Ichthyosis, xeroderma	Aphthous ulcers
	Seborrheic dermatitis	Acne
	HIV-associated gingivitis	Psoriasis
	Papular pruritic eruption (Ofuji disease)	
	Fixed drug reactions	Hypersensitivity reactions
	Black nail discoloration (zidovudine)	
	In-growing toenails (indinavir)	
	Hair changes	Hyperpigmentation
	Fat redistribution syndrome	

erythema multiforme, and SJS may occur. There is often an associated hepatitis with transient derangement of liver transaminases and mild anemia. Skin biopsy is nonspecific.

An acute decrease in the CD4+ count at seroconversion coincides with a surge in plasma HIV RNA levels to more than 1 million copies/mL. The decrease in the CD4+ count may be sufficient to allow opportunistic infections to occur. Because of the exceedingly high HIV viral load at this time, the patient is highly infectious should he or she engage in sexual activity. It is estimated that one quarter of HIV transmission occurs during this time. Attempts to eradicate HIV from the blood at this early stage to reduce the risk of transmission as a public health problem have been unsuccessful.

The severity of the seroconversion illness is related to the subsequent speed of development of AIDS. Without treatment, the median time to develop AIDS is approximately 8 years. This asymptomatic phase is called the "latent period." Many patients will be unaware of their HIV status during this time and may unwittingly pass on their infection.

SPECIFIC SKIN CONDITIONS IN HIV INFECTION

Virtually all dermatological conditions are more common and more severe in HIV infection. Unusually florid skin infections, neoplasias, drug reactions, and other unusual eruptions form the bulk of dermatological manifestations (Table 19.6). Early HIV-associated diseases include xerosis with pruritus, seborrheic dermatitis, and an itchy folliculitic dermatitis that may be fungal (*Malassezia furfur*), staphylococcal, or eosinophilic in etiology.

Seborrheic Dermatitis

This condition is probably the most common skin manifestation of HIV, occurring in up to 80% of all patients (Figure 19.3). It may be widespread and severe, and is often worse in late-stage HIV disease. Red scaly patches typically affect the hair-bearing areas of the skin such as the nasolabial folds, scalp, and flexures. Treatment is that of the underlying condition using HAART. Topical Oilatum® (Steiffel, Miami, FL) and topical or systemic imidazoles can be helpful.

Oral–Esophageal Candidiosis (Thrush)

Oral candidosis is a frequent manifestation that, in the absence of prior antibiotics, steroids, or immunosuppressive therapy, should immediately alert the clinician to the possibility of HIV infection. Severe disease may involve the posterior pharynx and esophagus, leading to dysphagia

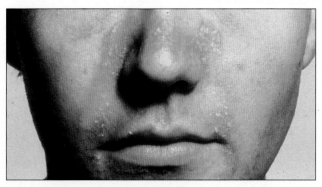

FIGURE 19.3: *Seborrheic dermatitis.*

and further weight loss. Less commonly, the patient may present with erythematous candidosis, which appears as a sore red smooth shiny tongue.

Candida albicans is normally sensitive to fluconazole (50 mg daily). In cases of nonresponse, antifungal drug sensitivity to imidazoles, caspofungin, and amphotericin should be requested from the microbiology reference lab. Endoscopy with biopsy should be performed to confirm the diagnosis and exclude the main differential diagnosis of cytomegalovirus (CMV) ulceration. Multiple copathologies with different types of pathogens are not uncommon in late-stage HIV and AIDS.

Oral Hairy Leukoplakia

Oral hairy leukoplakia is seen as adherent white plaques on the lateral margin of the tongue and is virtually pathognomonic of HIV infection. It is associated with EBV infection of the oral mucosa. It may be treated with acyclovir, although this is rarely indicated. Oral hairy leukoplakia and oral candidiosis in untreated patients predict progression to profound immune deficiency and development of AIDS within 1–2 years.

Molluscum Contagiosum

Molluscum contagiosum is an epidermal poxvirus infection that occurs in late-stage HIV disease. It is found in approximately 10% of AIDS patients. The lesions are usually 2- to 5-mm-diameter papules with a central umbilicus and tend to develop on the face, neck, and genitalia. The lesions usually disappear with treatment of the underlying HIV. Liquid nitrogen cryotherapy, topical retinoids, and cautery may be tried in cases of unsightly giant mollusca. The main differential diagnosis is disseminated cryptococcosis.

Herpes Simplex Virus Infections

Herpes simplex virus infection should be considered in any ulcerated or eroded lesion. These lesions can be painful, especially around the mouth and genitals. Recurrent, extensive, and troublesome herpes infections may occur in late-stage disease. Treatment is with high-dose acyclovir. Acyclovir resistance may develop, in which case cidofovir or foscarnet could be used as alternatives. An important differential is syphilis, which is more common in HIV. Syphilitic gumma produces painless lesions.

Varicella Zoster Virus

Shingles in an otherwise healthy person should act as an indicator for inquiry about risk factors for HIV infection. It can occur at any stage of the HIV natural history but is more frequent with failing immunity. In patients with a low CD4+ count (<100 cells/mm^3), the eruption may affect multiple dermatomes and is often florid. Persistent, recurrent, or disseminated varicella zoster disease may also occur.

Diagnosis is confirmed by viral culture, biopsy for characteristic inclusion bodies, or electron microscopy. Treatment is with high-dose (10 mg/kg tds) IV acyclovir. Specialist help should be sought in the management of ophthalmic shingles because of the risk of permanent loss of sight. The response to treatment and the risks of postherpetic neuralgia appear to be similar to those in the HIV-negative population.

Human Papillomavirus

Human papillomavirus infection is frequent among HIV-positive gay men. The disease may be extensive and difficult to manage. Lesions on the hands and feet (especially periungual) are also common and may attain considerable size, requiring surgery. Lesions usually improve on commencement of HAART. Human papillomavirus vaccination reduces the risk of infection and oncogenic transformation.[4]

Cryptococcosis

Cutaneous cryptococcosis is caused by *Cryptococcus neoformans* (the etiological agent of cryptococcal meningitis) and occurs in very-late-stage disease (CD4+ <50 cells/mm^3). It looks similar to molluscum. Serum cryptococcal antigen test is useful in the diagnosis. Treatment is with fluconazole.

Crusted Scabies

A severe variant of *Sarcoptes scabiei* infection producing a hyperkeratotic eruption (crusted scabies) may occur in advanced HIV. The infestation is often heavy, and patients are highly infectious. Uniquely in HIV infection, the face and neck can be affected. Paradoxically, the patient may not complain of severe itch. Treatment is with permethrin lotion. Ivermectin may also be of benefit, but the side effects should be weighed.

Psoriasis

Psoriasis is associated with severe flares in HIV infection, leading some to speculate on an infective etiology of this inflammatory condition. Treatment is with standard therapies. Treatment of the HIV will often improve the psoriasis.

Bacillary Angiomatosis

Bacillary angiomatosis is more common in HIV-infected individuals than are other bacterial infections such as syphilis and infections due to *Staphylococcus aureus* (folliculitis, cellulitis, and abscesses).

Bacillary angiomatosis is due to the cat-scratch bacillus *Bartonella henselae*. Lesions range from solitary superficial red–purple lesions resembling Kaposi sarcoma to multiple subcutaneous nodules or hyperpigmented plaques. Lesions are painful and bleed readily. Disseminated infection leads to fevers, lymphadenopathy, and hepatosplenomegaly. Diagnosis is with Warthin–Starry silver staining for aggregates of intracellular bacilli.

Eosinophilic Folliculitis

Eosinophilic folliculitis, also known as pustular pruritic eruption or Ofuji disease, is more common in persons of dark skin types and increases in frequency with advancement of immunosuppression. It is associated with a raised IgE and eosinophilia. The cause is not known. Itchy follicular papules and pustules affect the face, chest, and back. Treatments are often unsatisfactory but include topical steroids, phototherapy, and antihistamines.

Kaposi Sarcoma

Kaposi sarcoma is caused by human herpesvirus 8 (HHV-8), which is transmitted primarily through saliva. It is more common in men who have sex with men. The disease may be indolent or fulminant. Rapid clinical deterioration usually ensues with visceral involvement. It usually presents as painless purple macules, papules, nodules, and plaques affecting the limbs, face, and oral mucosa (especially the hard palate). The differential diagnosis includes bacillary angiomatosis and pyogenic granuloma. Prognosis depends on the CD4+ count. There is a wide range of therapies depending on the extent of the disease. The widespread use of HAART has resulted in a decline in the incidence of the disease. Combination therapy itself can result in regression of mucocutaneous lesions and even visceral disease and so is an important cornerstone of management.

ADVERSE DRUG REACTIONS

Adverse drug reactions are common in HIV and include both acute (e.g., abacavir HSR) and chronic (e.g., fat redistribution syndrome) reactions. Predictable reactions include drug side effects that occur in most patients who take a drug or combination of drugs. These are drug and dose dependent and not dependent on host factors. Other drug reactions previously thought to be idiosyncratic are now known to be genetically determined.

Nevirapine rash is a common side effect that begins within 2–4 weeks of starting this treatment. If severe, it may result in SJS. Recently, the human leukocyte antigen HLA-DRB1*01 has been found to be linked to rash associated with this class of drug.[5] Pharmacogenetic screening is now part of routine clinical practice in HIV medicine since the introduction of HLA compatibility testing prior to initiation of abacavir.

Abacavir Hypersensitivity Reaction

Abacavir (Ziagen) is a nucleoside analogue reverse transcriptase inhibitor licensed for the treatment of HIV. It is frequently used as a first-line drug because of its once-daily formulation and favorable lipid (fat redistribution syndrome) profile. It is an active component of coformulations Kivexa (with lamivudine) and TRIZIVIR (with lamivudine plus zidovudine). Abacavir HSR occurs in 5%–8% of patients during the 6 weeks of therapy, with a median onset of 11 days.[6,7] It usually presents with fever (80%) and rash (70%). Less common symptoms include nausea, vomiting, pruritus, malaise, diarrhea, abdominal pain, and fatigue. Numbness of the skin; puffiness of the throat, face, and neck; swollen glands; conjunctivitis; mouth ulcers; and low blood pressure may also occur.

Symptoms of the HSR to abacavir are nonspecific and may mimic influenza, the key difference being the presence of GI symptoms with abacavir. Symptoms worsen with continued use of the drug. Rapid reversal of symptoms occurs on discontinuation of abacavir.

An abacavir HSR may be life threatening; therefore, all patients prescribed this should be made familiar with the symptoms and should know to notify their doctor immediately if they develop any of these. More severe and even fatal reactions have been reported in patients rechallenged with abacavir after stopping the drug. Subsequent rechallenge with abacavir is therefore absolutely contraindicated.

Abacavir hypersensitivity is strongly associated with an HLA-B*5701 allele. Testing for the HLA B*5701 haplotype reduced the incidence of HSRs to zero in a randomized trial of nearly 2000 patients.[8] All patients should therefore be screened for this allele prior to commencing therapy.

The HLA B*5701 allele appears to be more common in white Caucasians and least common in black Africans infected with HIV (and in whom dermititis is often more difficult to distinguish). It is recommended that genetic testing should be routine for people of all ethnicities to reduce the instances of misdiagnosis of hypersensitivity in which abacavir is inappropriately withdrawn from patients who could have benefited from it.

Immune Restoration Inflammatory Syndrome

Immune restoration inflammatory syndrome (IRIS) is an adverse consequence of the restoration of pathogen-specific immune responses in HIV-infected patients during the initial months of HAART. The inflammatory syndrome reflects the restoration of a previously impotent immune system as it mounts an excessive response against organisms that were already present, but dormant, in the body.

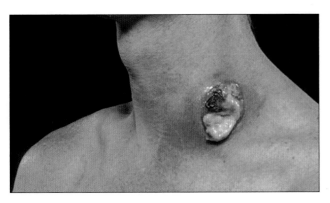

FIGURE 19.4: Suppurative mycobacterial adenopathy as an immune restoration inflammatory syndrome reaction following commencement of highly active antiretroviral therapy.

The immune restoration can have various manifestations, including lymph-node inflammation associated with *Mycobacterium avium-intracellulare* complex (Figure 19.4); eye inflammation (uveitis or vitritis) associated with CMV; worsening of tuberculosis, cryptococcosis, or toxoplasmosis symptoms; and elevated liver enzymes associated with hepatitis B or C co-infection.

The incidence of IRIS is greatest in patients with advanced immune suppression (CD4+ count <100 cells/mm^3) at the start of therapy. Immune restoration reactions are associated with larger viral load reductions (2.5 log or greater) or CD4+ cell increases after starting HAART. Starting an anti-HIV treatment with a combination that included a ritonavir-boosted protease inhibitor was also associated with an increased risk of IRIS.[9]

Because flare-ups indicate improvement of immune function following antiretroviral therapy, antiretroviral therapy is continued in all but the most serious cases. Even then it is usually only stopped temporarily until the patient's condition has stabilized. Antiinflammatory medications may help decrease symptoms during the intense inflammatory phase, but routine use of corticosteroid therapy is generally avoided. There have been anecdotal reports of successful management of reactions using pentoxifylline, thalidomide, and the asthma medication montelukast, but in most cases reactions resolve on their own without any additional treatment.

REFERENCES

1. Gottlieb MS, Schroff R, Schanker HM, et al. Pneumocystis carinii pneumonia and mucosal candidiasis in previously healthy homosexual men: evidence of a new acquired cellular immunodeficiency. N Engl J Med. 1981; 305:1425–31.
2. UNAIDS AIDS epidemic update, December 2007 [cited March 2008]. Available from: www.unaids.org.
3. Bunker CB, Staughton RCD. HIV-associated disease: dermatology. In: Gazzard BG, editor. AIDS Care Handbook. London: Mediscript, 2002.
4. Koutsky LA, Ault KA, Wheeler, CM, et al. A controlled trial of a human papillomavirus type 16 vaccine. N Engl J Med 2002; 347:1645–1.
5. Vitezica ZG, Milpied B, Lonjou C, et al. HLA-DRB1*01 associated with cutaneous hypersensitivity induced by nevirapine and efavirenz. AIDS 2008; 22:540–1.
6. Hetherigton S, McGuirk S, Powell G, et al. Hypersensitivity reactions during therapy with nucleoside reverse transcriptase inhibitor abacavir. Clin Ther 2001; 23:1603–14.
7. Hermandez JE, Cutrell A, Edwards M, et al. Clinical risk factors for hypersensitivity reactions to abacavir: restrospective analysis of over 8,000 subjects receiving abacavir in 34 clinical trials. In: Program and abstracts of the 43rd Interscience Conference on Antimicrobial Agents and Chemotherapy, Chicago, September 14–17, 2003. Washington DC: American Society for Microbiology, 2003:339. Abstract.
8. Mallal S, Phillips E, Carosi G, et al. HLA-B*5701 screeening for hypersensitivity to abacavir. N Engl J Med 2008; 358:568–79.
9. Manabe YC, Campbell JD, Sydnor E, Moore RD. Immune reconstitution inflammatory syndrome: risk factors and treatment implications. J Acquir Immune Defic Syndr 2007; 46:456–62.

CHAPTER 20

Graft Versus Host Disease

Jasna Lipozenčić

Ronni Wolf

THE SKIN is a major target organ for both acute and chronic graft versus host disease (GVHD) after stem cell transplantation (SCT). Although SCT is a life-saving measure and the treatment of choice for many patients with various hematologic malignancies, a high incidence of complications and a transplantation-associated mortality of approximately 30% are to be expected. GVHD is the major cause of morbidity and mortality at any time following SCT. The acute form occurs during the first 100 days after transplantation in up to 50% of graft recipients, whereas chronic GVHD develops in approximately 30%–50%, usually within 100–500 days following allogenic SCT. Target organs in GVHD can be all of those with lymphoid cells as well as epithelial structures, especially the skin, liver, gastrointestinal (GI) tract, lung, eyes, and neuromuscular system. Early diagnosis of GVHD can be difficult because drug reactions, viral infections, and cutaneous reactions to radiation therapy may have similar clinical and histological similarities. Histological findings of GVHD correlate poorly with clinical severity of the disease and have a limited role in predicting disease stage and progression.[1–4] The skin manifestations, histopathologic features, prophylaxis, and therapy of acute and chronic GVHD are presented in this chapter.

PATHOPHYSIOLOGY OF GVHD

GVHD is the result of a complex interaction of associative inflammation, endotoxicity, and activation of alloreactive cells. Cytotoxic donor T lymphocytes are mediators and effectors in GVHD. Proinflammatory cytokines in the cells of the donor and the recipient play an important role in the pathogenesis of GVHD. In acute GVHD, there are increased serum concentrations of tumor necrosis factor-α (TNF-α), interferon-γ (IFN-γ), interleukin 1 (IL-1), IL-2, and IL-6, but they are not specific for GVHD because bacterial infections show similar findings. The only correlation has been found between elevated IL-2 receptor (IL-2R) and severe GVHD.[5–7] Prophylactic administration of monoclonal anti–TNF-α antibodies in a patient with histocompatibility leukocyte antigen (HLA)-identical SCT in twins significantly alleviated acute GVHD.[8]

GVHD is in direct correlation with HLA incompatibility between donor and recipient.[9] Even in HLA-identical related SCT without prophylactic immunosuppression, GVHD occurs in 30%–50% of cases and has a severe course in 10%–20% of cases because of so-called HLA minor antigens.[10] HLA incompatibility between donors and patients increases the incidence of GVHD. The age of patients as well as difference in sex between donor and recipient are also risk factors, such as when there are two different HLA antigens and Y-chromosome–associated minor antigens.[4] In HLA-identical SCT, the incidence of GVHD is less than 25% in patients younger than 30 years with acute GVHD, but this number rises to 80% in patients older than 50 years.[11,12] The incidence of chronic GVHD is also higher in adults than in children.[4]

HLA incompatibility, age, and gender are not the only factors responsible for GVHD.[13–15] A three-phase model may explain the pathophysiology of GVHD. Phase I is "toxic" and lasts for approximately 60 days, whereas phase II begins with "lichenoid" symptoms before the 30th day and lasts until approximately the 100th day. Phase III starts near the 80th day and is characterized by "sclerodermiform" symptoms and cell infiltrate. There is interaction between different cell populations in both donor and recipient as well as between mediators of inflammation, and the result is cell death (apoptosis) in target organs of GVHD. Chronic GVHD often develops from acute GVHD through costimulation of cytokine production, and end-cell apoptosis through endotoxins is intensified. In this phase, there is hypersensitivity of macrophages through Th1-cytokine (INF-γ) stimulation. In acute GVHD, there is activation of Th1 cytokines with the production of proinflammatory mediators (TNF-α, IL-1), accompanied by organ-specific destruction and Th1 activation.

Risk factors for GVHD are genetic polymorphism in the promoter region of inflammatory (TNF-α) and anti-inflammatory (IL-10) cytokines. In chronic GVHD, there is the added risk factor of a former acute GVHD and the subsequent activation of Th2 cells and cytokine production. The chronicity of GVHD is due to alloreactive T cells having increased the production of IL-4 or IFN-γ, which induces collagen synthesis through fibroblasts.[4]

ACUTE GVHD

Acute GVHD begins 2–6 weeks after transplantation (median 3 weeks). In one study, GVHD took place after allogenic SCT in 35% of patients with HLA-identical donors, and the disease course was severe in 10%–20% of these cases (erythroderma, toxic epidermolysis). Acute GVHD is manifested on skin, liver, and the GI tract, as well as the lymphatic system, bone marrow, and the mucosa of the mouth and respiratory system. Development of "hyperacute" GVHD has been described as occurring 7–14 days after SCT.[11,12]

Skin Manifestations of Acute GVHD

The skin is the target organ of acute GVHD in more than 90% of cases. Early manifestations of acute GVHD include generalized pruritus, dysesthesia, painful palms of the hands and soles of the feet, or edema and erythema of the ears.[13] A maculopapular eruption first appears on the face, palms, and soles, followed by presentation on the shoulders and abdomen and then the whole body. These eruptions cannot be distinguished from a drug eruption or viral exanthema, either clinically or histologically. Exanthemas are variable and can be purpuric, follicular, morbilliform, or scarlatiniform. Perifollicular papular reactions indicate progression in a severe course, being characteristic of GVHD.[4]

Erythema on the palms, soles, and ears is typical in GVHD (Figure 20.1). Exanthemas with progression to erythroderma and blisters with a positive Nikolsky phenomenon are signs of a severe course. The most severe cases are those with bullous GVHD that include toxic epidermal skin and mucosal necrolysis and septicemia. Toxic epidermal necrolysis (TEN) has been reported in 6% of patients with a very high mortality. In this phase of GVHD, it is not easy to distinguish the epidermal necrolysis of SCT from that of drug-induced TEN. Hyperacute GVHD with TEN has been reported to begin 8 days after bone-marrow transplant.[14]

Mucosal reactions present as xerostomia, symptomatic of salivary gland dysfunction and pain upon eating as well as mucosal hypersensitivity. Mucosal reactions found in the mouth in acute GVHD can be fine papular white lesions, whitish lichenoid-reticular signs, or desquamative erosions.

In the progressive stage of acute GVHD, there are fingernail changes with periungual erythemas, hyperkeratosis, onycholysis, pigmentations, and hemorrhagia of the nail plates.

Extracutaneous Manifestations

The liver and the GI tract can be target organs after allogenic SCT. GI manifestations are present in 30%–50% of cases of acute GVHD.[15] They appear early or shortly after the skin manifestations and include diarrhea,

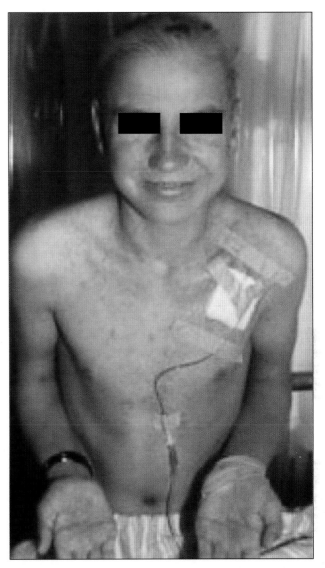

FIGURE 20.1: *Graft versus host disease, acute stage. There is erythema on the face and palms. (Photo courtesy of Ivan Dobrić, MD, PhD, Zagreb, Croatia.)*

vomiting, anorexia, malabsorption, abdominal pain, ileus, and colon hematuria, all of which are signs of a severe course. Liver disorders (bilirubin, alcal phosphatase, γ-glytamyltranspeptidase) with hepatomegaly are the second most prevalent manifestations after those of the skin, and are found in 40%–60% of cases.[15]

Clinical Stages of Acute GVHD

Acute GVHD severity has been graded by the pattern of organ involvement and clinical performance status, using a system introduced more than 30 years ago:[16] clinical stage and percentage of skin lesions, GI disorders, volume of diarrhea (mL/day), and value of bilirubin.[4,6,16] For example, stage I is characterized by a maculopapular exanthema (<25% body size), bilirubin 2–3 mg/dL, and diarrhea of 500–100 mL/day, whereas stage IV is characterized by bullous manifestations with TEN in the skin, bilirubin >15 mL/dL, and pain or ileus.[4,6,16,17] In acute GVHD, the "grade" survival is correlated with GVHD severity in grade (specifically, >90% survival in grade I, ~60% in grades II and III, and 0% in grade IV).

The International Bone Marrow Transplant Registry has adopted a new severity index for grading acute GVHD, based on objective parameters of target organs.[17] It has been proposed that the Severity Index enhances design and interpretation of clinical trials in the current era of allogeneic blood and bone-marrow transplantation.[17]

Histological Changes of Acute GVHD

Prophylaxis depends upon the degree of severity of acute GVHD and on histomorphologic changes resulting from GVHD. The dynamism of GVHD makes the histologic picture unstable, and it characteristically changes during the course of illness due to its being influenced by many other factors. Histological findings of the skin in early acute GVHD show focal basal cell degeneration of the epidermis and sometimes sparse perivascular lymphocytic infiltration in the upper dermis. In the late acute phase, there is a hypersensitivity reaction and activation of endothelial cells as well as penetration of T cells into the papillary dermis. The clinical signs include cytotoxic folliculitis and "satellite necrosis" because of the presence of T cells in the papillary dermis, lymphocytes in the epidermis, and hair follicles as well as necrosis of keratinocytes/apoptosis or necrosis.[4]

Histopathologic changes in acute GVHD have been described as grade I (vacuolization of basal cells of inflamed lymphocyte infiltrate in the upper dermis or epidermis), grade II (dyskeratosis of some keratinocytes, exocytosis of lymphocytes around necrotic keratinocytes in the epidermis ["satellite phenomenon"]), grade III (the beginning of late signs in the basal membrane zone with sparse necrosis in the epidermis), and grade IV (complete depletion of necrotic epidermis) (Figure 20.2).[4]

These histopathologic changes are not specific to GVHD, and similar ones can be found in viral exanthems, in drug eruptions, and post-chemotherapy. This is the reason for the need for optimal timing for skin biopsies: 24–48 hours after exanthema, before administering GVHD therapy, repeated biopsies in the early phase of acute GVHD, with paraffin block serial slices for focal GVHD with mostly follicular involvement.[15]

Differential Diagnosis

The clinical manifestations of viral exanthema and drug eruption are similar to dermal manifestations in the initial phase of GVHD. Bullous changes take place after total beam radiotherapy, accompanied by palmoplantar pain and stomatitis, some weeks later. Thus, it is imperative that the diagnosis is clear-cut, that clinical examinations are

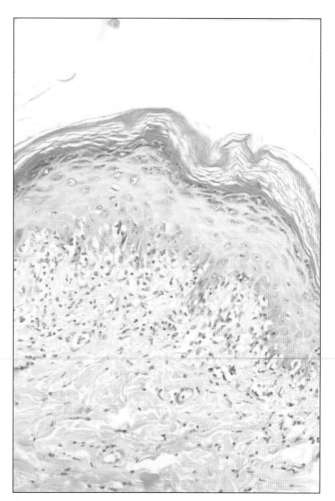

FIGURE 20.2: *Graft versus host disease, acute stage, stage II. Histological feature: rare subepidermal infiltrate of lymphocytes (with rare lymphocytes in lower epidermis), hydrops degeneration of basal layer of epidermis, and "satellite" cell necrosis. Hematoxylin and eosin, × 240. (Photo courtesy of Ivan Dobrić, MD, PhD, Zagreb, Croatia.)*

repeated, that biopsies are taken, and that microbiological findings are available. Increased values of liver enzymes or GI disorders can appear concomitantly with acute GVHD. Another cause for consideration are the side effects of immunosuppressive therapy.

Physicians need to recognize atypical early skin involvement in acute GVHD in patients after SCT so that they can promptly initiate appropriate treatment.[18] There is a suggestion of an association between acquired ichthyosis with GVHD.[19] Epidermodysplasia verruciformis in the setting of GVHD after SCT has also been described.[20]

Prognosis of Acute GVHD

The morbidity and mortality rates that determine prognosis in progressive acute GVHD are high after SCT. Whereas prognosis is good in cases of isolated skin GVHD or GVHD grade II when response to the first course of therapy is positive, it is grave in patients with refractory or severe GVHD. Even patients with GVHD grades II–IV have a low mortality rate if they react to initial therapy with complete remission. Fewer than 50% of patients with acute grades II–IV GVHD have long-term survival, so early diagnosis and therapy are essential. The most prevalent causes of death are infections, bleeding, and suppression of liver function.

CHRONIC GVHD

Chronic GVHD (100–500 days after SCT) is a multisystem disease, and between 30% and 50% of allogeneic transplantation patients develop it. The major risk factor for chronic GVHD is acute GVHD. Chronic GVHD can be either subclinical or clinical and either limited or extensive. Skin changes are local in 20% of cases and generalized in 80%. They can be progressive (32%) following acute GVHD as well as "de novo" (30%). Chronic GVHD can appear after ultraviolet radiation, trauma, or herpes zoster.[4]

Skin Manifestation of Chronic GVHD

Skin is the most frequently targeted organ in chronic GVHD.[4,13,15] The initial changes that take place, together with other early manifestations of chronic GVHD, include persistent face erythema with marked pigmentation, mouth dryness, and sensitivity to spicy food that can be associated with oral pain. Because skin changes can appear rapidly after sun exposure, sunscreens are vital for these patients. One fifth of them have a localized skin form of GVHD and rarely exhibit liver symptoms. The dermal expression is mostly lichen ruber planus (LRP), lichen sclerosus et atrophicus, or skin lesions linear to or along Blaschko lines; circumscript scleroderma is rare (3%). Generalized forms seen in disseminated GVHD are erythema, desquamation, telangiectasia, and pigmentation disorder. There are two chronic disseminated GVHD forms: lichenoid and sclerodermiform. The former is similar to LRP and characterized by livid-brown papules on the extremities (Figure 20.3). They are often present periorbitally, on the ears, hands, and soles, and lichenoid papular lesions are sometimes localized at the hair follicles. Generalized skin lesions and erythroderma are rare. Postinflammatory hyperpigmentation may appear after regression of the lesions, whereas hypopigmentation is uncommon. Pityriasis rosacea-like lesions in GVHD with rapid regression have been described as well.[4]

In addition to LRP, mucosal mouth lesions in chronic GVHD include Wickham striae, erosions, ulcerations or leukoplakia, painful erosions, and xerophthalmia similar to that found in sicca syndrome. Nail disturbances are seen in approximately 40% of patients, and they range from onycholysis, pterygium, and atrophy to total nail loss.

Sweat glands often show a disturbance of function until dehydration. Other changes include pigment loss in hair,

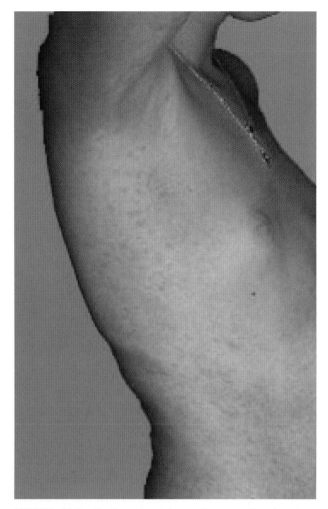

FIGURE 20.3: Graft versus host disease, chronic stage, lichenoid form. Papulous exanthema on the trunk. (Photo courtesy of Ivan Dobrić, MD, PhD, Zagreb, Croatia.)

cicatricial alopecia, poikiloderma with alopecia in sclerodermiform form, as well as vitiligo.

Sclerodermiform GVHD is a severe sequela of chronic GVHD that often occurs before LRP GVHD (Figure 20.4). It is a type of sclerosis of the dermis with localized morphea and generalized skin lesions that include contractures and ulcers with possible superinfections. This form is associated with HLA-A1-B1 and B2. Fasciitis is rare in chronic GVHD, as are eosinophilic fasciitis and cellulitis.[4]

Extracutaneous manifestations in chronic GVHD represent severe multisystem disease with involvement of the liver (30%), GI tract (diarrhea ~30%), lung (dyspnea, bronchitis), eyes (conjunctivitis, keratitis), and the neuromuscular system. Glomerulonephritis and arthritis are uncommon.

Clinical Stages of Chronic GVHD

Chronic GVHD can start subclinically (~30%) or display clinical symptoms (70%) that are either localized (20%)

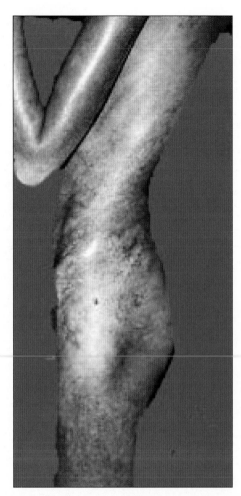

FIGURE 20.4: *Graft versus host disease, chronic stage, scleroderma form. Induration and hyperpigmentation of the skin. (Photo courtesy of Ivan Dobrić, MD, PhD, Zagreb, Croatia.)*

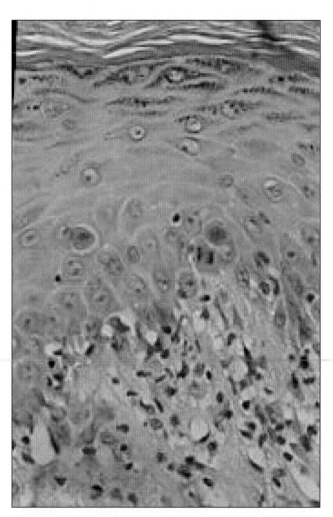

FIGURE 20.5: *Graft versus host disease, chronic stage lichenoid form. Histological feature: hypergranulosis and rare subepidermal bordered infiltrate of lymphocytes. Hematoxylin and eosin, ×200. (Photo courtesy of Ivan Dobrić, MD, PhD, Zagreb, Croatia.)*

or generalized (80%).[4] The traditional clinical grading system[11,12] is divided into three categories: subclinical grade I without evidence of GVHD but with positive histological findings; clinical grade II with limited disorders and localized skin lesion and liver dysfunction; and clinical grade III with extensive skin lesions, liver dysfunction, and hair loss accompanied by histological evidence of aggressive hepatitis, necrotic lesions, and cirrhosis in addition to other organ involvement, such as the eyes, oral mucosa, colon, and lung.[4,11,12]

Histological Changes in Chronic GVHD

As in acute GVHD, there are four histological forms:[4] 1) acanthosis, parakeratosis, hyperkeratosis, and hypergranulosis of the epidermis; 2) lichenoid GVHD with lichenoid infiltrate and melanophages, eosinophils, and plasma cells in the papillary dermis (Figure 20.5); 3) sclerodermiform GVHD with homogenous and swollen bundles of collagen and loss of appendages (Figure 20.6); and 4) atrophy of the epidermis (late phase). The lupus band test is positive in 86% of biopsies in chronic GVHD. There are no specific histologic parameters to differentiate between acute and chronic GVHD.

Differential Diagnosis

Differential diagnosis of chronic GVHD includes circumscribed and systemic scleroderma, lichenoid drug eruption, lupus erythematosus, pityriasis rosea, eosinophil fasciitis, Sjögren syndrome, rheumatoid arthritis, and primary biliary cirrhosis.

Prognosis of Chronic GVHD

Prognosis is more favorable, if the disease is limited to skin or liver involvement. In cases of more extensive disease in which multiple organs are affected and there is inadequate response to therapy, 80% of the patients will die. The prognosis of sclerodermiform GVHD is grave. Morbidity and mortality are highest in patients whose disease process had

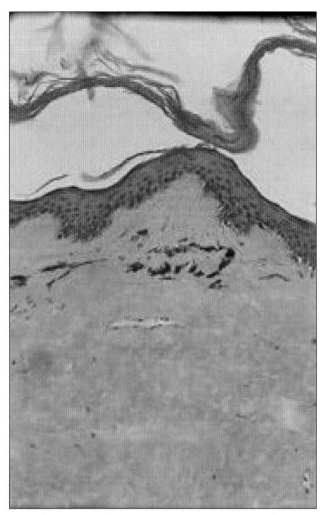

FIGURE 20.6: *Graft versus host disease, chronic stage, sclero-derma form. Histological feature: acellular dermis with swollen bundles of collagen and loss of structure in the interfascicular space and subepidermal melanophages. (Photo courtesy of Ivan Dobrić, MD, PhD, Zagreb, Croatia.)*

begun with acute GVHD and lowest in patients who had not undergone acute GVHD previously. The most prevalent causes of death are bacterial and viral infections.

PROPHYLAXIS AND THERAPY FOR GVHD

The most important factor in primary prophylaxis is choice of donors and histocompatibility. Drug prophylaxis is also essential.

Acute GVHD

Basic prophylaxis begins on the day of transplantation. It is initially intravenous and is followed by 6 months of oral cyclosporine A (CSA) in combination with methotrexate (MTX) or systemic corticosteroids instead of MTX. Tacrolimus is currently preferred over cyclosporine and some studies favor mycophenolate mofetil over MTX.[4] In vitro physical separation of immunocompetent T cells or

antilymphocyte or antithymocyte serum, as in vivo T-cell reducers, is used as well. Basic prophylaxis can decrease the incidence of acute GVHD but not of chronic GVHD. The therapeutic regimen for corticosteroid-resistant cases consists of cyclophosphamide, antithymocyte globulin, antilymphocyte globulin, pentostatin or monoclonal antibody against T lymphocytes or against immunosystem mediators (IL-2R, TNF-α).[4] The addition of other immunosuppressive therapeutic agents in GVHD comprises a risk for infections (fungal, viral) as well as associated Epstein–Barr virus lymphomas. Supportive therapy is fundamental for acute and chronic GVHD infections.[4]

Chronic GVHD

Skin lesions are the first manifestations in 90% of GVHD cases, but all target organs must be evaluated before therapy is administered. CSA and corticosteroids comprise the initial therapy. When an alternative therapy is needed due to resistance, mycophenolate mofetil with tacrolimus is one option, having shown a good effect in 50% of patients with drug-resistant chronic GVHD. In isolated skin GVHD, photochemotherapy with 8-methoxypsoralen is effective as is D-penicillamine and azathioprine as well as high-dose thalidomide. Acitretin and clofazimine can be given for sclerodermiform GVHD resistant to etretinate. Extracorporal photopheresis is also effective and has fewer side effects. Ultraviolet B phototherapy is considered adjuvant therapy in chronic GVHD.[4] Causal therapy is not yet available. Known side effects of therapy associated with immunosuppression involve the kidney and lead to liver and bone-marrow impairment as well as to tumors. The use of sunscreens is an important supplement to medication. Therapy for GVHD patients should be in the hands of hematologists and dermatologists.

MANAGEMENT OF GVHD

The influence of nonmyeloablative and ablative conditioning regimens on the occurrence of acute and chronic GVHD was recently evaluated in 137 patients.[21] Myeloablative regimens included intravenous bisulfan/cyclophosphamide ($n = 45$) and fludarabine/melphalan ($n = 29$). The nonmyeloablative group ($n = 63$) received fludarabine/idarubicin/cytarabine, cisplatin/fludarabine/idarubicin, and fludarabine/cyclophosphamide. The actuarial rate of grades II–IV acute GVHD was significantly higher in patients receiving ablative regimens (36%) compared with the nonmyeloablative group (12%). The cumulative incidence of chronic GVHD was higher in the ablative group (40%) compared with the nonmyeloablative group (14%).[21] The time of onset of GVHD and survival rate were analyzed in 395 patients with hematologic malignancies who underwent a nonmyeloablative regimen of 2 Gy total-body irradiation with or without fludarabine followed by postgrafting immunosuppression with mycophenolate mofetil and CSA. The cumulative incidences of grades II–IV acute GVHD and extensive chronic GVHD were 45% and 47%, respectively. High-dose corticosteroid treatment for acute or chronic GVHD was started at a median of 79 days and 30 days after transplantation, respectively.[22] When the donors were related, the cumulative incidence of nonrelapse mortality among patients with GVHD was 55% at 4 years when prednisone was started before day 50. The authors concluded that patients with early-onset GVHD after nonmyeloablative SCT from HLA-identical related donors might benefit from intensified primary immunosuppressive treatment.[22] The decision to treat immediately for GVHD without performing a skin biopsy provided the best patient outcomes.[23] When the prevalence of GVHD was 50% or higher (typical for allogeneic SCT), the best outcomes were obtained with treatment for GVHD and no skin biopsy. In populations with a prevalence of GVHD of 30% or less, obtaining a skin biopsy specimen to guide treatment was predicted to provide the best patient outcome.[23] The findings of a recent report showed that a better therapeutic approach would be to reduce the extent of immunosuppression and allow the patient's immune system the opportunity to reject the allograft donor T cells. The patients who responded to withdrawal of immunosuppression had a later onset of symptoms and a lower level of donor CD3+ T cells at the start of treatment.[24] Other investigators suggested that the patients with "composite" skin GVHD may benefit from an earlier, more aggressive immunosuppressive interventional strategy.[25] Imatinib showed a major impact on chronic myeloid leukemia treatment strategies. Indeed, GVHD involving the skin, liver, and digestive tract has been described in the syngeneic transplant setting, either with or without administration of prophylactic CSA: Complete remission was achieved with imatinib.[26]

CONCLUSIONS

GVHD is a devastating complication following SCT, and the prevention of GVHD should be the highest priority. Management of these patients should be multidisciplinary and involve hematologists and dermatologists. There are no known preventative measures for the causes of GVHD nor means of avoiding the side effects of immunosuppression that are often present in affected patients. Management is determined according to the stage of GVHD, and early diagnosis is of the essence.

ACKNOWLEDGMENT

Professor Ivan Dobrić, MD, PhD, Chief of the Dermatohistopathological Laboratory of the University Department of Dermatology and Venereology, School of Medicine and University Hospital Center, Zagreb, Croatia, provided the original figures of GVHD from his private collection.

REFERENCES

1. Kohler S, Hendrickson MR, Chao NJ, Smoller BR. Value of skin biopsies in assessing prognosis and progression of acute graft-versus-host disease. Am J Surg Pathol. 1997; 21:988–96.
2. Zhou Y, Barnett MJ, Rivers JK. Clinical significance of skin biopsies in the diagnosis and management of graft-vs-host disease in early postallogeneic bone marrow transplantation. Arch Dermatol. 2000; 136:717–21.
3. Vargas-Díez E, Fernández-Herrera J, Marin A, et al. Analysis of risk factors for acute cutaneous graft-versus-host disease after allogeneic stem cell transplantation. Br J Dermatol. 2003; 148:1129–34.
4. Karrer S. Cutaneous graft-versus-host disease. Hautarzt. 2003; 54:465–80; quiz 481–2.
5. Ferrara JL, Deeg HJ. Graft-versus-host disease. N Engl J Med. 1991; 324:667–74.
6. Thomas ED, Storb R, Clift RA, et al. Bone-marrow transplantation. N Engl J Med. 1975; 292:895–902.
7. Grimm J, Zeller W, Zander AR. Soluble interleukin-2 receptor serum levels after allogeneic bone marrow transplantations as a marker for GvHD. Bone Marrow Transplant. 1998; 21:29–32.
8. Holler E, Kolb HJ, Eissner G, Wilmanns W. Cytokines in GvH and GvL. Bone Marrow Transplant. 1998; 22:S3–S6.
9. Klingebiel T, Schlegel PG. GVHD: overview on pathophysiology, incidence, clinical and biological features. Bone Marrow Transplant. 1998; 21:S45–S49.
10. Goulmy E, Schipper R, Pool J, et al. Mismatches of minor histocompatibility antigens between HLA-identical donors and recipients and the development of graft-versus-host disease after bone marrow transplantation. N Engl J Med. 1996; 334:281–5.
11. Sullivan KM. Graft-versus-host disease. In: Thomas ED, Blume KG, Jorman SJ, editors. Hematopoietic cell transplantation. 2nd ed. Malden (MA): Blackwell Science Inc.; 1999. pp. 515–36.
12. Sullivan KM, Deeg HJ, Sanders J, et al. Hyperacute graft-versus-host disease in patients not given immunosuppression after allogeneic bone marrow transplantation. Blood. 1986; 67:1172–5.
13. Volc-Platzer B. Graft-versus-host disease. Hautarzt. 1992; 43:669–77.
14. Takeda H, Mitsuhashi Y, Kondo S, et al. Toxic epidermal necrolysis possibly linked to hyperacute graft-versus-host disease. J Dermatol. 1997; 24:635–41.
15. Heymer B. Clinical and diagnostic pathology of graft-versus-host disease. Berlin: Springer; 2002.
16. Glucksberg H, Storb R, Ferer A, et al. Clinical manifestations of graft-versus-host disease in human recipients of marrow from HLA-matched sibling donors. Transplantation. 1974; 18:295–304.
17. Rowlings PA, Przepiorka D, Klein JP, et al. IBMTR severity index for grading acute graft-versus-host disease: retrospective comparison with Glucksberg grade. Br J Haematol. 1997; 97:855–64.

18. Kuskonmaz B, Güçer S, Boztepe G, et al. Atypical skin graft-vs-host disease following bone marrow transplantation in an infant. Pediatr Transplant. 2007; 11:214–16.

19. Huang J, Pol-Rodriguez M, Silvers D, Garzon MC. Acquired ichthyosis as a manifestation of acute cutaneous graft-versus-host disease. Pediatr Dermatol. 2007; 24:49–52.

20. Kunishige JH, Hymes SR, Madkan V, et al. Epidermodysplasia verruciformis in the setting of graft-versus-host disease. J Am Acad Dermatol. 2007; 57:S78–S80.

21. Couriel DR, Saliba RM, Giralt S, et al. Acute and chronic graft-versus-host disease after ablative and nonmyeloablative conditioning for allogeneic hematopoietic transplantation. Biol Blood Marrow Transplant. 2004; 10:178–85.

22. Mielcarek M, Burroughs L, Leisenring W, et al. Prognostic relevance of 'early-onset' graft-versus-host disease following non-myeloablative haematopoietic cell transplantation. Br J Haematol. 2005; 129:381–91.

23. Firoz BF, Lee SJ, Nghiem P, Qureshi AA. Role of skin biopsy to confirm suspected acute graft-vs-host disease: results of decision analysis. Arch Dermatol. 2006; 142:175–82.

24. Chinnakotla S, Smith DM, Domiati-Saad R, et al. Acute graft-versus-host disease after liver transplantation: role of withdrawal of immunosuppression in therapeutic management. Liver Transpl. 2007; 13:157–61.

25. Bridge AT, Nelson RP, Schwartz JE, et al. Histological evaluation of acute mucocutaneous graft-versus-host disease in nonmyeloablative hematologic stem cell transplants with an observation predicting an increased risk of progression to chronic graft-versus-host disease. Am J Dermatopathol. 2007; 29:1–6.

26. Pelosini M, Galimberti S, Benedetti E, et al. Skin and stomach graft versus host disease after syngeneic BMT in CML: a case report. Leuk Res. 2007; 31:1603–4.

CHAPTER 21

Erythroderma/Exfoliative Dermatitis

Virendra N. Sehgal
Govind Srivastava

AN EXTREME STATE of skin irritation resulting in extensive erythema and/or scaling of the body in several skin disorders may ultimately culminate in erythroderma/exfoliative dermatitis. Largely, it is a secondary process; therefore, determining its cause is needed to facilitate precise management.[1] Its clinical pattern is fascinating and has been the subject of detailed studies: Its changing scenario in various age groups,[2–4] its presentation postoperatively, and its occurrence in human immunodeficiency virus (HIV)-positive individuals are vivid indicators. Several factors may be responsible for the causation of this extensive skin disorder. A detailed outline of a patient's history to elicit possible triggering events, namely, infection, drug ingestion, topical application of medicaments, and sun/ultraviolet light exposure, among other factors. It is also challenging to manage the condition, because the intricate process puts an extensive strain on an already compromised body system.[1,2,5,6] In addition, the original dermatosis may be masked by extensive erythema/scaling, thus making it difficult to obtain a clear-cut diagnosis. Its intriguing clinical expression in neonates/infants and children poses a serious emergent challenge for its life-threatening overture.[7,8]

DEFINITION

Erythroderma and exfoliative dermatitis are largely synonymous; however, erythroderma is the preferred term[1,9,10] and is currently in vogue. The former is characterized by extensive and pronounced erythema, coupled with perceptible scaling, whereas the latter is conspicuous by the presence of widespread erythema and marked scaling. Accordingly, 90% or more skin-surface involvement is considered as a salient prerequisite to make a clinical diagnosis of exfoliative dermatitis.[1,11] Some disorders in infants may initially be localized and then eventually develop into extensive erythema.[12]

INCIDENCE

It is hard to obtain a precise incidence for erythroderma/exfoliative dermatitis, as most reports are retrospective and do not address the issue of overall incidence. In surveys from India and The Netherlands, the annual incidence was recorded as variable at 35–0.9 per 100,000 skin patients.[1,13] A study based on an analysis of 138 consecutive erythroderma patients from South Africa found that 75% were black, 22.5% Indian, and 2.5% white.[6] A large number of patients were HIV positive, where a drug reaction was the most common cause, and men were affected 2–3 times more frequently.

The incidence as a function of age is usually variable, and any age group may be affected; however, affected (excluding hereditary disorders/atopic dermatitis) patients are usually older than 45 years,[1] with an average age of onset of 55 years. Erythroderma is a rather uncommon situation in the pediatric age group. A sample of 80 patients with erythroderma contained only 7 of the pediatric age group, of which only 3 belonged to 0–3 years and the other 4 to 4–13 years, equating to an incidence of 8.8%.[1,14,15] Male-to-female ratio was approximately equal, whereas age at onset varied according to its etiology. In a significant study comprising neonatal and infantile (up to 1 year) erythroderma, the composition was 30% in an immunodeficiency state, 24% in ichthyosis, 18% in Netherton syndrome, 20% had papulosquamous/eczematous dermatoses, and a further 8% were idiopathic.[16]

ETIOLOGY

Erythroderma/generalized exfoliative dermatitis possesses a wide spectrum of etiology, in both the pediatric and adult population (Tables 21.1 and 21.2a, b).

Erythroderma/exfoliative dermatitis may embrace or be caused by certain preexisting dermatosis, drug-induced malignancy, and miscellaneous/idiopathic disorders.[1,12]

Preexisting Dermatoses

Several dermatologic disorders or their therapy can result in exfoliative dermatitis (Tables 21.1 and 21.2a). This is the single most common cause of adult/pediatric exfoliative dermatitis in the majority of studies.[1,4,13,17–20] Psoriasis is the most common cause of exfoliative dermatitis among adults.[1,13] The causative disorders can be masked due to generalized erythema and/or scaling and have to be

TABLE 21.1: Erythroderma/Exfoliative Dermatitis in Children – Etiology

Cause(s)	Disease(s)/Syndrome(s)
Immunologic disorders	Omenn syndrome Graft versus host disease Cutaneous T-cell lymphoma Hypogammaglobulinemia DiGeorge syndrome
Metabolic/nutrition disorders	Kwashiorkor Renal failure Acrodermatitis enteropathica Cystic fibrosis dermatitis Leiner disease
Infections	Amino acid disorders Staphylococcal scalded skin syndrome Scarlet fever Neonatal candidiasis Toxic shock syndrome
Toxicities/drug reactions	Boric acid toxicity Drug-induced erythroderma/exfoliative dermatitis
Part component of various syndrome(s)	Netherton syndrome Sjögren–Larsson syndrome Keratitis–ichthyosis–deafness syndrome Ectodermal dysplasias Neutral lipid storage disease with ichthyosis Conradi–Hünermann syndrome Trichothiodystrophy
Cutaneous disorders	Atopic dermatitis Psoriasis vulgaris Ichthyosis–harlequin, lamellar, bullous Diffuse cutaneous mastocytosis Toxic epidermal necrolysis Pityriasis rubra pilaris Seborrheic dermatitis Crusted scabies

Data adapted from Sehgal VN, Srivastava G, Sardana K. Erythroderma/exfoliative dermatitis – a synopsis. Int J Dermatol. 2004; 43:39–47.

carefully looked.[21,22] In young children, the dermatoses form the main cause of erythroderma.

Drugs

Topical and systemic medications are notorious for precipitating erythroderma/exfoliative dermatitis. An apparent increase in the drug-induced instances may be directly proportional to the introduction of new drugs.[1,14,23–27] Apart from the well-known allopathic medicines, homeopathic, Unani, Ayurvedic, herbal, and common home remedies have been incriminated.[1,15] Many drug eruptions that commonly present as morbilliform, lichenoid, or urticarial forms may often progress to extensive erythema and exfoliation. The inventory of drugs causing erythroderma/exfoliative dermatitis is increasing; however, the most common are shown in Table 21.2b. Drug-induced erythroderma due to dapsone/antileprosy drug hypersen-

TABLE 21.2a: Dermatoses Frequently Resulting in Exfoliative Dermatitis in Adults

Common	Uncommon
Psoriasis	Candidiosis
Airborne contact dermatitis	Dermatophytosis
Seborrheic dermatitis	Mastocytosis
Atopic dermatitis	Lichen planus
Staphylococcal scalded skin syndrome	Reiter syndrome
	Toxic epidermal necrolysis
Phytophotodermatitis	Diffuse/erythrodermic mastocytosis
Photosensitive dermatitis	Sarcoidosis
Pityriasis rubra pilaris	Pemphigoid
Pemphigus foliaceus	Lupus erythematosus
Stasis dermatitis	Crusted (Norwegian) scabies
Ichthyosiform erythroderma	

Data adapted from Sehgal VN, Srivastava G, Sardana K. Erythroderma/exfoliative dermatitis – a synopsis. Int J Dermatol. 2004; 43:39–47.

sitivity may often mimic cutaneous T-cell lymphoma in terms of both clinical features and histopathology. Fortunately, it resolves after withdrawal of the offending drug(s) and the administration of supportive therapy.

Malignancies

One of the clinical expressions of reticuloendothelial neoplasms and internal blood vessel malignancies may be erythroderma. The latter invariably affect older individuals, and erythema/exfoliative dermatitis is considered to be a salient cutaneous marker of internal malignancy. Lymphomas in general and T-cell lymphoma (comprising mycosis fungoides and Sezary syndrome

TABLE 21.2b: Common Drugs Causing Exfoliative Dermatitis in Adults

Acetaminophen	Minocycline
Actinomycin-D	Nitrofurantoin
Allopurinol	Omeprazole
Arsenic	Para-amino salicylic acid
Barbiturates	Penicillin
Captopril	Phenothiazine
Chloroquine diphosphate	Phenytoin
Chlorpromazine	Quinidine
Cimetidine	Rifampicin
Dapsone	Streptomycin
Gold	Sulfadiazine
Hydantoin sodium	Sulfonylurea
Interferon	Tetracycline
Isoniazid/isonicotinic hydrazide	Thalidomide
Isotretinoin	Tolbutamide
Lithium	Vancomycin
Mercurials	

Data adapted from Sehgal VN, Srivastava G, Sardana K. Erythroderma/exfoliative dermatitis – a synopsis. Int J Dermatol. 2004; 43:39–47.

[its leukemia variant, in particular]) are often reported to present as exfoliative dermatitis. In adults they constitute more than 25%–40% of cases of malignancy-related erythrodermas.[4,13,14,28–31] Exfoliative dermatitis may precede, accompany, or follow T-cell lymphomas, and its appearance may be identical to that of benign erythroderma. An immunophenotypic study with the use of advanced antibody panels may be required to distinguish it from the benign form.[32] Reticular cell sarcoma, acute and chronic leukemia, and malignant histiocytosis are a few other implicated conditions. Carcinoma of the colon, lung, prostate, thyroid, fallopian tubes, larynx, and esophagus have also been alleged to cause the condition. An insidious, debilitating, progressive course, absence of a history of a previous skin disorder, and recalcitrant nature may warrant an exploration of the possibility of an underlying malignancy.[1,15,33–35]

Miscellaneous/Idiopathic Disorders

Hepatitis, irradiation, acquired immune deficiency syndrome (AIDS), graft versus host disease (GVHD), Ofuji papuloerythroderma, Omenn syndrome, and several cutaneous disorders can also cause the condition from infancy to old age.[1,15,36–38] Other cutaneous disorders causing erythroderma are discussed in the "Clinical Features/Connotation" section. Despite the best endeavors, a small proportion of patients remain in whom no clear-cut etiology can be defined; their disorders are classified as idiopathic. A sustained effort during the course of follow-up may lead to the precise definition of the etiology.[1,15]

PATHOGENESIS

The pathogenesis of the erythroderma/exfoliative dermatitis appears complex. It is surmised that the condition develops secondary to an intricate interaction of cytokines and cellular adhesion molecules; interleukin 1, 2, and 8; intercellular adhesion molecule 1; and the tumor necrotic factor.[39] These interactions result in a dramatic increase in the epidermal turnover rate, accelerated mitotic rate, and an increased absolute number of the germinative skin cells. The time required for cells to mature and travel through the epidermis is decreased and is manifested as an increased loss of epidermal material, together with a significant loss of protein and folate.[40] In contrast, the exfoliation of normal epidermis is much less and contains very little important viable material, such as nucleic acids, soluble proteins, or amino acids. Abel and colleagues[41] studied the immunophenotypic characteristics of benign (psoriasis, dermatitis, drug induced) and malignant (Sezary syndrome, mycosis fungoides) forms of erythroderma, and found them to be similar. In immunohistochemical studies,[42] the dermal infiltrate in patients with Sezary syndrome mainly showed a T-helper-2 cytokine profile, whereas benign reactive erythroderma showed a T-helper-1 cytokine profile, indicating that, although clinically similar, they have different underlying pathogenic mechanisms. In addition to these basic alterations, all earlier mentioned disorders have their own specific pathogenesis.

CLINICAL PRESENTATION/CONNOTATION

Exfoliative dermatitis starts as patch(es) of erythema accompanied by pruritus. The patch(es) enlarge and coalesce to form extensive areas of erythema, which eventually spread to cover all or most of the skin surface. Exfoliative dermatitis is also associated with profuse scaling, which has its onset 2–6 days after erythema with individual variations. The acute form is heralded by the formation of large scales, whereas the chronic form is recognized by small scales. The skin is conspicuously bright red, dry, scaly, hot, and indurated. Mild to severe pruritus is usually present. In addition, the nails become thick, lusterless, dry, brittle, and show ridging of the nail plate. Periorbital skin inflammation and edema cause ectropion and epiphora. Lymphadenopathy, hepatosplenomegaly, edema of the feet/ankles, and gynecomastia may also be observed. The basal metabolic rate is increased, and a catabolic state causes significant weight loss over time. At times, patients can slip into an irreversible hypothermia or hyperthermia. The former may result in ventricular bradycardia and hypotension. An increased peripheral blood flow may result in high-output cardiac failure. All body systems may be affected by these manifestations. The general picture is modified according to the nature of the underlying disorder.[1,15]

Cutaneous Disorder

Atopic Dermatitis. This condition is a well-conceived clinical cutaneous expression of atopy. It is a pruritic, eczematous dermatosis, the clinical manifestations of which chronically fluctuate with remissions and relapses. (Figure 21.1)

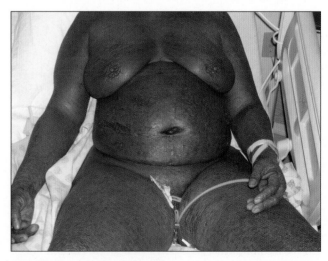

FIGURE 21.1: *Atopic dermatitis.*

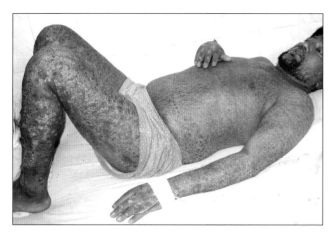

FIGURE 21.2: *Erythroderma/exfoliative dermatitis: psoriatic erythroderma.*

Most individuals with atopic dermatitis have an atopic diathesis identified through personal or family history of asthma, allergic rhinitis, and/or conjunctivitis and atopic dermatitis and/or predisposition to overproduction of immunoglobulin E (IgE) antibodies. Infants and children are most commonly affected. Erythema, exudation, papules, vesiculopapules, scales, and crust are its salient acute lesions. It may transform itself into erythroderma. Despite being widespread, the child is apparently well and thriving. Sparing of axilla and groins distinguishes it clinically from seborrheic dermatitis in typical cases.[1,15,43,44]

Psoriasis. Psoriasis is the most common underlying disorder, and its features may be present until the whole body develops exfoliative dermatitis. In a few cases, generalized pustular psoriasis may also be present. There may be a history of preceding plaque(s); treatment with tar, potent steroids, or psoralen plus UVA (PUVA) therapy; intermittent infections; or emotional stress.[1,15]

Congenital erythrodermic psoriasis is extremely uncommon, which is also true in infancy; however, its incidence is directly proportional to the increase in age. The clinical features of psoriasis are similar to those observed in adults with psoriatic erythroderma (Figure 21.2).[1,45] The prognosis of the condition is poor in infants and young children.[8,16]

Ichthyosis. Several syndromes with ichthyosis as an important component may be responsible for erythroderma in infants and children. Harlequin fetus, bullous ichthyosis, lamellar ichthyosis, and congenital ichthyosiform erythroderma (CIE) are its other clinical variants and are required to be taken cognizance of. A collodian membrane encasement is an essential part of both CIE and lamellar ichthyosis. In CIE, it is replaced with exfoliative erythroderma, whereas in lamellar ichthyosis it is followed by generalized ichthyosis with plate-like scales. Infants with

harlequin ichthyosis are born with generalized thick hyperkeratotic covering, which may prove fatal following acute respiratory distress. Bullous (epidermolytic hyperkeratosis) ichthyosis initially may present with widespread areas of denuded skin. Gradually, blistering diminishes and is replaced with ichthyosiform erythroderma with overt clinical features.[8,46]

Diffuse Cutaneous Mastocytosis. This condition is a well-appreciated rare entity in which the entire skin is heavily infiltrated with mast cells. Trivial injury, trauma, and pressure may cause extensive urtication and bullae formation. Unlike the adult-onset variety, cutaneous mastocytosis of infancy and childhood may regress spontaneously.[47]

Toxic Epidermal Necrolysis. This is a fascinating clinical expression wherein there is widespread blistering of the skin and/or mucous membrane. There is an extensive sloughing of the epidermis and dermis, and underneath the slough is "naked" and is attended by enormous exudation. There is a considerable loss of proteins and electrolytes. There is impaired thermoregulation and altered immunologic function; hence, patients are infection prone. This reaction pattern is mediated through the breakdown products or toxins of the microorganism, antibiotic medication administered to treat infective disorders, and/ or polysorbate toxicity. The condition is most frequently encountered in adults, but occasionally has been reported in infants.[48–50]

Pityriasis Rubra Pilaris. Erythroderma following pityriasis rubra pilaris (PRP) is fairly diagnostic, as it usually starts in childhood or adulthood[51,52] and the lesions occupy the hair follicle in the form of papules and/or plaques with "islands of sparing." Reddish follicular papules and/or plaques with thick, dry scales comprise its cardinal clinical expression (Figure 21.3). Invariably, it has an acute onset and is usually accompanied by pruritus. It is inherited as an autosomal dominant trait with variable expression and reduced penetrance. The familial form of PRP typically begins in early childhood with a gradual onset, and most of the familial cases are of type V (atypical juvenile type). The remainder of the familial cases belong to either type III (classic juvenile) or type IV (circumscribed juvenile).[49–54]

Seborrheic Dermatitis. This condition is a fairly common cause of erythroderma in children, less so in adults, and presents as erythematous moist, scaly lesions that occupy the seborrheic sites, namely scalp, axilla, neck, napkin, retroauricular area, and front and back of the chest. The scales are large, greasy, and yellow. It is amenable to various treatments.[4,12]

Crusted Scabies. Crusted or hyperkeratotic scabies is usually nonpruritic owing to impairment of the sensory nerves.

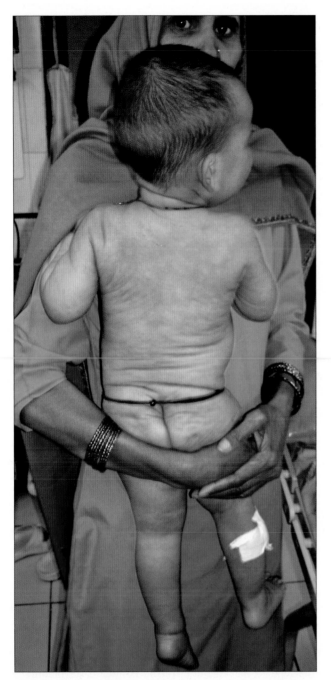

FIGURE 21.3: *Erythroderma/exfoliative dermatitis: developing in (juvenile) pityriasis rubra pilaris.*

It is characterized by sand-like, thick, tan crusts that flake off revealing underlining normal skin. The lesions are usually generalized. Fissures may be a constant source of fatal septic events. Crusted lesions are frequently encountered in immunocompromised HIV/AIDS and are a potential source of perpetuating the disease in the form of epidemics. The diagnosis is confirmed through the demonstration of *Sarcoptes scabiei*. A first- and second-generation screening test (enzyme-linked immunosorbent assay) followed by confirmation by western blot is mandatory to establish the diagnosis of HIV. The condition is amenable to specific topical and oral treatment.[38,55]

Immunologic Disorders

Omenn Syndrome/Familial Reticuloendotheliosis. This condition has infrequently been diagnosed in the recent past; nonetheless, the demonstration of abnormal histiocytic appearing cells in the skin, lymph nodes, spleen, and liver are significant. Erythroderma, failure to thrive, pronounced lymphadenopathy, and recurrent infections are the salient clinical features. Marked leukocytosis, eosinophilia, anemia, hypogammaglobulinemia, and depressed T-cell immunity are its other supplements. T lymphocytes CD4 5RO+ may be demonstrated at the molecular level,[16] and a skin biopsy may confirm the diagnosis[16,18] and help in differentiating it from Netherton syndrome and GVHD although it is mostly fatal. Cyclosporin and bone-marrow transplantation can be effective therapies.[12,56–58]

HypoGammaglobulinemia. An infant who is apparently normal at birth but who subsequently develops fever, diarrhea, and rapidly progressive generalized exfoliative dermatitis (erythroderma) may have hypogammaglobulinemia. Monthly replenishment by intravenous infusion of gamma globulin alleviates fever and erythema.[59]

GVHD. This condition is known to occur in infants who, unknowingly, are transfused with nonirradiated blood or have received small amount of maternal blood by placenta in utero. Usually these infants have primary immunodeficiency. Its clinical presentation is a nonspecific morbilliform eruption, which gradually progresses to erythroderma with epidermal sloughing.[12,60]

Cutaneous T-cell Lymphoma. Cutaneous T-cell lymphoma (CTCL) is a rare entity in children and is likely to be overlooked; however, in particular cases its features are lymphadenopathy, splenomegaly, and lymphocytosis. Sezary-like notched cells can be identified in the peripheral blood smear. In contrast to Omenn syndrome, the immunoglobulin G levels are elevated. Its histopathology is pathognomonic.[12,60]

DiGeorge Syndrome. This condition is an uncommon cause of erythroderma and is characterized by maculopapular/eczematous lesions that may progress to cover the whole of the skin surface. In severe combined immunodeficiency, the affected child often develops localized/widespread eczematous or seborrheic dermatitis.[61]

Metabolic/Nutritional Disorders

Kwashiorkor Cryoglobulins. This is a common form of routine malnutrition in both underdeveloped and developing countries. It may present with generalized erythema, edema, and increased skin fragility. Excessive protein loss may result in renal and/or hepatic failure in older children.[12]

Acrodermatitis Enteropathica. This condition is a well-recognized clinical entity in infants and children. The initial lesions are vesiculobullous, crusted, or psoriasiform in mostly perioral and perianal locations. It is usually accompanied by diarrhea, photophobia, and irritability. In addition to low serum zinc levels, serum alkaline phosphatase levels are also reduced, as this enzyme is zinc dependent. A similar condition may be observed in children with AIDS.[12,62]

Cystic Fibrosis Dermatitis. Initial presentation of this disease is quite different and is characterized by the development of severe, rapidly progressive, and unresponsive psoriasiform lesions. Pulmonary and gastrointestinal components complicate the condition later. The skin lesions may resolve following administration of pancreatic enzymes and nutritional supplements.[63]

Leiner Disease. This condition is composed of a group of disorders with similar presentations characterized by erythroderma, diarrhea, and failure to thrive. Ever since its first description, several innovations have been made, including that by Glover and colleagues,[59] who proved that some of the affected individuals with Leiner phenotype may have an associated immunodeficiency. Where the infant is apparently normal at birth and dermatitis and diarrhea make an early appearance, then the latter is severe and chronic. The dermatitis is associated with progressive erythema and erosions, which may ultimately become generalized. The condition does not respond to topical/oral medication. Adequate nutritional support along with hyperalimentation and individualized treatment may be helpful.[12,59,64]

Amino-Acid Disorders. Several reports have demonstrated the deficiency of various amino acids and their association with erythroderma. Maple syrup urine disease is an interesting example. Its treatment includes restriction of essential amino acids; otherwise, the severity of the dermatitis worsens with increased control on amino-acid intake.[65]

Infections

Staphylococcal Scalded Skin Syndrome. Unlike other erythrodermas in children, staphylococcal scalded skin syndrome (SSSS) onset is acute and accompanied by fever, systemic toxicity, and a positive Nikolsky sign. The erythema is generalized rapidly and progresses to sloughing and erosions. Histopathology examination often will distinguish it from toxic epidermal necrolysis. Occasionally, widespread staphylococcal pustulation resembling generalized candidiasis may develop in a healthy child; however, culture is usually positive for *Staphylococcus*. Accordingly, response to a relevant antimicrobial is ensured.[12,66]

Scarlet Fever. This condition forms an important differential diagnosis of rubella, toxic shock syndrome, severe staphylococcal infection, drug eruptions, mononucleosis, and exanthem subitum. The erythroderma is transient and successfully resolves following administration of penicillin/erythromycin.

Congenital Neonatal Candidosis. The initial lesions are in the form of a maculopapular eruption. Congenital candidosis gradually supervenes with the appearance of classical pustules, especially over the palms and soles. It spreads rapidly and often involves the umbilicus. The diagnosis is easy: either through the demonstration of mycelia/conidia in 10% potassium hydroxide mount or on Gram stain followed by positive culture of *Candida* spp. Sometimes systemic antifungals cause rapid resolution of the disease, and in the neonatal form of generalized cutaneous candidiasis the lesions start in the oral cavity or napkins area.[12,67]

Toxic Shock Syndrome. The clinical features of this condition include fever, hypertension, and diffuse macular blanching erythroderma, followed by desquamation of the palms and soles. Dysfunction of various organs or systems may be life threatening. Surgical wound infection of the skin, subcutaneous and/or soft tissue, and also of bone may be predisposing factor(s).[12,49]

TOXICITY AND DRUG REACTIONS

Boric Acid Toxicity

Maculopapular lesions progressing to erythema, edema, and desquamation are the salient clinical features of this condition, and the Nikolsky sign may be positive. Other features include alopecia, vomiting, diarrhea, fever, and irritability caused by inadvertent absorption of boric acid powder from the diaper area, where boric acid has been used as a dusting powder.[68]

Drug Induced

Drug-induced erythroderma in children is commonly observed with sulfonamide, isoniazid, streptomycin, nonsteroidal antiinflammatory drugs, and antiepileptic drugs; however, cases have also been recorded with Ayurvedic, Unani, homeopathic, and indigenous medications (Table 21.2b). A history of drugs for certain dermatoses/systemic disorders may be elicited prior to the onset of exfoliative dermatitis. Erythema is acute in onset and progresses to generalized exfoliation, which may resolve over the course of 2–6 weeks.[1] Topical preparations have caused generalization of the existing dermatoses in a proportion of cases. If the incriminating drug(s) is withdrawn and symptomatic treatment instituted, the prognosis is excellent.[49]

VARIOUS SYNDROMES

Trichothiodystrophy (Tay Syndrome)

The affected newborn may have collodion membrane and erythroderma with other features, including brittle, sparse hair, variable ichthyosis, and central nervous system manifestations. Erythroderma resolves itself during infancy.[12,69]

Netherton Syndrome

Infants and children affected with this disorder show a generalized exfoliative erythroderma. Trichorrhexis invaginata (bamboo hair) and atopy are its other features. The disease may be confused with generalized atopic dermatitis. A genetic linkage has been established to the SPINK-5 gene locus on chromosome 5q32 encoding the serum protease inhibitor LEKTI. This information may be useful in prenatal testing in any subsequent pregnancy of the mother of the affected child.[70]

Sjögren–Larsson Syndrome

Coincident with erythroderma occurring during infancy, the affected child has scaling, spasticity, and mental retardation. The diagnosis is made on the basis of enzyme assays on leukocytes, fibroblasts, or skin biopsy, which may reveal a deficiency of enzyme fatty alcohol oxidoreductase.[69]

Keratitis–Ichthyosis–Deafness

Keratitis–ichthyosis–deafness syndrome is a rare disorder in which the infant usually has diffusely thickened erythematous skin, which peels off in the course of the first week of life. Subsequently, atypical prominent follicular keratosis is identified over the head and extremities. In the following years or decades, keratoconjunctivitis with noticeable vascularization (pannus), along with neurosensory deafness, occurs.[71]

Ectodermal Dysplasias

Erythroderma is rather an uncommon feature of the disease, and other pathognomonic features help in the diagnosis of this disorder.[12]

Neutral Lipid Storage Disease with Ichthyosis (Dorfman–Chanarin Syndrome)

This condition resembles CIE. Demonstration of lipid vacuoles in the skin and elsewhere in the body supports its diagnosis. It may also have features such as cataract, myopathy, sensory-neural deafness, and growth retardation.[12,72]

Conradi–Hünermann Syndrome

This condition affects infants and is characterized by the presence of bands of ichthyosiform erythroderma along the lines of Blaschko. The bands resolve in due course, leaving behind follicular atrophoderma. Radiography shows an asymptomatic, focal, enchondral calcific strippling.[12,73]

HEMODYNAMIC/METABOLIC DISTURBANCES

The disease may cause an enormous aberration of body metabolism. The increased skin blood flow may cause hypothermia and profound heat loss. Compensatory hypermetabolism and an increased basal metabolic rate without any primary increase in thyroid activity may ensue. Excessive protein loss through scaling and leaking through skin, hemodilution due to the increased plasma column, and hypermetabolism may contribute to hyperalbuminemia and severe edema. High-output cardiac failure may occur at any time.[1,2,74]

HISTOPATHOLOGY

The histopathology of exfoliative dermatitis often reveals a nonspecific picture, consisting of orthokeratosis (hyperkeratosis, parakeratosis), acanthosis, and a chronic perivascular inflammatory infiltrate with or without eosinophilia. The clinicopathologic correlation in erythroderma is difficult, because the specific features of the dermatosis are masked by the nonspecific features of erythroderma.[10] In a study on Sezary syndrome, the diagnosis was established by the clonal population of T cells in the blood, despite a lack of diagnostic features on biopsy.[75] Others clinicians[76] advocated that the submission of multiple simultaneous biopsies from the affected skin enhanced the accuracy of the histopathologic diagnosis, and the cause could be identified in up to one half of cases. The stage of the disease can modify the histopathologic picture; in the acute stage, spongiosis and parakeratosis are prominent, whereas in the chronic stage acanthosis and elongated rete ridges are seen. Despite the uniformity of the clinical expression of erythroderma, diagnostic histopathologic features of the underlying disease are retained in the majority of patients.[77] Skin biopsies from characteristic clinical lesions may often confirm the diagnosis of psoriasis, PRP, ichthyosiform erythroderma, or pemphigus foliaceus.[1,48,78] Drug-induced exfoliative dermatitis may often reveal a lichenoid interface dermatosis histopathology.[79] In erythroderma due to

TABLE 21.3: Histological Clues to the Diagnosis of Erythroderma

Disease	Histologic clues
Psoriasis	Parakeratosis, Munro microabscess, suprapapillary plate thinning, squirting papillae, regular acanthosis
Cutaneous T-cell lymphoma (CTCL)/Sezary	Exocytosis of mononuclear cells, epidermotropism, Pautrier microabscesses
Drug reaction	Vascular change, necrotic keratinocytes
Actinic reticuloid	Hyperkeratosis, acanthosis, superficial and deep mixed dermal infiltrate with some atypical mononuclear cells
Pityriasis rubra pilaris	Alternating orthokeratosis and parakeratosis (vertically and horizontally) with or without keratotic plugging
Sarcoidosis	Dermal noncasketing epithelioid "naked" cell granulomas; occasional, giant cells surrounded by sparse lymphocytes
Contact dermatitis	Spongiosis, eosinophils within dermal infiltrate
Lymphoproliferative diseases	Interstitial pattern of atypical cells between collagen bundles
Scabies	Perivascular and interstitial infiltrates with eosinophils, scabetic mite/scybala/fecal pellets in stratum corneum
Dermatophytosis	Focal parakeratosis, hyphae in stratum corneum
Pemphigus	Supra basal intraepidermal cleavage, acantholytic keratinocytes, (acantholytic cells), direct immunofluorescence depicting IgG-bound cell surface, circulating antibodies
Pemphigoid	Subepidermal bulla with eosinophils
Acute graft versus host disease	Vacuolar change, satellite cell necrosis
Atopic dermatitis	Spongiosis, eosinophils within dermal infiltrate
Seborrheic dermatitis	Parakeratosis with neutrophils at lips of follicular ostia
Dermatomyositis/Subcutaneous lupus erythematosis	Vacuolar change, colloid bodies increased dermal mucin
Idiopathic subacute	Parakeratosis, spongiosis, epidermal hyperplasia, papillary dermal edema, superficial perivascular lymphohistiocytic infiltrate
Idiopathic chronic	Compact hyperkeratosis, psoriasiform hyperplasia, little spongiosis, papillary dermal thickening

Data adapted from Sehgal VN, Srivastava G, Sardana K. Erythroderma/exfoliative dermatitis – a synopsis. Int J Dermatol. 2004; 43:39–47.

lymphoma, the infiltrate may gradually become polymorphic until it acquires specific diagnostic features. This makes repeated skin biopsies, additional investigations of lymphocytes in peripheral blood, and sustained follow-up in dubious situations mandatory to permit the correct diagnosis.[76] Microscopic clues to the diagnosis of erythroderma, if reviewed systematically, can reveal the underlying diagnosis (Table 21.3).

Additional tests to increase the diagnostic specificity include immunophenotyping and direct immunofluorescence.[75]

INVESTIGATIONS/DIAGNOSIS

Mild anemia, leukocytosis, increased erythrocyte sedimentation rate, hypoalbuminemia, hyperglobulinemia, and hyperuricemia are frequent findings.[4,10,14,75] Increased IgE may be observed in erythroderma when caused by atopic dermatitis and drug reactions, although it has also been reported in other settings.[75] A decreased CD4+ T-cell count was observed in patients with erythroderma in the absence of HIV disease, as a consequence of sequestration of the lymphocytes in the skin.[81] Circulating Sezary cells at greater than 20% are indicative of Sezary syndrome, but at less than 10% are nonspecific findings in erythroderma. Immunophenotyping, flow cytometry, and, in particular, B-cell and T-cell gene rearrangement analysis may be helpful in confirming the diagnosis of lymphoma when it is strongly suspected.[3] Actinic retinoid is differentiated from Sezary syndrome by the increased CD8+ T cells in the latter and the nuclear contour index of peripheral blood lymphocytes.[75] A detailed guide to investigations is given in Table 21.4.

A detailed history of the sequence of events leading to the development of erythroderma/exfoliative dermatitis is a prerequisite in all patients. Often the clues obtained may help in the diagnosis and appropriate management. A thorough clinical examination is required to diagnose the etiology of exfoliative dermatitis and to allow appropriate urgent symptomatic treatment. An astute practitioner will

TABLE 21.4: Investigations/Laboratory Tests – Basic Investigations

- Weight, temperature, pulse, respiratory rate charting
- Fluid intake/output charting
- Complete hemogram, total and differential leukocyte counts, absolute platelet count, erythrocyte sedimentation rate
- Liver and kidney function tests, including serum electrolytes
- Histopathology
- Schedule urine macroscopy and microscopy
- Electrocardiogram (ECG) and chest radiograph

Disease-specific investigations:

- Skin scrapings/KOH (Norwegian scabies/Extensive tinea corporis)
- Patch test (after recovery, for suspected allergic contact dermatitis, photoallergic contact dermatitis, airborne contact dermatitis)
- Serum immunoglobulin E (atopic dermatitis)
- Serum and urine protein electrophoresis (multiple myeloma)
- Angiotensin-converting enzyme levels, serum calcium (sarcoidosis)
- Cultures may show bacterial overgrowth or the herpes simplex virus
- CD4+ T-cell count/CD8+ T cells
- Human immunodeficiency virus 1 and 2 testing, including western blot test, to exclude acquired immunodeficiency syndrome
- Immunology-antinuclear antibody, rheumatoid factor, anti-DNA
- Fine-needle aspiration cytology lymph nodes, bone-marrow examination (lymphoma/leukemia)
- Direct immunofluorescence (Pemphigus foliaceous, lichen planus, lupus erythematosus, graft versus host disease)
- Immunophenotyping, flow cytometry, and particularly, B-cell and T-cell gene rearrangement analysis – if lymphoma is strongly suspected
- Workup for occult malignancy, if suspected: chest radiograph, computed tomography scan and ECG, ultrasonography abdomen, stool for occult blood, mammography, sigmoidoscopy, prostate examination, cervical smear, as indicated

Data adapted from Sehgal VN, Srivastava G, Sardana K. Erythroderma/exfoliative dermatitis – a synopsis. Int J Dermatol. 2004; 43:39–47.

be able to identify the nature of the underlying dermatosis and proceed to confirm his or her suspicions. Histopathology is paramount and is rewarding in more than 50% of cases if a diligent effort is made. Fine needle aspiration cytology may be vital to distinguish between dermatopathic and malignant lymphadenopathy. In a recent development. Heteroduplex analysis of T-cell receptor gamma gene rearrangement can be used as an important diagnostic tool in skin biopsies to classify the underlying etiology of erythroderma.[82] T-cell clonality analysis may be useful for the diagnoses of cutaneous T-cell lymphoma in patients with erythroderma.[83]

MANAGEMENT

All cases should be considered as a dermatologic emergency and should preferably be hospitalized for treatment. Serious general medical problems may occur in due course if not appropriately treated. The initial management of all types of erythroderma is the same regardless of the etiology. The principle of management is to maintain skin moisture, avoid scratching, avoid precipitating factors, apply topical steroids, and treat the underlying cause and complications.[1,15,49,75] The patient requires a regulated environmental temperature, avoiding cooling and overheating. Together with general management, all unnecessary medication should be avoided. Cutaneous applications should be soothing and mild due to the already inflamed skin. Mild topical steroids/emollients after lukewarm washing can act as an antipruritic. Antihistamines (H1 receptor) can be administered to enhance the effect.

After the acute irritated state of the skin has improved, further treatment can be undertaken according to the etiology. Antimicrobials can be added to control secondary infections. Any hemodynamic or metabolic aberrations must be addressed appropriately. Each case requires regular monitoring of protein, electrolyte balance, circulatory status, and body temperature. Blood urea, serum electrolyte, and fluid balance should be monitored.

Erythroderma commonly resists therapy until the underlying disease is treated (e.g., phototherapy, systemic medications in psoriasis). The outcome is unpredictable in idiopathic erythroderma, and the course is marked by multiple exacerbations; prolonged glucocorticoid therapy is often needed. Appropriate inpatient/outpatient medications are influenced by the underlying etiology of erythroderma. For example, prednisone may be contraindicated in exfoliative dermatitis secondary to psoriasis, whereas retinoids are an excellent choice for this disease. Systemic steroids may be helpful in some cases, but should be avoided in suspected cases of psoriasis and SSSS.[84] Low-dose methotrexate or cyclosporin can be safely administered in erythrodermic psoriasis.[1,49] Carbamazepine is effective in the treatment of psoriatic erythroderma;[85] however, the same drug has caused exfoliative dermatitis/erythroderma in a few studies.[86] Similarly, methotrexate therapy for psoriasis has been reported to cause exfoliative dermatitis.[87]

The ideal treatment for erythrodermic cutaneous lymphoma is still elusive. Various modalities, such as systemic steroids, PUVA, total-body electron-beam irradiation, topical nitrogen mustard, systemic chemotherapy, and extracorporeal plasmapheresis, have been tried with variable results.[88] A proposed plan of treatment is given in Table 21.5.

Evaluation of infants and children suffering from erythroderma/exfoliative dermatitis is paramount. It not only assists in forming the precise treatment strategy, but also alleviates the anxiety of the child's carer who will be confronted with a dilemma. It is, therefore, imperative to arrive

TABLE 21.5: Treatment of Erythroderma

General	Specific (topical)	Specific (systemic)	Disease specific
-Inpatient care required -Adequate bed rest and sedation -Monitor fluid intake/electrolyte balance/temperature regulation -High protein diet/nutritional support -Discontinue all unnecessary medications	-Topical steroids (Triamcinolone acetonide cream 0.025%–1.0%) under wet dressing -Apply tap water wet dressings 2–3 hourly; gradually reduce frequency, followed by emollients application -Daily tepid bath may be soothing.	-Sedative antihistamine H_1 receptor (Hydroxyzine hydrochloride 25–50 mg orally every 4–6 h)/any other -Institute systemic antibiotics (to cover secondary infection by *Staphylococcus aureus*) -Systemic steroids (used with caution) – atopic dermatitis, seborrheic dermatitis; avoid in psoriasis and infections; taper down	Psoriasis – Methotrexate, retinoids, phototherapy Atopic dermatitis – Systemic steroids, antibiotics, antivirals Pityriasis rubra pilaris – Retinoids, methotrexate, systemic steroids Toxic epidermal necrolysis – Intravenous immunoglobulins Lymphoma – Extracorporeal phototherapy, PUVA, alkylating-agents Scabies – Permethrin 5%, Ivermectin 200 μg/kg

PUVA, psoralen plus UVA.
Data adapted from Sehgal VN, Srivastava G, Sardana K. Erythroderma/exfoliative dermatitis – a synopsis. Int J Dermatol. 2004; 43:39–47.

at a probable diagnosis based on the salient clinical features *vide supra* and relevant investigations. The differential diagnosis of erythroderma/exfoliative dermatitis in infants and children is intricate, bizarre, and extensive. Common causes of the disease should be considered in the first instance, and it is worthwhile to recapitulate atopic dermatitis, seborrheic dermatitis, toxicity/drug reactions, and infections as the most common causes of erythroderma.[1,2,49,75]

The basic management of erythroderma is supportive therapy and correction of the hematologic, biochemical, and metabolic imbalances. A regulated environmental temperature gives symptomatic relief to the affected patient. Liberal uses of emollients are useful in soothing the irritated skin. Low-potency topical corticosteroids are useful in only a few patients and may be ineffective or even harmful in other patients. The authors and other skeptics do have severe reservations.[1,49] The unfolding of underlying pathology may prove useful in defining an appropriate treatment.[74] Thus, a judicious individualized approach is required when treating erythroderma/exfoliative dermatitis in the pediatric age group.

Newer drugs such as rituximab,[89] tacrolimus,[90] infliximab,[91] and so forth can be tried after weighing the pros and cons and individual merits.

COMPLICATIONS AND PROGNOSIS

Exfoliative dermatitis is a complex disorder involving many factors, but the net outcome depends on the underlying disease. The disease course is rapid, if it results from drug allergy, lymphoma, leukemia, contact allergens, or SSSS.[1,3,75] The disease course is gradual if it results from the generalized spread of a primary skin disease (e.g., psoriasis or atopic dermatitis).[49,84] Drug-induced cases of

exfoliative dermatitis recover completely if initial medical management is promptly undertaken.[75] Despite skilled efforts, exfoliative dermatitis can sometimes prove fatal, especially in elderly patients. Secondary infection, dehydration, electrolyte imbalance, temperature dysregulation, and high-output cardiac failure are potential complications in all cases.

Postinflammatory hypopigmentation or hyperpigmentation may occur, especially in individuals with dark skin. Generalized vitiligo or pyogenic granuloma has also been recorded after exfoliative dermatitis.[88,92] Nevi and keloid formation are rare benign sequelae, as are alopecia and nail dystrophies.[8] In initial documented studies, the recorded death rate varied from 18% to 64%;[1,14,49,75] however, the mortality has been reduced due to advances in more rapid diagnosis and improved therapeutic regimens.

REFERENCES

1. Sehgal VN, Srivastava G. Exfoliative dermatitis – a prospective study of 80 patients. Dermatologica. 1986; 173:278–84.
2. Weismann K, Graham RM. Systemic disease and the skin. In: Champion RH, Burton JL, Burns DA, et al, editors. Textbook of dermatology, Vol. 3, 6th ed. Oxford: Blackwell Science; 1998. pp. 2703–58.
3. Sigurdsson V, Toonstra J, Hazemans-Boer M, et al. Erythroderma – a clinical and follow-up study of 102 patients with special emphasis on survival. J Am Acad Dermatol. 1996; 35:53–7.
4. Hasan T, Jansen CT. Erythroderma: a follow-up of fifty cases. J Am Acad Dermatol. 1983; 8:836–40.
5. Hisatomi K, Isomura T, Hirano A, et al. Post operative erythroderma after cardiac operation – possible role of depressed cell-mediated immunity. J Thorac Cardiovasc Surg. 1992; 104:648–53.

6. Morar N, Dlova N, Gupta AK, et al. Erythroderma – a comparison between HIV positive and negative patients. Int J Dermatol. 1999; 38:859–900.

7. Hoeger PH, Harper JI. Neonatal erythroderma: differential diagnosis and management of 'red baby.' Arch Dis Child. 1998; 79:186–91.

8. Sarkar R, Sharma RC, Koranne RV, et al. Erythroderma in children – a clinico-etiologic study. J Dermatol. 1999; 26:507–11.

9. King LE Jr. Erythroderma. Who, where, when, why and how. Arch Dermatol. 1994; 130:1503–7.

10. Botella-Estrada R, Sanmartin O, Oliver V, et al. Erythroderma. A clinical pathological study of 56 cases. Arch Dermatol. 1994; 130:1503–7.

11. Wong KS, Wong SN, Tham SN, et al. Generalized exfoliative dermatitis – a clinical study of 108 patients. Ann Acad Med Singapore. 1988; 17:520–3.

12. Spraker MK. Differential diagnosis of neonatal erythroderma. In: Harper J, Orange A, Prose N, editors. Textbook of pediatric dermatology. 1st ed. London: Blackwell Science Ltd; 2000. pp. 92–103.

13. Sigurdsson V, Steegmans PH, van Vloten WA. The incidence of erythroderma: a survey among all dermatologists in the Netherlands. J Am Acad Dermatol. 2001; 45:675–8.

14. Abrahams I, McCarthy JT, Sanders SL. 101 cases of exfoliative dermatitis. Arch Dermatol. 1963; 87:96–101.

15. Sehgal VN, Srivastava G, Sardana K. Erythroderma/ exfoliative dermatitis – a synopsis. Int J Dermatol. 2004; 43:39–47.

16. Pruszkowski A, Bodemer C, Fraitag S. Neonatal and infantile erythrodermas: a retrospective study of 51 patients. Arch Dermatol. 2000; 136:875–80.

17. King LE Jr., Dufresne RG Jr., Lovett GL, et al. Erythroderma review of 82 cases. South Med J. 1986; 79:1210–15.

18. Al-Dhalimi MA. Neonatal and infantile erythroderma: a clinical and follow-up study of 42 cases. J Dermatol. 2007; 34: 302–7.

19. Rym BM, Mourad M, Bechir Z, et al. Erythroderma in adults: a report of 80 cases. Int J Dermatol. 2005; 44:731–5.

20. Akhyani M, Ghodsi ZS, Toosi S, et al. Erythroderma: a clinical study of 97 cases. BMC Dermatol. 2005; 5:5.

21. Jaffer AN, Brodell RT. Exfoliative dermatitis. Erythroderma can be a sign of a significant underlying disorder. Postgrad Med. 2005; 117:49–51.

22. Rothe MJ, Bernstein ML, Grant-Kels JM. Life-threatening erythroderma: diagnosing and treating the "red man." Clin Dermatol. 2005; 23:206–17.

23. Gonzalo-Garijo MA, Perez-Calderon R, De Argila D, et al. Erythroderma to pseudoephedrine in a patient with contact allergy to phenylephrine. Allergol Immunopathol (Madr). 2002; 30:239–42.

24. Davies MG, Kersey PJ. Acute hepatitis and exfoliative dermatitis associated with minocycline. Br Med J. 1989; 298:1523–4.

25. Horiuchi Y. Propolis-induced erythroderma. J Dermatol. 2001; 28:580–1.

26. Gonzalo-Garijo MA, de Argila D. Erythroderma due to aztreonam and clindamycin. J Investig Allergol Clin Immunol. 2006; 16:210–11.

27. Antonov D, Grozdev I, Pehlivanov G, et al. Psoriatic erythroderma associated with enalapril. Skinmed. 2006; 5:90–2.

28. Dummer R, Foss F, Dreno B, et al. Clinical experience: practical management of five patients with cutaneous T-cell lymphoma (CTCL)-related symptoms. Semin Oncol. 2006; 33:26–32.

29. Vonderheid EC, Pena J, Nowell P. Sezary cell counts in erythrodermic cutaneous T-cell lymphoma: implications for prognosis and staging. Leuk Lymphoma. 2006; 47:1841–56.

30. Vonderheid EC. On the diagnosis of erythrodermic cutaneous T-cell lymphoma. J Cutan Pathol. 2006; 33:27–42.

31. Kameyama H, Shirai Y, Date K, et al. Gallbladder carcinoma presenting as exfoliative dermatitis (erythroderma). Int J Gastrointest Cancer. 2005; 35:153–5.

32. Vonderheid EC, Bernengo MG, Burg G, et al. Update on erythroderma cutaneous T-cell lymphoma – Report of International Society for Cutaneous Lymphomas. J Am Acad Dermatol. 2002; 46:95–106.

33. Faure M, Bertrand C, Manduit G, et al. Paraneoplastic erythroderma – apropos of a case. Dermatologica. 1985; 170:147–51.

34. Momm F, Pflieger D, Lutterbach J. Paraneoplastic erythroderma in a prostate cancer patient. Strahlenther Onkol. 2002; 178:393–5.

35. Fierro MT, Comessatti A, Quaglino P, et al. Expression pattern of chemokine receptors and chemokine release in inflammatory erythroderma and Sezary syndrome. Dermatology. 2006; 213:284–92.

36. Satoh H, Yamashita YT, Ohtsuka M, et al. Post-irradiation erythroderma. Clin Oncol. 2000; 12:336.

37. Lowenthal RM, Challis DR, Griffiths AE, et al. Transfusion-associated graft-versus-host disease: report of an occurrence following the administration of irradiated blood. Transfusion. 1993; 33:524–9.

38. Fuchs BS, Sapadin AN, Phelps RG, et al. Diagnostic dilemma: crusted scabies superimposed in psoriatic erythroderma in patient with acquired immunodeficiency syndrome. Skinmed. 2007; 6:142–4.

39. Wilson DC, Jester JD, King LE Jr. Erythroderma, an exfoliative dermatitis. Clin Dermatol. 1993; 11:67–72.

40. Hild DH. Folate loss from the skin in exfoliative dermatitis. Arch Intern Med. 1969; 123:51–7.

41. Abel EA, Lindae ML, Hoppe RT, et al. Benign and malignant forms of erythroderma: cutaneous immunophenotypic characteristics. J Am Acad Dermatol. 1988; 19:1089–95.

42. Sigurdsson V, Toonstra J, Bihari IC, et al. Interleukin-4 and interferon-gamma expression of the dermal infiltrate in patients with erythroderma and mycosis fungoides – an immunohistochemical study. J Cutan Pathol. 2002; 27:429–35.

43. Sehgal VN, Jain S. Atopic dermatitis: clinical criteria. Int J Dermatol. 1993; 32:628–37.

44. Eigenmann PA. Clinical features and diagnostic criteria of atopic dermatitis in relation to age. Pediatr Allergy Immunol. 2001; 12 Suppl 14:69–74.

45. Vasconcellos C, Dominques PP, Aoki V, et al. Erythroderma – analysis of 247 cases. Rev Saude Publica. 1995; 29:177–82.

46. Kumar S, Sehgal VN, Sharma RC. Common genodermatoses. Int J Dermatol. 1996; 35:685–94.

47. Valent P, Horny HP, Escribano L, et al. Diagnostic criteria and classification of mastocytosis – a consensus proposal. Leuk Res. 2001; 25:603–25.

48. Balistreri WF, Farrell MK, Bove KE. Lessons from the E-Ferol tragedy. Pediatrics. 1986; 3:503–6.

49. Sehgal VN, Srivastava G. Erythroderma/generalized exfoliative dermatitis in pediatric practice: an overview. Int J Dermatol. 2006; 45:831–9.

50. Sehgal VN, Srivastava G. A toxic epidermal necrolysis (TEN) Lyell's syndrome. J Dermatol Treat. 2005; 16:278–86

51. Sehgal VN, Srivastava G. Juvenile and adult (juvenile) pityriasis rubra pilaris. Int J Dermatol. 2006; 45:438–46.

52. Sehgal VN, Srivastava G, Dogra S. Adult onset pityriasis rubra pilaris: a focus on treatment dilemma. Indian J Dermatol Venereol Leprol. 2008; 74:311–21.

53. Gelmetti C, Schiuma AA, Cerri D, et al. Pityriasis rubra pilaris in childhood: a long-term study of 29 cases. Pediatr Dermatol. 1986; 3:446–51.

54. Sehgal VN, Jain S, Kumar S, et al. Familial pityriasis rubra pilaris (adult classic – I): a report of three cases in a single family. Skinmed. 2002; 1:161–4.

55. Funkhouser ME, Omohundro C, Ross A, et al. Management of scabies in patients with HIV disease. Arch Dermatol. 1993; 129:911–13.

56. Scheimberg I, Hoeger PH, Harper JI, et al. Omenn's syndrome: differential diagnosis in infants with erythroderma and immunodeficiency. Pediatr Dev Pathol. 2001; 4:237–45.

57. Puzenat E, Rohrlich P, Thierry P, et al. Omenn syndrome: a rare case of neonatal erythroderma. Eur J Dermatol. 2007; 17:137–9.

58. Meyer-Bahlburg A, Haas JP, Haase R, et al. Treatment with cyclosporine A in a patient with Omenn's syndrome. Arch Dis Child. 2002; 87:231–3.

59. Glover MT, Atherton DJ, Levinsky RJ. Syndrome of erythroderma, failure to thrive, and diarrhea in infancy – a manifestation of immunodeficiency. Pediatrics. 1988; 81:66–72.

60. Alain G, Carrier C, Beaumier L, et al. In utero acute graft-versus-host disease in a neonate with severe combined immunodeficiency. J Am Acad Dermatol. 1993; 29:862–5.

61. Llorente CP, Amors JT, Frutur FJO. Cutaneous lesions in severe combined immunodeficiency. Pediatr Dermatol. 1991; 8:314–21.

62. Sehgal VN, Jain S. Acrodermatitis enteropathica. Clin Dermatol. 2000; 18:745–8.

63. Darmstadt GL, Schmidt CP, Wechster DS. Dermatitis as presenting sign of cystic fibrosis. Arch Dermatol. 1992; 128:1358–64.

64. Goodyear HM, Harper JI. Leiner's disease associated with metabolic acidosis. Clin Exp Dermatol. 1989; 14:364–6.

65. Koch SE, Packman S, Koch TK, et al. Dermatitis in treated maple syrup urine disease. J Am Dermatol. 1993; 28:289–92.

66. Bass JW. The spectrum of staphylococcal disease. From Job's boils to toxic shock. Postgrad Med. 1982; 72:58–64.

67. Glassman BD, Muglia JJ. Widespread erythroderma and desquamation in a neonate. Congenital cutaneous candidiasis (CCC). Arch Dermatol. 1993; 129:899–902.

68. Kaufmann HJ, Held U, Salzberg R. Fatal transcutaneous resorption of boric acid in an infant. Dtsch Med Wochensch. 1962; 87:2374–8.

69. William ML, Shwayder TA. Ichthyosis and disorder of cornification. In: Schachner LA, Hansen RC, editors. Pediatric dermatology. Edinburgh: Churchill Livingstone; 1995. pp. 413–68.

70. Muller FB, Hausser I, Berg D, et al. Genetic analysis of a severe case of Netherton syndrome and application for prenatal testing. Br J Dermatol. 2002; 146:495–9.

71. Nazzaro V, Blanchet-Borden C, Lorette G, et al. Familial occurrence of KID (keratitis, ichthyosis, deafness) syndrome. Case reports. J Am Acad Dermatol. 1990; 23:385–8.

72. Srebrnik A, Tur E, Perluk C, et al. Dorfman–Chanarin syndrome – a case report and a review. J Am Acad Dermatol. 1987; 17:801–8.

73. Kalter DC, Atherton DJ, Clayton PT. X-linked dominant Conradi–Hunermann syndrome presenting as congenital erythroderma. J Am Acad Dermatol. 1989; 21:248–56.

74. Grice KA, Bettley FR. Skin water loss and accidental hypothermia in psoriasis, ichthyosis and erythroderma. Br Med J. 1967; 4:195–8.

75. Rothe MJ, Bialy TL, Grant-Kels, JM. Erythroderma. Dermatol Clin. 2000; 18:405–15.

76. Walsh NM, Prokopetz R, Tron VA, et al. Histopathology in erythroderma – review of a series of cases by multiple observers. J Cutan Pathol. 1994; 21:419–23.

77. Zip C, Murray S, Walsh NM. The specificity of histopathology in erythroderma. J Cutan Pathol. 1993; 20:393–8.

78. Tomasini C, Aloi F, Solaroli C, et al. Psoriatic erythroderma – a histopathologic study of 45 patients. Dermatology. 1997; 194:102–6.

79. Patterson JW, Berry AD 3rd, Darwin BS, et al. Lichenoid histopathologic changes in patients with clinical diagnosis of exfoliative dermatitis. Am J Dermatopathol. 1991; 13:358–64.

80. Sentis HJ, Willemze R, Scheffer E. Histopathologic studies in Sezary's syndrome and erythroderma mycosis fungoides: a comparison with benign forms of erythroderma. J Am Acad Dermatol. 1986; 15:1217–26.

81. Griffiths TW, Stevens SR, Cooper KD. Acute erythroderma as an exclusion criterion for idiopathic CD4+ T lymphocytopenia. Arch Dermatol. 1994; 130:1530–3.

82. Cherny S, Mraz S, Su L, et al. Heteroduplex analysis of T-cell receptors gamma gene re-arrangement as an adjuvant tool in diagnosis in skin biopsies from erythroderma. J Cutan Pathol. 2001; 28:351–5.

83. Cordel N, Lenormand B, Courville P, et al. Usefulness of cutaneous T-cell clonality analysis for the diagnosis of cutaneous T-cell lymphoma in patients with erythroderma. Arch Pathol Lab Med. 2005; 129:372–6.

84. Marks J. Erythroderma and its management. Clin Exp Dermatol. 1982; 7:415–22.

85. Smith KJ, Skelton HG. Accidental success of carbamazepine for psoriatic erythroderma. N Engl J Med. 1996; 26:1999–2000.

86. Troost RJ, Oranje AP, Lijnen RL, et al. Exfoliative dermatitis due to immunologically confirmed carbamazepine hypersensitivity. Pediatr Dermatol. 1996; 13:316–20.

87. Peters T. Exfoliative dermatitis after long-term methotrexate treatment of severe psoriasis. Acta Derm Venereol. 1999; 79: 391–2.
88. Mogavera HS. Exfoliative dermatitis. In: Provost TT, Farmer ER, editors. Current therapy in dermatology. 2nd ed. Philadelphia: Dekker; 1988. pp. 20–1.
89. Connelly EA, Aber C, Kleiner G, et al. Generalized erythrodermic pemphigus foliaceus in a child and its successful response to rituximab treatment. Pediatr Dermatol. 2007; 24:172–6.
90. Leonardi S, Rotolo N, Marchese G, et al. Efficacy and safety of tacrolimus ointment 0.03% treatment in a 1-month-old red baby: a case report. Allergy Asthma Proc. 2006; 27: 523–6.
91. Rongioletti F, Borenstein M, Kirsner R, et al. Erythrodermic, recalcitrant psoriasis: clinical resolution with infliximab. J Dermatol Treat. 2003; 14:222–5.
92. Torres JE, Sanchez JL. Disseminated pyogenic granuloma developing after an exfoliative dermatitis. J Am Acad Dermatol. 1995; 32:280–2.

CHAPTER 22

Acute, Severe Bullous Dermatoses

Snejina Vassileva

A VARIETY OF SKIN diseases may present with the appearance of blisters (Table 22.1). The skin reacts with the formation of vesicles or larger bullae to a number of external physical, chemical, and biological insults. Adverse reactions to systemic or topically applied drugs occupy an important place in the differential diagnosis of blistering eruptions. Bullous lesions can also occur as a manifestation of systemic diseases, as is the case of the bullae seen in diabetic patients. Atypical blistering forms of several inflammatory dermatoses exist, such as bullous lichen planus, bullous morphea, or bullous mycosis fungoides. In all these cases, blistering lesions are infrequent and temporary, in contrast to a group of chronic cutaneous disorders referred to as "bullous dermatoses," where vesiculobullous lesions are the main and characteristic clinical feature. Some bullous dermatoses are due to genetically determined loss of basic structural elements in the skin that maintain the cohesion between the keratinocytes in the epidermis, or between the epidermal layer and the dermis within the basement membrane zone (BMZ). The majority of bullous dermatoses, however, are acquired organ-specific autoimmune diseases in which the autoantibodies target structural proteins in the skin. These disorders constitute one of the major sources of morbidity and mortality in dermatology.

Acquired autoimmune bullous dermatoses are a heterogeneous group of uncommon but often debilitating diseases including pemphigus, bullous, and cicatricial pemphigoid (CP) and related entities, linear immunoglobulin A (IgA) disease (LAD), epidermolysis bullosa acquisita (EBA), and dermatitis herpetiformis (DH). Their histological classification is based on the level of the skin at which the cleft occurs and the mechanisms of blistering process. Intraepidermal acantholytic blisters, characteristic of pemphigus, result from autoantibody binding to desmosomal proteins leading to functionally impaired desmosomes and acantholysis. In the pemphigoid group of diseases, the autoantibodies are directed against different components of the dermal–epidermal junction, which results in subepidermal blistering. Several diagnostically relevant clinical signs and symptoms can be derived from the level of the cleft formation. Intraepidermal blisters, for instance, tend to be more flaccid and fragile and therefore rupture easily due to their thinner roof. In contrast, subepidermal blisters have a thick, "tense" roof and can remain intact even when firmly compressed.

Autoimmune bullous dermatoses are often misdiagnosed, and sometimes the delay in their diagnosis and institution of appropriate treatment can result in death.[1] Usually, in routine dermatologic practice, a careful clinical evaluation is sufficient to differentiate the transitory blisters of bacterial, viral, or parasitic origin, or those seen in the dermatitis/eczema group, or to orient the clinical diagnosis toward a possible immunobullous disease. Several clinical features, such as age of onset, family history, history of exposure to hazardous factors, known underlying systemic or other dermatologic diseases may provide clues as to the etiology of a blistering eruption.[2] A further step in the clinical recognition of bullous diseases takes into consideration the lesion morphology, distribution, evolution, and presence of characteristic clinical signs, such as the Nikolsky sign (i.e., lateral pressure in the vicinity of a blistering lesion produces detachment of the epidermis). The diagnosis of autoimmune bullous diseases, however, strictly relies on histological and immunologic criteria, the latter being provided by the results of the application of specialized immunohistology techniques.[3,4] Histological examination of a biopsy specimen from an early intact vesicle would discriminate among intraepidermal and subepidermal blister formation and the underlying histopathology patterns, but the direct and indirect immunofluorescence (DIF and IIF, respectively) techniques are essential in the diagnosis of immunobullous diseases. DIF reveals the type and location of the immunoreactants (immunoglobulins, complement components, fibrin, properdin) deposited *in vivo* in a patient's skin.[5] It is performed on biopsy specimens from normal-appearing skin immediately adjacent to a bullous lesion (perilesional skin). DIF on the patient's skin that has been separated through lamina lucida through incubation in a 1.0 M solution of NaCl allows further discrimination between the various subepidermal blistering diseases characterized by immune deposits in the lamina lucida or in the deeper layers of the BMZ. IIF is used for detecting circulating autoantibodies in the body fluids (blood, serum, blister fluid). Immunoelectron microscopy is a method combining the advantages of immunohistochemistry techniques and the resolution power of electron

TABLE 22.1: Causes of Blistering

Physical/Chemical
Friction
Pressure ulcers (decubitus ulcers)
Suction (vacuum) blisters
Thermal injury (burn, freezing)
Ultraviolet light irradiation
Carbon monoxide poisoning
Fracture blisters

Infectious
Impetigo contagiosa
Bullous impetigo/Staphylococcal scalded skin syndrome
Bullous erysipelas
Syphilis (pemphigus neonatorum)
Herpes simplex
Varicella-Zoster
Coxsackie (Hand–foot–mouth disease)
Dyshidrosiform tinea/Pompholyx

Parasitic
Scabies
Insect bites

Allergic/Immunologic
Contact dermatitis
Dyshidrosiform eczema/Pompholyx
Fixed drug eruption
Erythema exsudativum multiforme
Blistering drug eruptions
Stevens–Johnson syndrome/Toxic epidermal necrolysis
Coma-induced blisters
Bullous amyloidosis
Bullous lichen planus
Bullous morphea
Bullous allergic vasculitis
Bullous mastocytosis
Bullous pyoderma gangrenosum
Bullous mycosis fungoides
Leukemic bullae
Grover disease (transient acantholytic dermatosis)

Metabolic diseases
Porphyria (cutanea tarda, erythropoietic)
Pseudoporphyria (can be also drug induced)
Chronic renal failure (hemodialysis)
Bullosis diabeticorum
Pellagra

Autoimmune
Pemphigus
Pemphigoid
Linear immunoglobulin A disease
Epidermolysis bullosa acquisita
Bullous systemic lupus erythematosus
Dermatitis herpetiformis

Genetic/Hereditary
Hailey–Hailey disease
Darier disease
Epidermolysis bullosa hereditaria
Congenital bullous erythroderma
Kindler syndrome
Incontinentia pigmenti
Hydroa vacciniforme

microscopy that is used to identify the different ultrastructural binding sites of immunoglobulins and complement within the dermal–epidermal junction in the subepidermal blistering diseases.[6] Immunoblotting and immunoprecipitation are used to identify the antigen or antigens precipitated by the autoantibodies circulating in a patient's serum.[7] Enzyme-linked immunosorbent assay (ELISA) is used as a sensitive method for the detection of autoantibodies to the immunodominant epitopes in pemphigoid and pemphigus.

For several decades, a variety of both local and systemic therapies has become available that can be used to treat these diseases. Although the mortality from autoimmune bullous diseases has decreased significantly during the past several decades, they still represent one cause of morbidity in dermatology, and the common causes of death are often due to the complications of the therapeutic agents used. Suppression of autoantibody production and tissue binding is a main route in treating patients with autoimmune bullous dermatoses.

PEMPHIGUS

Pemphigus is a group of rare, life-threatening autoimmune blistering diseases characterized by widespread blistering and erosions of the skin and mucous membranes. It is mediated by pathogenic autoantibodies against desmosomal cadherins desmoglein 1 and desmoglein 3.[8] Because desmosomes constitute the main adhesion structure of the epidermis, binding of autoantibodies to their target antigens leads to loss of cell–cell adhesion between keratinocytes and intraepithelial blister formation, called acantholysis. Three major variants of pemphigus are currently recognized: pemphigus vulgaris, pemphigus foliaceus, and paraneoplastic pemphigus (PNP). These variants differ considerably in their clinical, histological, and immunological features and prognosis. Pemphigus vulgaris, also known as "deep" pemphigus, is characterized by blister formation above the basal-cell layer and is associated with antibodies against desmoglein 3, which is located in the lower portions of the epidermis and is found in both the skin and mucous membranes. In contrast, pemphigus foliaceus or "superficial" pemphigus is characterized by subcorneal acantholysis and antibodies against desmoglein 1, which is expressed in the upper epidermal layers and is found only in the skin. Pemphigus vulgaris affects both the skin and mucous membranes, mainly the oral mucosa, whereas in pemphigus foliaceus the lesions are confined to the skin. Several subtypes of both forms of pemphigus exist.

Before the advent of corticosteroids in the 1950s, pemphigus had been a deadly disease with mortality rates up to 90%–100% of affected patients within 2 years of onset.[9] The introduction of corticosteroids and immunosuppressive drugs has dramatically transformed what was almost invariably a fatal illness into one the mortality of which is

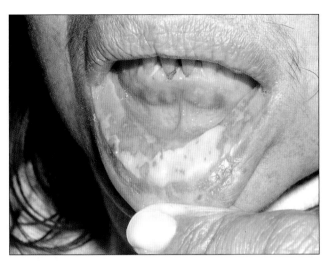

FIGURE 22.1: *Painful erosions on the lip mucosa in a patient with pemphigus vulgaris.*

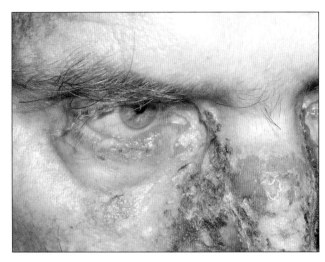

FIGURE 22.2: *Erosive lesions of lid margins and conjunctiva in a patient with mucocutaneous pemphigus vulgaris.*

now less than 10%.[10] Despite the advances in management and improved prognosis, pemphigus is still regarded as a chronic debilitating condition in which the patient's life is mainly endangered by the complications and side effects of the long-term treatment and not by the disease itself.

Pemphigus vulgaris is the most common and one of the most severe forms of pemphigus that still carries a grave prognosis. Although people from all races can be affected, pemphigus vulgaris is more prevalent in some ethnic groups (Ashkenazi Jewish, Japanese), and in some regions such as the Mediterranean and Balkan countries.[11] Individuals with certain human leukocyte antigen (HLA) allotypes are predisposed to the disease, although the susceptibility gene differs depending on ethnic origin;[12] thus, HLA-DRB1*0402 is associated with the disease in Ashkenazi Jews and DRB1*1401/04 and DQB1*0503 in non-Jewish patients of European or Asian descent. Pemphigus vulgaris most often affects middle-aged adults, the mean age of onset being between the age of 40 and 60 years. In the majority of cases, the disease starts from the oral mucosa and nasopharynx and in 50%–60% of patients may remain localized to these sites for months. Flaccid blisters that easily rupture by leaving painful erosions are characteristic of the mucosal variant of pemphigus vulgaris (Figure 22.1). The erosions show little or no tendency to heal, which results in decreased food intake and progressive loss of weight. There is usually a characteristic *foetor ex ore*. Other mucous membranes such as the conjunctiva (Figure 22.2), esophagus, and genital and anal mucosa may be involved.

Within various periods of time, cutaneous involvement develops in addition to the mucosal disease. The skin lesions are characterized by flaccid, peripherally extending bullae, arising on unchanged skin. The flexural areas, trunk, face, and scalp are most often affected (Figure 22.3). If left untreated, the disease shows a progressive course

with appearance of new bullous lesions and involvement of larger areas of skin. Individuals younger than 18 years can be rarely affected (pemphigus juvenilis, childhood pemphigus, adolescent pemphigus).[13] In the pediatric population, the disease has a similar course to that in adults.

Histopathologically, pemphigus vulgaris is characterized by acantholytic intraepidermal blister formation above the basal layer of keratinocytes (Figure 22.4). The immunologic hallmark of pemphigus vulgaris is the demonstration of in vivo bound and circulating immunoglobulin G (IgG) autoantibodies against the cell surface of keratinocytes. DIF reveals deposits of IgG on the epithelial cell surface throughout the epidermis, a diagnostic staining pattern found in practically all patients with active disease (Figure 22.5). The deposits are found in the perilesional and clinically normal skin and mucosa, but the best results are obtained from biopsy specimens from perilesional skin.

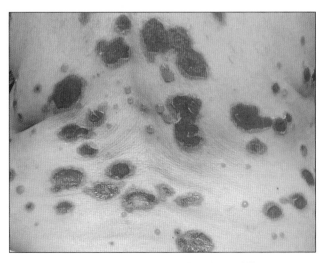

FIGURE 22.3: *Pemphigus vulgaris: few flaccid blisters on normal skin and large peripherally extending erosions.*

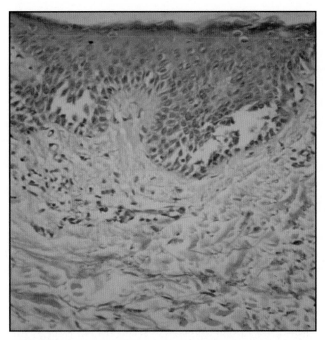

FIGURE 22.4: *Acantholysis with suprabasilar clefts in pemphigus vulgaris. Few acantholytic cells floating in the blister cavity.*

The presence of circulating autoantibodies can be detected and measured using various serologic assays including IIF, immunoblotting, and ELISA. IIF reveals serum IgG antibodies, which produce the characteristic epithelial cell surface fluorescence pattern on monkey esophagus (or human esophagus) as a substrate (Figure 22.6). Their titers correlate with the activity of the disease. Immunoblot analysis can detect autoantibody profiles that have been defined to be specific for each clinical phenotype of pemphigus.[14,15] Patients with mucosal involvement, with no or limited skin blisters (mucosal dominant phenotype of pemphigus vulgaris) demonstrate autoantibody binding to a 130 kd

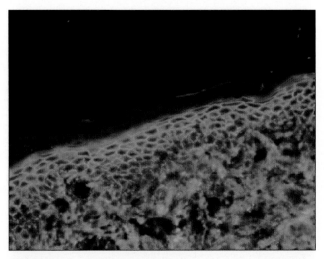

FIGURE 22.5: *Direct immunofluorescence on perilesional skin in pemphigus: intercellular fluorescence pattern with immunoglobulin G throughout the epidermis.*

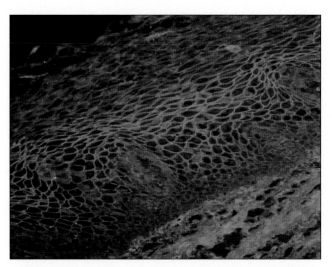

FIGURE 22.6: *Indirect immunofluorescence with pemphigus serum on human esophagus substrate: binding of immunoglobulin G antibodies on the epithelial cell surface (network epidermal fluorescence).*

protein (desmoglein 3), whereas patients with mucocutaneous involvement have autoantibodies that react with desmoglein 3 but also with desmoglein 1 (160 kd protein) (Figure 22.7). Patients with dominant skin disease have higher desmoglein 1 antibody titers than those with oral-dominant pemphigus vulgaris.[16] Therefore, the presence of desmoglein 1 antibodies in pemphigus vulgaris is predictive of a potentially more severe phenotype with extensive skin involvement.[17] A standardized ELISA is commercially available to measure autoantibody titers to both desmoglein 1 and 3.

Pemphigus vegetans is a rare clinical form of pemphigus vulgaris (1%–2% of patients) affecting the intertriginous areas, where hypertrophic, papillomatous, or verrucous vegetating lesions are present. Two types of pemphigus vegetans are distinguished: 1) the Neumann type, in which long-lasting (refractory) erosions in the folds are transformed into vegetating lesions (Figure 22.8); and 2) the Hallopeau type, characterized by the appearance of pustules, rapidly followed by formation of verrucous vegetating plaques with peripheral pustules resembling Figure 22.9.[18]

Pemphigus foliaceus is a rare variant of pemphigus characterized by subcorneal epidermal blisters and pathogenic IgG anti-desmoglein 1 autoantibodies.[19] Clinically, pemphigus foliaceus manifests with transient cutaneous superficial blisters that are fragile to the point that often only scaly, crusted erosions with erythema are found on physical examination (Figure 22.10). Lesions are typically in a seborrheic distribution – the central face, head, neck, and upper torso. Most often the disease remains localized for several years, but may progress to erythroderma (Figure 22.11). The fact that the mucous membranes are not affected is an important clinical feature that differentiates pemphigus foliaceus from pemphigus vulgaris. The absence of mucosal lesions in

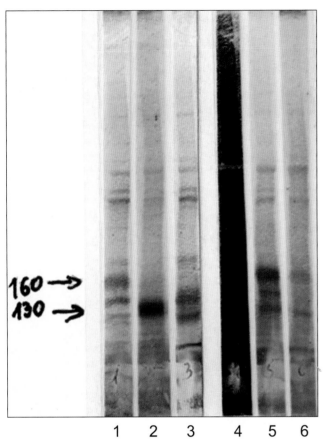

FIGURE 22.7: *Immunoblot analysis of pemphigus sera on epidermal extracts. Lanes 1 and 2: control sera from patients with pemphigus foliaceus and pemphigus vulgaris, respectively. Lanes 5 and 6: the antibodies bind to both the 160 kd and 130 kd antigens.*

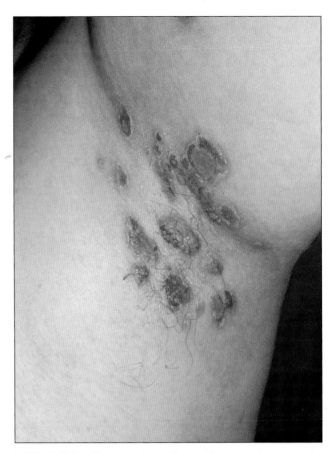

FIGURE 22.8: *Neumann type of pemphigus vegetans: vegetations arise at the places of persisting erosions.*

pemphigus foliaceus is explained by the compensatory presence of desmoglein 3 in the squamous mucosal epithelia.[20] DIF is similar to that in pemphigus vulgaris, but a stronger staining has been described in the upper epidermal portion. Circulating antiepithelial cell surface IgG antibodies are best detected by IIF using guinea pig lip substrate. By immunoblotting and ELISA, the antibodies in pemphigus foliaceus specifically bind to desmoglein 1.

An endemic subtype of pemphigus foliaceus, known as fogo selvagem (from the Portuguese "wild fire"), exists in certain regions of Brazil and other countries of South America.[21] Endemic pemphigus foliaceus differs from the nonendemic form of the disease in its geographic distribution, high familial incidence, and younger age of onset;[22] a higher incidence of severe generalized exfoliative forms is related to a greater morbidity and mortality in fogo selvagem. An endemic form of pemphigus foliaceus has also been recently described in Colombia[23] and Tunisia.[24] The endemic nature of the condition is thought to be precipitated by an immune response to an environmental antigen(s), currently not yet identified.

Pemphigus erythematosus, also referred to as pemphigus seborrhoicus, or Senear–Usher syndrome, is a rare subtype of pemphigus foliaceus that combines clinical and immunopathologic features of pemphigus and cutaneous systemic lupus erythematosus (SLE) (Figure 22.12). Usually the scalp, face, upper portions of the chest, and back are involved. The lesions of the face may show the typical butterfly distribution characteristic of SLE. In addition to the intercellular epidermal staining pattern, DIF in pemphigus erythematosus shows a band of immunoreactants at the dermal–epidermal junction.

PNP is the most severe variant of the disease, occurring in association with malignancies, mainly of B-cell lymphoproliferative origin. It was defined in 1990 on clinical, histological, and immunologic criteria.[25] The autoantibody response in PNP is directed against an antigen complex composed of desmogleins 1 and 3, as well as to desmosomal proteins of the plakin family, including desmoplakins I and II, envoplakin, periplakin, the 230 kd antigen of bullous pemphigoid (BP), and a yet not fully identified 170-kda antigen.[26,27,28] Clinical symptoms of PNP combine features of pemphigus, erythema multiforme, or Stevens–Johnson syndrome, BP, and lichen planus. Severe involvement of multiple mucous membranes is a major clinical

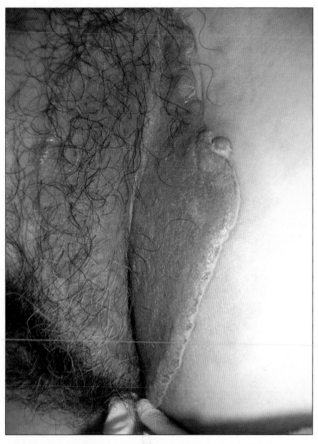

FIGURE 22.9: Hallopeau type of pemphigus vegetans: a solitary vegetating plaque resembling pyoderma vegetans.

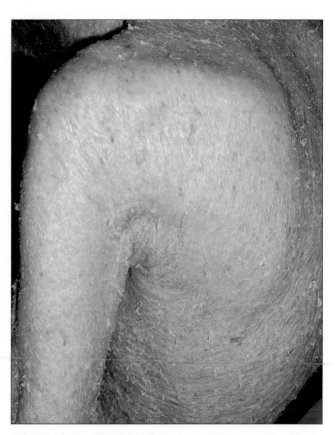

FIGURE 22.11: Pemphigus foliaceus: exfoliative erythroderma.

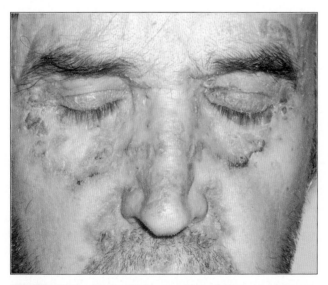

FIGURE 22.10: Nonendemic pemphigus foliaceus: scaly, erythematous plaques with few crusted erosions at the periphery, located in the seborrheic zones.

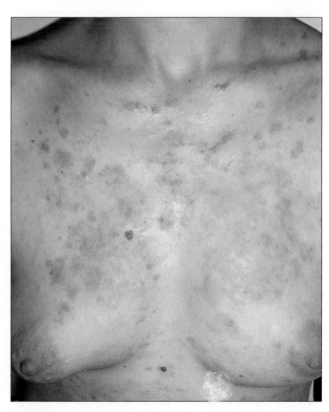

FIGURE 22.12: Pemphigus erythematosus: superficial crusted erosions with erythema and scaling on sun-exposed skin.

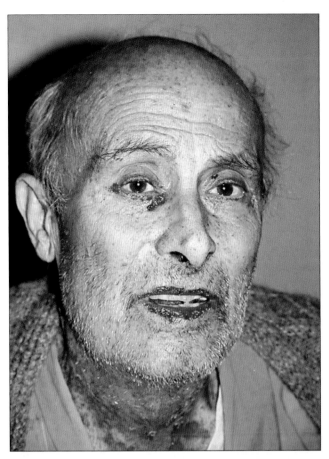

FIGURE 22.13: Paraneoplastic pemphigus: prominent involvement of the ocular, nasal, and oral mucosa, extending on the lips.

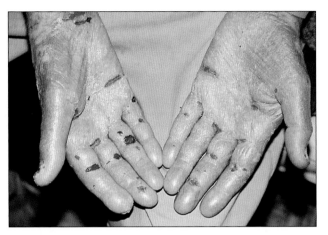

FIGURE 22.14: Palmoplantar blistering and targetoid lesions are suggestive of paraneoplastic pemphigus.

feature (Figure 22.13). Cutaneous lesions are polymorphic and may consist of flaccid but also tense blisters, morbilliform exanthema, lichenoid or psoriasiform changes, as well as palmoplantar target lesions (Figure 22.14).[29] DIF reveals deposits of immunoreactants in the intercellular (pemphigus-like) and/or linear BMZ (pemphigoid-like) pattern. By IIF, PNP antibodies react with the simple, columnar, and transitional epithelial tissue substrates (rat bladder substrate) in addition to the stratified squamous epithelium.[30]

Approximately 80% of reported cases with PNP are linked to non-Hodgkin's lymphoma, CLL, and Castleman disease, and less commonly Waldenström macroglobulinemia, T-cell lymphoma, thymoma, Hodgkin's disease, retroperitoneal sarcoma, reticulum cell sarcoma, round-cell liposarcoma, and inflammatory fibrosarcoma have been described.[31,32] Isolated reports on association with solid cancers exist.[33] The mortality rate in PNP is estimated to be more than 90%. Death is usually secondary to sepsis, gastrointestinal (GI) bleeding, multiple organ failure, or respiratory failure. Respiratory failure with features of bronchiolitis obliterans occurs in approximately 30%

of patients.[34] Recently, the term "paraneoplastic autoimmune multiorgan syndrome" was introduced to encompass the aggregate of signs and symptoms associated with the distinct morbid process affecting the skin, mucosa, and lungs in a heterogeneous group of patients with PNP.[35]

Drug-induced pemphigus, first recognized half a century ago, is attributed mainly to molecules that contain a thiol (–SH) group, such as D-penicillamine, captopril, and thiopronine, or a disulfide bond that readily releases SH groups, such as penicillin and cephalosporins.[36] It has been demonstrated that these drugs possess powerful acantholytic qualities in vitro.[37] Other drugs known to induce pemphigus contain an active amide group in their molecule.[38] In some cases, the disease disappears when the drug is withdrawn (drug-induced pemphigus), but it usually continues even after removal of the initiating agent (drug-triggered pemphigus). Some cases of pemphigus have been described after occupational contact with pesticides, which led to the description of "contact pemphigus" as a variant of environmentally induced disease.[39,40] Besides, pemphigus has been reported in association with several other autoimmune diseases, including SLE, myasthenia gravis, rheumatoid arthritis, and BP.

Systemic corticosteroids are the mainstay of treatment for pemphigus. Several corticosteroid regimens have been proposed in the literature, and there has been a debate on whether rapid institution of treatment and higher initial steroid dose are related to more favorable outcome. Usually prednisolone is administered at a dose of 40–60 mg daily in mild disease, and 60–100 mg daily in more severe cases, with or without other immunosuppressive agents, and is continued until there is cessation of appearance of new blistering lesions and healing of the majority of erosions.[41] The dosage is then reduced by one half until all of the lesions have cleared, followed by tapering to a minimum effective maintenance dosage. Because the disease has a chronic course, patients receiving long-term corticosteroid therapy frequently have serious side effects. Alternative or adjuvant therapies for patients who do not respond to or who experience complications from corticosteroids include immunosuppressive agents such as cyclophosphamide, azathioprine, cyclosporine, methotrexate, and mycophenolate mofetil, and immunomodulatory drugs and procedures such as dapsone, gold salts, and plasmapheresis.[42] Administration of high-dose intravenous immunoglobulins (2 g/kg/month) has been successfully employed in cases of pemphigus unresponsive to conventional immunosuppressive treatment.[43] Recently, a single cycle of rituximab, a monoclonal antibody directed against the CD20 antigen of B lymphocytes, has been demonstrated to effectively control severe pemphigus, but the potential long-term risks of this treatment need to be further assessed.[44]

Even with the use of corticosteroids and other immunosuppressive agents, there is still significant morbidity and mortality associated with pemphigus. A common cause of death is infection secondary to the immunosuppression required to treat the disease. Most deaths occur within the first few years of the disease. Unfortunately, many of the drugs used to treat this disease have serious side effects, and patients must be monitored closely for infection, renal and liver function abnormalities, electrolyte disturbances, hypertension, diabetes, anemia, and GI bleeding.[45]

AUTOIMMUNE SUBEPIDERMAL BULLOUS DERMATOSES

Autoimmune subepidermal blistering dermatoses include the pemphigoid group of diseases, LAD, EBA, and DH. With the exception of DH, all these disorders are characterized by circulating and tissue-bound autoantibodies against various components of the dermo-epidermal anchoring complex.[46] Anchoring complexes are specialized focal attachment sites within the cutaneous BMZ that play a crucial role in dermo-epidermal adhesion. Antibody binding to various proteins within this complex results in dermo-epidermal separation and tense blister formation. The dermo-epidermal anchoring complex consists of hemidesmosomes of the basal keratinocytes, anchoring filaments of the basement membrane, and anchoring fibrils of the papillary dermis. Structural proteins within this complex, described as autoantigens in various autoimmune bullous dermatoses, include BP antigen 180 (BP, pemphigoid gestationis, mucous membrane pemphigoid, LAD), BP230 (BP), $\alpha6\beta4$ integrin (mucous membrane pemphigoid), laminin 5 and 6 (mucous membrane pemphigoid), and type VII collagen (EBA and bullous SLE). Recent advances in the molecular characterization of BMZ components have led to a better understanding of the interaction between these molecules as well as the autoimmune response against these proteins.

PEMPHIGOID GROUP

The pemphigoid group of autoimmune bullous dermatoses is characterized by the production of autoantibodies targeting adhesion molecules that are part of the hemidesmosomes at the dermal–epidermal junction. Their immunohistological hallmark is the formation of subepidermal blister and deposits of immunoreactants, usually IgG and complement, along the BMZ. The pemphigoid group of bullous dermatoses comprises BP, mucous membrane (cicatricial) pemphigoid, pemphigoid gestationis, and lichen planus pemphigoides. Other recently identified rare forms of pemphigoid include p200 pemphigoid, p105 pemphigoid, and antilaminin 5 pemphigoid.

BP

BP is a subepidermal autoimmune bullous disease typically affecting elderly individuals older than 60 years. In 1953,[47] BP was first described as a separate disease from pemphigus vulgaris, and later studies in 1967[48] revealed the presence of in vivo bound and circulating autoantibodies directed against the BMZ of stratified epithelia. Two hemidesmosomal proteins, the BP antigen 230 (BP230), also termed BP antigen 1 (BPAG1) and the BP antigen 180 (BP180), also termed BP antigen 2 (BPAG2) or type XVII collagen, have been identified as the targets of the autoantibodies in BP.[49,50] A passive-transfer mouse model of BP strongly suggests that antibodies directed against the BP180 protein are of primary pathogenic importance in the development of the disease (Liu et al, 1993).

BP is believed to be the most common autoimmune blistering disease in Western European countries, with an estimated incidence of 6–7 cases per 1 million population per year in France[51] and Germany[52] and even higher in the United Kingdom.[53] The disease appears to be rarer in the Far East.[54] Historically, BP has been thought to be of better prognosis than pemphigus.[55] Over the past decade, however, several large European studies demonstrated that, even with treatment, patients with BP have a prognosis as grim as a diagnosis of end-stage heart disease, with more than 40% of patients dying within 12 months.[56-58] Much of the mortality may be related to the age and the general condition of patients. In a retrospective study from Scotland, 48% of patients with BP died within 2 years of diagnosis, particularly from respiratory diseases.[59] Treatment with corticosteroids and other immunosuppressive agents may also play a role. It has been suggested that patients with circulating antibodies to BPAG2 tend to have a poorer prognosis due to a more severe disease requiring higher doses of systemic steroids.[60,61]

Clinically, BP is characterized by a polymorphic eruption consisting of large, tense blisters on erythematous or normal-appearing skin, urticaria-like patches and plaques,

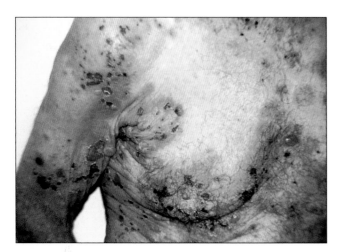

FIGURE 22.15: *Bullous pemphigoid in an elderly man: tense blisters on inflammatory background, involving the flexural surfaces and lateral trunk.*

and eczematous plaques. Usually, the eruption is intensely pruritic. There might be a prodromal period of generalized pruritus that lasts for months without any skin manifestations.[62] The eruption is usually widespread, with a predilection for the flexural surfaces of the arms and legs, lower abdomen, and the lateral aspects of the trunk (Figure 22.15). Localized forms also occur. In rare occasions, BP may affect mucosal surfaces such as the mouth, but scarring is not observed. Rarely, BP may occur in children.[63]

BP has been described in association with carcinoma at various sites, as well as with sarcoma, melanoma, and lymphoproliferative disorders; however, case–control studies did not confirm the significance of this association, which seems to be most likely related to the old age of the patients.[64] Thus, unless abnormalities are found on physical examination, exhaustive investigations to rule out malignant disease are not recommended. Association of BP with a variety of other autoimmune disorders (such as rheumatoid arthritis, Hashimoto thyroiditis, dermatomyositis, SLE, and autoimmune thrombocytopenia) was, but evidence for such an increased incidence was not, revealed by large controlled studies regarding such a relationship.[65] In some cases BP has been thought to be induced by physical injury (burn, radiotherapy, ultraviolet irradiation)[66] or by systemic or topical medications.[67]

The diagnosis of BP relies on the histology findings of subepidermal blistering accompanied by eosinophilic infiltration in the superficial dermis, and on the results of IF testing. Linear IgG and C3 deposition at the BMZ are observed on DIF of perilesional skin (Figure 22.16). IIF reveals circulating IgG anti-BMZ antibodies in patients' serum that react with the epidermal side of 1.0 M NaCl split skin as a substrate (Figure 22.17). Autoantibodies against the NC16A domain of BP180 are identified by ELISA.

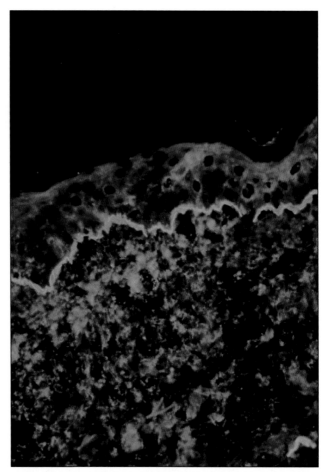

FIGURE 22.16: *Bullous pemphigoid: direct immunofluorescence on perilesional skin showing linear C3 at the basement membrane zone.*

Treatment of BP consists of corticosteroids, administered at lower doses (0.5–0.75 mg/kg/day) than those used to treat pemphigus, alone or in combination with steroid-sparing agents such as azathioprine, mycophenolate mofetil, or tetracycline. These drugs are usually started simultaneously, followed by a gradual tapering of the prednisone and continuation of the steroid-sparing agent until clinical remission is achieved. Methotrexate may be used in patients with severe disease who are unable to tolerate prednisone. Plasma exchange therapy may be considered in refractory cases. Because most morbidity and mortality are secondary to treatment, there is now a tendency to treat patients with less aggressive regimens. In mild cases, potent topical corticosteroids may be sufficient. The disease is self-limited, and approximately one half of treated cases will remit within 6 years.[68]

Mucous Membrane (Cicatricial) Pemphigoid

Mucous membrane pemphigoid, previously known as CP, is a rare but well-defined variant of pemphigoid,

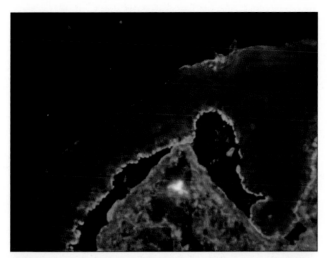

FIGURE 22.17: Bullous pemphigoid: indirect immunofluorescence on salt-split skin substrate reveals binding of antibodies to the roof of the blister.

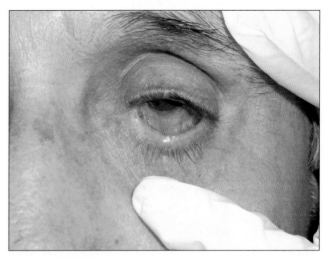

FIGURE 22.19: Ocular cicatricial pemphigoid: conjunctival erosions on the lower lid with multiple synechiae.

characterized by erosive, scarring subepidermal blistering lesions of mucosal surfaces, particularly of the oral mucosa and ocular membranes, and less often, the skin. Depending on the mucosal surface that is mainly affected, patients with mucous membrane pemphigoid may first present to the ophthalmologist, dermatologist, dentist, gastroenterologist, gynecologist, otolaryngologist, or to the primary care physician. The oral mucosa is almost always affected, followed by other mucosae (eye, nose, pharynx, larynx, esophagus, genitalia, anus) and rarely the skin. Desquamative gingivitis is the most common oral manifestation (Figure 22.18), but nonhealing ulcers on buccal mucosa and soft and hard palates are not rare. Bullae quickly rupture, leaving slowly healing erosions, followed by scarring and adhesions between the various structures of the oral cavity involved. Laryngeal involvement may lead to a sore throat,

hoarseness, and possible loss of speech. Supraglottic stenosis secondary to erosions, scarring, and edema may necessitate a tracheostomy as the airway is further compromised. Esophageal erosions and scarring can lead to the formation of strictures, with dysphagia, odynophagia, and weight loss. Ocular CP is characterized by progressive subconjunctival cicatrization that leads to decreased vision, photosensitivity, scarring, and fibrosis that can eventually cause blindness (Figure 22.19). The course of the disease is usually slow but progressive and may be punctuated by periods of explosive inflammatory activity. There is a 2:1 preponderance for women; the average age of onset of CP is reported to be 65 years, but this does not take into account the observation that most cases of CP are relatively advanced at the time of diagnosis.[69]

A less frequently encountered variant of CP, referred to as Brunsting–Perry benign pemphigoid, is characterized by vesiculobullous lesions and scarring confined to the head and neck areas.[70]

Pemphigoid Gestationis

Pemphigoid gestationis, previously known as "herpes gestationis," is a pregnancy-specific autoimmune subepidermal blistering dermatosis that usually develops in the second or third trimester and clinically presents with severely pruritic urticarial lesions that progress to large tense bullae (Figure 22.20). The estimated incidence of the disease ranges between 1 in 10,000 and 1 in 50,000 pregnancies,[71] with only 14% of the cases developing postpartum.[72]

Pemphigoid gestationis is characterized by linear deposition of C3 along the BMZ on DIF and by the presence of circulating IgG autoantibodies directed toward the transmembrane 180 kd protein BPAG2. Epitope mapping of the antigen showed that pemphigoid gestationis and BP autoantibodies bind to a common antigenic site within

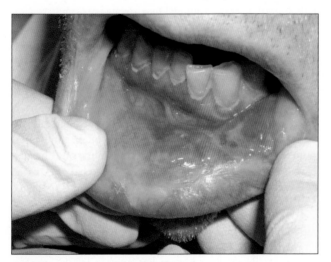

FIGURE 22.18: Bleeding erosions on the gingival and lip mucosa in cicatricial pemphigoid.

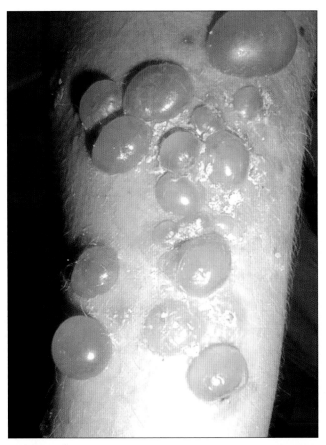

FIGURE 22.20: *Tense blisters with clear fluid over the inner aspect of the forearms in a patient with pemphigoid gestationis.*

the noncollagenous domain (NC16A) of BPAG2.[73] The exact pathogenesis of pemphigoid gestationis is still largely unknown, but it has been postulated that the disease is primarily related to an allogeneic reaction against the fetoplacental unit, triggered by an aberrant expression of *major* histocompatibility complex class II molecules in the placenta. The result is an autoimmune response directed against the chorioamniotic cells but cross-reacting with BPAG2 in the skin. Hormonal factors have also been implicated in the pathogenesis of the disease as flares have been reported with menses or use of oral contraceptives.

LAD

LAD is an autoimmune subepidermal blistering disease defined by the presence of linear deposits of IgA at the dermal–epidermal junction. It was first recognized as a separate entity from DH in 1979,[74] based on the finding of in vivo bound IgA anti-BMZ antibodies and the lack of an associated gluten-sensitive enteropathy. Currently, there is compelling evidence that the IgA autoantibodies in LAD are directed against heterogeneous antigen targets in the BMZ and ultrastructurally localize to the lamina lucida, anchoring fibrils, or the lamina densa.[75] The major

LAD antigens identified by immunoblot analysis in dermal and/or epidermal tissue extract include BP180 (and its breakdown products, the 97 kd and 120 kd antigens) and BP230, a 285 kd antigen, and collagen VII.[76–79]

LAD can occur at any age, but there are two peaks of onset: in adults between 40 and 60 years old, and in children of preschool age. Although the childhood variant has been formerly considered as a distinct entity termed "chronic bullous disease of childhood," both forms of LAD have identical immunopathologic features and are currently regarded as one and the same disease process. The estimated incidence of LAD in studies from Western Europe varies from 0.22 to 0.5 per million.[80–82] It has been reported to be more common in women than in men.[83]

Although in the majority cases LAD is "idiopathic," there have been a number of triggering factors reported, including trauma, ultraviolet exposure, infections, and a wide range of drugs, such as vancomycin, penicillin, antiepileptics, captopril, diclofenac, and sulfonamides.[84] Drug-induced LAD tends to resolve after discontinuation of the offending drug and is associated with a lower morbidity;[85] however, some more severe cases mimicking erythema multiforme, Stevens–Johnson syndrome, and toxic epidermal necrolysis have been described.[86–88] Other important systemic associations of LAD include autoimmune diseases, such as inflammatory bowel disease, SLE, dermatomyositis, rheumatoid arthritis, and acquired hemophilia. Besides, a relationship between LAD and lymphoid but also nonlymphoid malignant diseases has been reported, including Hodgkin disease, non-Hodgkin's lymphoma, chronic lymphatic leukemia, multiple myeloma, and plasmocytoma, but also visceral malignant tumors such as bladder, breast, esophageal, uterine, ovarian, thyroid, and renal cell carcinoma.[89]

The clinical features of LAD can be heterogeneous. The cutaneous eruption is characterized by large, tense bullae, which may arise on normal skin or on erythematous bases, and urticarial plaques. Arciform or annular blister arrangement at the periphery of the lesions that show a tendency to heal in the center is a characteristic feature of LAD, described as the "cluster of jewels" sign (Figure 22.21). Lesions are usually generalized, with some tendency to grouping but, in contrast to DH, no symmetry is present. Common areas of involvement include the lower trunk and limbs, especially the inner thighs and pelvic regions; the latter distribution is more typical for childhood LAD. Pruritus may be severe or entirely absent. Mucous membrane involvement is frequent, reported in 60%–80% of patients;[90] rarely mucosal involvement can be the sole clinical manifestation.

The diagnosis of LAD is based on the histology, which invariably shows a subepidermal blister with a superficial dermal infiltrate of neutrophils, and on the DIF finding of linear IgA along the BMZ. The IIF of patient's serum can be either negative or detect low levels of IgA anti-BMZ

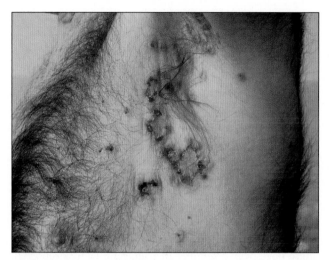

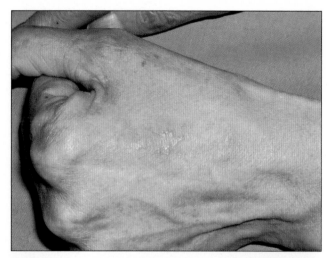

FIGURE 22.21: *Adult linear immunoglobulin A dermatoses: annular lesions with tense blisters at the periphery ("cluster of jewels" sign).*

FIGURE 22.22: *Classical epidermolysis bullosa acquisita: atrophy and milia are observed at the sites of healing mechanobullous lesions.*

antibodies that would react with the epidermal, dermal, or both sides of the blister when tested on saline-separated skin as a substrate.

The aim of treatment in LAD is to suppress disease activity with the minimum treatment possible. In the majority of cases there is spontaneous remission between 3 and 6 years after disease onset; therefore, it is important not to overtreat the disease. Dapsone is the empiric therapy of choice in managing LAD; occasionally, low-dose oral corticosteroids are needed as an adjuvant. There are reports of successful treatment of LAD with macrolide antibiotics.[91] Immunosuppressive agents such as mycophenolate mofetil and cyclosporine have been used with a variable success. Successful use of IVIG therapy has been reported in patients with progressive LAD that was unresponsive to dapsone, systemic corticosteroids, and systemic antibiotics.[92]

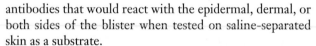

EBA

EBA is an acquired autoimmune bullous dermatosis characterized by subepidermal blisters, and tissue-bound and circulating antibodies directed against sublamina densa of the epithelial basement membranes.[93] The patient's antibodies recognize type VII collagen, which is the major component of anchoring fibrils, the structures that connect lamina densa of the BMZ to the papillary dermis.[94] It was first described by Elliott[95] more than 100 years ago as an acquired form of epidermolysis bullosa, with clinical features highly reminiscent of the inherited forms of dystrophic epidermolysis bullosa, in which a hereditary defect in the gene encoding for type VII collagen results in paucity of anchoring fibrils and skin fragility. In 1971, Roenick and colleagues[96] established the first diagnostic criteria for EBA as an adult-onset disease closely resembling heredi-

tary dystrophic epidermolysis bullosa and characterized by spontaneous or trauma-induced blisters that heal with scars and milia. In addition to this "classical" mechanobullous form, however, several inflammatory subtypes of EBA were described that can be clinically indistinguishable from BP or CP,[97–100] and LAD, and can, therefore, remain underdiagnosed. EBA is a chronic disease that is difficult to treat and for which there is no cure.[101] It is associated with significant morbidity resulting from involvement of various skin and mucosal surfaces.

The exact incidence and prevalence of EBA is unknown, but it seems to be a rare disease. The results from few available studies showed an incidence of 0.22 cases per million people per year in Germany,[102] 0.26 per million per year in France, 0.23 per million per year in Kuwait,[103] to a slightly higher incidence of 0.5 per million per year in Singapore.[104] It appears that EBA is slightly more common in women and in blacks.[105] The mean age of onset is in persons in their 40s; the disease occurs infrequently in elderly persons and even less often in children.

The clinical features of EBA are heterogeneous. The "classical" form presents as a noninflammatory mechanobullous disease with acral distribution. Due to the extreme mechanical fragility of the skin, blisters occur under minor trauma over the back of the hands, knuckles, elbows, knees, sacral area, and feet. Healing occurs with scarring and milia formation (Figure 22.22).

Approximately one half of patients with EBA present with widespread inflammatory vesiculobullous eruption mimicking BP. There is often prominent involvement of the trunk and flexural skin (Figure 22.23). In contrast to classical EBA, skin fragility is not prominent and scarring and milia formation may be minimal or absent. In some cases, overlapping between both the classical and the BP-like forms may exist, or can be seen in evolution.

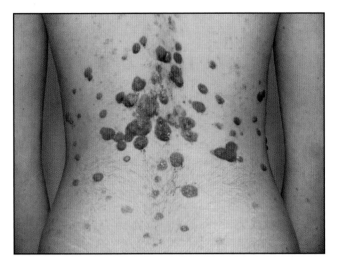

FIGURE 22.23: Inflammatory epidermolysis bullosa acquisita: widespread blistering eruption involving the trunk.

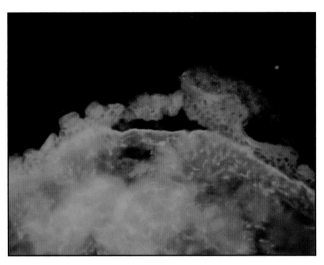

FIGURE 22.24: Epidermolysis bullosa acquisita: indirect immunofluorescence on salt-split skin substrate reveals binding of antibodies to the floor of the blister.

Another group of patients with EBA may have predominant involvement of the mucous membranes that can result in irreversible complications similar to those seen in CP, including blindness and esophageal strictures. Tracheal involvement and upper airway obstruction requiring tracheotomy have been described.[106] EBA has been reported in association with a number of other systemic diseases, including SLE, inflammatory bowel disease, amyloidosis, multiple myeloma, autoimmune thyroiditis, diabetes mellitus, acquired hemophilia, and multiple endocrinopathy syndromes.[107] The most frequent association is with inflammatory bowel disease. A recent study showed that sera from patients with Crohn disease reacted by immunoblot analysis with type VII collagen, which exists in both the skin and the gut.[108] In addition, paraneoplastic cases of EBA in association with lymphoproliferative malignancies have been reported.[109]

DIF of perilesional skin reveals linear deposits of IgG and more rarely, C3 at the BMZ. On IIF, in the serum of 10%–30% of patients, circulating IgG anti-BMZ antibodies are present that bind to the dermal side of a salt-split skin substrate (Figure 22.24). In patients who lack serum anti-BMZ antibodies, DIF on salt-split skin sections is helpful to discriminate EBA from BP by demonstrating deposits of immunoreactants at the dermal side of the blister.[110] Using direct immunoelectron microscopy, the IgG and/or C3 deposits were found to localize to the sublamina densa region of dermal–epidermal junction.[111] By immunoblotting (or immunoprecipitation), EBA autoantibodies bind to 290 kd and 145 kd proteins, which represents the full-length α chain of type VII collagen or its amino-terminal globular NC1 domain, respectively.[94] A sensitive ELISA for the detection of autoantibodies to type VII collagen using recombinant protein is also available.[112]

Treatment for EBA is challenging and is often unsatisfactory. Mild cases follow a chronic time course, whereas aggressive disease is often difficult to control and is associated with a significant mortality rate. Systemic corticosteroids, used as standard treatment for EBA, often in combination with cyclophosphamide, azathioprine, or methotrexate, may be ineffective in some cases. Some therapeutic success has been reported with colchicine, dapsone, photopheresis, infliximab, or high-dose intravenous immunoglobulin.[113]

DERMATITIS HERPETIFORMIS

Dermatitis herpetiformis (DH), also known as Duhring disease, is an uncommon subepidermal blistering disease characterized by an intensely pruritic cutaneous eruption, typical IF findings, and association with a gluten-sensitive enteropathy. Since its initial description in 1884 by Louis Duhring,[114] DH has been confounded for decades with BP under the term Duhring–Brocq disease. Through the 1960s to 1970s, however, several clinical and IF features, typical for DH and not found in other immunobullous diseases, were identified that led to the current concept of DH as a distinct immunobullous disorder, strongly related to celiac disease (CD) in the spectrum of the gluten-sensitive disorders.[115–117] DH and CD have a common immunogenetic background, sharing a strong association with certain major histocompatibility complex antigens, such as HLA-B8, HLA-DR3, and HLA-DQw2. First-degree relatives of patients with DH frequently develop CD. Immunohistologically, DH is characterized by granular deposits of IgA and complement C3 in the papillary dermis of uninvolved skin.[118] Recently, it has been found that epidermal and tissue transglutaminases, cytosolic enzymes involved in cell envelope formation during keratinocyte

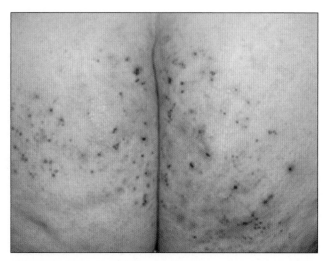

FIGURE 22.25: *Dermatitis herpetiformis: symmetric pruritic polymorph eruption on the buttocks.*

differentiation, are the major autoantigens recognized in the skin lesions of DH and targeted by the circulating IgA antibodies to endomysium (intermyofibril substance of smooth muscle) found in the serum of patients with DH and CD.[119,120]

Clinically, DH presents with an intensely itchy cutaneous eruption involving symmetrically the extensor surfaces, including elbows, knees, shoulders, sacrum, and buttocks. The eruption is polymorphic and consists of urticarial plaques, erythematous papules, and vesicles, often grouped in a herpetiform pattern (Figure 22.25). As the vesicles are heavily excoriated, only small erosions, crusting, and postinflammatory pigment changes can be seen in evolution. The scalp and face are often affected. Mucosal surfaces are usually spared, although oral lesions have been frequently described earlier, probably due to confusion of the disease with pemphigoid or LAD. The onset of DH is usually in the second or third decade, but may occur at any age. A diet overloaded with gluten or iodides (seafood) can often precipitate a flare of the eruption. The eruption runs a chronic course, with flares and remissions, especially if unrecognized or left untreated. Patients from both genders may be affected, but there seems to be a slightly higher male preponderance.

DH and CD show an uneven geographic distribution, with higher incidence rates in Europe or in populations with European descent. In Sweden and Finland, the incidence is between 0.86 and 1.45 in 100,000 per year. In Anglo-Saxon and Scandinavian populations, the prevalence is between 10 and 39 per 100,000.[121] In contrast, DH is extremely rare in Orientals and is uncommon in Asians and Afro-Caribbeans.[122] Morbidity in DH is mainly related to the intense pruritus, scratching, discomfort, and insomnia, as well as to the risk of superimposed bacterial or viral infections. Systemic complications include complications of the associated gluten-sensitive enteropathy, which is now

accepted to be present in practically all patients with DH, despite the fact that most of them may have only subclinical GI disease. Symptoms related to the gluten-sensitive enteropathy are milder than those seen in patients with CD without skin findings but may include malnutrition, weight loss, abdominal pain, dyspepsia (they can even mimic peptic ulcer disease), and perforation. Deficiency states (such as folate deficiency, iron deficiency anemia, and B12 deficiency), neurologic disturbances, bone disease, infertility, chronic fatigue, and premature dental loss may all be seen.

Patients with DH, similarly to those with CD, have a higher incidence of associated autoimmune disorders, including thyroid disorders, atrophic gastritis, type I diabetes, pernicious anemia, Addison disease, vitiligo, and various connective tissue disorders.[4] Besides, patients with DH, like patients with CD, are at an increased risk for developing GI lymphoma of T-cell lineage, usually described as enteropathy-associated T-cell lymphomas.[4,123] Therefore, when DH is diagnosed, examinations for possible signs and symptoms of such associations is necessary.[124]

The diagnosis of DH is based on clinical, histologic, and IF criteria. Histologic examination of an early vesicle

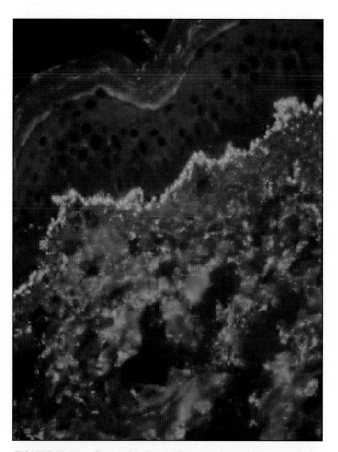

FIGURE 22.26: *Dermatitis herpetiformis: direct immunofluorescence on perilesional skin showing granular immunoglobulin A deposits at the dermal–epidermal junction, more intense in the tips of the dermal papillae.*

lesion shows subepidermal blister formation with collections of neutrophils forming microabscesses in the dermal papillae. DIF of perilesional uninvolved skin shows granular deposition of IgA and complement C3 along the BMZ, mostly confined to the tips of the dermal papillae (Figure 22.26). IIF of patients' sera shows IgA-antiendomysial antibodies on monkey esophagus as a substrate; however, no anti-BMZ antibodies are present in DH. Serum antibodies to tissue transglutaminase are detected using ELISA.

The treatment of DH is aimed to combat both the skin and GI symptoms. The most common medications used to treat DH are dapsone and sulfapyridine. Administration of dapsone with a starting dose of 50–100 mg daily is usually followed by a dramatic response, with disappearance of the pruritus within 24 hours; this rapid response helps to confirm the diagnosis. Common side effects of dapsone therapy that should be carefully monitored include hemolysis, methemoglobinemia, and agranulocytosis; dapsone is contraindicated in patients with glucose-6-phosphate dehydrogenase deficiency. In patients who do not tolerate dapsone, the cutaneous eruption can be alternatively controlled by sulfapyridine 0.5–2.0 g daily (to a maximum dose of 4.0 g daily) or with sulphamethoxypyridazine 0.5–1.0 g daily; however, sulfonamides do not influence the GI changes. Similar to the treatment of CD, treatment of DH should always include a gluten-free diet for a lifetime, which may result in remission of both the skin lesions and the bowel disease. The results of a retrospective study of 487 patients with DH showed a protective role for a strict gluten-free diet against development of lymphoma in DH patients.[125]

REFERENCES

1. Fine JD. Management of acquired bullous skin diseases. N Engl J Med. 1995; 30:1475–84.
2. Powell AM, Black M. A stepwise approach to the diagnosis of blisters in the clinic. Clin Dermatol. 2001; 19:598–606.
3. Harman KE. New laboratory techniques for the assessment of acquired immunobullous disorders. Clin Exp Dermatol. 2002; 27:40–6.
4. Mihai S, Sitaru C. Immunopathology and molecular diagnosis of autoimmune bullous diseases. J Cell Mol Med. 2007; 11:462–81.
5. Vassileva S. Immunofluorescence in dermatology. Int J Dermatol. 1993; 32:153–61.
6. Prost C, Labeille B, Chaussade V, et al. Immunoelectron microscopy in subepidermal autoimmune bullous diseases: a prospective study of IgG and C3 bound in vivo in 32 patients. J Invest Dermatol. 1987; 89:567–73.
7. Pas HH. Immunoblot assay in differential diagnosis of autoimmune blistering skin diseases. Clin Dermatol. 2001; 19:622–30.
8. Amagai M. Pemphigus: autoimmunity to epidermal cell adhesion molecules. Adv Dermatol. 1996; 11:319–52.
9. Seidenbaum M, David M, Sandbank M. The course and prognosis of pemphigus. A review of 115 patients. Int J Dermatol. 1988; 27:580–4.
10. Bystryn JC, Steinman NM. The adjuvant therapy of pemphigus. An update. Arch Dermatol. 1996; 132:203–12.
11. Tsankov N, Vassileva S, Kamarashev J, et al. Epidemiology of pemphigus in Sofia, Bulgaria. A 16-year retrospective study (1980–1995). Int J Dermatol. 2000; 39:104–8.
12. Bystryn JC. Pemphigus. Lancet. 2005; 366:61–73.
13. Kanwar AJ, Kaur S. Pemphigus in children. Int J Dermatol. 1991; 30:343–6.
14. Amagai M, Tsunoda K, Zillikens D, et al. The clinical phenotype of pemphigus is defined by the antidesmoglein autoantibody profile. J Am Acad Dermatol. 1999; 40:167–70.
15. Ding X, Aoki V, Mascaro JM, et al. Mucosal and mucocutaneous (generalized) pemphigus vulgaris show distinct autoantibody profiles. J Invest Dermatol. 1997; 109:592–6.
16. Ishii K, Amagai M, Hall RP, et al. Characterization of autoantibodies in pemphigus using antigen-specific enzyme-linked immunosorbent assays with baculovirus-expressed recombinant desmogleins. J Immunol. 1997; 159:2010–17.
17. Harman KE, Gratian MJ, Bhogal BS, et al. A study of desmoglein 1 autoantibodies in pemphigus vulgaris: racial differences in frequency and the association with a more severe phenotype. Br J Dermatol. 2000; 143:343–8.
18. Lever WF. Pemphigus and pemphigoid. Springfield IL: Charles C. Thomas; 1965. 266 pp.
19. Stanley JR, Klaus-Kovtun V, Sampaio SAP. Antigenic specificity of fogo selvagem autoantibodies is similar to North American pemphigus foliaceus and distinct from pemphigus vulgaris autoantibodies. J Invest Dermatol. 1986; 87:197–201.
20. Shirakata Y, Amagai M, Hanakawa Y, et al. Lack of mucosal involvement in pemphigus foliaceus may be due to low expression of desmoglein 1. J Invest Dermatol. 1998; 110:76–8.
21. Diaz LA, Sampaio SAP, Rivitti EA, et al. Endemic pemphigus foliaceus (fogo selvagem). I. Clinical features and immunopathology. J Am Acad Dermatol. 1989; 20:657–9.
22. Friedman H, Campbell I, Rocha-Alvarez R, et al. Endemic pemphigus foliaceus (fogo selvagem) in native Americans from Brazil. J Am Acad Dermatol. 1995; 32:949–56.
23. Abreu-Velez AM, Hashimoto T, Bollag WB, et al. A unique form of endemic pemphigus in northern Colombia. J Am Acad Dermatol. 2003; 49:599–608.
24. Bastuji-Garin S, Souissi R, Blum L, et al. Comparative epidemiology of pemphigus in Tunisia and France: unusual incidence of pemphigus foliaceus in young Tunisian women. J Invest Dermatol. 1995; 104:302.
25. Anhalt GJ, Kim SC, Stanley JR, et al. Paraneoplastic pemphigus: an autoimmune mucocutaneous disease associated with neoplasia. N Engl J Med. 1990; 323:1729–35.
26. Amagai M, Nishikawa T, Nousari HC, et al. Antibodies against desmoglein 3 (pemphigus vulgaris antigen) are present in sera from patients with paraneoplastic pemphigus and cause acantholysis in vivo in neonatal mice. J Clin Invest. 1998; 102:775–82.
27. Hashimoto T, Amagai M, Watanabe K, et al. Characterization of paraneoplastic pemphigus autoantigens by immunoblot analysis. J Invest Dermatol. 1995; 104:829–34.

28. Joly P, Thomine E, Gilbert D, et al. Overlapping distribution of autoantibody specificities in paraneoplastic pemphigus and pemphigus vulgaris. J Invest Dermatol. 1994; 103:65–72.

29. Wade MS, Black MM. Paraneoplastic pemphigus: a brief update. Austral J Dermatol. 2005; 46:1–10.

30. Helou J, Allbritton J, Anhalt GJ. Accuracy of indirect immunofluorescence testing in the diagnosis of paraneoplastic pemphigus. J Am Acad Dermatol. 1995; 32:441–7.

31. Robinson ND, Hashimoto T, Amagai M, et al. The new pemphigus variants. J Am Acad Dermatol. 1999; 40:649–72.

32. Anhalt GJ. Paraneoplastic pemphigus: the role of tumours and drugs. Br J Dermatol. 2001; 144:1101–4.

33. Niimi Y, Kawana S, Hashimoto T, et al. Paraneoplastic pemphigus associated with uterine carcinoma. J Am Acad Dermatol. 2003; 48:569–72.

34. Nousari HC, Deterding R, Wojtczack H, et al. The mechanism of respiratory failure in paraneoplastic pemphigus. N Engl J Med. 1999; 340:1406–10.

35. Nguyen VT, Ndoye A, Bassler KD, et al. Classification, clinical manifestations, and immunopathological mechanisms of the epithelial variant of paraneoplastic autoimmune multiorgan syndrome. Arch Dermatol. 2001; 137:193–206.

36. Brenner S, Bialy-Golan A, Ruocco V. Drug-induced pemphigus. In: Kanitakis J, Vassileva S, Woodley D, editors. Diagnostic immunohistochemistry of the skin. London: Chapman & Hall; 1998. pp. 84–93.

37. Ruocco V, De Angelis E, Lombardi ML. Drug-induced pemphigus. II. Pathomechanisms and experimental investigations. Clin Dermatol. 1993; 11:507–13.

38. Wolf R, Brenner S. An active amide group in the molecule of drugs that induce pemphigus: a casual or causal relationship? Dermatology. 1994; 189:1–4.

39. Tsankov N, Stransky L, Kostowa M, et al. Induced pemphigus caused by occupational contact with Basochrom. Derm Beruf Umwelt. 1990; 38:91–3.

40. Tsankov N, Kazandjieva J, Gantcheva M. Contact pemphigus induced by dihydrodiphenyltrichlorethane. Eur J Dermatol. 1998; 8:442–3.

41. Harman KE, Albert S, Black MM. Guidelines for the management of pemphigus vulgaris. Br J Dermatol. 2003; 149:926–37.

42. Bystryn JC, Jiao D, Natow S. Treatment of pemphigus with intravenous immunoglobulin. J Am Acad Dermatol. 2002; 47:358–63.

43. Ahmed AR. Intravenous immunoglobulin therapy in the treatment of patients with pemphigus vulgaris unresponsive to conventional immunosuppressive treatment. J Am Acad Dermatol. 2001; 45:679–90.

44. Joly P, Mouquet H, Roujeau JC, et al. A single cycle of rituximab for the treatment of severe pemphigus. N Engl J Med. 2007; 357:545–52.

45. Bickle KM, Roarck TR, Hsu S. Autoimmune bullous dermatoses: a review. Am Fam Physician. 2002; 65:1861–70.

46. Schmidt E, Zillikens D. Autoimmune and inherited subepidermal blistering diseases: advances in the clinic and the laboratory. Adv Dermatol. 2000; 16:113–57.

47. Lever WF. Pemphigus. Medicine. 1953; 32:1–123.

48. Jordon RE, Beutner EH, Witebsky E, et al. Basement zone antibodies in bullous pemphigoid. JAMA. 1967; 200:751–8.

49. Stanley JR, Hawley-Nelson P, Yuspa SH, et al. Characterization of bullous pemphigoid antigen: a unique basement membrane protein of stratified squamous epithelia. Cell. 1981; 24:897–903.

50. Labib RS, Anhalt GJ, Patel HP, et al. Molecular heterogeneity of bullous pemphigoid antigens as detected by immunoblotting. J Immunol. 1986; 136:1231–5.

51. Bernard P, Valliant L, Labeille B, et al. Incidence and distribution of subepidermal autoimmune bullous skin diseases in three French regions. Arch Dermatol. 1995; 131:48–52.

52. Zillikens D, Wever S, Roth A, et al. Incidence of autoimmune subepidermal blistering dermatoses in a region of Central Germany. Arch Dermatol. 1995; 131:957–8.

53. Khumalo N, Kirtschig G, Middleton P, et al. Interventions for bullous pemphigoid (Review). Cochrane Database Syst Rev. 2005, 3. Art. No.: CD002292.

54. Korman NJ. Bullous pemphigoid: the latest in diagnosis, prognosis, and therapy. Arch Dermatol. 1998; 134:1137–41.

55. Swerlick RA, Korman NJ. Bullous pemphigoid: what is the prognosis? J Invest Dermatol. 2004; 122:xvii–xviii.

56. Venning VA, Wojnarowska F. Lack of predictive factors for the clinical course of bullous pemphigoid. J Am Acad Dermatol. 1992; 26:585–9.

57. Rzany B, Partscht K, Jung M, et al. Risk factors for lethal outcome in patients with bullous pemphigoid: low serum albumin level, high dosage of glucocorticosteroids, and old age. Arch Dermatol. 2002; 138:903–8.

58. Joly P, Roujeau JC, Benichou J, et al. A comparison of oral and topical corticosteroids in patients with bullous pemphigoid. N Engl J Med. 2002; 346:321–7.

59. Gudi VS, White MI, Cruickshank N, et al. Annual incidence and mortality of bullous pemphigoid in the Grampian Region of North-east Scotland. Br J Dermatol. 2005; 153:424–7.

60. Tanaka M, Hashimoto T, Dykes PJ, Nishikawa T. Clinical manifestation in 100 Japanese bullous pemphigoid cases in relation to autoantigen profiles. Clin Exp Dermatol. 1996; 21:23–7.

61. Bernard P, Bedane C, Bonnetblanc JM. Anti-BP180 autoantibodies as a marker of poor prognosis in bullous pemphigoid: a cohort analysis of 94 elderly patients. Br J Dermatol. 1997; 136:694–7.

62. Lamb PM, Abell E, Tharp M, et al. Prodromal bullous pemphigoid. Int J Dermatol. 2006; 45:209–14.

63. Kuenzli S, Grimaître M, Krischer J, et al. Childhood bullous pemphigoid: report of a case with life-threatening course during homeopathy treatment. Pediatr Dermatol. 2004; 21:160–3.

64. Venning VA, Wojnarowska F. The association of bullous pemphigoid and malignant disease: a case control study. Br J Dermatol. 1990; 123:439–45.

65. Venning VA, Wojnarowska F, Welch K. Bullous pemphigoid and autoimmunity. J Am Acad Dermatol. 1993; 29:181–4.

66. Vassileva S, Mateev G, Balabanova M, Tsankov N. Burn-induced bullous pemphigoid. J Am Acad Dermatol. 1994; 30:1027–8.

67. Vassileva S. Drug-induced pemphigoid: bullous and cicatricial. Clin Dermatol. 1998; 16:379–89.

68. Bickle KM, Roark TR, Hsu S. Autoimmune bullous dermatoses: a review. Am Fam Physician. 2002; 65:1861–70.
69. Tauber L. Autoimmune diseases affecting the ocular surface. In: Holland EJ, Mannis MJ, editors. Ocular surface disease. Medical and surgical management. New York: Springer-Verlag; 2002. pp. 113–27.
70. Michel B, Bean SF, Chorzelski T, Fedele CF. Cicatricial pemphigoid of Brunsting-Perry: immunofluorescent studies. Arch Dermatol. 1977; 113:1403–5.
71. Kroumpouzos G, Cohen LM. Specific dermatoses of pregnancy: an evidence-based systematic review. Am J Obstet Gynecol. 2003; 188:1083–92.
72. Jenkins RE, Hern S, Black MM. Clinical features and management of 87 patients with pemphigoid gestationis. Clin Exp Dermatol. 1999; 24:255–9.
73. Guidice GJ, Emery DJ, Zelickson BD, et al. Bullous pemphigoid and herpes gestationis autoantibodies recognize a common non-collagenous site on the BP180 ectodomain. J Immunol. 1993; 151:5742–50.
74. Jablonska S, Chorzelski TP. Dermatose à IgA linéaire. Ann Dermatol Venereol. 1979; 106:651.
75. Allen J, Wojnarowska F. Linear IgA disease: the IgA and IgG response to dermal antigens demonstrates a chiefly IgA response to LAD285 and a dermal 180-kDa protein. Br J Dermatol. 2003; 149:1055–8.
76. Zhou S, Ferguson DJP, Allen J, Wojnarowska F. The localization of target antigens and autoantibodies in linear IgA disease is variable: correlation of immunogold electron microscopy and immunoblotting. Br J Dermatol. 1998; 139: 591–7.
77. Zone J, Taylor T, Meyer L, et al. The 97 kDa linear IgA bullous disease antigen is identical to a portion of the extracellular domain of the 180 kDa bullous pemphigoid antigen, BPAg2. J Invest Dermatol. 1998; 110:207–10.
78. Hashimoto T, Ishiko A, Shimizu H, et al. A case of linear IgA bullous dermatosis with IgA anti-type VII collagen autoantibodies. Br J Dermatol. 1996; 134:336–9.
79. Ghohestani R, Nicolas J, Kanitakis J, et al. Linear IgA bullous dermatosis with IgA antibodies exclusively directed against the 180- or 230-kDa epidermal antigens. J Invest Dermatol. 1997; 108:854–8.
80. Wojnarowska F. What's new in linear IgA disease? J Eur Acad Dermatol Venereol. 2000; 14:441–3.
81. Zillikens D, Wever S, Roth A, et al. Incidence of autoimmune subepidermal blistering dermatoses in a region of central Germany. Arch Dermatol. 1995; 131:957–8.
82. Bernard P, Vaillant L, Labeille B, et al. Incidence and distribution of subepidermal autoimmune bullous skin diseases in three French regions. Bullous Diseases French Study Group. Arch Dermatol. 1995; 131:48–52.
83. Wojnarowska F, Marsden RA, Bhogal BS, Black MM. Chronic bullous disease of childhood, childhood cicatricial pemphigoid, and linear IgA disease of adults. A comparative study demonstrating clinical and immunopathologic overlap. J Am Acad Dermatol. 1988; 19:792–805.
84. Tonev S, Vassileva S, Kadurina M. Depot sulfonamid associated linear IgA bullous dermatosis with erythema multiforme-like clinical features. J Eur Acad Dermatol Venereol. 1998; 11:165–8.
85. Nousari H, Kimyai-Asadi A, Caeiro J, et al. Clinical, demographic, and immunohistologic features of vancomycin-induced linear IgA bullous disease of the skin. Report of 2 cases and review of the literature. Medicine. 1999; 78:1–8.
86. Tonev S, Vassileva S, Kadurina M. Depot sulfonamid associated linear IgA bullous dermatosis with erythema multiforme-like clinical features. J Eur Acad Dermatol Venereol. 1998; 11:165–8.
87. Argenyi ZB, Bergfeld WF, Valenzuela R, et al. Linear IgA bullous dermatosis mimicking erythema multiforme in adults. Int J Dermatol. 1987; 26:513–17.
88. Bachot N, Wechsler J, Demoule A, Roujeau JC. Amiodarone related linear IgA bullous dermatosis. J Am Acad Dermatol. 2003; 49:e2.
89. Godfrey K, Wojnarowska F, Leonard J. Linear IgA disease of adults: association with lymphoproliferative malignancy and possible role of other triggering factors. Br J Dermatol. 1990; 123:447–52.
90. Kelly SE, Frith PA, Millard PR, et al. A clinicopathological study of mucosal involvement in linear IgA disease. Br J Dermatol. 1988; 119:161–70.
91. Cooper SM, Powell J, Wojnarowska F. Linear IgA disease: successful treatment with erythromycin. Clin Exp Dermatol. 2002; 27:677–9.
92. Khan IU, Bhol KC, Ahmed AR. Linear IgA disease bullous dermatosis in a patient with chronic renal failure: response to intravenous immunoglobulin therapy. J Am Acad Dermatol. 1999; 40:485–8.
93. Gammon WR, Briggaman RA. Epidermolysis bullosa acquisita and bullous systemic lupus erythematosus. Diseases of autoimmunity to type VII collagen. Dermatol Clin. 1993; 11:535–47.
94. Woodley DT, Briggaman RA, O'Keefe EJ, et al. Identification of the skin basement-membrane autoantigen in epidermolysis bullosa acquisita. N Engl J Med. 1984; 310:1007–13.
95. Elliott GT. Two cases of epidermolysis bullosa. J Cutan Genitourin. 1895; 13:10.
96. Roenigk HH Jr., Ryan JG, Bergfeld WF. Epidermolysis bullosa acquisita. Report of three cases and review of all published cases. Arch Dermatol. 1971; 103:1–10.
97. Dahl MG. Epidermolysis bullosa acquisita – a sign of cicatricial pemphigoid? Br J Dermatol. 1979; 101:475–84.
98. Gammon WR, Briggaman RA, Wheeler CE Jr. Epidermolysis bullosa acquisita presenting as an inflammatory bullous disease. J Am Acad Dermatol. 1982; 7:382–7.
99. Gammon WR, Briggaman RA, Woodley DT, et al. Epidermolysis bullosa acquisita – a pemphigoid-like disease. J Am Acad Dermatol. 1984; 11:820–32.
100. Caux F, Kirtschig G, Lemarchand-Venencie F, et al. IgA-epidermolysis bullosa acquisita in a child resulting in blindness. Br J Dermatol. 1997; 137:270–5.
101. Woodley DT, Chen M, O'Toole E, Chan L. Epidermolysis bullosa acquisita. In: Kanitakis J, Vassileva S, Woodley D, editors. Diagnostic immunohistochemistry of the skin. London: Chapman & Hall; 1998. pp. 114–22.
102. Zillikens D, Wever S, Roth A, et al. Incidence of autoimmune subepidermal blistering dermatoses in a region of central Germany. Arch Dermatol. 1995; 131:957–8.

103. Nanda A, Dvorak R, Al-Saeed K, et al. Spectrum of autoimmune bullous diseases in Kuwait. Int J Dermatol. 2004; 43:876–81.

104. Wong SN, Chua SH. Spectrum of subepidermal immunobullous disorders seen at the National Skin Centre Singapore: a 2-year review. Br J Dermatol. 2002; 147:476–80.

105. Gammon WR. Epidermolysis bullosa acquisita. Semin Dermatol. 1988; 7:218–24.

106. Wieme N, Lambert J, Moerman M, et al. Epidermolysis bullosa acquisita with combined features of bullous pemphigoid and cicatricial pemphigoid. Dermatology. 1999; 198:310–13.

107. Hallel-Halevy D, Nadelman C, Chen M, Woodley DT. Epidermolysis bullosa acquisita update and review. Clin Dermatol. 2001; 19:712–18.

108. Chen M, O'Toole EA, Sanghavi J, et al. The epidermolysis bullosa acquisita antigen (type VII collagen) is present in human colon and patients with Crohn's disease have autoantibodies to type VII collagen. J Invest Dermatol. 2002; 118:1059–64.

109. Radfar L, Fatahzadeh M, Shahamat Y, Sirois D. Paraneoplastic epidermolysis bullosa acquisita associated with multiple myeloma. Spec Care Dentist. 2006; 26:159–63.

110. Gammon WR, Kowalewski C, Chorzelski TP, et al. Direct immunofluorescence studies of sodium chloride-separated skin in the differential diagnosis of bullous pemphigoid and epidermolysis bullosa acquisita. J Am Acad Dermatol. 1990; 22:664–70.

111. Yaoita H, Briggaman RA, Lawley TJ, et al. Epidermolysis bullosa acquisita: ultrastructural and immunological studies. J Invest Dermatol. 1981; 76:288–92.

112. Chen M, Chan LS, Cai X, et al. Development of an ELISA for rapid detection of anti-type VII collagen autoantibodies in epidermolysis bullosa acquisita. J Invest Dermatol. 1997; 108:68–72.

113. Chen M, Hallel-Halevy D, Nadelman C, et al. Epidermolysis bullosa acquisita. In: Hertl M, editor. Autoimmune diseases of the skin, pathogenesis, diagnosis, management. Vienna: Springer-Verlag; 2001. pp. 99–122.

114. Jordon RE, Chorzelski TP, Beutner EH. Clinical significance of autoantibodies in bullous pemphigoid. In: Beutner EH, Chorzelski TP, Beutner EH, editors. Autosensitization in pemphigus and bullous pemphigoid. Springfield IL: Charles C. Thomas; 1970. pp. 91–9.

115. Nicolas MEO, Krause PK, Gibson LE, Murray JA. Dermatitis herpetiformis. Int J Dermatol. 2003; 42:588–600.

116. Rose C, Zillikens D. Dermatitis herpetiformis Duhring. In: Hertl M, editor. Autoimmune diseases of the skin, pathogenesis, diagnosis, management. Vienna: Springer-Verlag; 2001. pp. 85–98.

117. Alonso-Llamazares J, Gibson LE, Rogers III RS. Clinical, pathologic, and immunopathologic features of dermatitis herpetiformis: review of the Mayo Clinic experience. Int J Dermatol. 2007; 46:910–19.

118. Van Der Meer JB. Granular deposits of immunoglobulins in the skin of patients with dermatitis herpetiformis. An immunofluorescent study. Br J Dermatol. 1969; 81:493–503.

119. Dieterich W, Laag E, Bruckner-Tuderman L, et al. Antibodies to tissue transglutaminase as serologic markers in patients with dermatitis herpetiformis. J Invest Dermatol. 1999; 113:133–6.

120. Sardy M, Karpati S, Peterfy F, et al. Comparison of a tissue transglutaminase ELISA with the endomysium antibody test in the diagnosis of gluten-sensitive enteropathy. Z Gastroenterol. 2000; 38:357–64.

121. Cotell S, Robinson ND, Chan LS. Autoimmune blistering skin diseases. Am J Emerg Med. 2000; 18:288–99.

122. Banfield CC, Allen J, Wojnarowska F. Dermatitis herpetiformis and linear IgA disease. In: Kanitakis J, Vassileva S, Woodley D, editors. Diagnostic immunohistochemistry of the skin. London: Chapman & Hall; 1998. pp. 105–13.

123. Sigurgeirsson B, Agnarsson BA, Lindelof B. Risk of lymphoma in patients with dermatitis herpetiformis. Br Med J. 1994; 308:13–15.

124. Reunala T, Collin P. Diseases associated with dermatitis herpetiformis. Br J Dermatol. 1997; 136:315–18.

125. Lewis HM, Renaula TL, Garioch JJ, et al. Protective effect of gluten-free diet against development of lymphoma in dermatitis herpetiformis. Br J Dermatol. 1996; 135:363–7.

CHAPTER 23

Emergency Management of Purpura and Vasculitis, Including Purpura Fulminans

Lucio Andreassi

Roberta Bilenchi

PURPURIC LESIONS are the clinical expression of the passage of erythrocytes from the vascular compartment to the extravascular one, generally following damage related to permeabilization of the walls of small vessels. At times, they are the only clinical feature, at other times the sign of a more complex morbid process and the expression of a serious condition, as in the systemic vasculitides.

The clinical spectra of vasculitides are broad, with a variety of conditions ranging from mainly cutaneous involvement with a relatively benign course, such as leukocytoclastic vasculitis, to situations in which the cutaneous involvement is less evident but an integral part of a process that could progress to a critical situation requiring emergency treatment. Acute pulmonary insufficiency or renal blockage, as an expression of a systemic vasculitis, is relatively frequent in intensive care units.[1,2] Central and peripheral nervous system involvement, cardiac failure, and intestinal ischemia, as complications or first presenting signs of systemic vasculitides, are clinical conditions commonly encountered in current practice.[3-5] Purpura fulminans (PF), often associated with disseminated intravascular coagulation (DIC), is a dramatic condition that must be identified correctly and differentiated from purpura simplex.[6]

Purpuras and vasculitides are medical emergencies that require rapid diagnosis, identification of the causal factors, and initiation of a treatment, which is often aggressive but must be carried out as early as possible.[7] Particularly important in this regard are some situations occurring in Henoch–Schönlein purpura (HSP), Wegener granulomatosis (WG), Churg–Strauss syndrome (CSS), polyarteritis nodosa (PAN), microscopic polyangiitis (MPA), Kawasaki disease (KD), and PF (Table 23.1).

Dermatologists may encounter situations involving the evolution or complications of pathologies with initial cutaneous involvement or be called to assist with the diagnosis and management of emergency patients; therefore, knowledge of the disease entities included in the group of purpuras and vasculitides, particularly of the conditions that could progress to emergency situations, must be an integral part of the dermatologist's training. The aim of this chapter is to call attention to purpuras and vasculitides that can present as or evolve into emergency situations and to the procedures for managing these patients.

CLINICAL PRESENTATION AND PATHOGENESIS

HSP is an immunoglobulin A (IgA)-mediated leukocytoclastic vasculitis characterized by antiseptic lesions with perivascular infiltrates, fibrinoid necrosis, and vascular occlusion caused by platelet thrombi. The disease occurs mainly in children, sometimes following an upper respiratory tract infection, and has an acute onset distinguished by cutaneous manifestations on the buttocks and extensor surfaces of the extremities and by general symptoms such as discomfort, headache, fever, polyarthralgia, and abdominal

TABLE 23.1: Purpuras and Vasculitides Potentially Evolving into Emergency Situations

Disease	Possible conditions requiring emergency treatment
Henoch–Schönlein purpura	Abdominal and renal complications
Wegener granulomatosis	Pulmonary and renal involvement
Churg–Strauss syndrome	Hemoptysis and respiratory failure, myocardial infarction, myocarditis, renal failure
Polyarteritis nodosa	Renal insufficiency, cardiomyopathy, gastrointestinal bleeding, bowel perforation
Microscopic polyangiitis	Deterioration of renal function and respiratory failure
Kawasaki disease	Cardiac involvement in the acute stage; development of coronary artery aneurysms later in the course
Purpura fulminans	Disseminated intravascular coagulation

pain. In most cases, HSP resolves without leaving any negative traces, but in some cases kidney involvement can progress to renal insufficiency.[8]

The cutaneous involvement begins with a symmetric macular erythematous rash on the lower extremity, which rapidly evolves into purpura. Initially, the eruption may be limited to the malleolar skin but usually extends to the dorsal surface of the legs, buttocks, and ulnar side of the upper extremities. Within 12–24 hours, the macules turn into palpable dark red purpuric lesions, sometimes merging into vast ecchymosis-like patches. In children younger than 2 years, the cutaneous involvement may be dominated by marked edema on the scalp, periorbital region, hands, and feet. The intensity of the edema, attributed to the intestinal loss of proteins, is related to the severity of the vasculitis. Palpable purpura occurs in all cases of HSP and is almost always the first presenting sign, whereas articular involvement and possible renal and abdominal involvement appear later.[9]

In the criteria recently proposed by the European League against Rheumatism (EULAR) for the classification of childhood vasculitides, a prerequisite for the diagnosis of HPS is palpable purpura associated with another clinicopathological feature, such as diffuse abdominal pain, tissue deposits of IgA, arthritis or arthralgia, renal involvement shown by hematuria, or proteinuria.[10] The cutaneous manifestations are crucial for an early preliminary diagnosis, which must then be confirmed.

WG is a multisystemic disease characterized by necrotizing granulomas of the respiratory apparatus, disseminated vasculitis, and glomerulonephritis. Both sexes can be affected, usually in middle age, although there are occasional cases of children and people older than 70 years. The etiology is unknown, although numerous studies support an autoimmune origin.[11,12]

An autoimmune etiology of WG is suggested by the almost constant presence of granular pattern antineutrophil cytoplasmic antibodies (c-ANCA), the levels of which are correlated with the severity of the disease and are predictive of relapses. The frequent finding of IgA and IgE, the possible association with human leukocyte antigen (HLA) HLA-B8 and HLA-DR2, and the efficacy of immunosuppressive therapy are further elements supporting an autoimmune origin.[13] Protease 3 (PR-3), an enzyme stored in the azurophilic granules of neutrophils and monocytes, seems to be the main target of c-ANCA. Another enzyme, a myeloperoxidase (MPO) contained in the azurophilic granules, could play a role because it is activated by perinuclear pattern antineutrophil cytoplasmic antibodies (p-ANCA), found in a small number of patients.[14] In vitro studies have shown that ANCA are able to activate leukocyte degranulation and the release of toxic radicals and lysosomal enzymes responsible for a cytokine-mediated inflammatory process.[15] In vivo studies have not provided direct evidence of the responsibility of ANCA in the pathogenesis of WG.[16] The role of an infectious agent has been hypoth-

esized on the basis of the good results of sulfamethoxazole-trimethoprim treatment of early signs of the disease.[17] The histopathological features seen in recent lesions confirm the hypothesis of an immune-mediated pathogenesis because they document an involvement of neutrophils and endothelial cells as possible targets and promoters of the inflammation. Indeed, we know that endothelial damage and neutrophil activation can produce mediators of inflammation that lead to the recruitment of monocytes and T cells able to increase the endothelial damage.

Clinically, the disease begins with the classic triad of respiratory tract involvement, systemic vasculitis of the small vessels, and focal glomerulonephritis, although the clinical pattern is not always complete. Upper respiratory tract involvement occurs in more than 70% of patients, with manifestations in the nasal mucosa, which is affected by an inflammatory process with hemorrhage, necrosis, and ulceration that can even lead to destruction of the septal cartilage and deformation of the nasal profile. Lower respiratory tract involvement occurs in approximately 50% of cases, with pulmonary, nodular, and cavity lesions, a frequent cause of hemoptysis. Nephropathy in the initial phases occurs in approximately 20% of patients, with a rapid increase later in the course. The joints, eye, and nervous system can be compromised to variable degrees according to the progression of the disease.

The clinical picture is rarely dominated by cutaneous lesions, the initial frequency of which is relatively low but can rise to more than 50% in the advanced phases of the disease. The first and most typical signs are papulonecrotic lesions located mainly on the elbows, knees, and buttocks, sometimes preceded by an erythematous, edematous, or vesicular inflammatory phase. Subcutaneous nodules and ulcerative lesions with the appearance of pyoderma gangrenosum can be found at the onset and in the later phases. Purpuric manifestations involving extensive skin areas, associated or not with erythematous and vesicular lesions, are observed more frequently in the late phases of WG but can sometimes be present at onset and are an important sign for diagnostic purposes.[18]

The diagnosis of WG generally follows histopathological examination of a tissue fragment taken from the nasal mucosa and is generally based on the demonstration of granulomatosis and vasculitis. The detection of ANCA and the identification of their pattern (i.e., cytoplasmic or perinuclear) are useful diagnostic complements and can contribute to a more complete classification, which naturally requires instrumental and functional examinations of the respiratory apparatus and kidneys.

CSS is a severe necrotizing vasculitis of the small vessels usually associated with asthma and eosinophilia, which is why it is also called allergic granuloma.[19] The onset of the syndrome is often ambiguous, with the appearance of mainly asthmatic or rhinitic respiratory symptoms that can precede the visceral, neurological, and cutaneous involvement by some years. Classically, there are three phases: the initial one characterized by allergic rhinitis, nasal polyposis, sinusitis, and asthma; the intermediate one with recurrent episodes of pneumonia and gastroenteritis associated with circulating eosinophilia; and the final one in which respiratory involvement prevails. In the final phase, there may also be digestive apparatus involvement with the appearance of hematic diarrhea, urinary apparatus involvement with hematuria, articular involvement with arthralgia, and heart and peripheral nervous system involvement. The latency between the appearance of the first symptoms and the advanced phase is 3 years on average. Death is generally due to a granulomatous infiltration of the heart or vasculitis of the coronary arteries.[20]

Cutaneous involvement in CSS occurs in approximately 70% of cases and is often late and polymorphic, with purpuric maculopapular lesions on the extremities, mainly the acral parts. More rarely, there are cutaneous and subcutaneous nodules on the head and extremities. The cutaneous lesions do not differ from those found in other forms of vasculitis and are characterized by purpuric manifestations, nodules, and polymorphic-like erythematous patches, with possible progression to necrosis.[21,22]

Histologically, there is a leukocytoclastic vasculitis in the initial phase, followed by the formation of a palisading granuloma around the foci of collagen degeneration, with the presence of nuclear dust.[23] The granuloma presents basophilic or eosinophilic staining, according to the predominance of neutrophils or eosinophils in the infiltrate. The process can involve both small vessels of the dermis and larger vessels of the subcutis, although the finding of vasculitis is not constant. At times, it is possible to observe deposits of C3 and fibrin in the vessel wall.[24]

CSS falls into the group of ANCA-vasculitides including WG and microscopic angiitis, often with poorly defined borders between the different entities.[25,26] ANCA, circulating antibodies directed against antigenic constituents of the cytoplasm of polymorphonuclear neutrophils, seem to play an important role in the pathogenesis of the disease. In vitro studies have shown that various types of antigenic stimuli (such as drugs, viruses, and bacteria) increase the serum levels of tumor necrosis factor-α (TNF-α) and interleukin-1, with activation of polymorphonuclear neutrophils and transfer of PR-3 from the intracytoplasmic azurophilic granules to the cell membrane. The interaction of PR-3 with circulating ANCA causes the subsequent degranulation of polymorphonuclear neutrophils and tissue damage. Recent studies suggest that ANCA are more involved in the vasculitic manifestations, such as glomerulonephritis, whereas the eosinophilic infiltration and the associated cytotoxicity could be responsible for the cardiomyopathy. If confirmed, these results would support an individual stratification in accordance with the clinical pattern.[27]

PAN is a multisystemic vasculopathy of medium and small arteries (and sometimes arterioles), mainly involving the skin, kidneys, nerves, and gastrointestinal (GI) tract. It

can develop after a phase characterized by aspecific symptoms, such as discomfort, fever, weight loss, and muscular and/or articular pain. Cutaneous involvement is frequent with purpuric lesions, livedo reticularis, nodules, ulcers, and gangrene.

The most frequent cutaneous signs are painful nodules of variable size and number, located mainly on the lower extremities, particularly the legs. The nodules are usually the first cutaneous sign; they appear after a more or less long benign course and develop with multiple flares leaving a pigmentary or livedoid residue with characteristic reticular pattern. The livedo reticularis is more evident in some areas, such as the legs, feet, buttocks, and shoulder blades, and can persist as the only evidence of vascular damage.[28]

The pathogenetic mechanisms leading to the vascular damage are probably heterogeneous and involve the intervention of immune complexes, ANCA, adhesion molecules, cytokines, and antibodies against endothelial cells. The immune complexes are the result of previous infections and act via the activation of complement able to attract neutrophils. ANCA play an important role in inducing endothelial damage but are not always present in PAN. Various adhesion molecules (lymphocyte function-associated antigen 1, intercellular adhesion molecule 1, endothelial cell leukocyte adhesion molecule 1) are able to favor contact between neutrophils and endothelial cells and to initiate the cascade of events leading to vasculitis.

In approximately 10% of subjects with PAN, there is a contemporaneous hepatitis B virus (HBV) infection. In these patients, circulating immune complexes, formed by HBV antigens and relative antibodies, could play an important role in the pathogenesis of the vasculitic lesions.[29,30]

MPA is a systemic necrotizing vasculitis frequently associated with glomerulonephritis and pulmonary involvement. Considered the microscopic form of PAN, it acquired clinical autonomy in 1994 after the consensus conference aimed at redefining the classification of small-vessel vasculitides.[31] Involvement of the small vessels, including arterioles, capillaries, and venules, is absent in PAN but is typical of MPA. In pathogenetic terms, MPA, along with WG and CSS, belongs to the group of small-vessel vasculitides linked to the role of ANCA. Anti-MPO p-ANCA antibodies, present in MPA and absent in PAN, help to differentiate the two disease entities.[32] The absence of granulomas and the lack of upper respiratory tract involvement help to distinguish MPA from WG, although the distinction is not always easy.[33]

MPA generally has a rapid and progressive course, and a timely diagnosis can be important for effective treatment. In this regard, the finding of cutaneous signs may be useful for the purposes of the histological examination. They present as erythematous or purpuric macules, mainly located on the extremities and are observed in more than 50% of cases.[34] The cutaneous histopathology of MPA is characterized

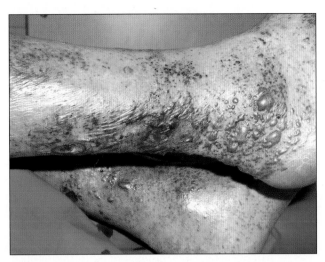

FIGURE 23.1: Purpura fulminans and disseminated intravascular coagulation in a 71-year-old man suffering from leg ulcers and diabetes. Note the multiple hemorrhagic bullae.

by a necrotizing vasculitis with a moderate neutrophilic infiltrate affecting the papillary and middle dermis and the subcutaneous tissue. The detection and titration of ANCA could be useful for diagnostic and prognostic purposes.[35]

KD, a vasculitic syndrome of unknown origin described in 1967, is characterized by an eruption associated with fever of relatively brief duration. Initially thought to be a benign self-resolving process, it was later related to a series of deaths from myocardial infarction due to thrombotic occlusion of aneurismatic coronary arteries. Exceptional in adolescents and adults, KD is typically a childhood disease with a higher incidence in Asian populations, particularly in Japan and China.[36]

The etiology of KD is unknown, although the idea of an infectious origin is attractive. This origin is suggested by the self-resolving course, lack of relapses, fever, exanthema, and adenopathy, all typical of an infectious disease. Direct attempts to isolate an infectious agent have proven negative. It is possible that KD is the result of an immune response induced by different microbial agents. This hypothesis is supported by the frequent isolation of infectious microorganisms in individual cases and the similarities to other syndromes caused by multiple agents, such as aseptic meningitis.[37]

The inflammatory infiltrate found in KD, characteristic of a vasculitis, can involve blood vessels throughout the organism. In autopsies, aneurysms have been found in arteries in many regions (e.g., the celiac, mesenteric, femoral, iliac, and renal arteries).[38]

The diagnosis is based on fever persisting for at least 5 days and alterations of the extremities, characterized in the acute phase by palmoplantar edema and in the subacute phase by desquamation of the fingertips, hands, and feet. Other typical signs are polymorphic exanthema, bilat-

eral hyperemic conjunctivitis without secretion, redness of the lips and oral cavity, fissuration of the lips, strawberry tongue, and hyperemia of the pharynx and oral cavity. A usually unilateral laterocervical lymphadenopathy is also frequently observed.[39]

Cardiovascular symptoms may be evident as early as the acute phase of KD, and they are the main cause of long-term morbidity and mortality. In this phase, the pericardium, myocardium, endocardium, valves, and coronary arteries can be involved. Cardiac function shows anomalies such as tachycardia and myocardial contractile deficit, a cause of insufficiency and shock.[40]

Coronary artery aneurysms develop in 15%–25% of untreated persons and can lead to myocardial infarction, sudden death, or ischemic cardiac disease.[41,42] Various point systems are available to identify children at high risk of coronary arteriopathy.[43]

PF, a disease generally associated with sepsis, is found most frequently in children. The clinical pattern is often dominated by shock with hypotension and hypovolemia, clinically distinguished by a weak and frequent pulse, anxiety, pallor, cold sweating, and cyanotic lips. The cutaneous lesions consist of purpuric patches that rapidly evolve into peripheral hemorrhagic necrosis, sometimes preceded by bulla formation. PF is almost always associated with or progresses to DIC, an expression of thrombocytopenia with increased production of thrombin and fibrinolysis (Figures 23.1 and 23.2).

The lesions in PF are generally considered the result of a Schwartzman-like reaction. The Schwartzman phenomenon occurs when a dose of endotoxin is intravenously (IV) injected into animals previously inoculated subcutaneously with a small dose of the same endotoxin. The reaction occurs within a few hours at the site of the first inoculation and is characterized by an inflammatory event

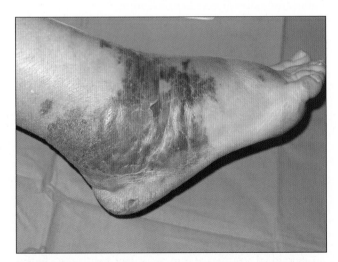

FIGURE 23.2: Cellulitis with signs simulating purpura fulminans in a 56-year-old woman. The clinical presentation was dominated by the appearance of purpuric patches, hemorrhagic bullae, and fever.

that rapidly progresses to necrosis. The Schwartzman phenomenon cannot be explained by an immune mechanism and is probably due to a toxic effect. In PF (at least in the forms associated with sepsis), the vascular lesions are considered the result of a necrotizing inflammatory process caused by infectious agents. Meningococcus is the most frequent cause of PF, but other infectious agents have been recorded, such as *Pneumococcus* and *Staphylococcus*.[44,45] A malignant tumor, a possible triggering factor in PF, has been found in a significant number of cases.[46]

In PF lesions, there is extensive coagulation in the small vessels, with fibrin thrombi and a modest inflammatory component. This feature differentiates PF from other vasculitides such as HSP, characterized by an accentuated inflammatory component.[47]

PF is associated with marked hematic alterations, particularly low concentrations of fibrinogen, coagulation factors, and platelets, due to consumption of platelets and extended prothrombin and partial thromboplastin times. Fibrinogen-degradation products tend to increase, and the concentrations of proteins C and S and antithrombin III (AT III) tend to decrease. DIC often develops under these conditions; it is the consequence of anomalous thrombin activation leading to the conversion of fibrinogen to fibrin, as well as of the activation and consumption of platelets. These coagulation alterations are believed to be related to systemic anomalies, particularly activation of protein C, which are congenital or induced by pathological conditions.[48]

MANAGEMENT AND TREATMENT

The treatment of patients affected by purpuras and vasculitides, in critical or emergency conditions, is based on general reanimation techniques and case-specific measures. Useful general procedures are those aimed at improving the hemodynamic and hydroelectrolytic imbalance and correcting eventual coagulation anomalies, which could require specific drugs in addition to substantial plasma and/or whole-blood infusions.

Systemic vasculitides associated with circulating ANCA are characterized by frequent renal parenchyma involvement, represented by a necrotizing glomerulonephritis, which translates into acute renal insufficiency. The presence in the blood of autoantibodies with an important role in the pathogenesis of the lesions has prompted the use of plasmapheresis, on the assumption that rapid removal of the autoantibodies and, at the same time, coagulation factors and mediators of inflammation could strongly affect the progression of the disease (Table 23.2).[49,50]

Corticosteroids are the most important category of immunosuppressor drugs used in the treatment of systemic vasculitides. They can be useful in all forms of vasculitides but are the first-line agents in several forms, such as WG, CSS, and PAN. Corticosteroids can be used alone

TABLE 23.2: Drugs and Procedures Used in the Treatment of Emergencies Related to Purpuras and Vasculitides

Drugs and procedures	Indications
Plasmapheresis	ANCA-associated systemic vasculitides
Corticosteroids	All vasculitides; first-line treatment in WG, CSS, PAN
Cyclophosphamide	Associated with corticosteroids in WG, CSS, PAN
Azathioprine and methotrexate	Used as maintenance therapy in patients with WG, CSS, PAN
Intravenous immunoglobulins	First-line treatment in Kawasaki disease; potential alternative treatment for ANCA-associated systemic vasculitides
Infliximab	Able to induce clinical remission in acute or active ANCA-associated vasculitides
Rituximab	Active in refractory or relapsed ANCA-associated WG

ANCA, antineutrophil cytoplasmic antibodies; WG, Wegener granulomatosis; CSS, Churg–Strauss syndrome; PAN, polyarteritis nodosa.

in the less severe forms but are usually combined with cyclophosphamide in the severe forms. Other immunosuppressors, such as azathioprine and methotrexate, are used as maintenance therapy in the remission phases of the disease.[51]

The appearance of IV immunoglobulins (IVIg) has further expanded the therapeutic arsenal for systemic vasculitides. At high doses, IVIg can interfere with the immune system at various levels, being indicated in various pathologies based on inflammation–immune mechanisms. IVIg have proven particularly useful for KD, but their use (alone or associated with corticosteroids or other immunosuppressor) has also proven successful in the ANCA-associated vasculitides.[52]

New prospects in the treatment of systemic vasculitides have recently been provided by the introduction of biological drugs, particularly infliximab, etanercept, and rituximab. In association with conventional therapy, infliximab, an anti-TNF chimeric monoclonal antibody, has been able to induce clinical remission in various systemic vasculitides,[53] whereas the efficacy of etanercept has been modest. Rituximab, a genetically chimeric murine–human CD20 antigen expressed on the surface of B lymphocytes, is more promising as it has proven effective against refractory or relapsed ANCA-associated WG.[54]

HSP

The management and therapy of HSP patients must take into account various factors such as age, possible renal involvement, and the presence of complications such as nervous system involvement. HSP is generally a benign disease with a good prognosis, characterized in more than 80% of patients by a single episode lasting a few weeks, with relapses in 10%–20% of cases and chronic forms, particularly renal insufficiency, in 5% of cases. For this reason, the usefulness of always adopting a systemic therapy has been placed in doubt, particularly treatment with steroids, because placebo-controlled prospective studies have shown their limited efficacy.[55] Prophylactic steroid therapy is unable to prevent renal and gastrointestinal (GI) complications but is indicated in the treatment of abdominal pain, subcutaneous edema, and nephritis.[56] Prednisone, at 1 mg/kg/day for 2 weeks followed by a lower dose for another 2 weeks, has been shown to improve the GI and articular involvement and to reduce the severity of renal involvement. Other immunosuppressors (e.g., azathioprine, cyclophosphamide, cyclosporin, and mycophenolate mofetil) can be combined with steroids, although their use is controversial in view of the low efficacy recorded in clinical trials.[57] Similar conclusions have been made about other drugs, such as IVIg, vitamin E, and other antioxidants.[58] Plasmapheresis deserves separate mention because it has proven effective in delaying the progression of renal damage.[59]

WG

The use of conventional immunosuppressors has led to significant improvement of the course and prognosis of WG, although there are still serious limitations due to possible cytotoxic side effects and frequent relapses after the suspension of treatment. Many doubts remain about the use of biological therapies, whereas there is great hope concerning the possible development of drugs that will interfere with specific targets with an important role in maintaining the autoimmune response (e.g., ANCA).[60,61]

The standard treatment of WG involves the combination of cyclophosphamide and corticosteroids until remission and then maintenance therapy with azathioprine or methotrexate. Complete remission or marked improvement compatible with a normal social life is recorded in 90% of cases, although relapses are frequent (50%) and the drugs have high toxicity. Replacing cyclophosphamide with methotrexate after remission is achieved may be advantageous in view of its low toxicity, and it could be used as the first-line agent in association with corticosteroids.[62] All the previously mentioned drugs induce immunosuppression with the consequent risk of opportunistic infection, above all *Pneumocystis jiroveci* pneumonia, although this can be prevented by sulfamethoxazole–trimethoprim treatment, especially during remission. This drug has also been used satisfactorily to reduce relapses, above all in patients with limited, not very aggressive forms.

WG has also been the subject of trials to assess the efficacy of biological drugs, especially by means of anti-TNF-α agents, likely involved in the pathogenesis of WG.

Etanercept, a soluble TNF receptor fusion protein, is not very effective, inducing long-lasting remissions in only a minority of the treated patients,[63] whereas infliximab, a chimeric monoclonal antibody against TNF, seems to merit further investigation.[64] The results obtained with rituximab, a chimeric monoclonal antibody against CD20, are more interesting because it causes depletion of B cells in the blood within 6–12 months. By this mechanism, rituximab seems to recreate the tolerance to ANCA antigens, at least in some WG patients.[65]

WG can also be treated with other drugs, including leflunomide, mycophenolate mofetil, and deoxyspergualin. Leflunomide inhibits de novo synthesis of pyrimidine, necessary for the function of activated T lymphocytes. Its use in WG can control relapses in a high number of subjects.[66] Mycophenolate mofetil is an inhibitor of inosine monophosphate dehydrogenase, an essential enzyme for purine synthesis and thus for the proliferation and function of lymphocytes. Its use in the maintenance of remission in subjects treated with corticosteroids and cyclophosphamide has not proven very effective, and it requires further evaluation.[67] Deoxyspergualin, of unclear mechanism of action, has proven effective in WG patients unresponsive to conventional therapies.[68]

CSS

Corticosteroids are the first-line agents in the treatment of CSS. They can be used according to the standard procedures, but some authors suggest high IV doses, especially in emergency situations. The response is usually dramatic: The eosinophilia is normalized, the asthma regresses, and the muscle enzyme levels return to normal. After the result has been obtained, the steroids can be gradually tapered to a minimal dose able to control the disease. If the corticosteroids are not sufficient to control the disease, it may be necessary to combine cyclophosphamide (the use of which is always advisable) and steroids in life-threatening cases. Methotrexate could also be helpful to control CSS and can be associated with steroids.[69]

In severe cases, particularly when steroids and cyclophosphamide do not induce remission, anti-TNF agents such as infliximab and etanercept can be used, although they could increase the risk of infections. In this regard, prophylactic treatment with sulfamethoxazole–trimethoprim may be appropriate. An alternative could be the use of recombinant interferon-α (IFN-α).[70] More recently, encouraging results have been obtained with rituximab, but the data must be confirmed by larger trials.[71,72]

IV gammaglobulins could be a valid alternative in patients unresponsive to conventional treatment, especially those presenting with myocardiopathy and neuropathy. The mechanism of action of this therapy is still unclear and requires further investigation, but this does not diminish the practical efficacy of the treatment.[73]

PAN

First, the systemic forms must be distinguished from the limited forms and the idiopathic forms from the HBV-related forms. That said, the treatment of PAN depends on the severity of the clinical features, quantified by the degree of involvement of the affected organs. In particular, it is necessary to assess the extent of proteinuria and creatininemia, the severity of eventual cardiomyopathy and GI signs, and the nervous system involvement. In general, corticosteroids associated with cyclophosphamide represent the standard treatment of PAN, whereas antiviral agents and plasmapheresis are necessary in HBV-related cases.[74,75]

In patients with a relatively benign prognosis, corticosteroids alone may be sufficient. Prednisone, commonly used in the treatment of PAN, must be administered until regression of the symptoms, generally after approximately 1 month. The dose can then be tapered to a level able to control the disease, after which the minimal dose must be maintained for 9–12 months.

Cyclophosphamide is generally associated when the disease is refractory to treatment with steroids alone, during relapses, and generally in all severe cases. Pulsed IV administration is the most common procedure, but oral administration can be used when it is unsuccessful. The association of cyclophosphamide with steroids for more than 1 year should be avoided.

In HBV-related cases, plasmapheresis is considered the treatment of choice, because it can remove the viral components, including circulating immune complexes. Antiviral agents, such as IFN-α2b and lamivudine, are obviously important in such cases, possibly in combination. Naturally, corticosteroids are always indicated in PAN.[76,77] On exceptional occasions, HBV-related PAN may show a fulminant onset, requiring treatment with prednisone combined with pulsed IV cyclophosphamide and lamivudine.[78]

MPA

As in other forms of vasculitis, the initial treatment of MPA consists of the induction of remission with prednisone and cyclophosphamide. The initial dose of prednisone is 1 mg/kg/day for 1 month or at least until significant improvement is observed. This dose is followed by a weekly decrease to the maintenance dose, which can be continued for long periods, possibly on alternate days. The initial cyclophosphamide dose is 1.5–2 mg/kg/day, but higher doses may be required (possibly IV) in emergency situations (e.g., in capillaritis with pulmonary hemorrhage).[79] After remission, it is necessary to establish a maintenance regimen, continuing the prednisone and replacing the cyclophosphamide with azathioprine or methotrexate, both at relatively low doses. Alternative drugs to be combined with prednisone in the maintenance phase are methotrexate, cyclosporin, and mycophenolate mofetil.[80] *Pneumocystis carinii* and *Pneumocystis jiroveci* infections are prevented by sulfamethoxazole–trimethoprim administered 3 times a week.

KD

The treatment of acute KD is aimed at reducing inflammation in the walls of the coronary arteries and preventing thrombosis, whereas long-term therapy in individuals with coronary aneurysms is aimed at preventing ischemia and myocardial infarction. The acute phase procedures, often carried out in emergency conditions, are based on the earliest possible administration of aspirin and IVIg.[81]

Although aspirin is an important antiinflammatory and has antiplatelet aggregation activity, its use alone does not seem to reduce the frequency of coronary alterations. During the acute phase of KD, it is administered at 80–100 mg/kg/day in association with IVIg, which potentiates the antiinflammatory effect. Aspirin is administered at high doses until fever subsides, generally after 2–3 days, and is then used at 3–5 mg/kg/day for antiplatelet aggregation until the patient is free of the risk of coronary alterations.[82]

The mechanism of action of IVIg is still unknown, but administration leads to rapid lowering of the fever and resolution of the clinical signs of KD in most patients. The prevalence of coronary disease drops from 20%–25% in children treated with aspirin alone to 2%–4% in those treated with IVIg and aspirin in the first 10 days of the disease. IVIg treatment is also indicated in patients diagnosed after the 10th day of the disease if the fever persists, because the antiinflammatory effect could be helpful.[83] Occasionally, some patients may not respond to the initial IVIg infusion or show only a partial response. These subjects are usually treated with an additional IVIg infusion, but its efficacy must still be demonstrated.[84]

The use of corticosteroids in acute KD is controversial and still under investigation. According to recent studies, IV administration of methylprednisolone as an adjuvant of conventional therapy with IVIg and aspirin seems to improve the prognosis.[85] Another drug used in the acute phase of KD is pentoxifylline, which is well tolerated, practically without toxicity, and perhaps able to further reduce the risk of coronary aneurysms.[86] Other drugs have been used along with corticosteroids in patients unresponsive to conventional treatment, including cytotoxic agents such as cyclophosphamide and anti-TNF-α monoclonal antibodies. Among these, infliximab is particularly promising, but its use requires additional evaluation.[87]

PF

PF patients often present in a critical condition and must be treated in an intensive care unit, where appropriate procedures to deal with shock can be carried out. Such procedures, particularly treatment of hypovolemia by infusions

TABLE 23.3: Anticoagulant Substances Used in the Treatment of PF

Drugs	Indications
Heparin	Mainly as a bolus followed by an infusion; low-molecular-weight heparins in the prophylaxis of relapse
Protein C	First line in PF due to protein C deficiency; adjuvant hemostatic support in PF-associated meningococcemia
Antithrombin III	May be reduced in PF, and its replacement has been shown to normalize levels and reverse disseminated intravascular coagulation
Tissue plasminogen activator	To be used for PF unresponsive to conventional treatment
Epoprostenol	Has been used to treat PF from sepsis in infants and neonates
Dextran	May be used in PF patients who fail to respond to plasma and heparin therapy

PF, purpura fulminans.

of plasma and physiological solution, correction of the acid–base imbalance, and assisted ventilation, combined with appropriate antibiotic therapy, have considerably reduced the mortality due to PF. The efficacy of the treatment, both quoad vitam and to prevent or limit the possible necrotic evolution of acral lesions, largely depends on the precocity of treatment. The role of dermatologists can be decisive in this regard because they can identify PF and its possible infectious origin on the basis of the first presenting symptoms. The problem is to distinguish a PF from a vasculitis with cutaneous involvement, and this is not always easy to do. Acral involvement, hemorrhagic bullae, a tendency to necrosis, and hypovolemic shock are all suggestive of PF.[88]

Some laboratory tests can be helpful for diagnostic and therapeutic purposes. The blood levels of prothrombin fragments 1 and 2, the D-dimer test, the AT III level, fibrin- and fibrinogen-degradation products, the platelet count, the prothrombin time, and the levels of other coagulation factors can all provide useful indications.[89]

The availability of tests to investigate more thoroughly the coagulation system has led to the isolation and synthesis of new drugs that affect the coagulation process at various levels. These drugs have been added to the traditional therapeutic arsenal and deserve a brief discussion regarding PF treatment (Table 23.3).

Although one of the oldest anticoagulant drugs, heparin can still play a role in the treatment of PF.[90] It must be administered as early as possible, even though there are some reservations, because it can cause thrombocytopenia and bleeding and there are no validated dosage schedules to use in all cases. Administration as a bolus followed by slow infusion seems to be the most reliable procedure,[91]

but there are reports of relapses due to too early suspension.[92] The introduction of low-molecular-weight heparins is interesting in this regard, but further investigation is required.[93]

Protein C, an important physiological anticoagulant factor, is a vitamin K–dependent protease activated by thrombin. Its activated form, along with protein S (which acts as a cofactor), degrades factor Va to factor VIIIa.[94] Its blood level is a useful reference to determine the quantity and timing of administration.[95] The clinical course is the most important parameter for the establishment of when protein C infusion will be useful and if it can be suspended. Protein C is the first-line agent in cases of neonatal PF associated with homozygote protein C deficiency.[96] It is administered by continuous or intermittent IV infusion until normalization and stabilization of the coagulation parameters.[97]

AT III is a glycoprotein produced by the liver with a powerful inhibitory effect on the cascade of reactions involved in coagulation. Although its name indicates activity against thrombin, it interferes with virtually all the enzymes of coagulation and is particularly active when administered with heparin, with which it forms an anticoagulation complex. It is indicated for the prevention and treatment of thromboembolic processes due to AT III deficiency, of which two forms are known: those due to an absolute lack of the factor (type I) and those due to an inadequately functioning AT III (type II).[98]

Absolute or functional AT III deficiencies, such as those occurring during a surgical intervention, pregnancy, childbirth, sepsis, polytrauma, and/or other pathological conditions associated with acute consumption coagulopathy and which can lead to DIC, are elective conditions for the use of AT III, although the efficacy of this treatment has recently been placed in serious doubt.[99] AT III can be diminished during PF, and the restoration of normal levels by infusion could help to improve the clinical course.[100]

Plasminogen activators, essential to convert plasminogen to plasmin and to initiate fibrinolysis, include urokinase, streptokinase, and various substances of tissue and vascular origin, particularly tissue plasminogen activator (t-PA), a human enzyme now obtained with the recombinant DNA technique (rt-PA). rt-PA, currently used in the treatment of myocardial infarction and ischemic stroke, has recently been applied successfully in the treatment of peripheral thromboses caused by physical agents[101] and in the treatment of PF.[102] rt-PA is able to activate fibrinolysis without unpleasant hemodynamic consequences. It is administered by infusion at 0.25–0.5 mg/kg/h, and treatment can be prolonged if necessary.[103] The possible risk of bleeding has raised some doubts about the use of rt-PA in PF, and it has been suggested that it be adopted only in forms unresponsive to conventional treatment.[104]

Epoprostenol is generally used to inhibit platelet aggregation during renal dialysis, especially when there is a high risk of hemorrhagic problems following heparin use. It is also used to treat primary pulmonary hypertension refractory to other treatments, generally together with other anticoagulants. Because its half-life is only approximately 3 minutes, it must be administered by continuous IV infusion. Because it is a potent vasodilator, its side effects include hot flashes, headache, and hypotension. In PF from sepsis, it has been used in children and neonates at 5–20 ng/kg/min without significant collateral effects.[105,106]

Dextrans are glucose polymers of variable molecular weight used as plasma substitutes and as antithrombotics because they are able to reduce platelet aggregation. The rheological effect produced by these molecules is due to their ability to adhere to the endothelial surface (reducing the reactivity between the cell and vessel surfaces), to hemodilution, to reduction of cell aggregation, and to increased platelet rigidity with consequent reduced adhesive ability and aggregation. These activities are translated into improved flow in the microcirculation and increased oxygen transport. Dextran with a molecular weight of 40 has been used in PF as an adjuvant of other treatments, particularly heparin therapy.[107]

The management of PF patients must be based on general reanimation procedures and identification of the causal factor, particularly recognition of an infectious agent and administration of an appropriate antibiotic. In meningococcal sepsis, the most frequent event (especially in children), the first-line antibiotic is penicillin; however, in cases in which the nature of the sepsis is unclear, a third-generation cephalosporin, such as cefotaxime, can be used from the beginning. Subsequent strategies are aimed at correcting and restoring the altered coagulation mechanisms. In this context, the use of the drugs reported in Table 23.3 must be weighed and based on the clinical and laboratory findings in the individual cases.

CONCLUSIONS

Systemic vasculitides can frequently evolve into emergency conditions and sometimes present a critical situation from their onset. The latter occurs most frequently in PF, whereas progress to a critical situation is observed in HSP, WG, CSS, PAN, MPA, and KD. The management of such patients may require the dermatologist because the correct interpretation of cutaneous lesions, an integral part of the clinical pattern, can provide substantial help in identifying the nature and phase of the disease. Dermatological assistance may be essential in the treatment of lesions largely involving the skin.

The clinical features in an emergency situation requiring treatment in an intensive care unit mainly include abdominal and renal complications in HSP; pulmonary and renal involvement in WG; hemoptysis, respiratory and renal failure, myocarditis, and myocardial infarction in CSS; renal insufficiency, cardiomyopathy, and GI bleeding and perforation in PAN; deterioration of renal function and respiratory failure in MPA; and cardiac involvement in the acute phase and subsequent development of coronary aneurysms in KD. The emergency situation can be particularly serious in PF, a disease that frequently evolves into DIC, a dramatic condition often culminating in death.

When present, dermatological signs can be decisive in arriving at the correct diagnosis and treatment. Purpuric lesions mainly situated on the lower extremities, associated with polyarthralgia and abdominal pains, are almost always sufficient for a diagnosis of HSP. Acral inflammatory manifestations, sometimes associated with polymorphic exanthema and laterocervical lymphadenopathy in a child with persistent high fever, reliably indicate a diagnosis of KD; however, it can be more difficult to interpret cutaneous lesions in conditions suspected to be WG, CSS, PAN, or MPA. The histological examination and other hematochemical data can provide other useful information for a diagnosis. PF deserves special consideration because it can assume different clinical signs as a result of a meningococcal infection, especially in children, or as the evolution of a vascular pathology in adults. In both situations, necrotizing purpuric lesions are decisive for an accurate diagnosis.

The management and treatment of emergencies caused by systemic vasculitides must be carried out in an intensive care unit, where the patient can benefit from procedures aimed at improving the pulmonary ventilation and cardio-circulatory conditions and normalizing the hemodynamic and hydroelectrolytic imbalance. In this context, infusions of plasma (or its substitutes) and of whole blood may be useful. Regarding the use of specific drugs, corticosteroids are the first-line agents in WG, CSS, and PAN, diseases in which the association of cyclophosphamide can complete the emergency procedure. IVIg are fundamental in KD, where they can drastically reduce the onset of cardiological complications. Other drugs, such as azathioprine, methotrexate, and the most recent biological drugs, are more suitable for the prevention of relapses. The correction of coagulation alterations, fundamental in PF, requires much attention because it must be carried out with drugs such as heparin, protein C, AT III, and plasminogen activators, the use of which demands accurate monitoring of laboratory parameters and, above all, proven clinical experience.

REFERENCES

1. Cruz BA, Ramanoelina J, Mahr A, et al. Prognosis and outcome of 26 patients with systemic necrotizing vasculitis admitted to the intensive care unit. Rheumatology. 2003; 42:1183–8.
2. Semple D, Keogh J, Forni L, Venn R. Clinical review: vasculitis on the intensive care unit-part 1: diagnosis. Crit Care. 2005; 9:92–7.
3. Younger DS. Vasculitis of the nervous system. Curr Opin Neurol. 2004; 17:317–36.

4. Specker C. Das Herz bei rheumatologischen Erkrankungen. Internist (Berl). 2007; 48:284–9.

5. Passam FH, Diamantis ID, Perisinaki G, et al. Intestinal ischemia as the first manifestation of vasculitis. Semin Arthritis Rheum. 2004; 34:431–41.

6. Davis MD, Dy KM, Nelson S. Presentation and outcome of purpura fulminans associated with peripheral gangrene in 12 patients at Mayo Clinic. J Am Acad Dermatol. 2007; 57: 944–56.

7. Slobodin G, Hussein A, Rozenbaum M, Rosner I. The emergency room in systemic rheumatic diseases. Emerg Med J. 2006; 23:667–71.

8. Roberts PF, Waller TA, Brinker TM, et al. Henoch-Schönlein purpura: a review article. South Med J. 2007; 100:821–4.

9. Trapani S, Micheli A, Grisolia F, et al. Henoch Schonlein purpura in childhood: epidemiological and clinical analysis of 150 cases over a 5-year period and review of literature. Semin Arthritis Rheum. 2005; 35:143–53.

10. Ozen S, Ruperto N, Dillon MJ, et al. EULAR/PReS endorsed consensus criteria for the classification of childhood vasculitides. Ann Rheum Dis. 2006; 65:936–41.

11. Mohammad AJ, Jacobsson LT, Mahr AD, et al. Prevalence of Wegener's granulomatosis, microscopic polyangiitis, polyarteritis nodosa and Churg-Strauss syndrome within a defined population in southern Sweden. Rheumatology. 2007; 46:1329–37.

12. Mahr A, Guillevin L, Poissonnet M, Aymé S. Prevalences of polyarteritis nodosa, microscopic polyangiitis, Wegener's granulomatosis, and Churg-Strauss syndrome in a French urban multiethnic population in 2000: a capture-recapture estimate. Arthritis Rheum. 2004; 51:92–9.

13. de Lind van Wijngaarden RA, van Rijn L, Hagen EC, et al. Hypotheses on the etiology of antineutrophil cytoplasmic autoantibody associated vasculitis: the cause is hidden, but the result is known. Clin J Am Soc Nephrol. 2008; 3:237–52.

14. Talor MV, Stone JH, Stebbing J, et al. Antibodies to selected minor target antigens in patients with anti-neutrophil cytoplasmic antibodies (ANCA). Clin Exp Immunol. 2007; 150:42–8.

15. Lamprecht P, Gross WL. Current knowledge on cellular interactions in the WG-granuloma. Clin Exp Rheumatol. 2007; 25:S49–51.

16. Kallenberg CG, Heeringa P, Stegeman CA. Mechanisms of disease: pathogenesis and treatment of ANCA-associated vasculitides. Nat Clin Pract Rheumatol. 2006; 2:661–70.

17. DeRemee RA. Trimethoprim-sulphamethoxazole for the treatment of Wegener's granulomatosis. Rheumatology. 2003; 42:396.

18. Ben Ghorbel I, Dhrif AS, Miled M, Houman MH. Atteintes cutanées révélatrices d'une granulomatose de Wegener. Presse Med. 2007; 36:619–22.

19. Keogh KA, Specks U. Churg-Strauss syndrome: clinical presentation, antineutrophil cytoplasmic antibodies, and leukotriene receptor antagonists. Am J Med. 2003; 115:284–90.

20. Lhote F. Syndrome de Churg et Strauss. Presse Med. 2007; 36:875–89.

21. Tomassini C, Seia Z. Churg-Strauss sindrome. G Ital Dermatol Venereol. 2004; 139:485–91.

22. Davis MD, Daoud MS, McEvoy MT, Su WP. Cutaneous manifestations of Churg-Strauss syndrome: a clinicopathologic correlation. J Am Acad Dermatol. 1997; 37:199–203.

23. Kawakami T, Soma Y, Kawasaki K, et al. Initial cutaneous manifestations consistent with mononeuropathy multiplex in Churg-Strauss syndrome. Arch Dermatol. 2005; 141:873–8.

24. Jennette JC, Falk RJ. The role of pathology in the diagnosis of systemic vasculitis. Clin Exp Rheumatol. 2007; 25(1 Suppl 44):S52–6.

25. Haubitz M. ANCA-associated vasculitis: diagnosis, clinical characteristics and treatment. Vasa. 2007; 36:81–9.

26. Ozaki S. ANCA-associated vasculitis: diagnostic and therapeutic strategy. Allergol Int. 2007; 56:87–96.

27. Pagnoux C, Guilpain P, Guillevin L. Churg-Strauss syndrome. Curr Opin Rheumatol. 2007; 19:25–32.

28. Díaz-Pérez JL, De Lagrán ZM, Díaz-Ramón JL, Winkelmann RK. Cutaneous polyarteritis nodosa. Semin Cutan Med Surg. 2007; 26:77–86.

29. Janssen HL, van Zonneveld M, van Nunen AB, et al. Polyarteritis nodosa associated with hepatitis B virus infection. The role of antiviral treatment and mutations in the hepatitis B virus genome. Eur J Gastroenterol Hepatol. 2004; 16:801–7.

30. Guillevin L, Mahr A, Callard P, et al. French Vasculitis Study Group. Hepatitis B virus-associated polyarteritis nodosa: clinical characteristics, outcome, and impact of treatment in 115 patients. Medicine. 2005; 84:313–22.

31. Pagnoux C, Guilpain P, Guillevin L. Polyangéite microscopique. Presse Med. 2007; 36:895–901.

32. Kallenberg CG. Antineutrophil cytoplasmic autoantibody-associated small-vessel vasculitis. Curr Opin Rheumatol. 2007; 19:17–24.

33. Guillevin L, Durand-Gasselin B, Cevallos R, et al. Microscopic polyangiitis: clinical and laboratory findings in eighty-five patients. Arthritis Rheum. 1999; 42:421–30.

34. Kawakami T, Kawanabe T, Saito C, et al. Clinical and histopathologic features of 8 patients with microscopic polyangiitis including two with a slowly progressive clinical course. J Am Acad Dermatol. 2007; 57:840–8.

35. Seishima M, Oyama Z, Oda M. Skin eruptions associated with microscopic polyangiitis. Eur J Dermatol. 2004; 14:255–8.

36. Lane SE, Watts R, Scott DG. Epidemiology of systemic vasculitis. Curr Rheumatol Rep. 2005; 7:270–5.

37. Newburger JW, Takahashi M, Gerber MA, et al. Diagnosis, treatment, and long-term management of Kawasaki disease: a statement for health professionals from the Committee on Rheumatic Fever, Endocarditis, and Kawasaki Disease, Council on Cardiovascular Disease in the Young, American Heart Association. Pediatrics. 2004; 114:1708–33.

38. Naoe S, Takahashi K, Masuda H, Tanaka N. Kawasaki disease. With particular emphasis on arterial lesions. Acta Pathol Jpn. 1991; 41:785–97.

39. Royle J, Burgner D, Curtis N. The diagnosis and management of Kawasaki disease. J Paediatr Child Health. 2005; 41:87–93.

40. Gouveia C, Brito MJ, Ferreira GC, et al. Kawasaki disease. Rev Port Cardiol. 2005; 24:1097–113.

41. Kato H, Sugimura T, Akagi T, et al. Long-term consequences of Kawasaki disease. A 10- to 21-year follow-up study of 594 patients. Circulation. 1996; 94:1379–85.

42. Levy DM, Silverman ED, Massicotte MP, et al. Longterm outcomes in patients with giant aneurysms secondary to Kawasaki disease. J Rheumatol. 2005; 32:928–34.

43. Daniels SR, Specker B, Capannari TE, et al. Correlates of coronary artery aneurysm formation in patients with Kawasaki disease. Am J Dis Child. 1987; 141:205–7.

44. Schellongowski P, Bauer E, Holzinger U, et al. Treatment of adult patients with sepsis-induced coagulopathy and purpura fulminans using a plasma-derived protein C concentrate (Ceprotin). Vox Sang. 2006; 90:294–301.

45. Vincent JL, Nadel S, Kutsogiannis DJ, et al. Drotrecogin alfa (activated) in patients with severe sepsis presenting with purpura fulminans, meningitis, or meningococcal disease: a retrospective analysis of patients enrolled in recent clinical studies. Crit Care. 2005; 9:R331–43.

46. Lee JH, Song JW, Song KS. Diagnosis of overt disseminated intravascular coagulation: a comparative study using criteria from the International Society versus the Korean Society on Thrombosis and Hemostasis. Yonsei Med J. 2007; 48:595–600.

47. Franchini M. Pathophysiology, diagnosis and treatment of disseminated intravascular coagulation: an update. Clin Lab. 2005; 51:633–9.

48. DeLoughery TG. Critical care clotting catastrophies. Crit Care Clin. 2005; 21:531–62.

49. Gaskin G, Pusey CD. Plasmapheresis in antineutrophil cytoplasmic antibody-associated systemic vasculitis. Ther Apher. 2001; 5:176–81.

50. Jayne DR, Gaskin G, Rasmussen N, et al. Randomized trial of plasma exchange or high-dosage methylprednisolone as adjunctive therapy for severe renal vasculitis. J Am Soc Nephrol. 2007; 18:2180–8.

51. Jayne D, Rasmussen N, Andrassy K, et al. A randomized trial of maintenance therapy for vasculitis associated with antineutrophil cytoplasmic autoantibodies. N Engl J Med. 2003; 349:36–44.

52. Jayne DR, Chapel H, Adu D, et al. Intravenous immunoglobulin for ANCA-associated systemic vasculitis with persistent disease activity. QJM. 2000; 93:433–9.

53. Booth A, Harper L, Hammad T, et al. Prospective study of TNFalpha blockade with infliximab in anti-neutrophil cytoplasmic antibody-associated systemic vasculitis. J Am Soc Nephrol. 2004; 15:717–21.

54. Keogh KA, Ytterberg SR, Fervenza FC, et al. Rituximab for refractory Wegener's granulomatosis: report of a prospective, open-label pilot trial. Am J Respir Crit Care Med. 2006; 173:180–7.

55. Ronkainen J, Koskimies O, Ala-Houhala M, et al. Early prednisone therapy in Henoch-Schönlein purpura: a randomized, double-blind, placebo-controlled trial. J Pediatr. 2006; 149:241–7.

56. Dillon MJ. Henoch-Schönlein purpura: recent advances. Clin Exp Rheumatol. 2007; 25(1 Suppl 44):S66–8.

57. Zaffanello M, Brugnara M, Franchini M. Therapy for children with Henoch-Schonlein purpura nephritis: a systematic review. ScientificWorldJournal. 2007; 7:20–30.

58. Lamireau T, Rebouissoux L, Hehunstre JP. Intravenous immunoglobulin therapy for severe digestive manifestations of Henoch-Schönlein pur pura. Acta Paediatr. 2001; 90:1081–2.

59. Shenoy M, Ognjanovic MV, Coulthard MG. Treating severe Henoch-Schönlein and IgA nephritis with plasmapheresis alone. Pediatr Nephrol. 2007; 22:1167–71.

60. Lamprecht P, Till A, Steinmann J, et al. Current state of biologicals in the management of systemic vasculitis. Ann NY Acad Sci. 2007; 1110:261–70.

61. Yazici Y. Vasculitis update, 2007. Bull NYU Hosp Jt Dis. 2007; 65:212–14.

62. Wung PK, Stone JH. Therapeutics of Wegener's granulomatosis. Nat Clin Pract Rheumatol. 2006; 2:192–200.

63. Wegener's Granulomatosis Etanercept Trial (WGET) Research Group. Etanercept plus standard therapy for Wegener's granulomatosis. N Engl J Med. 2005; 352:351–61.

64. Mukhtyar C, Luqmani R. Current state of tumour necrosis factor {alpha} blockade in Wegener's granulomatosis. Ann Rheum Dis. 2005; 64 Suppl 4:31–6.

65. Antoniu SA. Treatment options for refractory Wegener's granulomatosis: a role for rituximab? Curr Opin Investig Drugs. 2007; 8:927–32.

66. Metzler C, Miehle N, Manger K, et al. Elevated relapse rate under oral methotrexate versus leflunomide for maintenance of remission in Wegener's granulomatosis. Rheumatology. 2007; 46:1087–91.

67. Langford CA, Talar-Williams C, Sneller MC. Mycophenolate mofetil for remission maintenance in the treatment of Wegener's granulomatosis. Arthritis Rheum. 2004; 51:278–83.

68. Schmitt WH, Birck R, Heinzel PA, et al. Prolonged treatment of refractory Wegener's granulomatosis with 15-deoxyspergualin: an open study in seven patients. Nephrol Dial Transplant. 2005; 20:1083–92.

69. Hellmich B, Gross WL. Recent progress in the pharmacotherapy of Churg-Strauss syndrome. Expert Opin Pharmacother. 2004; 5:25–35.

70. Arbach O, Gross WL, Gause A. Treatment of refractory Churg-Strauss-Syndrome (CSS) by TNF-alpha blockade. Immunobiology. 2002; 206:496–501.

71. Kaushik VV, Reddy HV, Bucknall RC. Successful use of rituximab in a patient with recalcitrant Churg-Strauss syndrome. Ann Rheum Dis. 2006; 65:1116–17.

72. Koukoulaki M, Smith KG, Jayne DR. Rituximab in Churg-Strauss syndrome. Ann Rheum Dis. 2006; 65:557–9.

73. Taniguchi M, Tsurikisawa N, Higashi N, et al. Treatment for Churg-Strauss syndrome: induction of remission and efficacy of intravenous immunoglobulin therapy. Allergol Int. 2007; 56:97–103.

74. Colmegna I, Maldonado-Cocco JA. Polyarteritis nodosa revisited. Curr Rheumatol Rep. 2005; 7:288–96.

75. Guillevin L, Pagnoux C. Therapeutic strategies for systemic necrotizing vasculitides. Allergol Int. 2007; 56:105–11.

76. Takeshita S, Nakamura H, Kawakami A, et al. Hepatitis B-related polyarteritis nodosa presenting necrotizing vasculitis in the hepatobiliary system successfully treated with lamivudine, plasmapheresis and glucocorticoid. Intern Med. 2006; 45:145–9.

77. Deléaval P, Stadler P, Descombes E, et al. Life-threatening complications of hepatitis B virus-related polyarteritis nodosa developing despite interferon-alpha2b therapy: successful treatment with a combination of interferon, lamivudine, plasma exchanges and steroids. Clin Rheumatol. 2001; 20:290–2.

78. Lau CF, Hui PK, Chan WM, et al. Hepatitis B associated fulminant polyarteritis nodosa: successful treatment with pulse cyclophosphamide, prednisolone and lamivudine following emergency surgery. Eur J Gastroenterol Hepatol. 2002; 14:563–6.

79. Langford CA. Small-vessel vasculitis: therapeutic management. Curr Rheumatol Rep. 2007; 9:328–35.

80. Hoffman GS, Langford CA. Can methotrexate replace cyclophosphamide in the treatment of a subset of Wegener's granulomatosis and microscopic polyangiitis? Nat Clin Pract Rheumatol. 2006; 2:70–1.

81. De Rosa G, Pardeo M, Rigante D. Current recommendations for the pharmacologic therapy in Kawasaki syndrome and management of its cardiovascular complications. Eur Rev Med Pharmacol Sci. 2007; 11:301–8.

82. Durongpisitkul K, Gururaj VJ, Park JM, Martin CF. The prevention of coronary artery aneurysm in Kawasaki disease: a meta-analysis on the efficacy of aspirin and immunoglobulin treatment. Pediatrics. 1995; 96:1057–61.

83. Newburger JW, Takahashi M, Burns JC, et al. The treatment of Kawasaki syndrome with intravenous gamma globulin. N Engl J Med. 1986; 315:341–7.

84. Marasini M, Pongiglione G, Gazzolo D, et al. Late intravenous gamma globulin treatment in infants and children with Kawasaki disease and coronary artery abnormalities. Am J Cardiol. 1991; 68:796–7.

85. Sundel RP, Baker AL, Fulton DR, Newburger JW. Corticosteroids in the initial treatment of Kawasaki disease: report of a randomized trial. J Pediatr. 2003; 142:611–16.

86. Furukawa S, Matsubara T, Umezawa Y, et al. Pentoxifylline and intravenous gamma globulin combination therapy for acute Kawasaki disease. Eur J Pediatr. 1994; 153:663–7.

87. Weiss JE, Eberhard BA, Chowdhury D, Gottlieb BS. Infliximab as a novel therapy for refractory Kawasaki disease. J Rheumatol. 2004; 31:808–10.

88. Carey MJ, Rodgers GM. Disseminated intravascular coagulation: clinical and laboratory aspects. Am J Hematol. 1998; 59:65–73.

89. Toh CH, Downey C. Back to the future: testing in disseminated intravascular coagulation. Blood Coagul Fibrinolysis. 2005; 16:535–42.

90. Feinstein DI. Diagnosis and management of disseminated intravascular coagulation: the role of heparin therapy. Blood. 1982; 60:284–7.

91. Ewing CI, David TJ, Davenport PJ. Heparin for uncontrolled disseminated intravascular coagulation in meningococcal septicaemia. J R Soc Med. 1989; 82:762–3.

92. Hjort PF, Rapaport SI, Jorgensen L. Purpura fulminans. Report of a case successfully treated with heparin and hydrocortisone. Review of 50 cases from the literature. Scand J Haematol. 1964; 61:169–92.

93. Oguma Y, Sakuragawa N, Maki M, et al. Treatment of disseminated intravascular coagulation with low molecular weight heparin. Research Group of FR-860 on DIC in Japan. Semin Thromb Hemost. 1990; 16 Suppl:34–40.

94. Smith OP, White B. Infectious purpura fulminans: caution needed in the use of protein C. Br J Haematol. 1999; 106:253–4.

95. Sen K, Roy A. Management of neonatal purpura fulminans with severe protein C deficiency. Indian Pediatr. 2006; 43:542–5.

96. Müller FM, Ehrenthal W, Hafner G, Schranz D. Purpura fulminans in severe congenital protein C deficiency: monitoring of treatment with protein C concentrate. Eur J Pediatr. 1996; 155:20–5.

97. de Kleijn ED, de Groot R, Hack CE, et al. Activation of protein C following infusion of protein C concentrate in children with severe meningococcal sepsis and purpura fulminans: a randomized, double-blinded, placebo-controlled, dose-finding study. Crit Care Med. 2003; 31:1839–47.

98. Kaiserman D, Whisstock JC, Bird PI. Mechanisms of serpin dysfunction in disease. Expert Rev Mol Med. 2006; 8: 1–19.

99. Afshari A, Wetterslev J, Brok J, Møller A. Antithrombin III in critically ill patients: systematic review with meta-analysis and trial sequential analysis. BMJ. 2007; 335:1248–51.

100. Darmstadt GL. Acute infectious purpura fulminans: pathogenesis and medical management. Pediatr Dermatol. 1998; 15:169–83.

101. Twomey JA, Peltier GL, Zera RT. An open-label study to evaluate the safety and efficacy of tissue plasminogen activator in treatment of severe frostbite. J Trauma. 2005; 59: 1350–4.

102. Spronk PE, Rommes JH, Schaar C, Ince C. Thrombolysis in fulminant purpura: observations on changes in microcirculatory perfusion during successful treatment. Thromb Haemost. 2006; 95:576–8.

103. Zenz W, Zoehrer B, Levin M, et al. Use of recombinant tissue plasminogen activator in children with meningococcal purpura fulminans: a retrospective study. Crit Care Med. 2004; 32:1777–80.

104. Baines P, Carrol ED. Recombinant tissue plasminogen activator in children with meningococcal purpura fulminans– role uncertain. Crit Care Med. 2004; 32:1806–7.

105. Winrow AP. Successful treatment of neonatal purpura fulminans with epoprostenol. J R Soc Med. 1992; 85:245.

106. Stewart FJ, McClure BG, Mayne E. Successful treatment of neonatal purpura fulminans with epoprostenol. J R Soc Med. 1991; 84:623–4.

107. Roderick P, Ferris G, Wilson K, et al. Towards evidence-based guidelines for the prevention of venous thromboembolism: systematic reviews of mechanical methods, oral anticoagulation, dextran and regional anaesthesia as thromboprophylaxis. Health Technol Assess. 2005; 9:1–78.

CHAPTER 24

Emergency Management of Connective Tissue Disorders and Their Complications

Kristen Biggers

Noah Scheinfeld

COLLAGEN VASCULAR diseases are complex multi-organ states of pathologic dysfunction. The collagen vascular diseases that most commonly result in emergency situations include systemic lupus erythematosus (SLE), dermatomyositis (DM), and scleroderma. This chapter will review emergency management of connective tissue disorders and their complications. In particular, the clinical and laboratory aids required for diagnosis, therapy, and prognosis will be reviewed. Because we assume that the reader has a basic understanding of the diseases, the chapter does not review them.

SLE

SLE is a complex state of systemic dysregulation that can affect any organ system (see Figure 24.1). The noted writer Flannery O'Connor died at the age of 39, after surgery led to a reactivation and intensification of lupus that resulted in fatal kidney failure. As lupus can be a systemic disease, the most serious emergency management pertaining to it includes cardiovascular, pulmonary, hematologic, neurological, renal, and gastrointestinal (GI) dysfunctions.[1] The prevalence of SLE for 15- to 44-year-old white women has been estimated to be between 18.3 and 40 cases per 100,000 and twice that for 15- to 44-year-old black women.[2] The American College of Rheumatology has established a standard for the diagnosis of SLE, based on the patient having 4 of 11 criteria, including positive titers for various antibodies (Table 24.1).[3]

CARDIOVASCULAR DYSFUNCTION AND SLE

Background

There are manifold intersections of cardiovascular dysfunction and SLE. In patients with long-standing lupus, the most common causes of death are due to cardiovascular events.

The basis for cardiovascular disease in patients with lupus is complex and seems to involve a combination of inflammatory and immune mechanisms. In patients with SLE, oxidized lipid levels (such as oxidized low-density lipoprotein and proinflammatory high-density lipoprotein) are increased, adhesion molecules are upregulated, and cytokines (such as monocyte chemotactic protein-1, tumor necrosis factor-α, interferon-γ, interleukin-1, and interleukin-12) are upregulated. These oxidized lipids deposit in the walls of coronary vessels. Autoantibodies bind to the oxidized lipids, forming immune complexes, which provide a basis for the development of atherosclerosis.

The most common cardiac pathology in SLE patients is pericarditis with a reported prevalence of 60%. Valvular, myocardial, and coronary vessel lesions can also be manifested in SLE patients.[4] Atherosclerotic cardiovascular disease is common and is related to increased antiphospholipid antibodies.[4] Patients with lupus nephritis are at an increased risk for developing hypertension.[4] Antiphospholipid syndrome can result in ventricular dysfunction, intracardiac thrombi, myxomas, and pulmonary hypertension. The coronary arteries are not immune from the effects of vasculitis associated with lupus.

Diagnosis

Laboratory testing and imaging studies are utilized in the diagnosis of lupus-related cardiac disease, as in other cardiac diseases. Elevated lipid or C-reactive protein levels can be seen in patients with cardiac abnormalities associated with SLE. Mild pericarditis, valvular lesions, and

TABLE 24.1: Antibodies Associated
with Systemic Lupus Erythematosus

Antinuclear antibody (ANA)
Anti-double-stranded DNA (anti-dsDNA)
Anti-Smith (anti-Sm) antibody
Anti-anionic phospholipids antibodies
Mostly anti-cardiolipin (aCL)
Anti-β2 glycoprotein 1 antibodies
Anti-C1Q antibodies
Anti-Ro (SSa) antibody
Anti-La (SSb) antibody

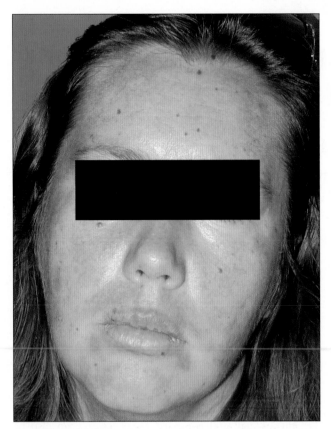

FIGURE 24.1: *Classic malar and facial erythema of systemic lupus erythematosus.*

myocardial dysfunctions can be detected with echocardiography, a technique that is both sensitive and specific.

Therapy

Patients with SLE and cardiovascular disease are approached similarly as non-SLE patients with heart disease. Lifestyle changes are recommended, including dietary and exercise counseling. Risk factors, such as increased lipid levels, are targeted for reduction. Because patients with SLE are predisposed to clotting, it has been suggested that they should be placed on more aggressive anticoagulant therapy. All patients with SLE should take aspirin prophylactically, and more potent anticoagulants should be added to the treatment regimen as needed.

Course and Prognosis

Cardiovascular events in patients with SLE are less severe due to advances in therapy.

PULMONARY DYSFUNCTION AND SLE

Background

SLE is associated with respiratory pathology in all anatomic locations, including the pleura, pulmonary parenchyma, airways, vessels, and respiratory muscles. These disease processes can occur in one area of the respiratory system or in multiple places simultaneously. Pulmonary symptoms can wax and wane, further increasing the morbidity and mortality associated with lupus.

In SLE, the most common respiratory complaints are attributed to pleural disease, a pathology that affects up to 35% of patients.[5,6] As in cardiovascular disease, lupus autoantibodies form immune complexes that are deposited in the pleura, resulting in injury. Other pulmonary disorders associated with SLE patients include acute lupus pneumonitis, alveolar hemorrhage pleural disease, pneumonia, diffusion impairments, diffuse alveolar hemorrhage, acute lupus pneumonitis, thrombosis, and pulmonary hypertension.[4,7] Sudden-onset dyspnea and fever are characteristic of acute lupus pneumonitis and alveolar hemorrhage, which also results in hypoxemia and a chest x-ray demonstrating patchy alveolar infiltrates.[7,8] Patients affected by diffuse alveolar hemorrhage (1%–5% of patients with SLE)[9,10] have a 50%–90% risk of death attributed to the acute decrease in hemoglobin levels.[4,7,11,12] SLE therapy, including glucocorticoids or immunomodulatory agents, increases a patient's risk for developing pneumonia.[13,14]

Pulmonary physiology is adversely affected in patients with SLE.[15] In a study comparing the lung function of 70 nonsmoking, non-lupus patients with 70 age-matched, nonsmoking SLE patients showed normal lung function in 83% of subjects in the control group and only 33% in SLE patients.[15] Diffusion capacity of carbon monoxide in the lung (DLCO) is the most common adversely affected pulmonary function test and can be decreased even in the absence of a concomitant restrictive lung disease.[15,16] As in vessels throughout the body, antiphospholipid antibodies can be deposited in the pulmonary vessels, causing thrombosis[17,18] that results in fatal pulmonary hypertension, unresponsive to therapy.

Diagnosis

Imaging studies, including computed tomography (CT) and magnetic resonance imaging (MRI), are useful in developing a diagnosis of lung disease in patients with SLE.[19,20] Additional diagnostic information can be gained from pulmonary function tests and lung biopsy.

Therapy

Corticosteroids are the mainstays of treatment for SLE patients with pulmonary disease. Cyclophosphamide (500–1000 mg/m^2 intravenously [IV] every 4 weeks) can be used in resistant cases. This therapy has been reported to be especially effective in treating interstitial lung disease.[21,22] Steroid-sparing agents such as azathioprine and methotrexate are useful in some situations.[3] Extremely resistant cases may benefit from plasmapheresis or IV immunoglobulin (IVIg). Recently, rituximab has been shown to increase the effectiveness of traditional therapy when used as an adjunct in patients who are unresponsive to traditional therapy alone.

Course and Prognosis

The course of SLE associated with neuropsychiatric conditions can be extended and complex. The prognosis of SLE associated with neuropsychiatric conditions is not good and is a negative prognostic indicator for the morbidity and mortality associated with SLE.

HEMATOLOGIC DYSFUNCTION AND SLE

Background

Vasculitis and thrombosis are common manifestations of SLE. In addition to making antiphospholipid antibodies, patients with lupus can make antiplatelet antibodies that precipitate thrombocytopenia.[4]

Diagnosis

The antiphospholipids produced in patients with SLE include anticardiolipin antibodies, lupus anticoagulants, and anti-β2 glycoprotein-1–specific antibodies.[23,24] Lupus anticoagulant levels can be assessed via blood titers.[23,24] If a patient is suspected of having a thrombus, imaging studies can be performed to confirm.

Therapy

Hematologic dysfunction in lupus is treated symptomatically with immunosuppressives for vasculitis and anticoagulants for thrombosis. Nonsteroidal therapy includes azathioprine and methotrexate.[3] Thrombocytopenia caused by anti-deoxyribonucleic acid (anti-DNA) antibodies can be treated with IVIg.[25]

Course and Prognosis

Increased risk of thrombotic events is especially dangerous in pregnant women and can be fatal for both the mother and the fetus.

NEUROLOGICAL DYSFUNCTION AND SLE

Background

Rarely, SLE is associated with neuropsychiatric conditions including organic brain syndrome, seizures, cerebrovascular accidents, strokes, psychosis, peripheral neuropathy, and achorea.[4] Even less common neuropsychiatric manifestations are aseptic meningitis, pseudotumor cerebri, Guillain–Barré syndrome, athetosis, and cerebral venous sinus thrombosis.[4] Many neurologic disorders in SLE are related to the deposition of antiphospholipid and anti-ribonucleoprotein (anti-RNP) antibodies.[26] Raynaud

phenomenon and livedo reticularis are associated with an increased risk of neuropsychiatric manifestations in patients with SLE.[27]

Diagnosis

In patients with SLE-associated neuropsychiatric disorders, a spinal tap can be performed and may show increased cell counts, increased protein levels, and increased immunoglobulins in the cerebrospinal fluid.[28] Less invasive diagnostic techniques can be utilized to detect cranial bleeds, thrombosis, vasculitis, and inflammation, and include CT, MRI, and transcranial Doppler monitoring.[28]

Therapy

In patients with SLE, neuropsychiatric complications are controlled by treating the underlying pathology, as in the other organ systems mentioned previously.[4] IVIg and plasmapheresis are often used sooner in neuropsychiatric conditions associated with SLE than when other organ systems are affected due to the severe complications that can result if insufficiently treated.[4]

Course and Prognosis

Patients with SLE associated with neuropsychiatric conditions resistant to IVIg and/or plasmapheresis therapy can be emergently administered pulsed high dose intravenous methylprednisolone to bring the disease rapidly under control.[29,30]

RENAL DYSFUNCTION AND SLE

Background

The most common systemic complication of SLE is renal disease,[1,31–33] the manifestations of which include focal proliferative, diffuse proliferative, or membranous glomerulonephritis.[34] Anti-DNA antibodies form complexes with double-stranded DNA polynucleotide antigens that deposit in the small vessels of the kidney, which is the major cause of lupus nephritis. Type III sensitivity reactions, during which antibodies bind with fixed antigens to form a complex, may also play a role in lupus nephritis. It has also been hypothesized that sensitized T cells may contribute to renal pathology in lupus patients.

Diagnosis

The presence of proteinuria (>0.5 g/d) or cellular casts is required to diagnose renal involvement in patients with SLE, as defined by the American College of Rheumatology.[34] Lupus nephritis and renal dysfunction can be further complicated by the presence of antiphospholipid antibodies, low complement (C3) levels, thrombocytopenia, anemia, or hypertension, and death may result.[35] Immune complexes composed of DNA double-stranded polynucleotide antigens and anti-DNA antibodies may be found in patients with lupus nephritis and may be elevated. In addition to serum testing, a renal biopsy may be performed to diagnose focal proliferative, diffuse proliferative, or membranous glomerulonephritis.[34]

Therapy

As in most patients with lupus, corticosteroids are the mainstay of treatment for patients with lupus nephritis with the addition of mycophenolate mofetil (MMF) and azathioprine to the therapeutic regimen.[36–38] IV cyclophosphamide (0.5 g/m^2) may be necessary for refractory renal disease or in patients with diffuse proliferative lupus nephritis. When this treatment is selected, cyclophosphamide is infused monthly for 6 months, and then every several months for a full year following remission.[39]

Course and Prognosis

In patients who meet the criteria for SLE-associated renal disease, their survival is largely determined by their creatinine levels.[1,31–33] Patients with SLE-associated renal disease may suffer from end-stage renal disease and require dialysis.

GI DYSFUNCTION AND SLE

Background

GI dysfunction is common in patients with SLE, and over a lifetime affects 60%–70% of those patients. The liver is particularly susceptible in patients with lupus and antiphospholipid syndrome. Portal hypertension, cirrhosis, biliary cirrhosis, autoimmune hepatitis, Budd–Chiari syndrome, hepatic infarct, and hepatic-veno-occlusive disease are all possible associated conditions. Other GI manifestations include vasculitis throughout the GI tract, oral ulcers, dysphagia, intestinal infarction or bleeding, splenic infarction, and acute pancreatitis. Corticosteroids used to treat SLE can have adverse effects on the GI tract by causing spontaneous hemorrhage.

Diagnosis

Lupus patients can present with abdominal pain, anorexia, hemorrhage, nausea, and vomiting. Clinical testing may yield little as far as symptom etiology.

Therapy

Patients with chronic symptoms can be treated with corticosteroids or anticoagulants. Those with an acute presentation should be assessed quickly, as emergent surgery is usually the treatment of choice. Exploratory surgery is often required in patients with suspected peritoneal collections or

TABLE 24.2: Maternal Antibodies

Anti-Ro(SS-A)
Anti-La(SS-B)
U1-RNP

GI perforations. In cases of perforation or bowel ischemia, the affected area should be surgically resected as the first step in treatment.

Course and Prognosis

Lupus patients with acute GI symptoms can rapidly progress to life threatening status without immediate intervention.

NEONATAL LUPUS ERYTHEMATOSUS

Background

Women with lupus have several autoantibodies (Table 24.2) that are capable of crossing the placenta. A pregnant woman with lupus can pass these antibodies on to her fetus, resulting in neonatal lupus erythematosus (NLE). After delivery, the infant can present with dermatologic signs similar to those in adults with SLE. Pathology specific to infants with NLE include characteristic dermatologic manifestations (raccoon eyes) and congenital heart block.[21]

Diagnosis

M-mode fetal echocardiograms and Doppler ultrasounds performed between 18 and 24 weeks gestation can be useful in detecting atrioventricular (AV) heart block or atrial arrhythmia in a fetus with NLE. If a heart block is detected, these studies can also determine the degree of the block (1st, 2nd, or 3rd) as well as any valvular (especially tricuspid) regurgitation or other congenital anatomic cardiac anomalies.

Pregnant women with lupus should receive fetal echocardiograms throughout their pregnancies to facilitate the early identification of heart block.

Therapy

When a first- or second-degree AV block has been identified in a fetus with NLE, corticosteroids can be administered to the mother in an attempt to eliminate the heart block. The reversal of third-degree heart block with corticosteroids is highly unlikely.

Course and Prognosis

Unfortunately, completely unremarkable echocardiograms can change in 1 week to an echocardiogram demonstrating

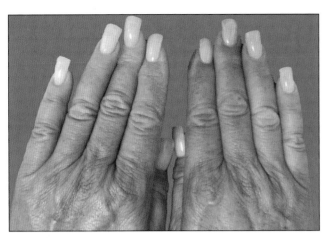

FIGURE 24.2: *Gottron sign of dermatomyositis: reddish plaques on the joints and on the fingers.*

TABLE 24.3: Dermatomyositis Antibodies[43]

Antibodies associated with dermatomyositis	Antibodies overlapping with other collagen vascular diseases
Antisynthetase	Anti-Ku
Anti–Mi-2	Anti–PM-Scl
Anti-SRP	Anti–U1 RNP
	Anti-Ro

Data adapted from (43).

DM

cardiomyopathy or third-degree AV block without warning. Only 80% of infants with NLE-related first-degree heart block survive the first year. Of those children who do survive, the majority of them will need a pacemaker.

DM is an inflammatory myopathy, the nature of which is idiopathic. The manifestations of this disease include progressive symmetrical proximal muscle weakness and dermatologic manifestations (e.g., Gottron papules, heliotrope eruption) (see Figure 24.2).[40] Additional organ systems affected in systemic DM are the GI tract, lungs, and blood vessels.[41,42] The systemic manifestations are responsible for emergent situations in patients with DM.[42] Ricky Bell, a football player, who was a standout running back for the University of Southern California Trojans, and played for Tampa Bay and San Diego in the National Football League, died from heart failure caused by DM.

To be diagnosed with DM, a person must present with at least 3 of the following clinical criteria: 1) muscle weakness; 2) muscle biopsy pathology; 3) elevated creatine kinase, aldolase, lactate dehydrogenase, aspartate aminotransferase, or alanine aminotransferase, all of which point to muscle involvement; 4) a triad of electromyographic abnormalities; or 5) skin eruption.[43] In all manifestations of the disease, creatine kinase levels may be used to track the progression of or the response to treatment of DM.[43] Specific serum antibody levels can be drawn to aid in the diagnosis of DM (Table 24.3).

Muscle involvement may be tracked using electromyography, ultrasonography, or MRI.[44] Additionally, a muscle biopsy can be performed to assess muscle involvement and will show immune-mediated necrosis and regenerating fibers. On skin biopsy, mucin in the background of interface dermatitis is commonly seen histologically.[45]

GI TRACT AND DM

Background

DM can affect much of the GI tract, especially the esophagus and intestines. Esophageal disease is common in patients with DM (15%–50%) and most often stems from problems associated with weakness of the cricopharyngeal striated muscles or dysfunction of the lower esophagus.[46] Of all patients with DM, approximately 30% of them will die from complications associated with aspiration pneumonia.[46] Less frequently (and especially in young patients with DM), ulceration, perforation, or hemorrhage may occur in the GI tract as a result of vasculopathy in that area.[47]

Diagnosis

DM can cause inflammation in the GI tract, leading to patients presenting with reflux esophagitis, abdominal pain, and cycles of constipation alternating with diarrhea.[48] A traditional GI workup, including CT, MRI, colonoscopy, and barium studies are used, as in other GI diseases, to assess the severity of disease.[49]

Treatment

Surgical intervention and immunosuppressives are the standard of care for treating GI disease in DM. IVIg may be successful in treating resistant esophageal disease that might otherwise be life threatening.[50–52]

Course and Prognosis

The pharyngeal muscle weakness in patients with DM causes loss of control of foods and can result in aspiration. Due to the aspiration risk, these patients may be placed on a feeding tube.[53] Patients with esophageal muscle weakness do not respond well to therapy; therefore, they have a poor prognosis.[46,53]

PULMONARY SYSTEM AND DM

Background

Pulmonary disease is a fairly common occurrence in patients with DM (15%–30%), and in 50% of these patients

TABLE 24.4: Antisynthetase Antibodies

Anti-Jo
Anti–PI-7
Anti–PI-12
Anti-O
Anti-EJ
Anti-KS

it is the first presenting sign of the disease.[49] The majority of DM patients presenting with respiratory disease (60%) have an insidious onset. Others (25% of patients) have an acute onset of signs, and 15% of patients have an infraclinical onset that presents as an incidental finding on exam. Patients with amyopathic DM can have fatal pulmonary diseases or pulmonary complications.[54]

Pulmonary inflammation is the leading pathology in lung diseases in patients with DM.[49] Respiratory muscle weakness leads to hypoventilation and esophageal muscle weakness leads to aspiration, both of which result in inflammatory processes.[49] Additionally, the treatment for DM itself, usually immunosuppressive therapies, can leave the patient susceptible to opportunistic infections or hypersensitivity pneumonitis.[49]

Pulmonary diseases associated with DM include pulmonary hypertension,[48] pneumothorax, pneumomediastinum, interstitial lung disease, and subcutaneous emphysema.[55]

Diffuse alveolar damage, respiratory bronchiolitis, bronchiolitis obliterans, and pneumonia (desquamative interstitial and nonspecific interstitial) are all interstitial pulmonary diseases caused by fibrosing alveolitis in DM.[54]

Diagnosis

Patients with DM and associated pulmonary disease may present with the symptoms of exertional dyspnea and nonproductive cough, as well as the clinical sign of bibasilar fine crackling rales.[54] Because pulmonary physiology can be affected, further studies should include pulmonary function testing, which demonstrate decreased DLCO and a restrictive pattern.[54] A high-resolution CT scan should be performed with the pulmonary function tests as part of the initial workup.

Antisynthetase antibodies (Table 24.4) can be seen in DM patients with pulmonary disease.[43] Patients with an acute onset of interstitial pulmonary fibrosis and dramatic polymyositis that is resistant to therapy should be considered for antisynthetase syndrome.[55,56] This often fatal syndrome can be seen in patients with DM and antisynthetase antibodies who also suffer from fever, interstitial pulmonary fibrosis, Raynaud phenomenon, arthritis, and mechanic's

hand.[56] Additionally, patients with pulmonary fibrosis may express the myositis antibody, anti-Se.[43]

Therapy

As in patients with other forms of DM, corticosteroids remain the treatment of choice for patients suffering from pulmonary disease.[57] High-dose IV corticosteroids can be administered in severe cases with acute onset. If corticosteroids fail to alleviate symptoms, methotrexate can be added to the regimen or administered alone as a second-line agent.[58] Azathioprine, cyclophosphamide, chlorambucil, cyclosporine, MMF, or chlorambucil can be used as third-line treatments.[58] Interstitial pulmonary disease in DM responds well to cyclosporin A therapy.[59–61] IVIg and rituximab may be used in resistant cases.[50–52]

Pulmonary function tests and CT scans should be repeated regularly to assess treatment effectiveness and progression of disease.

Course and Prognosis

Unfortunately, for patients with pulmonary symptoms in the context of DM, their prognosis is poor.[49] Pulmonary fibrosis results in interstitial lung disease and pulmonary hypertension, both of which are often fatal. The chronic respiratory insufficiency resulting from interstitial lung disease is fatal in 30%–66% of patients.[48]

CARDIOVASCULAR DISEASE AND DM

Background

Although cardiac disease is rarely a complication of DM, when it presents, it is usually fatal.[48] Inflammatory myositis can result in cardiac dysfunction as can vasoconstriction from vasculitis.[62]

Diagnosis

When a patient with DM presents with cardiac symptoms, the same tests should be performed as would be on any patient presenting with cardiac symptoms. These standard cardiac tests should reveal the location and degree of involvement of heart muscle. Cardiac disease is more common in patients who produce the antibody to signal recognition particle (anti-SRP antibody).[43] Additional testing could include blood-vessel biopsies. A biopsy of a vessel affected by DM should demonstrate scarring in the vessel wall, with or without associated fibrosis.

Treatment and Prognosis

For those patients who suffer from DM-associated cardiac disease, few treatment options are available, and those

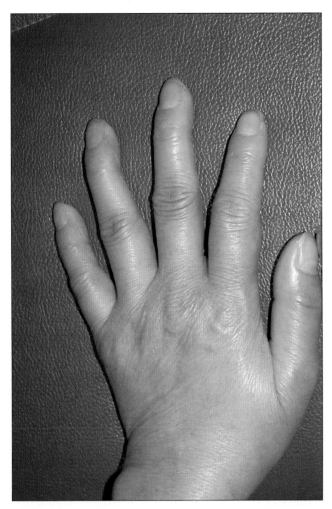

FIGURE 24.3: *Scleroderma of the hand demonstrating sclerodactyly.*

that are available are usually unable to alleviate disease. Having pulmonary and cardiac symptoms simultaneously greatly increases a patient's risk of fatality.[48] Neurological symptoms can appear in children with DM due to inflammatory changes in the blood vessels.[47] These vasculitis-associated conditions include stroke, hemiparesis, seizures, and pseudoseizures.[47]

SCLERODERMA (SYSTEMIC SCLEROSIS)

Scleroderma, by definition, is a systemic disease and can have adverse affects on the GI, renal, and pulmonary systems. The respiratory system is most commonly the location for pathology that can be emergently life threatening in patients with systemic sclerosis (SS).[63,64] In fact, Paul Klee (the noted Swiss artist who had scleroderma) died of scleroderma-related pulmonary fibrosis that led to respiratory failure. It can affect the skin and lead to hardening of the skin, nail fold changes, calcinosis, and sclerodactyly (Figure 24.3).

PULMONARY DISEASE AND SCLERODERMA

Background

Pulmonary fibrosis, a normal manifestation of scleroderma, results in interstitial fibrosis of the lungs. Vasculidities resultant from SS and interstitial fibrosis can both lead to the development of pulmonary hypertension, as seen in 5%–50% of patients with scleroderma.[65,66]

Diagnosis

Patients present with dyspnea on exertion as their initial manifestation of pulmonary hypertension. Clinically, pulmonary hypertension is tested, while the patient is exercising and is defined as an increase in mean pulmonary arterial pressure to greater than 25 mm Hg.[65]

Therapy

Early stages of scleroderma-related pulmonary hypertension are treated as is hypertension in most disease states, with vasodilators. While the vascular damage is still reversible, calcium channel blockers and prostanoids (prostaglandin E1 and iloprost) are the treatments of choice and have been shown to be effective early in the disease process.[66–68] With progression of pulmonary hypertension, patients with scleroderma may benefit from IV epoprostenol, a prostanoid analog.[69] A newer, more stable compound, treprostinil, is administered subcutaneously[65] and is more effective than epoprostenol at relieving pulmonary symptoms and decreasing arterial pressure and vascular resistance.[70] Bosentan, an oral endothelin antagonist, and sildenafil, an oral cyclic guanosine 3′, 5′-monophosphate phosphodiesterase type five (cGMP PDE5) inhibitor, have been effective in relieving the symptoms of pulmonary hypertension in patients with scleroderma.[71,72] A significant relief of symptoms and adverse effects associated with pulmonary hypertension has been observed when a combination therapy including bosentan, iloprost, and sildenafil is administered to scleroderma patients.

For pulmonary fibrosis, immunosuppressives are the treatment of choice. In cases of severe pulmonary fibrosis, 100 mg/d doses of cyclophosphamide have been shown to improve both forced vital capacity and overall survival.[73–75] Some investigators believe, however, that corticosteroids have no positive effect on lung function.[74]

Course and Prognosis

In patients with scleroderma-related pulmonary disease, their initial symptom of dyspnea on exertion increases in severity. Such patients usually end up suffering from right-sided heart failure, which further increases symptoms.[65]

RENAL DISEASE AND SCLERODERMA

Background

The most common systemic manifestation in scleroderma, occurring in 25% of patients, involves the renal system.[42] Renal crisis is more prevalent in scleroderma patients whose symptoms include the presence of anti-ribonucleic acid (RNA) polymerase III antibody in the serum, rapidly progressive skin thickening,[76] pericardial effusion, arrhythmias, and anemia.[77] Additionally, the treatment for SS, corticosteroids, especially cyclosporine, can precipitate renal crisis.[77] Renal crisis presents within the first 4 years of diagnosis of scleroderma in the majority of patients (75%), rarely occurring in patients suffering from SS for many years.[78]

Patients with SS develop narrowed arteries and arterioles.[77] This phenomenon greatly impacts upon the kidneys and can result in renal crisis.[77] A positive-feedback loop occurs that significantly restricts the blood flow to the kidneys. Initially, collagen deposits in arteriole walls, decreasing their diameter and limiting blood flow to the kidneys. The juxtaglomerular apparatus recognizes the postglomerular decrease in blood pressure and releases renin.[77] This release of renin activates the renin–angiotensin system, resulting in increased secretion of angiotensin II. Angiotensin II causes vasoconstriction of the afferent and efferent arterioles in the kidney. This vasoconstriction further limits blood flow, leading to ischemia and renal crisis.[77]

Diagnosis

There are recognized diagnostic criteria for renal crisis in patients with scleroderma. Patients usually present with a dramatic spike in arterial blood pressure with concomitant symptoms of headaches, visual disturbances, and seizures, and signs of thrombocytopenia, microangiopathic hemolytic anemia, accelerated oliguric renal failure, pericardial effusion, and congestive heart failure.[76] The diagnostic criteria for hypertensive scleroderma renal crisis are elevated serum creatinine, proteinuria, hematuria, thrombocytopenia, and hemolysis.[76] The majority of patients (90%) present with hypertension,[76] and nearly all of them have elevated renin plasma levels.[77]

Therapy

The only effective treatment for people in renal crisis is an angiotensin-converting enzyme (ACE) inhibitor to help dampen the effects of the increased plasma renin levels.[78]

Course and Prognosis

Although ACE inhibitors have been shown to decrease mortality and morbidity associated with renal crisis,[79] some patients may require dialysis. In general, renal crisis is viewed as an indicator of poor prognosis in patients with SS.

MIXED CONNECTIVE TISSUE DISEASE

Background

Patients with symptoms that overlap those of SLE, SS, and DM are classified as having a mixed connective tissue disease.

Diagnosis

The presence of anti-uridine-rich RNA-small nuclear ribonucleoprotein (snRNP) antibodies is required to diagnose a patient with mixed connective tissue disease. As would be expected, pulmonary disorders in patients with mixed connective tissue disease resemble those seen in patients with lupus, DM, and scleroderma. These disorders include interstitial fibrosis (20%–65%), pleural effusion (50%), pulmonary hypertension (10%–45%), and pleurisy (20%). Other less common pulmonary features of MCTD include pulmonary vasculitis, thromboembolism, aspiration pneumonia, miscellaneous infections, hemorrhage, obstructive airway disease, respiratory failure (hypoventilatory), and diaphragm muscle weakness.

Treatment

As in patients with DM, corticosteroids are the gold standard for treatment of pulmonary symptoms in patients with mixed connective tissue disease.

Course and Prognosis

The prognosis for patients with pulmonary hypertension in the setting of mixed connective tissue disease is similar to those with pulmonary hypertension associated with other collagen vascular disorders: grim. Despite aggressive treatment, usually symptomatic relief is briefly attained before the disease contributes to the patient's mortality.

CONCLUSIONS

Because collagen vascular diseases are widely systemic, effecting many organ systems, their successful treatment is as complex as the diseases themselves. Most important to treatment success is early recognition and proper diagnosis. Early therapy may prevent possible life-threatening emergencies in the future. Because many patients may initially present with dermatologic manifestations, it is important for the physician to look beyond the patient's primary complaint to the possible outcomes of systemic manifestations.

REFERENCES

1. Cervera R, Khamashta MA, Font J, et al. Morbidity and mortality in systemic lupus erythematosus during a 5-year period. A multicenter prospective study of 1000 patients. Medicine. 1999; 78:167–75.
2. Siegel M, Lee SL. The epidemiology of systemic lupus erythematosus. Semin Arthritis Rheum. 1973; 3:1–54.
3. Brasington RD, Kahl LE, Ranganathan P, et al. Immunologic rheumatic disorders. J Allergy Clin Immunol. 2003; 111:S593–S601.
4. Boumpas DT, Austin HA, Fessler BJ, et al. Systemic lupus erythematosus: emerging concepts: Part I. Renal, neuropsychiatric, cardiovascular, pulmonary and hematologic disease. Ann Intern Med. 1995; 122:940–50.
5. Swaak AJ, Van Den Brink HG, Smeenk RJ, et al. Systemic lupus erythematosus: clinical features in patients with a disease duration of over 10 years, first evaluation. Rheumatology (Oxford). 1999; 38:953–8.
6. Jacobsen S, Petersen J, Ullman S, et al. A multicentre study of 513 Danish patients with systemic lupus erythematosus: i. Disease manifestations and analyses of clinical subsets. Clin Rheumatol. 1998; 17:468–77.
7. Wiedmann HP, Matthay RA. Pulmonary manifestations of systemic lupus erythematosus. J Thorac Imag. 1992; 7:1–18.
8. Boulware DW, Hedgpeth MT. Lupus pneumonitis and anti-SSA(Ro) antibodies. J Rheumatol. 1989; 16:479–81.
9. Santos-Ocampo AS, Mandell BF, Fessler BJ. Alveolar hemorrhage in systemic lupus erythematosus: presentation and management. Chest. 2000; 118:1083–90.
10. Barile LA, Jara LJ, Medina-Rodriguez F, et al. Pulmonary hemorrhage in systemic lupus erythematosus. Lupus. 1997; 6:445–8.
11. Mulherin D, Bresnihan B. Systemic lupus erythematosus. Clin Rheumatol. 1994; 7:31–57.
12. Schwab EP, Schumacher HR Jr., Freundlich B, Callegari PE. Pulmonary alveolar hemorrhage in systemic lupus erythematosus. Semin Arthritis Rheum. 1993; 23:8–15.
13. Cervera R, Khamashta MA, Font J, et al. Morbidity and mortality in systemic lupus erythematosus during a 10-year period: a comparison of early and late manifestations in a cohort of 1,000 patients. Medicine (Baltimore). 2003; 82:299–308.
14. Noel V, Lortholary O, Casassus P, et al. Risk factors and prognostic influence of infection in a single cohort of 87 adults with systemic lupus erythematosus. Ann Rheum Dis. 2001; 60:1141–4.
15. Andonopoulos AP, Constantopoulos SH, Galanopoulou V, et al. Pulmonary function of nonsmoking patients with systemic lupus erythematosis. Chest. 1988; 94:312–15.
16. Traynor AE, Corbridge TC, Eagan AE, et al. Prevalence and reversibility of pulmonary dysfunction in refractory systemic lupus: improvement correlates with disease remission following hematopoietic stem cell transplantation. Chest. 2005; 127:1680–9.
17. Somers E, Magder LS, Petri M. Antiphospholipid antibodies and incidence of venous thrombosis in a cohort of patients with systemic lupus erythematosus. J Rheumatol. 2002; 29:2531–6.

18. Ruiz-Irastorza G, Egurbide MV, Ugalde J, et al. High impact of antiphospholipid syndrome on irreversible organ damage and survival of patients with systemic lupus erythematosus. Arch Intern Med. 2004; 164:77–82.
19. Bankier AA, Kiener HP, Wiesmayr MN, et al. Discrete lung involvement in systemic lupus erythematosus: CT assessment. Radiology. 1995; 196:835–40.
20. Fenlon HM, Doran M, Sant SM, et al. High-resolution chest CT in systemic lupus erythematosus. AJR Am J Roentgenol. 1996; 166:301–7.
21. Heffernan MP, Do JH, Mehta J. Antinuclear antibodies in dermatology. Semin Cutan Med Surg. 2001; 20:2–13.
22. Eiser AR, Shanies HM. Treatment of lupus interstitial lung disease with intravenous cyclophosphamide. Arthritis Rheum. 1994; 37:428–31.
23. Bertolaccini ML, Khamashta MA. Laboratory diagnosis and management challenges in the antiphospholipid syndrome. Lupus. 2006; 15:172–8.
24. McNeil HP, Chesterman CN, Krilis SA. Anticardiolipin antibodies and lupus anticoagulants comprise separate antibody subgroups with different phospholipid binding characteristics. Br J Haematol. 1989; 73:506–13.
25. Strand V. New therapies for systemic lupus erythematosus. Rheum Dis Clin North Am. 2000; 26:389–406.
26. Brey RL, Escalante A. Neurological manifestations of antiphospholipid antibody syndrome. Lupus. 1998; 7: S67.
27. Takashi Y. Livedo reticularis and central nervous system involvement in systemic lupus erythematosus. Arch Dermatol. 1986; 122:66–70.
28. Amigo MC, Khamashta MA. Antiphospholipid syndrome in systemic lupus erythematosus. Rheum Dis Clin North Am. 2000; 26:331–48.
29. Kimberly RP, Lockshin MD, Sherman RL, et al. High dose intravenous methylprednisolone pulse therapy in systemic lupus erythematosus. Am J Med. 1981; 70:817–24.
30. Mackworth-Young CG, David J, Morgan SH, Hughs GR. A double blind placebo controlled trial of intravenous methylprednisolone in systemic lupus erythematosus. Ann Rheum Dis. 1988; 47:496–502.
31. Fries JF, Weyl S, Hellman HR. Estimating prognosis in disease activity. Am J Med. 1974; 57:561–6.
32. Seleznick MJ, Fries JF. Variables associated with decreased survival in systemic lupus erythematosus. Semin Arthritis Rheum. 1991; 21:73–80.
33. Alarcon GS, McGwin G, Bastian HM, et al. Systemic lupus erythematosus in three ethnic groups VIII. Predictors of early mortality in the LUMINA cohort. Arthritis Care Res. 2001; 45:191–202.
34. Golbus J, McCune WJ. Lupus nephritis. Classification, prognosis, immunopathogenesis, and treatment. Rheum Dis Clin North Am. 1994; 20:213–42.
35. Ginzler EM, Felson DT, Anthony JM, Anderson JJ. Hypertension increases the risk of renal deterioration in systemic lupus erythematosus. J Rheumatol. 1993; 20:1694–700.
36. Briggs WA, Choi MJ, Scheel PJ. Successful mofetil treatment of glomerular disease. Am J Kidney Dis. 1998; 31: 213–17.

37. Ho A, Madger L, Petri M. The effect of azathioprine/mycophenolate on systemic lupus erythematosus activity. Arthritis Rheum. 1998; 41:S281.

38. Pashinian N, Wallace DJ, Klinenberg JR. Mycophenolate mofetil for systemic lupus erythematosus. Arthritis Rheum. 1998; 41:S110.

39. Ortmann RA, Klippel JH. Update on cyclophosphamide for systemic lupus erythematosus. Rheum Dis Clin North Am. 2000; 26:363–75.

40. Dourmishev LA, Dourmishev AL, Schwartz RA. Dermatomyositis: cutaneous manifestations of its variants. Int J Dermatol. 2002; 41:625–30.

41. Sunkureddi P, et al. Signs of dermatomyositis. Hosp Physician. 2005; 41–4.

42. Katsambas A, Stefanaki C. Life-threatening dermatoses due to connective tissue disorders. Clin Dermatol. 2005; 23:238–48.

43. Targoff IN. Laboratory testing in the diagnosis and management of idiopathic inflammatory myopathies. Rheum Dis Clin North Am. 2002; 28:859–90.

44. Callen J. Dermatomyositis. Lancet. 2000; 355:53–7.

45. Kovacs SO, Kovacs CS. Dermatomyositis. J Am Acad Dermatol. 1998; 39:899–920.

46. Marie I, Hachulla E, Hantron PY, et al. Polymyositis and dermatomyositis: short term and long term outcome, and predictive factors of prognosis. J Rheumatol. 2001; 28:2230–7.

47. Ramanan AV, Feldman BM. Clinical features and outcomes of juvenile dermatomyositis and other childhood onset myositis syndromes. Rheum Dis Clin North Am. 2002; 28:833–57.

48. Yazici Y, Kagen LJ. Clinical presentation of the idiopathic inflammatory myopathies. Rheum Dis Clin North Am. 2002; 28:823–32.

49. Callen JP, Wortmann RL. Dermatomyositis. Clin Dermatol. 2006; 24:363–73.

50. Dalakas MC. Controlled studies with high-dose intravenous immunoglobulin in the treatment of dermatomyositis, inclusion body myositis and polymyositis. Neurology. 1998; 51:S37–S45.

51. Rutter A, Luger TA. High dose intravenous immunoglobulins: an approach to treat severe immune mediated and autoimmune diseases of the skin. J Am Acad Dermatol. 2001; 44:1010–24.

52. Marie I, Hachulla E, Levesque H, et al. Intravenous immunoglobulins as treatment of life threatening esophageal involvement in polymyositis and dermatomyositis. J Rheumatol. 1999; 26:2706–9.

53. Oddis CV. Idiopathic inflammatory myopathy: management and prognosis. Rheum Dis Clin North Am. 2002; 28:979–1001.

54. Sontheimer RD. Dermatomyositis: an overview of recent progress with emphasis on dermatologic aspects. Dermatol Clin. 2002; 20:387–408.

55. Jansen TL, Barrera P, Van Engelen BG, et al. Dermatomyositis with subclinical myositis and spontaneous pneumomediastinum with pneumothorax: case report and review of the literature. Clin Exp Rheumatol. 1998; 16:733–5.

56. Dourmishev LA, Dourmishev AL, Schwartz RA. Dermatomyositis: cutaneous manifestations of its variants. Int J Dermatol. 2002; 41:625–30.

57. Dawkins MA, Jorizzo JL, Walker FO, et al. Dermatomyositis: a dermatology based case series. J Am Acad Dermatol. 1998; 38:397–404.

58. Villalba L, Adams EM. Update on therapy for refractory dermatomyositis and polymyositis. Curr Opin Rheumatol. 1996; 8:544–51.

59. Maeda K, Kimura R, Komuta K, et al. Cyclosporine treatment for polymyositis/dermatomyositis: is it possible to rescue the deteriorating cases with interstitial pneumonitis? Scand J Rheumatol. 1997; 26:24–9.

60. Nawata Y, Kurasawa K, Takabayashi K, et al. Corticosteroid resistant interstitial pneumonitis in dermatomyositis/polymyositis: prediction and treatment with cyclosporine. J Rheumatol. 1999; 26:1527–33.

61. Sauty A, Rochat T, Schoch OD, et al. Pulmonary fibrosis with predominant CD8 lymphocytic alveolitis and anti-Jo-1 antibodies. Eur Respir J. 1997; 10:2907–12.

62. Caro I. Dermatomyositis. Semin Cutan Med Surg. 2001; 20:38–45.

63. Simenon CP, Armadans L, Fonollosa V. Survival prognostic factors and markers of morbidity in Spanish patients with systemic sclerosis. Ann Rheum Dis. 1997; 56:723–8.

64. Hesselstrand R, Scheja A, Akeson A. Mortality and causes of death in a Swedish series of systemic sclerosis patients. Ann Rheum Dis. 1998; 57:682–6.

65. Matucci-Cerinic M, D'Angelo S, Denton CP, et al. Assessment of lung involvement. Clin Exp Rheumatol. 2003; 21:S19–S23.

66. Denton CP, Black CM. Pulmonary hypertension in systemic sclerosis. Rheum Dis Clin North Am. 2003; 29:335–49.

67. Righi A, Cerinic MM. New treatments in scleroderma: the rheumatologic perspective. J Eur Acad Dermatol Venereol. 2002; 16:431–2.

68. Wax D, Garofano R, Barst RJ. Effects of long-term infusion of prostacyclin on exercise performance in patients with pulmonary hypertension. Chest. 1999; 116:914–20.

69. Badesch DB, Tapson VF, McCoon MD, et al. Continuous intravenous epoprostenol for pulmonary hypertension due to scleroderma spectrum of disease. A randomized controlled trial. Ann Intern Med. 2000; 132:425–34.

70. Simonneau G, Barst RJ, Galie N, et al. Continuous subcutaneous infusion of treprostinil, a prostacyclin analogue, in patients with pulmonary arterial hypertension: a double blind, randomized, placebo controlled trial. Am J Respir Crit Care Med. 2002; 165:800–4.

71. Channick RN, Simonnea G, Sitbon O, et al. Effects of the dual endothelin-receptor antagonist bosentan in patients with pulmonary hypertension: a randomized placebo controlled study. Lancet. 2001; 358:1119–23.

72. Rubin LF, Badesch DB, Barst RJ. Bosentan therapy for pulmonary hypertension. N Engl J Med. 2002; 346:896–903.

73. Silver EM, Warrick JH, Kinsella MB, et al. Cyclophosphamide and low dose prednisone therapy in patients with systemic sclerosis (scleroderma) with interstitial lung disease. J Rheumatol. 1993; 20:838–44.

74. White B, Moore W, Wingley F, et al. Cyclophosphamide is associated with pulmonary function and survival benefit

in patients with scleroderma and alveolitis. Ann Intern Med. 2000; 132:947–54.

75. Pakas I, Ioannides JP, Malagari K, et al. Cyclophosphamide with low or high dose prednisolone for systemic sclerosis lung disease. J Rheumatol. 2002; 29:298–304.

76. Steen VD, Mayes MD, Merkel PA. Assessment of kidney involvement. Clin Exp Rheumatol. 2003; 21:S29–S31.

77. Steen VD. Scleroderma renal crisis. Rheum Dis Clin North Am. 2003; 29:315–33.

78. Steen VD, Medsger TA Jr. Long term outcomes of scleroderma renal crisis. Ann Intern Med. 2000; 17; 600–3.

79. Petri M. Hopkins lupus cohort. 1999 Update. Rheum Dis Clin North Am. 2000; 26:199–213.

CHAPTER 25

Skin Signs of Systemic Infections

Jana Kazandjieva

Georgeta Bocheva

Nikolai Tsankov

MANY SYSTEMIC infections have cutaneous presentations that sometimes are unspecific. These cutaneous signs and symptoms may be helpful in making the proper diagnosis, prescribing the appropriate therapy, and assisting in prevention. Some clinical manifestations of systemic infections highlight the possible infectious etiology for unusual cutaneous lesions.

Bacterial systemic infections may be more common in remote areas of the world; these same bacterial diseases also may be seen, however, in travelers or immigrants from these areas. Some of these infections, such as plague and melioidosis, are potential biological weapons used for bioterrorism.

MELIOIDOSIS

Melioidosis is a highly invasive and resistant infection caused by the gram-negative bacterium *Burkholderia pseudomallei*, which is synonymous with the old nomenclature *Pseudomonas pseudomallei*.

The first reported cases of *P. pseudomallei* were initially known as Whitmore disease. In 1911, a British pathologist, Captain Alfred Whitmore, described a case of pneumonia in a young boy in Burma, where *P. pseudomallei* was isolated as the causative agent.[1] The term "melioidosis" was subsequently used in 1921. It is derived from the Greek word "melis" meaning "a distemper of donkeys," because it resembles glanders, which causes mainly pulmonary disease in asses.[2] This infection is endemic in Southeast Asia and North and Central Australia, and peaks during the monsoon seasons.[3] The disease in those regions often causes septicemia and death. Melioidosis also occurs sporadically in temperate countries and is mostly imported by travelers.[4]

Melioidosis contributes from 20% to 40% of deaths due to community-acquired septicemia in Northeast Thailand, especially in rice farmers.[5] In Singapore, the disease is uncommon, even though a significant percentage of the population has been exposed to *B. pseudomallei*.[6] The overall mortality rate remains near 45%, despite antibiotic therapy. Before the antibiotic era, 95% of patients died.[2]

B. pseudomallei is distributed in soil and surface water; thus, infection can be spread via inoculation though cutaneous abrasions. Inhalation or ingestion of contaminated bacilli materials is less frequent. Melioidosis is strongly associated with diabetes mellitus (50% of Asian patients), and is 4 times more common in men than in women.

Clinical Features

Clinical manifestations develop after an incubation period, which varies from a few days to several months or years. Patients develop high fever and rigors, as well as occasional confusion, stupor, jaundice, and diarrhea. The clinical spectrum includes five possible forms of presentations: acute fulminant septicemia (fatal within days); subclinical form;[7] subacute and chronic presentations (more likely associated with skin involvement); and relapsing–remitting course of the disease (requiring prolonged antibiotic treatment).[8]

The disease can be localized or disseminated with multiorgan involvement. Any organ can be involved in melioidosis with rapid development of small abscesses, which tend to coalesce to form larger abscesses, especially in lungs (50% of the cases), skin and subcutaneous tissues, bones and joints, liver, spleen, kidney, and brain.

Most commonly, melioidosis presents as an acute pulmonary infection, causing fulminant necrotizing pneumonia, septicemia, and death, or as an indolent cavitary disease, and mild bronchitis.[2] Severe melioidosis is usually seen in immunocompromised patients (with diabetes mellitus or renal failure).[5] Metastatic infection can remain latent for years. Common laboratory findings include anemia, neutrophil leukocytosis, coagulopathy, and renal and hepatic abnormalities.[9]

Cutaneous Manifestations

Very rarely, melioidosis can be demonstrated as a subacute form with cutaneous manifestations only.[10-12] Skin involvement, seen in 10%–20% of the patients with melioidosis, varies greatly. Patients often receive pustules and cutaneous abscesses, associated with lymphangitis, cellulitis, or regional lymphadenitis.[9,13,14] Draining sinuses from lymph nodes or bone may develop. Abscesses may ulcerate[15] and sometimes can form ecthyma gangrenosum–like lesions, or even progress to necrotizing fasciitis.[9,16] The most common cutaneous manifestation in children is acute suppurative parotitis. Severe urticaria has been described in one case of pulmonary melioidosis.[17] There are also some case reports of melioidosis, associated with cutaneous polyarteritis nodosa and porphyria cutanea tarda.[18,19] In acute septicemia, patients may develop non-specific flushing, cyanosis, and a pustular eruption.[20]

Differential Diagnosis

Because of the variety of skin presentations many infectious diseases must be considered: fungal infections, tuberculosis, and atypical mycobacterial infections. Cat scratch disease, tularemia, and lymphogranuloma venereum have similar clinical and histological presentations. Staphylococcal and streptococcal infections should be also considered.

Treatment

The treatment of melioidosis includes intensive care, draining of abscesses, and antibiotic therapy. Usually *B. pseudomallei* antibiogram shows resistance to aminoglycosides, polymyxins, fluoroquinolones, and many β-lactams (the older generation penicillins and cephalosporins); nevertheless, the bacillus is highly susceptible to amoxicillin/clavulanic acid, tetracyclines, and chloramphenicol. The treatment of melioidosis requires multiple antibiotics combination. Resistance to a single antibiotic may occur during the treatment. A course of antibiotics is recommended for at least 2 months, but may require prolonged antibiotic therapy to prevent complications, including osteomyelitis, sepsis, and (rarely) rupture of mycotic aneurysm.[21]

The localized cutaneous form of melioidosis can be successfully treated with combinations of amoxicillin/clavulanic acid (60 mg/kg/day orally three times daily) and tetracycline (40 mg/kg/day orally three times daily) or trimethoprim/sulfamethoxazole. Systemic involvement requires an extra use of intravenous (IV) ceftazidime (120 mg/kg/day twice daily) for 2–4 weeks, plus the oral combination described above for the subclinical forms of melioidosis.[15]

TYPHOID FEVER

Salmonella infections in humans include gastroenteritis, typhoid fever, bacteremia, and localized infection. Localized infection is a complication commonly affecting bones and joints, although subcutaneous, splenic,[22] breast, and intraperitoneal abscesses[23–27] have been described.

Typhoid fever is a systemic febrile disease caused by *Salmonella typhi*, a flagellated, gram-negative bacillus belonging to the Enterobacteriaceae family. The infection occurs most often during traveling to endemic regions (with 18 times greater risk compared with the other) such as: the Indian subcontinent, Southeast and Far-East Asia, the Middle East, Africa, and Central and South America.[28] Small endemics can occur sporadically as the result of food handlers who are carriers of *S. typhi*. Worldwide typhoid fever remains a health threat. Reported cases now are fewer than 500 per year.[29] The case-fatality rate is reduced to 2% by using the appropriate antibiotics and improvements in supportive care; nevertheless, in some developing countries, the case-fatality rate is higher – approximately 30%.[30]

S. typhi affects only humans during ingestion of food or water contaminated with the feces of patients with active diseases, or people who are asymptomatic carriers. The incubation period ranges from 5 to 21 days.[31] The severity of disease is in parallel with the amount of bacteria ingested. The illness is usually characterized by nonspecific manifestations.

Clinical Features

Typhoid fever classically presents with prolonged fever, headache, paradoxical bradycardia, and gastrointestinal symptoms, including abdominal pain,[32] and a rose-colored eruption. Many extraintestinal manifestations of *S. typhi* infection, such as osteomyelitis, intraabdominal abscess, urinary tract infection, and meningitis, have been described.[33] Fever, which is seen in 98%–100% of patients, is the most common finding. The classic relative bradycardia (Faget sign) and the presence of rose spots[34] are the clues to the diagnosis. Laboratory findings in this infection are also nonspecific – thrombocytopenia, proteinuria, elevated transaminases, and relative leukopenia.[35]

Initially, patients present with diarrhea and abdominal pain. Other associated signs, less commonly found, are a nonproductive cough, constipation, meningismus, deafness, confusion, and weight loss. Asymptomatic hepatitis is common. Severe kidney and liver failure with marked jaundice has also been described. Pancreatitis can occur in typhoid fever, ranging from enzyme abnormalities to pancreatic abscesses requiring surgery.[36]

Early diagnosis and treatment of typhoid fever allows prevention of the complications and spread of the infection. Complications may occur involving any organ and system. Splenic abscess represents nearly 30% of complicated *Salmonella* abdominal infection of untreated typhoid fever.[32,37] Other complications are intestinal hemorrhage and perforation. Perforation classically occurs in Peyer patches of the terminal ileum. Other less common complications include toxic myocarditis, hepatitis, cholecystitis, polymyositis, mild bronchitis, and toxic confusional state.[35] Typhoid fever may affect the kidneys, leading to nephrotic syndrome.[29,36]

A chronic carrier state may occur in up to 3% of treated patients. Patients with cholelithiasis are at greater risk for persistence of *S. typhi*.

Cutaneous Manifestations

In 30%–50% of patients,[35] so-called rose spots are described as a cutaneous classical manifestation. The spots are caused by bacterial embolization, and bacterial cultures taken from the rose spots may be positive. Lesions are characterized as pink blanching papules, 2–4 mm in diameter, localized mainly on the mid-trunk, developing often between the 7th and 12th day of infection.

Subcutaneous abscesses may rarely occur as a localized skin and soft-tissue complication due to *S. typhi* bacteremia. *Salmonella* bacteremia increases among the patients with acquired immune deficiency syndrome (AIDS), in whom these abscesses are found.[38] Abscess formation in most described cases are secondary and usually do not ulcerate. Most reported cases of subcutaneous abscesses were due to *Salmonella* species other than *S. typhi*.[37,38] A unique case of cutaneous ulceration occurred as a clinical manifestation of *S. typhi* infection in a nonimmunocompromised patient with complete absence of systemic signs.[39]

Another possible skin presentation is pustular dermatitis. Purpura or skin petechiae are rare, and are described mainly in the setting of *Salmonella* endocarditis.[33] A patient with cutaneous leukocytoclastic vasculitis associated with abdominal lesions developed during typhoid fever but without endocarditis was reported.[37]

Differential Diagnosis

The differential diagnosis of typhoid fever includes other systemic febrile illnesses: brucellosis, tularemia, leptospirosis, tuberculosis, rickettsial disease, viral hepatitis, mononucleosis, AIDS, and cytomegalovirus infection.[35] Additional infections to consider include malaria, dengue fever, and schistosomiasis. Noninfectious etiologies, such as lymphoma, leukemia, or adverse drug reaction, can also cause prolonged fever.

Treatment

Antimicrobial therapy is necessary. Worldwide, chloramphenicol was the most commonly used antibiotic for typhoid fever. Unfortunately, resistance to chloramphenicol is increasing, especially in Southeast Asia. Amoxicillin and trimethoprim/sulfamethoxazole are also efficacious in the treatment of acute infection and the carrier state, but a high incidence of resistance is reported, too.

Fluoroquinolones (e.g., oral ciprofloxacin 500 mg twice daily for 10 days) are currently the drugs of choice for typhoid fever.[40] They have the lowest incidence of both relapse and development of a chronic carrier state. The third-generation cephalosporins (e.g., IV ceftriaxone 2 g/d for 5 days, especially for patients with cholelithiasis) are also effective for treatment of typhoid fever.

LEPTOSPIROSIS

Leptospirosis is a spirochetal infection caused by pathogenic *Leptospira* species. The spirochetes have hooked ends, and because of that Stimson named them *Spirochaeta interrogans* for their resemblance to a question mark.[41] Within the species of *Leptospira interrogans*, 200 serovars are recognized.

Leptospirosis is presumed to be the most widespread zoonosis in the world,[42] with many wild and domestic animal reservoirs. Leptospirosis causes clinical illness in both humans and animals. Human infection is typically due to exposure to infected animal urine, by direct contact or indirect exposure through water or soil.[43] The usual portal of entry is damaged skin or the conjunctiva. Inhalation of water or aerosols may result in infection of the respiratory tract.[44] Rarely, infection may follow animal bites.[45,46]

The incidence of infection is significantly higher in tropical countries because of warm and humid conditions, allowing the much longer survival of leptospires.[47,48] The disease is seasonal, with peaks (in the summer) in temperate regions and (in rainy seasons) in areas with warm climates. Cases of leptospirosis also follow floods and hurricanes.[49,50] Within the United States, the highest incidence was found in Hawaii.[51] Leptospirosis is highly endemic in Malaysia[52,53] and Nicaragua.[54–57]

Some occupational groups have a significant risk for leptospirosis. The infection was recognized early on in sewer workers (first reported in the 1930s),[58–61] then in fish workers (86% of all cases in northeast Scotland) and coal miners.[62] More recently, fish farmers have been shown to be at higher risk,[63] particularly for infection with *L. icterohaemorrhagiae*,[64] because of the high mortality rate associated with the *L. icterohaemorrhagiae* serogroup.

Clinical Features

The spectrum of human leptospirosis is extremely wide, ranging from subclinical infection to a severe multiorgan infection with high mortality rate. Leptospirosis mainly affects liver and kidney. The classical syndrome of Weil disease represents only the most severe presentation. This syndrome, demonstrated by icteric leptospirosis with renal failure, was first reported by Adolf Weil in Heidelberg.[65] In humans, severe leptospirosis is frequently caused by serovars of the *L. icterohaemorrhagiae* serogroup. Thus, in Europe, serovars *L. icterohaemorrhagiae* and *L. copenhageni*, carried by rats, are usually responsible for leptospiral infection.

The clinical manifestation of leptospirosis is biphasic, with an acute or septicemic phase lasting about a week, followed by the immune phase, characterized by antibody production and excretion of leptospires in the urine.[66,67] Most of the complications of leptospirosis are associated with tissue invasion of leptospires during the immune phase of the infection.

The majority of cases are subclinical and mild. A smaller proportion of anicteric leptospirosis is presented as a febrile illness, with chills, severe headache (with retro-orbital pain and photophobia), myalgia, abdominal pain, conjunctival suffusion, and (rarely) a skin eruption. In addition, aseptic meningitis may be found in 25% of all cases. Some anicteric form of the disease challenged this view and demonstrated severe anicteric leptospirosis.[68] The mortality is almost nil in anicteric form, but 2.4% of the anicteric patients in a Chinese outbreak received massive pulmonary hemorrhage and death.[69]

The icteric form of the disease affects between 5% and 10% of all patients with leptospirosis.[70] Icteric leptospirosis is more severe, often rapidly progressive, with a high mortality rate, and ranges between 5% and 15%. The jaundice occurring in leptospirosis is not associated with hepatocellular necrosis. Serum bilirubin, transaminase, and alkaline phosphatase level elevations are usually minor.

Leptospirosis is a common cause of acute renal failure (ARF), which occurs in 16%–40% of cases.[71–73] Serum amylase level is often significantly increased in association with ARF,[74,75] but clinical signs of pancreatitis are rare. Thrombocytopenia occurs in more than 50% of cases, is usually associated with multiorgan involvement, and is a predictor for ARF development.[76,77] Thrombocytopenia in leptospirosis is transient and does not result from disseminated intravascular coagulation.[78,79]

Pulmonary involvement can be the major manifestation of leptospirosis in some cases.[80–82] The severity of respiratory disease is unrelated to the presence of jaundice.[83] Pulmonary signs and symptoms may present with cough, dyspnea, hemoptysis (from mild to severe), and adult respiratory distress syndrome. Intraalveolar hemorrhage may be found, even in the absence of pulmonary symptoms, and may be severe, causing death.[84–86] Radiographic abnormalities are most commonly noted in the first week of the disease, presented by alveolar infiltrates.

Cutaneous and Mucosal Manifestations

The skin eruption in the anicteric form of leptospirosis is often transient, lasting less than 24 hours. Petechial, ecchymotic, or purpuric skin lesions may occur in leptospirosis. Conjunctival suffusion is seen in the majority of patients and in the presence of scleral icterus is thought to be pathognomonic for Weil disease.[87] Bacterial causes of erythema nodosum, in particular leptospirosis, also should be considered.[88] A rare complication of leptospirosis may be Kawasaki syndrome.[89,90]

Recently, a case of anicteric leptospirosis, presenting with respiratory insufficiency and acquired ichthyosis, was described.[91] The sudden appearance of ichthyosis, especially in adults, has been considered a marker of systemic disease. Acquired ichthyosis may be associated with malignant disease and autoimmune disorders, as well as systemic infections (like the association of leptospirosis and ichthyosis mentioned earlier in this chapter).

Differential Diagnosis

The multiorgan involvement of leptospirosis may be confused with other tropical infections – malaria, dengue, enteric fever, typhoid fever, and melioidosis. Influenza should be considered in mild anicteric cases.

Treatment

Treatment of leptospirosis varies depending on the duration and severity of the symptoms. Patients with mild, flu-like symptoms are treated only symptomatically. The management of icteric leptospirosis requires admission and treatment of the patients in an intensive care unit. Patients with ARF need dialysis. Cardiac monitoring is also necessary during the first few days.

Recently, the antimicrobial susceptibility of 13 Leptospira isolates (from Egypt, Thailand, Nicaragua, and Hawaii) to 13 antimicrobial agents has been studied. Leptospires were susceptible to penicillin G, cefotaxime, ceftriaxone, and fluoroquinolones (moxifloxacin, ciprofloxacin, and levofloxacin). Tetracyclines had the highest MIC90s (minimum inhibitory concentration required to inhibit the growth of 90% of organisms).[92] Leptospiral infection can be successfully treated by penicillin G or doxycycline. IV penicillin should be given at a dosage of 8 million units/day for 7–10 days.[93,94] A treatment regimen of oral doxycycline is 100 mg twice daily; for short-term prophylaxis – doxycycline 200 mg once weekly.[95]

PLAGUE

The plague is a synonym of an old and forgotten infection, often used today with a totally different meaning – as a curse, trouble, harassment, and so forth. Globally, the World Health Organization reports 1000–3000 cases of plague naturally occurring worldwide every year. In 2006, a total of 13 human plague cases were reported in the United States. This is the largest number of cases reported in a single year in the United States since 1994.[96]

The discovery of *Yersinia pestis* is fascinating. The microbe causing the disease was invisible and unknown until 1894, when Alexandre Yersin described it. Yersin was sent to Hong Kong to conduct research on a bubonic plague epidemic that was sweeping through China. Yersin arrived in Hong Kong on June 15, 1894. Seven days later, while

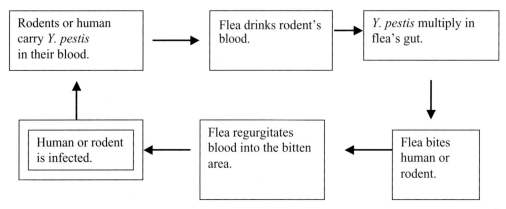

FIGURE 25.1: *Usual path of plague transmission.*

working in a small bacteriological research laboratory set up for him, he isolated the plague bacillus.

The Japanese bacteriologist Shibasaburo Kitasato (1852–1931) had arrived a shortly before Yersin in Hong Kong. Within a few days, he also found a bacillus and announced it to the world via telegraph. Kitasato published his findings in Japanese and English at the same time that Yersin published his discovery in French. People in various parts of the world credited one or the other with the discovery, depending on which journals they had read. Yersin named the organism *Pasteurella pestis* after his teacher Pasteur, but since 1970, the bacillus has been known as *Yersinia pestis*.

Plague is an infectious disease of animals and humans caused by the bacterium *Y. pestis*. *Y. pestis* is a non–spore-forming, gram-negative coccobacillus measuring 1.5 × 0.75 µm. The genome of *Y. pestis* has been sequenced, including the three virulence plasmids, pPst, pLcr, and pFra.[97] *Y. pestis* belongs to the group of bacilli with low resistance to environmental factors. Sunlight, high temperatures, and desiccation have a destructive effect, and ordinary disinfectants such as Lysol® and preparations containing chlorine kill it in 1–10 minutes. *Y. pestis* circulates particularly in rodents in the natural foci of infection found on all continents except Australia. Plague is spread from one rodent to another by flea ectoparasites and to humans either by the bite of infected fleas or when handling infected hosts (Figure 25.1). At least 30 types of fleas and more than 200 species of mammals in 73 genera serve as reservoirs.[98]

The plague has had three pandemic waves.[99] The first certain plague pandemic, known as Justinian's plague, was recorded in the 6th century CE. The epidemic spread over Asia, Africa, and Europe and claimed nearly 100,000,000 victims.

The second plague pandemic is the well-known "Black Death" of the 14th century. It caused 50 million deaths, half of them in Asia and Africa and the other half in Europe, where a quarter of the population succumbed. The third

plague pandemic began in Canton and Hong Kong in 1894. It was carried by rats aboard the swifter steamships and spread rapidly throughout the world. Plague entered 77 ports on five continents. The last great outbreak of plague occurred in the early 1900s in India, killing more than 20 million people.

There is a well-known classification of the clinical presentation of plague. Three types of plague are differentiated: bubonic, pneumonic, and septicemic.

Bubonic Plague

The classic form of infection is the bubonic plague (Greek *boubon* = groin). It is transmitted only by a flea bite and is not spread from person to person. The incubation period varies from 1 to 8 days.

Clinical Features. The illness begins with fever, chills, and pain in the area of the lymph nodes.

Cutaneous Manifestations. The characteristic sign is the painful, swollen, and warm to the touch lymph node – a "bubo" – which occurs in the groin, axilla, and/or cervical region. Bubo location is primarily a function of the region of the body in which an infected flea inoculates the plague bacillus. Buboes are usually 1–10 cm in diameter and may suppurate and rupture. Nausea, vomiting, and/or diarrhea are common as systemic manifestations of the infection. This form may progress to secondary pneumonic plague or secondary septicemic plague. Bubonic plague has a 1%–15% death rate in treated cases and a 40%–60% death rate if left untreated.

Differential Diagnosis. A wide differential diagnosis could be made with cat scratch disease, ulceroglandular tularemia, staphylococcal or streptococcal adenitis, mycobacterial infection, lymphogranuloma venereum, chancroid, primary genital herpes, and even a strangulated inguinal hernia.

Pneumonic Plague

Pneumonic plague is the deadliest form. It is caused by inhaling the bacteria and transmitting it. The transmission requires close contact with an infected person. The incubation period is up to 6 days.

Clinical Features. The pneumonic plague begins with fulminant fever, malaise, myalgias, headache, and gastrointestinal symptoms. The death rate for pneumonic plague is 100% if not treated within the first 24 hours of infection.

Cutaneous Manifestations. Patients in the terminal stages often develop large ecchymoses on the back – "the Black Death."

Differential Diagnosis. The differential diagnosis is made with any case of severe gram-negative pneumonia, community-acquired pneumonia (bacterial, *Mycoplasma*, *Legionella*, *Chlamydia*), viral pneumonia (influenza, respiratory syncytial virus, cytomegalovirus, hantavirus), Q fever, inhalational anthrax, tularemia, or ricin poisoning. Recently, an outbreak of pneumonic plague in a remote diamond mine in the Democratic Republic of the Congo has been registered. The multidisciplinary team of epidemiologists, physicians, and logisticians from Médecins Sans Frontières confirmed 136 cases of pneumonic plague, 57 of them fatal.[100]

Septicemic Plague

Septicemic plague is caused by flea bites or is a result of bubonic or pneumonic plague. It is not spread from person to person, and occurs when plague bacteria multiply in the blood. In this form, lymph nodes usually do not enlarge. It is not contagious and has a 40% death rate in treated cases and 100% in untreated cases.

Clinical Features. The clinical picture includes acute fever, chills, prostration, abdominal pain, nausea, vomiting, and internal bleeding.

Cutaneous Manifestations. Purpuric skin lesions and gangrene of the distal digits (acral necrosis) are common. Rose-colored purpuric lesions give rise to the nursery rhyme "Ring around the rosy."[101]

In all forms, skin lesions may occur at the site of flea bite (papules, vesicles, pustules), and petechiae and ecchymoses may occur during hematogenous spread. Ecthyma gangrenosum has been reported in several patients as a rare skin sign.[102]

Differential Diagnosis. Differential diagnosis should be made with gram-negative sepsis, meningococcemia, rickettsiosis, malaria, and appendicitis.

There are no widely available, rapid diagnostic tests for plague. Blood, bubo aspirates, and sputum should be stained with Giemsa stain. Smears typically show the bacillus to have a bipolar or "safety pin" appearance. *Y. pestis* is slow growing in cultures of blood, bubo aspirate, sputum, and skin lesions. Direct fluorescent antibody testing for *Y. pestis* capsular (F1) antigen may be helpful. Several serologic tests are also available (passive hemagglutination, enzyme-linked immunosorbent assay). A single titer of more than 1:10 is positive for plague if the patient has not been vaccinated previously. With paired sera 4–6 weeks apart, a fourfold increase in titer is considered confirmatory.

Treatment for Plague

The patients have to be isolated. The preferred treatment is streptomycin (1 g intramuscularly [IM], 12 h) or gentamicin (5 mg/kg IM or IV once daily, or 2 mg/kg loading dose followed by 1.7 mg/kg IM or IV). Alternative therapeutic regimens are courses with doxycycline (100 mg every 12 h or 200 mg once per day), ciprofloxacin (400 mg every 12 h), or chloramphenicol (25 mg/kg every 6 h, max 4 g/d). The treatment's duration is 10 days. In pregnant women, gentamicin is the preferred choice.

As prevention, close physical contact is restricted to proximity of no less than 2 m to a person who is symptomatic with plague. All health care personnel must take precautions – wear goggles, gloves, gowns, and possibly masks. In endemic areas, personal protective measures such as use of insecticides and insect repellents are recommended for reducing the incidence of infection.[103]

Commercial plague vaccine dates back to 1896. At that time killed bacteria were first used by Greer Laboratories in its production. Nowadays, no vaccines are currently in production.

Plague may be rare today, but doctors should be educated about the characteristic clinical signs of this infection. First because the bacillus is easily aerosolized and second because the symptoms are not likely to arouse suspicion until an epidemic is evident. Its potential usage as a bioweapon should not be overlooked.[104]

REFERENCES

1. Whitmore A, Kriswhnaswami CS. An account of the discovery of a hitherto undescribed infective disease occuring among the population of Rangoon. Indian Med Gaz. 1912; 47: 262–7.
2. Ip M, Osterberg LG, Chau PY, et al. Pulmonary melioidosis. Chest. 1995; 108:1420–4.
3. Dance DAB. Melioidosis: the tip of the iceberg? Clin Microbiol Rev. 1991; 5:52–60.
4. Dance DAB, Smith MD, Aucken HM, et al. Imported melioidosis in England and Wales. Lancet. 1999; 353:208–12.

5. Chaowagul W, White NJ, Dance DAB, et al. Melioidosis: a major cause of community-acquired septicemia in northern Thailand. J Infect Dis. 1989; 159:890–9.

6. Tan A, Ang BSP, Ong YY. Melioidosis: epidemiology and antibiogram of cases in Singapore. Singapore Med J. 1990; 31:335–7.

7. Nigg C. Serologic studies on subclinical melioidosis. Chest. 1995; 108:1420–4.

8. Silbermann MH, Gyssens IC, Enditz HP, et al. Two patients with recurrent melioidosis after prolonged antibiotic therapy. Scand J Infect Dis. 1997; 29:199–201.

9. Walsh AL, Wuthiekanun V. The laboratory diagnosis of melioidosis. Br J Biomed Sci. 1996; 53:249–53.

10. Tran D, Tan HH. Cutaneous melioidosis. Clin Exp Dermatol. 2002; 27:280–2.

11. Thng TG, Seow CS, Tan HH, Yosipovitch G. A case of non-fatal cutaneous melioidosis. Cutis. 2003; 72:310–12.

12. Ezzedine K, Malvy D, Steels E, et al. Imported melioidosis with an isolated cutaneous presentation in a 90-year-old traveller from Bangladesh. Bull Soc Pathol Exot. 2007; 100: 22–5.

13. Maccanti O, Pardelli R, Tonziello A, et al, Melioidosis in a traveller from Thailand: case report. J Chemother. 2004; 16:404–7.

14. Svensson E, Welinder-Olsson C, Claesson BA, Studahl M. Cutaneous melioidosis in a Swedish tourist after the tsunami in 2004. Scand J Infect Dis. 2006; 38:71–4.

15. Teo L, Tay YK, Mancer KJ. Cutaneous melioidosis. J Eur Acad Dermatol Venereol. 2006; 20:1322–4.

16. Wang YS, Wong CH, Kurup A. Cutaneous melioidosis and necrotizing fasciitis caused by Burkholderia pseudomallei. Emerg Infect Dis. 2003; 9:1484–5.

17. Steck WD, Byrd RB. Urticaria secondary to pulmonary melioidosis. Report of a case. Arch Dermatol. 1969; 99:80–1.

18. Choonhakarn C, Jirarattanapochai K. Cutaneous polyarteritis nodosa: a report of a case associated with melioidosis (Burkholderia pseudomallei). Int J Dermatol. 1998; 37:433–6.

19. Fung WK, Tam SC, Ho KM, et al. Porphyria cutanea tarda and melioidosis. Hong Kong Med J. 2001; 7:197–200.

20. Chaowagul W. Melioidosis; a treatment challenge. Scand J Infect Dis Suppl. 1996; 101:14–16.

21. Steunmetz I, Stosiek P, Hergenrother D, et al. Melioidosis causing a mycotic aneurysm. Lancet. 1996; 347:1564–5.

22. Sharr MM. Splenic abscess due to Salmonela agona. Br Med J. 1972; 1:546.

23. Vellodi C. Subcutaneous Salmonella abscess – an unusual manifestation of salmonellosis. J R Soc Med. 1990; 83: 190.

24. Molina M, Ortega G, Pérez Garcia A, Pretel L. Cutaneous abscesses caused by Sallmonella. Enferm Infecc Microbiol Clin. 1990; 8:259–60.

25. Shamiss A, Thaler M, Nussinovitch N, et al. Multiple Salmonella enteritidis led abscesses in a patient with systemic lupus erythematosus. Postgrad Med J. 1990; 66:486–8.

26. Indrisano JP, Simon GL. Facial Salmonella abscess. Ann Intern Med. 1989; 110:171.

27. Nice CS, Panigrahi H. Cutaneous abscess caused by Salmonella enteritidis: an unusual presentation on salmonellosis. J Infect. 1993; 27:204–5.

28. Mermin JH, Townes JM, Gerber M, et al. Typhoid fever in the United States, 1985–1994. Arch Intern Med. 1998; 158:633–8.

29. Ryan CA, Hargrett-Bean NT, Blake PA. Salmonella typhi infections in the United States, 1975–1984: increasing role of foreign travel. Rev Infect Dis. 1989; 11:1–7.

30. Hook EW. Typhoid fever today. N Engl J Med. 1984; 310:116–18.

31. Hornick RB, Greiseman SE, Woodward TE, et al. Typhoid fever: pathogenesis and immunological control. New Engl J Med. 1970; 283:686–91.

32. Miller SI, Hohmann EL, Pegues DA. Salmonella (including Salmonella typhi). In: Mandell GL, Benett JE, Dolin R, editors. Principles and practice of infectious diseases. 4th ed. New York: Churchill Livingstone; 1995. pp. 2013–32.

33. Cohen JI, Bartlett JA, Corey GR. Extra-intestinal manifestations of Salmonella infections. Medicine. 1987; 66:349–88.

34. Hoffman TA, Ruiz CJ, Counts GW, et al. Waterborne typhoid fever in Dade County, Florida. Am J Med. 1975; 59:481–7.

35. Mandal BK. Salmonela infections. In: Cook GC, editor. Manson's tropical disease. 2nd ed. London: WB Saunders Ltd.; 1996. pp. 849–64.

36. Khan M, Coovadia Y, Sturm AW. Typhoid fever complicated by acute renal failure and hepatitis: case reports and review. Am J Gastroenterol. 1998; 93:1001–3.

37. Lambotte O, Debord T, Castagné C, Roué R. Unusual presentation of typhoid fever: cutaneous vasculitis, pancreatitis, and splenic abscess. J Infect. 2001; 42:161–2.

38. Sperber SJ, Schleupner CJ. Salmonellosis during infection with human immunodeficiency virus. Rev Infect Dis. 1987; 9:925–34.

39. Marzano AV, Mercogliano M, Borghi A, et al. Cutaneous infection caused by Salmonella typhi. JEADV. 2003; 17: 575–7.

40. Rowe B, Ward LR, Threlfall EJ. Multidrug-resistant Salmonella typhi: worldwide epidemic. Clin Infect Dis. 1997; 24:106–9.

41. Stimson AM. Note of an organism found in yellow-fever tissue. Public Health Rep. 2000; 22:541.

42. World Health Organization. Leptospirosis worldwide. 1999; 72:237–42.

43. Phraisuwan P, Whitney EA, Tharmaphornpilas P, et al. Leptospirosis: skin wounds and control strategies, Thailand, 1999. Emerg Infect Dis. 2002; 8:1455–9.

44. Silverstein CM. Pulmonary manifestation of leptospirosis. Radiology. 1953; 61:327–34.

45. Luzzi GA, Milne LM, Waitkins SA. Rat-bite acquired leptospirosis. J Infect. 1987; 15:57–60.

46. Gollop JH, Katz RC, Rudoy RC, Sasaki DM. Rat-bite acquired leptospirosis. West J Med. 1993; 159:76–7.

47. Everard JD, Everard COR. Leptospirosis in the Caribbean. Rev Med Microbiol. 1993; 4:114–22.

48. Ratnam S. Leptospirosis: an Indian perspective. Indian J Med Microbiol. 1994; 12:228–39.

49. Epstein PR, Pena OC, Racedo JB. Climate and disease in Colombia. Lancet. 1995; 346:1243–4.

50. Levett PN. Leptospirosis. Clin Microbiol Rev. 2001; 14:296–326.

51. Centers for Disease Control and Prevention. Summary of notifiable diseases, United States. Morb Mortal Wkly Rep. 1994; 43:1–80.
52. Tan DC. Occupational distribution of leptospiral (SEL) antibodies in Malaysia. Med J Malaysia. 1973; 27:253–7.
53. Centers for Disease Control and Prevention. Outbreak of acute febrile illness among participants in EcoChallenge Sabah 2000-Malaysia. Morb Mortal Wkly Rep. 2000; 49:816–17.
54. Brandling-Benett AD, Pinheiro F. Infectious diseases in Latin America and the Caribbean: are they really emerging and increasing? Emerg Infect Dis. 1996; 2:59–61.
55. Centers for Disease Control and Prevention. Outbreak of acute febrile illness and pulmonary hemorrhage – Nicaragua. Morb Mortal Wkly Rep. 1995; 44:841–3.
56. Levett PN. Leptospirosis: re-emerging or re-discovered disease? J Med Microbiol. 1999; 48:417–18.
57. Trevejo RT, Rigau-Perez JG, Ashford DA, et al. Epidemic leptospirosis associated with pulmonary hemorrhage – Nicaragua, 1995. J Infect Dis. 1998; 178:1457–63.
58. Alston JM. Leptospiral jaundice among sewer-workers. Lancet. 1935; i:806–9.
59. Failey NH. Weil's disease among sewer workers in London. BMJ. 1934; 2:10–14.
60. Johnson DW, Brown HE, Derrick EH. Weil's disease in Brisbane. Med J Aust. 1937; 1:811–18.
61. Stuart RD. Weil's disease in Glasgow sewer workers. BMJ. 1939; i:324–6.
62. Waitkins SA. Leptospirosis as an occupational disease. Br J Ind Med. 1986; 43:721–5.
63. Robertson MH, Clarke IR, Coghlan JD, Gill ON. Leptospirosis in trout farmers. Lancet. 1981; ii:626–7.
64. Gill ON, Coghlan JD, Calder IM. The risk of leptospirosis in United Kingdom fish farm workers. J Hyg. 1985; 94:81–6.
65. Weil A. Ueber eine eigentümliche, mit Milztumor, Icterus und Nephritis einhergehende akute Infektionskrankheit. Dtsche Arch Klin Med. 1886; 39:209–32.
66. Kelley PW. Leptospirosis. In Gorbach SL, Bartlett JG, Blacklow NR, editors. Infectious diseases. 2nd ed. Philadelphia: WB Saunders; 1998. pp. 1580–7.
67. Turner LH. Leptospirosis I. Trans R Soc Trop Med Hyg. 1967; 61:842–55.
68. Thomas JH, Stephens DP. Leptospirosis: an unusual presentation. Crit Care Resusc. 2006; 8:186.
69. Wang C, John L, Chang T, et al. Studies on anicteric leptospirosis. I. Clinical manifestations and antibiotic therapy. Clin Med J. 1965; 84:283–91.
70. Heath CW, Alexander AD, Galton MM. Leptospirosis in the United States: 1949–1961. N Engl J Med. 1965; 273:857–64, 915–22.
71. dos Santos VM, dos Santos JA, Sugai TA, dos Santos LA. Weil's syndrome. Rev Cubana Med Trop. 2003; 55:44–6.
72. Abdulkader RCRM. Acute renal failure in leptospirosis. Renal Fail. 1997; 19:191–8.
73. Winearls CG, Chan L, Coghlan JD et al. Acute renal failure due to leptospirosis: clinical features and outcome in six cases. Q J Med. 1984; 53:487–95.
74. Edwards CN, Everard COR. Hyperamylasemia and pancreatitis in leptospirosis. Am J Gastroenterol. 1991; 86:1665–8.
75. O'Brien MM, Vincent JM, Person DA, Cook BA. Leptospirosis and acute pancreatitis: a report of ten cases. Pediatr Infect Dis J. 1998, 17:436–8.
76. Turgut M, Sunbul M, Bayirli D, et al. Thrombocytopenia complicating the clinical course of leptospiral infection. J Int Med Res. 2002; 30:535–40.
77. Edwards CN, Nicholson GD, Everard CO. Thrombocytopenia in leptospirosis. Am J Trop Med Hyg. 1982; 31:827–9.
78. Edwards CN, Nicholson GD, Hassel TA, et al. Thrombocytopenia in leptospirosis: the absence of evidence for disseminated intravascular coagulation. Am J Trop Med Hyg. 1986; 35:352–4.
79. Nicodemo AC, Duarte MI, Alves VA, et al. Lung lesions in human leptospirosis: microscopic, immunohistochemical, and ultrastructural features related to thrombocytopenia. Am J Trop Hyg. 1997; 56:181–7.
80. Teglia OF, Battagliotti C, Villavicencio R, et al. Leptospiral pneumonia. Chest. 1995; 108:874–5.
81. O'Neil KM, Leland S, Richman Lazarus AA. Pulmonary manifestations of leptospirosis. Rev Infect Dis. 1991; 13:705–9.
82. Martinez MA, Damia AD, Villanueva RM, et al. Pulmonary involvement in leptospirosis. Eur J Clin Microbiol Infect Dis. 2000; 19:471–4.
83. Hill MK, Sanders CV. Leptospiral pneumonia. Semin Respir Infect. 1997; 12:44–9.
84. Dive AM, Bigaignon G, Reynaert M. Adult respiratory distress syndrome in Leptospira icterohaemorrhagiae infection. Intensive Care Med. 1987; 13:214.
85. Allen PS, Raftery S, Phelan D. Massive pulmonary haemorrhage due to leptospirosis. Intensive Care Med. 1989; 15:322–4.
86. Alani FSS, Mahoney MP, Ormerod LP, et al. Leptospirosis presenting as atypical pneumonia, respiratory failure and pyogenic meningitis. J Infect. 1993; 27:281–3.
87. Van Thiel PH. The leptospirosis. Universitaire Pers: Leiden; The Netherlands. 1948.
88. Derham RLJ. Leptospirosis as a cause of erythema nodosum. BMJ. 1976; 2:403–4.
89. Humphry T, Sanders S, Stadius M. Leptospirosis mimicking MLNS. J Pediatr. 1977; 91:853–4.
90. Wong ML, Kaplan S, Dunkle LM, et al. Leptospirosis: a childhood disease. J Pediatr. 1977; 90:532–7.
91. Othman N, Intan HI, Yip CW, et al. Severe leptospirosis with unusual manifestation. J Trop Pediatr. 2007; 53:55–8.
92. Ressner RA, Griffith ME, Beckius ML, et al. Antimicrobial susceptibilities of geographically diverse clinical human isolates of Leptospira. Antimicrob Agents Chemother. 2008; 52:2740–4.
93. Edwards CN, Nicholson GD, Hassell TA, et al. Penicillin therapy in icteric leptospirosis. Am J Trop Med Hyg. 1988; 39:388–90.
94. Kadurina M, Bocheva G, Tonev S. Penicillin and semisynthetic penicillins in dermatology. Clin Dermatol. 2003; 21:12–23.
95. McClain JBL, Ballou WR, Harrison SM, Steinweg DL. Doxycycline therapy for leptospirosis. Ann Intern Med. 1984; 100:696–8.

96. Human plague–four states, 2006. MMWR Morb Mortal Wkly Rep. 2006; 55:940–3.

97. Rollins SE, Rollins SM, Ryan ET. Yersinia pestis and the plague. Am J Clin Pathol. 2003; 119 Suppl:S78–85.

98. Kant S, Nath LM. Control and prevention of human plague. Indian J Pediatr. 1994; 61:629–33.

99. Tsankov N. Plague, epidemiology, clinics and therapy. XV EADV Congress, Rhodes, October 4–8, 2006.

100. Weir E. Plague: a continuing threat. CMAJ. 2005; 172: 1555.

101. Mee C. How a mysterious disease laid low Europe's masses. Smithsonian. 1990; 20:66–79.

102. Welty TK, Grabman J, Kompare E. Nineteen cases of plague in Arizona: a spectrum including ecthyma gangrenosum due to plague and plague in pregnancy. Western J Med. 1985; 142:641–6.

103. Lazarus AA, Decker CF. Plague. Respir Care Clin N Am. 2004; 10(1):83–98.

104. Branda JA, Ruoff K. Bioterrorism. Clinical recognition and primary management. Am J Clin Pathol. 2002; 117 Suppl:S116–23.

CHAPTER 26

Skin Signs of Systemic Neoplastic Diseases and Paraneoplastic Cutaneous Syndromes

Kyrill Pramatarov

THE SKIN MAY reflect many visceral diseases, malignancies included. Sometimes, the skin may even give a clue to the underlying neoplasm. The French dermatologist Delacrétaz has definded the term "paraneoplasia:"

Cutaneous paraneoplastic syndromes are non-metastatic manifestations on the skin as a result of the existence of a malignant visceral tumor and/or disease of the lymphoma group, especially leukaemias. The close relation between the dermatosis and tumor is confirmed by the phenomenon of disappearance or not at all influenced skin disease, if the malignant tumor is eliminated by operation, irradiation or cytostatics. The recurrence of the skin changes (dermatosis) indicates a relapse of the tumor or metastases.[1]

The paraneoplastic signs or syndromes may precede, appear parallel to, or follow the appearance of the internal malignancy. There are many classifications of the paraneoplastic signs and syndromes, utilizing a variety of criteria: Some of them are based on the morphology of skin changes, others are based on the frequency of the association of dermatosis/visceral malignancy. The paraneoplastic signs and syndromes may be divided into two groups: indirect associations and direct associations with parallel evolutions corresponding to the paraneoplastic syndrome.[2] The pathogenesis of the development of paraneoplasias include:

- peptides, mediators, and hormones released from the tumor;
- immunological defense reactions induced by the tumor antigens and appearing after cross-reaction with the structures of the skin;
- deposits of immunocomplexes of tumor antigens and antibodies;[3] and
- various cytokines and possibly growth factors.[4]

Metastases to skin are more specific signs of internal cancer. Sister Mary Joseph nodule (Figure 26.1) may be considered more as metastases from an intraabdominal malignancy. Clinically, Sister Mary Joseph nodule is an indurate nodule or plaque. The surface of the nodule is sometimes ulcerated with exudation of purulent or mucosal discharge. Occasionally, the lesions form a tumor. Sister Mary Joseph nodules are signs of an advanced intraabdominal malignancy. They appear as a sign of previously diagnosed neoplasia. The primary malignancy is localized in the gastrointestinal or genital tract, mainly as gastric adenocarcinoma, but also adenocarcinoma of the ovary, colon, pancreas, prostate, or liver.[5]

DERMATOSES HIGHLY ASSOCIATED WITH MALIGNANCY

Acanthosis Nigricans Maligna

Besides malignant acanthosis nigricans, there is a benign form that may develop under various circumstances – endocrinopathy and drug-induced forms. It may also be clinical presentation of congenital conditions.

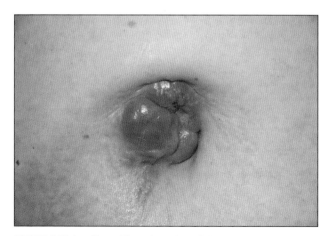

FIGURE 26.1: Sister Mary Joseph nodule.

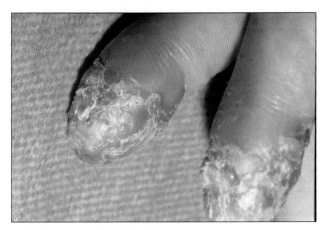

FIGURE 26.2: *Bazex syndrome (Photo courtesy of V. Benea, MD).*

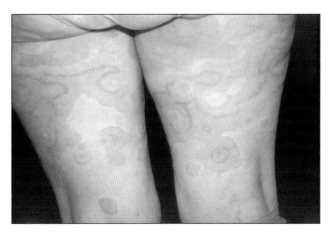

FIGURE 26.3: *Erythema gyratum repens.*

In the malignant form, some epidermal growth factors produced by the tumor cells are responsible for the clinical appearance. Clinically, malignant acanthosis nigricans is characterized by brown verrucous plaques. They are located symmetrically on the back of the neck, groin, and axillae. Similar lesions, but mostly darkly pigmented papules, appear on the lips, eyelids, nipples, and the anogenital area.

There is an extreme form that is always a clinical sign of an internal malignancy. Brown thickening of the skin over the dorsa of fingers or the palms may occur also. Oral lesions may be present, as well. Malignant acanthosis nigricans is associated with adenocarcinoma of the gastrointestinal tract, cancer of the lung, gynecological tumors, and lymphomas.[6,7]

Bazex Syndrome

Bazex syndrome (acrokeratosis paraneoplastica) is usually associated with carcinoma of the upper digestive tract, including neoplasms of the lower lip, tongue, tonsils, esophagus, and pharyngolaryngeal region (Figure 26.2).The upper part of the respiratory tract (the upper third of the lung, especially) also may be involved with malignancy in this syndrome. Other tumors have been reported also: cancer of the prostate, bladder, and lower part of the leg, and some hematologic malignancies. The skin lesions appear in several phases. Initially, they may resemble dermatitis, psoriasis, or lupus erythematosus. They begin with erythema and scaling and appear on the fingers and toes. Rarely vesicles, bullae, and crusts are present. The lesions are not itchy or painful. The nails are hypertrophic with onycholysis. Sometimes, paronychia is present. Similar changes appear on the nose and conchae of the ears. In the later stages of the disease, the skin of the body is also involved. Pityriasiform scaling appears on the surfaces of the hands and feet. This scaling and a livid erythema appear on the skin of the arms, legs, and trunk,

and (in severe cases) an erythroderma may be present. The skin changes may even become hyperkeratotic on the skin of the hands and feet.[8,9]

Erythema Gyratum Repens

Erythema gyratum repens is a paraneoplastic syndrome of unknown etiology. The lesions of this syndrome consist of erythematous concentric rings that form the classic woodgrain appearance (Figure 26.3). They may be flat or raised. The skin changes are localized on the trunk, arms, and thighs and proximal aspects of the extremities. The feet, hands, and face are usually not affected. The rings spread outward in a serpiginous pattern. The lesions are itchy, and the pruritus may be severe.[10]

The pathogenesis is still obscure. Immunological pathogenesis of erythema gyratum repens is possible because granular deposits of immunoglobulin G and C3 have been detected at the basement membrane zone of both involved and uninvolved skin.[11] In 82% of erythema gyratum repens patients, there is internal malignancy of the lung, breast, stomach, and/or esophagus. Regression of the skin legions usually occurs with treatment of the underlying cancer. Other diseases such as tuberculosis, CREST (calcinosis, Raynaud phenomenon, esophageal dysmotility, sclerodactyly, and telangiectasia) syndrome, and sclerodactyly also have been reported in association with erythema gyratum repens.[12]

Muir–Torre Syndrome

Muir–Torre syndrome is a rare autosomal dominant disorder. The skin lesions of Muir–Torre syndrome consist of sebaceous epithelioma, adenoma, or carcinoma and multiple keratoacanthomas. The skin changes may precede the appearance of the internal malignancies, but more often they occur later. The internal malignancies are multiple. They are less aggressive, and metastases rarely occur. The tumors are mostly colorectal cancers. In 50% of patients, tumors of the genitourinary tract, breast, and/or upper gastrointestinal tract are detected.[13,14]

The Sign of Leser–Trelat

The sign of Leser–Trelat presents with numerous seborrheic keratoses, known as seborrheic warts or verrucae senilis. They are common in elderly people, but the sign of Leser–Trelat must be considered as a paraneoplastic sign, if there is a sudden increase in the number or size of previous existing keratoses and if their appearance is associated with an internal malignancy.[15] The lesions are itchy. Association of the sign of Leser–Trelat with malignant acanthosis nigricans is quite possible, and this association supports the hypothesis of the paraneoplastic nature of the sign. There are no histological differences between common seborrheic keratosis and those with malignancy.

The pathogenesis of the sign is unclear. Probably, a tumor-secreted growth factor plays a role in its appearance. In most patients with the sign of Leser–Trelat, adenocarcinoma of the stomach is detected. The reported cases with the sign of Leser–Trelat had malignancy of the breast, colon, and/or rectum; less frequently, they had cancer of the duodenum, esophagus, pancreas, ovary, uterus, cervix, prostate, and/or gallbladder. The associated malignant diseases have an aggressive course; thus, the sign of Leser–Trelat is a poor prognostic sign. Association of the sign of Leser–Trelat has been reported with many hematologic disorders, such as mycosis fungoides, lymphoma, leukemia, and melanoma.[16]

Necrolytic Migratory Erythema (Glucagonoma Syndrome)

Necrolytic migratory erythema (glucagonoma syndrome) is strongly associated with the glucagon-secreting pancreatic islet cell tumor. Skin changes are erythematous, scaly, and then crusted. Blisters can appear after pustular evolution due to bacterial or mycotic superinfection. The lesions are often confluent and painful. The skin changes are localized on sites of friction and pressure, such as feet and legs, but also on buttocks, groins, and the pubic area. Additionally, mucocutaneous lesions such as atrophic glossitis, cheilitis, stomatitis, balanoposthitis, or vulvovaginitis can appear. Because the condition is associated with pancreatic tumors, high blood sugar levels are expected. The erythrocyte sedimentation rate is high. The amounts of free amino acids and of free fatty acids are low.[17]

Sweet Syndrome

Sweet syndrome (acute febrile neutrophilic dermatosis) can occur without other pathologic processes, but most commonly it might be associated with malignancy. In 85% of cases, malignancy-associated Sweet syndrome is a marker of hematologic neoplasm. The hematologic malignancies include acute myeloid leukemia, Hodgkin disease, non-Hodgkin lymphoma, myelodysplastic syndrome, myeloproliferative disease, and chronic myelogenous leukemia.[18]

The idiopathic form presents with tender plaques or nodules located on the face, hands, and/or upper extremities. The skin is erythematous and livid. The diameter of the lesions varies. Fever accompanies the skin changes, and neutrophilia is detected. The condition responds promptly to corticosteroids. There is a difference in the skin signs between the idiopathic form and malignancy-related ones. The latter are more severe, vesicular, bullous, or ulcerative. Other dermatoses can appear in the malignancy-related variant, such as pyoderma gangrenosum, erythema nodosum, or erythema multiforme. In the paraneoplastic form, the mucous membranes can be affected as well. The extracutaneous involvement is more frequent: musculoskeletal signs and symptoms, involvement of the eyes, and glomerulonephritis. In the paraneoplastic variant, there is absence of neutrophilia, which is common in the idiopathic form.[19]

Other Genodermatoses

Besides Muir-Torre syndrome, there are several autosomal dominant tumor-associated genodermatoses. These include Gardner syndrome, Peutz–Jeghers syndrome, and Cowden syndrome. In Gardner syndrome, multiple epidermoid cysts, fibromas, and primary osteoma of the skin (which are associated with cancer of the colon) are present. In Peutz–Jeghers syndrome, multiple perioral and mucosal lentigines are observed. The skin changes are present beginning in early childhood, but later the patients develop tumor of the testis, ovaries, pancreas, and/or gastrointestinal tract. In Cowden syndrome, multiple trichilemmomas, trichoepitheliomas, hemangiomas, and oral and acral papules appear in association with breast and thyroid cancer or tumors of the gastrointestinal tract.[3]

Paraneoplastic Pemphigus

Paraneoplastic pemphigus is a mucocutaneous blistering disease associated with malignancy and caused by Hodgkin disease, non-Hodgkin lymphoma, chronic lymphocytic leukemia, and/or Castleman disease, as well as Waldenstrom macroglobulinemia, T-cell lymphoma, thymoma, retroperitoneal sarcoma, and/or reticulum cell sarcoma. Reports on association with solid cancers are isolated.[20,21]

DERMATOLOGY DISORDERS THAT MAY BE ASSOCIATED WITH MALIGNANCY

Pyoderma Gangrenosum

Pyoderma gangrenosum begins as a papule or pustule that later develops into an erythematous nodule. These nodules form an ulcer with irregular borders. The lesions have a

TABLE 26.1: Dermatologic Diseases and Disorders in Associations of Malignancy

Skin disorder	Related malignancy	References
Porphyria cutanea tarda	Hepatocellular carcinoma	Federman et al.[30]
Amyloidosis	Multiple myeloma	Zappasodi et al.[19]
Ichthyosis acquisita	Multiple myeloma, non-Hodgkin lymphoma, Hodgkin disease	Zappasodi et al.[19]
Granuloma annulare	Non-Hodgkin lymphoma, Hodgkin disease, solid tumors	Cohen[31]
Sarcoidosis	Solid tumors of cervix, liver, lung, uterus, testicles, melanoma; leukemias, lymphomas, myeloma	Cohen[31]
Papuloerythroderma of Ofuji	T-cell lymphomas, hepatocellular carcinoma	Schepers et al.[32] Nishijima[33]
Bullous pemphigoid	Non-Hodgkin lymphoma	Zappasodi et al.[19]
Relapsing polychondritis	Adenocarcinoma of bladder, breast, bronchus, colon, lung, pancreas, prostate, rectum, vocal cords; leukemias, lymphomas, myeloma	Cohen[31]
Systemic lupus erythematosus	Solid tumors of breast, cervix, ovary, brain, colon, biliary tract, kidney, pancreas, stomach, rectum, thymus, urinary bladder; leukemias, lymphomas, myeloma, nonmelanoma skin cancer	Cohen[31]
Erythromelalgia	Myeloproliferative disease	Zappasodi et al.[19]
Subcorneal pustular dermatosis	Multiple myeloma, non-Hodgkin lymphoma	Zappasodi et al.[19]
Dermatitis herpetiformis	Non-Hodgkin lymphoma	Zappasodi et al.[19]
Linear immunoglobulin A dermatosis	Multiple myeloma, non-Hodgkin lymphoma	Zappasodi et al.[19]
Erythroderma and exfoliative dermatitis	Hodgkin disease, non-Hodgkin lymphoma	Zappasodi et al.[19]
Pityriasis lichenoides et varioliformis acuta	Mycosis fungoides	Kempf et al.[34]
Eosinophilic fasciitis	T-cell malignant neoplasm	Chan et al.[35]
Scleroderma	Ovarian cancer	Vottery et al.[36]
Pityriasis lichenoides chronica	Oncocytoma renis	Lazarov et al.[37]

necrotic base, and hemorrhagic exudates may be present. The lesions are painful and have a predilection for lower extremity involvement. The sign of pathergy is present, and lesions develop after minor trauma.[19]

Pyoderma gangrenosum is associated in approximately 50% of patients with such systemic diseases as ulcerative colitis, Crohn disease, and inflammatory arthritis.[22] In 7% of cases, hematologic malignancies, most commonly leukemias and multiple myeloma, are detected.[19] When the condition is associated with hematologic disorders, bullae may also be seen on the face.[23]

Dermatomyositis

Dermatomyositis is an inflammatory myopathy with characteristic skin manifestations. The diagnostic criteria of dermatomyositis include symmetrical proximal muscle weakness, inflammatory myopathy, elevation of serum levels of muscle enzymes, electromyographic evidence of myopathy, and typical cutaneous findings of dermatomyositis. The prevalence of malignancy in dermatomyositis ranges from 3% to 60%.[24] Dermatomyositis may precede, occur concurrently with, or develop after the malignancy. The most expected tumors associated with dermatomyositis are cancers of the ovary, stomach, lung, and/or breast.[25]

Clubbing

Digital clubbing is associated with a disabling lung disease, mostly pulmonary emphysema, but also with chronic bronchitis, hepatic cirrhosis, and inflammatory intestinal diseases. It is characterized by an increase in the diameter of the distal phalanges and alterations to the fingernails. The disorder is classified into five phases. It begins with an increase and fluctuation of the ungual bed and, in the last phase, increase of the extremity with thickening of the distal phalange and longitudinal striations are observed.[26] Digital clubbing is associated with bronchogenic cancer, and in this paraneoplastic form the bones are not usually changed.[27]

Tripe Palms

Tripe palms present with brown thickening of the skin of the palms, resembling pig intestine; hence, the name. The epidermal ridges are broadened, and the sulci are deep. These changes are associated with internal malignancy and usually appear with acanthosis nigricans.[28]

Hypertrichosis Lanuginose

This paraneoplastic sign occurs in women, mostly. The face is affected mainly. Less frequently, hypertrichosis is observed on the neck, trunk, arms, and legs. It must be differentiated from hirsutism and hypertrichosis, which occur because of androgens produced by some endocrinologic disorders. Hypertrichosis lanuginose appears with cancer of the lung and/or colon.[3]

The vasculitides, which are a heterogenous group of diseases, are associated with cancer in approximately 5% of the patients. Most commonly, patients with paraneoplastic vasculitis have such hematologic malignancies as hairy cell leukemia and lymphomas. Vasculitis reported in association with hematologic malignancies includes leukocytoclastic vasculitis and polyarteritis nodosa.[19,29]

OTHER DERMATOLOGIC DISEASES ASSOCIATED WITH MALIGNANCIES

Numerous additional dermatologic diseases and disorders have been reported in associations of malignancy (Table 26.1).

Additionally, dermographism and pruritus must be considered as common paraneoplastic signs without any particular associations with malignancies.

REFERENCES

1. Delacretaz J. Nouveaux syndromes paraneoplasiques cutanes. Med Hyg Geneve. 1967; 25:1005–6.
2. Vlckova-Laskovska MT, Balabanova-Stefanova MG, Caca-Biljanovska NG. Cutaneous paraneoplastic syndromes. Bull CEEDVA. 2004; 6:13–16.
3. Balo-Banga JM, Vajda A. Paraneoplastic disorders and syndromes of the skin. Bull CEEDVA. 2004; 6:4–12.
4. Thomas I, Schwartz R. Cutaneous paraneoplastic syndromes: uncommon presentations. Clin Dermatol. 2005; 23:593–600.
5. Powell F, Cooper A, Massa M, et al. Sister Mary Joseph's nodule: a clinical and histologic study. J Am Acad Dermatol. 1984; 10:610–15.
6. Andreev V, Boyanov L, Tsankov N. Generalized acanthosis nigricans. Dermatologica. 1981; 163:19–24.
7. Balo-Banga JM, Racz I, Szalay F, et al. Ein mit Castleman-to-Rhino Hamarton einhergehende paraneoplastischer Symptomenkomplex. Z Hautkr. 1990; 65:761.
8. Wareing MJ, Vaughan-Jones SA, McGibbon DH. Acrokeratosis paraneoplastica: Bazes syndrome. J Laryng Otolog. 1996; 110:899–900.
9. Sarkar B, Knecht R, Sarkar C, et al. Bazex syndrome acrokeratosis paraneoplastica. Eur Archiv Oto-Rhino-Laringol. 1998; 255:205–10.
10. Eubanks LE, McBurney E, Reed R. Erythema gyratum repens. Am J Med Sci. 2001; 321:302–5.
11. Holt PJA, Davies MG. Erythema gyratum repens – an immunologically mediated dermatosis. Br J Dermatol. 1977; 96:343–7.
12. Gantcheva M, Tsankov N, Pramatarov K. Erythema gyratum repens without internal malignancy. J Eur Acad Dermatol Venereol. 1995; 5:67–9.
13. Lynch MT, Linch PM, Pester J, et al. The cancer family syndrome: rare cutaneous phenotypic linkage of Torre's syndrome. Arch Intern Med. 1981; 141:607–11.
14. Suspiro A, Fidalgo P, Crovo M, et al. The Muir-Torre syndrome: a rare variant of hereditary nonpolyposis colorectal cancer associated with hMSH2 mutation. Am J Gastroenterol. 1998; 93:1572–4.
15. Rampen HJ, Schwengle LE. The sign of Leser – Trelat: does it exist. J Am Acad Dermatol. 1989; 21:50–5.
16. Schwartz RA. The sign of Leser – Trelat. J Am Acad Dermatol. 1996; 35:88–95.
17. Santacroce L, Gagliardi Abraham M. Clucagonoma e Medicine. Endocrinology 2007 Feb 9
18. Cohen PR, Talpaz M, Kurzrock R. Malignancy-associated Sweet's syndrome: review of the world literature. J Clin Oncol. 1988; 6:1887–97.
19. Zappasodi P, Del Forno C, Corso A, et al. Mucocutaneous paraneoplastic syndromes in hematologic malignancies. Int J Dermatol. 2006; 45:14–20.
20. Anhalt GJ. Paraneoplastic pemphigus: the role of tumors and drugs. Br J Dermatol. 2001; 144:1101–4.
21. Vassileva S, Drenovska K, Serafimova D, et al. Paraneoplastic pemphigus: report of two cases associated with chronic lymphocytic leukemia. Bull CEEDVA. 2004; 6:17–22.
22. Callen JP, Woo TY. Vesiculopustular eruption in a patient with ulcerative colitis. Arch Dermatol. 1985; 121:399–403.
23. Kurzrock R, Cohen PR. Mucocutaneous paraneoplastic manifestations in hematologic malignancy. Am J Med. 1995; 92:207–16.
24. Maoz CR, Langevitz P, Livneh A, et al. High incidence of malignancies in patients with dermatomyositis and polymyositis: an 11-year analysis. Semin Arthritis Rheum. 1998; 27:319–24.
25. Bernard P, Bonnetblanc JM. Dermatomyositis and malignancy. J Invest Dermatol. 1993; 100:128–32.
26. Sridhar KS, Lobo CF, Altman RD. Digital clubbing and lung cancer. Chest. 1998; 114:1535–7.
27. Macedo AG, Fusari VC, Paes del Almeida JR, et al. Digital clubbing as the initial diagnosis of bronchogenic cancer. Anais Brasil Dermatol. 2004; 79:457–62.
28. Breathnach SM, Wells GC. Acantosis nigricans: tripe palms. Clin Exp Dermatol. 1980; 5:181–9.
29. Sanchez-Guerrero J, Gutierrez-Urena S, Vidaller A, et al. Vasculitis as a paraneoplastic syndrome: report of 11 cases and review of the literature. J Rheumatol. 1990; 17:1458–62.
30. Federman D, Brescia G, Horne M, et al. Cutaneous manifestation of malignancy. Postgrad Med Online. 2004; 115:1–13.
31. Cohen P. Granuloma annulare, relapsing polychondritis, sarcoidosis, and systemic lupus erythematosus: conditions whose dermatologic manifestation may occur as hematologic malignancy – associated mucocutaneous paraneoplastic syndromes. Int J Dermatol. 2006; 45:70–80.
32. Schepers C, Malvehy J, Azon-Masoliver A, et al. Papuloerythroderma of Ofuji: a report of 2 cases including the first European case associated with visceral carcinoma. Dermatology. 1996; 193:131–5.

33. Nishijima S. Papuloerythroderma associated with hepatocellular carcinoma. Br J Dermatol. 1998; 139:1115–16.

34. Kempf W, Kutzner H, Kettelhack N, et al. Paraneoplastic pityriasis lichenoides in cutaneous lymphoma: case report and review of the literature on paraneoplastic reactions of the skin in lymphoma and leukemia. Br J Dermatol. 2005; 152:1327–31.

35. Chan LS, Hanson CA, Cooper KD. Eosinophilic fasciitis as a paraneoplastic syndrome. Arch Dermatol. 1991; 127:862–5.

36. Vottery R, Biswas G, Deshmukh C, et al. Scleroderma and dermographism in a case of carcinoma ovary. Indian J Dermatol Venereol Leprol. 2005; 71:429–30.

37. Lazarov A, Lalkin A, Cordoba M, et al. Paraneoplastic pityriasis lichenoides chronica. J Eur Acad Dermatol Venereol. 1999; 12:189–90.

CHAPTER 27

Burn Injury

Samuel H. Allen

ACUTE INJURY caused by burns produces some of the most horrendous and harrowing deformities encountered by persons working in the emergency and health care services. These injuries have a high mortality and, should the patients survive, they will carry with them the lifelong scars – physical, psychological, and emotional.

Worldwide, injury caused by fire is a major cause of morbidity, especially in sub-Saharan Africa where open fires are used to heat food and water. Sadly, most of these injuries occur in toddlers.

In the developed world, house fires and industrial accidents are the major culprits causing burn injury. In the United States alone, more than 500,000 people are seen in emergency departments each year as a result of burn injury; more than 50,000 are admitted to hospital, and more than 5000 deaths per year are attributed to the burn injury.

Approximately 50% of household and domestic burn injuries result from hot-water scalding and fires that occur in the kitchen. Most are managed outside hospital practice. Highest rates of burn-related injury and death are observed in children younger than 5 years and elderly persons older than 75 years.[1] Since the introduction of gas-fired central heating and the tightening of health and safety laws, the incidence of these events has become less commonplace.

Heat energy is transmitted through radiation, conduction, and convection. Thermal injury usually occurs as a result of fire, but chemicals, electricity, and radiation can also cause burn injury. It is the direct effect of the flames' heat that causes the greatest harm. When the skin's integument is destroyed the essential function of the skin is lost, leading to profound fluid loss as well as inflammation and pain. To compound the injury, the burn is often associated with other injuries arising from the accident such as shock, smoke and debris inhalation, and blunt trauma. Superheated air may cause direct thermal injury leading to upper airway edema and obstruction of the respiratory tract. More than 50% of fire-related deaths are the result of smoke inhalation.

PATHOPHYSIOLOGY

A burn is caused by the coagulative destruction of the skin and mucous membranes, leading to blistering and local inflammatory changes. Large injury is associated with systemic shock and organ hypoperfusion that is compounded by the pathological fluid loss. After resuscitation, the patient attains a hypermetabolic state associated with gluconeogenesis, insulin resistance, and increased protein catabolism. Late complications can arise from tissue edema and swelling, which in turn may lead to compartment syndrome, superimposed infection, and contractures. Wound infection is often associated with multidrug-resistant organisms as a result of prior use of broad-spectrum antibiotics. Psychological sequelae are common and include posttraumatic stress disorder, depression, and body image disorder.

CLINICAL AND LABORATORY AIDS REQUIRED FOR DIAGNOSIS

In most cases of burn injury the diagnosis and etiology are self-evident. Even so, it is important to try to establish the time of the injury as this will have implications in the management and anticipation of complications. What may be less clear is the extent – and depth – of the injury.

Extent of Burn

A rapid and usefully accurate estimate of the body surface area of the injury can be calculated using the Rule of Nines (Figure 27.1).[2]

Calculation of body surface area differs in children. For children younger than 1 year, the head surface area represents approximately 18% of total surface area and the legs 14%. Therefore, for children older than 1 year, one should add 0.5% to the leg area and subtract 1% from the head surface area for each additional year until adult values are attained. Alternatively, the Lund and Browder[3] chart can be used to estimate body surface area in children. For a wide age range, the area of the palm plus palmer aspect of the digits represents 1% of the total body area.

Depth of Burn

Accurate assessment of the burn depth is important in making decisions about dressings and timing of surgery. The depth may not always be clear from the initial assessment.

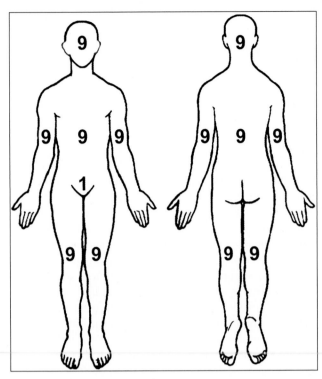

FIGURE 27.1:   Rule of Nines.[2]

Depth of burn was previously classified as first-, second-, or third-degree burn but is now more accurately described as an epidermal, superficial, or deep partial-thickness or full-thickness burn (Figure 27.2).

Epidermal Burns. By definition, these burns affect only the epidermis. The lesion is typified by sunburn. Erythema and pain are present. Blistering is unusual in this type of injury. The skin adnexae that contain regenerating keratinocytes within the sweat glands and hair follicles are preserved, so the lesion normally heals within a week without scarring. Supportive therapy is all that is required. Regular analgesia and intravenous fluids may be required if there is extensive injury and/or signs of heat stroke.

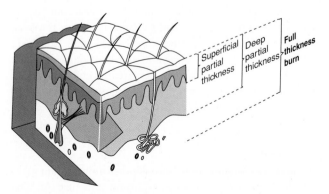

FIGURE 27.2:   Classification of injury according to depth of burn.

Superficial Partial-Thickness Burns. These burns affect the superficial dermis (papillary layer) and epidermis. The lesion has a red or mottled appearance with associated swelling and blister formation. Scalding typically causes this type of lesion. The skin often has a weeping or wet appearance and may be hypersensitive, even to air. Exposure of the superficial nerves makes these injuries extremely painful. Healing is usually complete within 2 weeks depending on the density of skin adnexae. Thin hairless skin (e.g., inner arm and eyelids) will heal more slowly than thick or hairy skin (e.g., scalp or face) because it contains fewer hair follicles or sweat glands that contain the regenerating keratinocytes.

Deep Partial-Thickness Burns. Damage to the deep dermis, which is the reticular layer containing the superficial parts of the hair follicles and sweat and sebaceous glands, is often the most difficult to assess and treat. Initial lesions may appear superficial, even with blanching on pressure, but on reexamination 48 hours later show fixed capillary staining. Fewer skin adnexae – hence islands of regeneration – are present at this depth, so healing is slower. The exposed dermis is pale white–yellow and insensate because sensory nerves in the dermis are destroyed. Blistering is common, and there is no capillary refill. Lesions heal with scarring. If injuries are extensive or in functional or cosmetically sensitive areas they are better excised to a viable depth and then skin-grafted for best functional recovery. Healing takes between 3 and 8 weeks.

Full-Thickness Burns. In full-thickness burns, all regenerative tissues are destroyed such that healing may only naturally occur from the edges of the wound. Consequently, healing usually results in considerable contraction. The skin may vary in appearance between appearing dark, charred, and leathery to appearing translucent, mottled, or waxy white. Occasionally, the injury may be missed, being mistaken for unburnt skin. All full-thickness burn injuries should be excised and grafted unless they are small (<1 cm in diameter) or in an area that would not compromise function. Analgesia to pinprick signifies a deep dermal or full-thickness injury.

The clinical features of epidermal, partial-, and full-thickness burns are shown in Table 27.1. A so-called fourth-degree burn exhibits destruction of the subcutaneous fat, muscle, and sometimes bone. Such injury requires major reconstruction and often amputation.

THERAPY

The chances of surviving a complex major burn injury are better now than ever before. Patients should be managed on a specialized burn unit or center with experience in managing these types of injury. This management usually

TABLE 27.1: Clinical Features of Epidermal, Partial-, and Full-Thickness Burns

Depth	Color	Blisters	Capillary refill	Sensation
Epidermal	Pink or red	No	Present	Sore
Superficial partial thickness	Pink or red	+/−	Present	Painful
Deep partial thickness	Red or pale	+/−	no	+/−
Full thickness	White	No	no	No

involves a multidisciplinary effort involving the surgical team, specialist nursing, microbiology, dieticians, physiotherapy, and psychology. It is important that the wound is reviewed regularly until healing is ensured. Factors such as the local or systemic inflammatory response, wound infection, dehydration, cooling, and nutritional support will influence the outcome.

Immediate Management: Airway, Breathing, and Circulation

Initial management of the burned patient requires an urgent assessment of the airway, breathing, and circulation (ABC) of the injured person, an assessment of his or her level of consciousness, and rapid fluid replacement.

All clothing should be removed unless adherent to the burn victim's flesh (in which case it should be cooled and soaked with water for formal debridement later). Jewelry such as rings and wristwatches should be removed to prevent later complications arising from edema of the extremities. Recent burn injury should be actively cooled with copious amounts of tepid water for up to 20 minutes. Extra caution should be taken in children as their greater surface area-to-weight ratio may lead to hypothermia. The patient should be nursed in a bed with warm, dry, clean linens to prevent hypothermia. Any blisters should be left intact. Antiseptic creams should not be applied.[4]

Inhalation injury should be suspected if there is burn to the face, neck, and/or lips; hoarseness; or evidence of carbon particles (produced by combustion) at the mouth or in the sputum. Inhalation injury is more likely if the victim is found in an enclosed space or if the injury occurred as a result of an explosion.

Smoke inhalation usually consists of carbon monoxide (CO) and/or cyanide poisoning combined with a severe chemical pneumonitis. Modern building construction materials yield significant amounts of cyanide. A carboxyhemoglobin level greater than 10% in a burn victim would be indicative of inhalation smoke injury.

Anoxia is the first complication to consider. Causes are laryngeal obstruction, pulmonary edema, contracted burned skin encircling the chest, carboxyhemoglobin, anemia, and shock. The airway above the glottis is particularly susceptible to obstruction from heat-induced edema. Inhalation injury may be subtle and often does not appear in the first 24 hours, mandating that patients be observed and have blood gases monitored for at least 24 hours prior to discharge.

Acute inhalation injury requires transfer to a specialist unit for endotracheal intubation and mechanical ventilation.

Management on the Burn Unit

Fluid Replacement. A flow sheet outlining the patient's management should be commenced and kept with the patient on arrival on the burn unit. Baseline determination for the major burn patient is shown in Table 27.2. Ideally, the patient should be weighed on admission to the unit, and a full survey of the extent of other injuries should be taken. This will often involve a radiological survey.

The burn represents a large fistula leaking water, electrolytes, and protein. The rate of daily water loss through the breached skin averages 0.30 mL/cm² burned area. If not done already, large-caliber intravenous lines must be established. Any adult with more than 20% burns (i.e., two whole upper limbs or one whole leg) or a child with more than 10% burns (i.e., one whole upper limb, excluding erythema) will require circulatory volume support. A burn patient will require 2–4 mL of Ringer's lactate or colloid solution per kilogram body weight per percent partial- or full-thickness body surface burns in the first 24 hours. In children, plasma equal to the child's plasma volume should be given for every 15% of skin burned. The intravenous fluid rate is adjusted to give one half of the estimated fluid

TABLE 27.2: Baseline Determination for the Major Burn Patient

- Blood: complete blood count, blood type and cross-match, carboxyhemoglobin, serum glucose, electrolytes
- Pregnancy test in women of child-bearing age
- Arterial blood gases
- X-ray: chest x-ray, other x-rays as indicated by injuries
- Time of injury
- Patient's weight
- Estimate of burn injury: extent (% body surface area) and depth of injury
- Comorbidities and medication

volume replacement within the first 8 hours after the burn injury and the remainder in the subsequent 16 hours. Fluid requirement calculations for infusion rates are based on time from injury, not from the time fluid resuscitation is initiated. The amount of fluid given should be adjusted according to the individual patient's response to maintain a urinary output of 0.5–1 mL/kg/h (adult) or 1–1.5 mL/kg/h (in children). The goal is to maintain vital organ function while avoiding the complications of inadequate or excessive fluid infusion that can lead to increased tissue edema.

Blood pressure may be difficult to obtain and may be unreliable. Arterial line blood-pressure monitoring is therefore preferable in the intensive care or burn unit setting with cardiac monitoring for signs of dysrhythmia. Electrolyte, acid–base, and fluid balance will need to be meticulously monitored with hourly urine output for which the patient will require urinary catheterization. If there are signs of nausea, vomiting, or abdominal distension, or if burn involves more than 20% of the total body surface area, nasogastric tube insertion will be required. Blood transfusion is rarely needed.

CO Poisoning. The diagnosis of CO poisoning should be assumed in any injured person found in a smoke-filled environment. Patients with CO levels less than 20% usually have no physical symptoms. Higher CO levels can cause headache, nausea, confusion, coma, and/or death.

CO dissociates very slowly from hemoglobin, but this can be increased by breathing high-flow oxygen via a non-rebreathing mask. Arterial blood gas determinations should be obtained at baseline, but arterial pO_2 does not reliably predict CO poisoning. Therefore, 100% oxygen should be administered after baseline carboxyhemoglobin levels have been taken.

Severely burned patients may be agitated or anxious from hypoxemia or hypovolemia rather than from pain. The patient may then respond better to oxygen or increased fluid administration rather than to narcotic analgesics or sedatives that may mask other signs of hypoxemia or hypovolemia. Narcotics, analgesics, and sedatives should be administered in small, frequent doses by the intravenous route only.

Hyperbaric oxygen therapy has been used in the treatment of major burn injury. To be effective, hyperbaric oxygen therapy must be started within 24 hours of the burn (and preferably sooner). It is particularly useful in cases of concomitant smoke inhalation and CO or cyanide poisoning.

Airway Management. Stridor is an indication for immediate endotracheal intubation. Circumferential burn to the neck can lead to swelling of the tissues around the airway and will usually require intubation. If oxygen and humidification are not adequate, positive-pressure ventilation may be needed.

Elevation of the head and chest by 20–30 degrees reduces neck and chest wall edema. Chest wall escharotomy (burn incised into subcutaneous fat) may be required in the case of a full-thickness burn of the torso, leading to restriction of the chest wall motion. Local anesthesia is not required because the skin is rendered insensate.

Nutritional Support. The average sodium loss is 0.03 mmol/cm², and the protein loss is similar to dilute plasma, about 30 g/L. Extensively burned patients will require approximately one-and-a-half times the calories and 2–3 times the protein needed in health. Feeding may be commenced via the nasogastric tube within 24 hours after the burn injury. If oral feeding is not possible, potassium should be administered by mouth or intravenously to prevent ileus.

Wound Management

Superficial Partial-Thickness Burns. A moist, infection-free environment facilitates the process of reepithelialization. In the case of a superficial partial-thickness injury, an antimicrobial cream plus an occlusive dressing should be applied. Hypafix applied directly to superficial wounds can be useful to preserve mobility and allow washing of the affected part with the dressing intact. It should be soaked in oil (such as olive oil) for an hour before removal and changed at least twice weekly until the wound has healed. Alternatively, tulle gras or a silicone dressing such as Mepitel can be applied, with or without a silver sulfadiazine cream or Acticoat and gauze.[5]

The wound should be cleaned, dressed, and reviewed on alternate days to optimize healing. Antimicrobial cream should be applied using the aseptic method with sterile gloves to avoid inoculation of potentially pathogenic organisms into the wound. Facial burns heal well and may be left exposed. Any burn that has not healed within 2 weeks should be referred for reassessment.

Deep Partial-Thickness Burns. These injuries are the most difficult to treat and assess. Some deep partial-thickness injuries will heal if the wound environment is optimized to encourage endogenous healing. Other injuries will require excision and grafting.

Delay in reepithelialization beyond 3 weeks is associated with hypertrophic scarring. Therefore, all injuries that show no sign of healing by 10 days should be referred to a specialist burn unit for consideration of grafting. Either the depth has been assessed incorrectly or the wound environment has become compromised.

A number of bioengineered skin substitutes have been designed to promote healing. TransCyte, for example, contains nonviable allogenic fibroblasts that produce cytokines that have been shown to improve healing in vitro. In a systematic review, such agents were at least as safe as biological skin replacements or topical agents.[6] Bioengineered skin substitutes, however, tend to be expensive and need to be applied by trained staff in theatre.

Surgery

With major burns, the goal of therapy is geared toward preservation of life and limb. Wounds that are obviously deep at presentation must be referred early before tissue necrosis triggers multiple organ failure or leads to sepsis. In such cases, more superficial burns may be treated with dressings until healing occurs or fresh donor sites become available.

The best time for surgery is within 5 days of injury to minimize blood loss. The burn eschar is shaved tangentially or excised to deep fascia. The aim is to remove the nonviable burnt skin while leaving a bed of viable tissue to allow for regranulation.

The ideal covering is split-skin autograft from unburnt areas. Thickness is usually tailored to the depth of the excision for good cosmesis. Donor sites are often harvested adjacent to the injury to optimize the color match. Unmeshed sheet graft is preferred for the best cosmetic result and is used for the hands and face.

Where donor sites are sparse, or the wound bed is likely to bleed profusely, the graft is perforated with a mesher to allow expansion. Although this improves graft "take" where the wound is bleeding after tangential excision, the mesh pattern is permanent and unsightly.

Rotation of the donor site may be used where unburnt split-skin donor sites are in short supply, or else the excised wound is covered with a temporary cover until donor sites have regenerated for reharvest. Examples of temporary cover include cadaveric allograft from an unrelated donor, xenograft (pigskin is most commonly used), cultured epithelial autograft, or a number of synthetic products.

Cultured epithelial autografts permit greater use of available donor sites. Cultured cells can be applied as sheets (available after 3 weeks) or in suspension (available within 1 week). The development of synthetic products (such as Integra dermal regeneration template) has enabled surgeons to shave extremely large burns and still achieve physiological closure with potentially lower mortality than was previously possible. These products can be used in combination with mesh graft to improve the final cosmetic result.

Role of Antimicrobials

Unless soiled at the time of injury, an acute burn injury is usually sterile because the heat from the initial burn is sufficient to kill most skin bacteria. Antibiotics, therefore, should not be routinely commenced following a burn injury but should be reserved for the treatment of secondary infection.

TABLE 27.3: Criteria for Referral to a Burns Center

- Deep burns involving:
  - 10% or more of the total body surface area in adults, or
  - 5% or more of the total body surface area in children
- Burns to the face, eyes, ears, hands, feet, genitalia, perineum, inner joint surfaces
- Inhalation injury
- Significant chemical and electrical burns, including lightning injury
- Burn injury with any of the following:
  - Major preexisting illness such as diabetes that could complicate management and recovery
  - Suspected child abuse and neglect
  - Concomitant injury

Wounds should be swabbed regularly for bacterial growth and culture sensitivities. The choice of antimicrobials, if indicated, should be based on these results, along with the results of screening swabs, for example, for methicillin-resistant *Staphylococcus aureus* (MRSA).

Tetanus toxoid should be administered. Human antitetanus immunoglobulin should be considered if treatment has been delayed or the wound is heavily contaminated with soil or feces.

COURSE AND PROGNOSIS

A rough calculation of the survival probability can be made using the formula:

100 – (age in years + area of burn, as a percentage)

For example, a 25-year-old man with a 30% burn can expect a 45% [100 – (25 + 30)] survival.

Optimum treatment of the wound reduces morbidity and reduces mortality. It also shortens the time to healing and return to normal function and thus reduces the need for plastic surgery.

CRITERIA FOR REFERRAL TO A BURN UNIT

Although not all the patients in the categories in Table 27.3 will require transfer to a specialized burn unit, consultation with the appropriate center should take place at presentation to plan further management and anticipate possible complications.

Full-thickness injuries have no regenerative elements left. Unless they are very small, they will take weeks to heal and undergo severe contraction. They should be referred for surgery as early as possible.

COMPLICATIONS

The number and complexity of complications will depend on the premorbid state of the patient as well as the extent and type(s) of injury.

Compartment Syndrome

Raised intracompartmental pressure due to progressive tissue damage and inflammation can impede compartmental blood flow leading to ischemia and anoxic necrosis. Fasciotomy and nerve decompression (requiring clinical vigilance and close liaison with the surgical team) should be undertaken prior to the onset of irreversible damage.

Infection

Unless there is debris in the wound, the thermal energy from the burn will kill the commensal flora of the skin. The routine use of broad-spectrum antibiotics on admission is therefore not recommended, unless the wound involves areas with a high bacterial load, such as the perineum or feet, or where the wound has been soiled.

Exposed devitalized flesh provides a warm, moist culture medium, and a sterile wound can quickly become colonized when the skin has lost its integument. Even so, it will normally take approximately 5 days for an infection or significant colonization to become established in a previously sterile site.

If a wound infection is suspected or the patient develops any signs of sepsis (raised temperature, raised C-reactive protein, raised white cell or neutrophil count), then wound swabs and blood cultures should be taken before embarking on "blind" antimicrobial therapy. The choice of antibiotics will depend on the unit guidelines based on the local endemic resistance pattern and cost. Close liaison with the microbiologist is essential to avoid inappropriate prescribing.

The emergence of multiresistant organisms (including resistant *Pseudomonas* spp., *Acinetobacter baumannii*, MRSA, and vancomycin-resistant *Enterococcus*) within burn units has become an increasing problem. The overall attributable mortality rate for these organisms is high, and once established, eradication from the burn unit can be difficult because of their ubiquitous nature and ability to survive for prolonged periods on inanimate surfaces.

Thromboembolic Disease

Burn injury, coupled with fluid loss and a prolonged period of rest in a warm environment, will increase plasma fluid viscosity. Prophylaxis with a low-molecular-weight heparin is recommended but can be delayed until after initial debridement and shave excision procedures. The clinical team should be mindful of late thromboembolic complications such as deep vein thrombosis or pulmonary embolus. D-dimers will be of limited use in the context of a recuperating burn patient, and diagnosis will rely on Doppler ultrasound or venogram. Treatment will be as for a general surgical patient with a target international normalized ratio of 2.5, range 2–3.

OTHER TYPES OF BURN INJURY

Chemical Burns

Chemical burns may result from exposure to acids, alkalis, and petroleum products. Alkali burns tend to be deeper and more serious than acid burns.

Management involves washing the burn with copious amounts of running water for at least 20–30 minutes (longer for alkali burns). Certain chemicals will produce toxic products with only a small amount of water, so it is important to use a copious amount of water to dilute the effects of the chemical. If the toxic chemical is in powder form then the powder should be brushed away before irrigation with water.

Ocular chemical injury requires continuous irrigation for at least 8 hours in the case of alkali burns.

Electrical Burns

Electrical burns account for approximately 3% of burn patients attending specialized centers. These burns are arbitrarily classified as high- or low-tension injuries depending on the voltage, with high-tension burns resulting from shocks of greater than 1000 volts. Most electrical burns, however, are the result of low-tension domestic appliances. Other sources of current are overhead high-voltage power lines and rail electrification, including the "third rail." These overhead power lines pose a threat not only to workers but also to sports enthusiasts involved in pursuits such as fly-fishing, kite-flying, hang-gliding, and parachuting.[7,8] Removal of bodies from overhead cables will require electrical isolation at the point of recovery.

Electric shock will cause reflex muscle contraction. Thus, when navigating his or her way out of a smoke-filled room, a firefighter will have been trained to feel the way with the back of a hand rather than the palm, so that if an exposed live wire is encountered the shock will produce a repulsion of the limb rather than a grasp reflex.

The severity of electrical burn injury is related to the voltage, duration of contact, and thickness and wetness of the skin.

Electrical burns are often more serious than they appear on the surface. Any organ between the entry and exit point can be injured. High-voltage contact results in significant rhabdomyolysis with myoglobinuria and subsequent risk of renal failure. Death may occur as a result of cardiac stunning.

The histology of a skin injury shows a distinctive vertical elongation of the nuclei of the cells of the basal layer.

The superficial epidermal cells may show similar changes. Dermal–epidermal separation may be present with elongated degenerated cytoplasmic processes from the basal cells protruding into this space.

Lightning Strike

Approximately 100 deaths occur every year from a lightning strike in the United States. Millions of volts are conducted through a channel of approximately 1-cm diameter in less than a few milliseconds. Although 90% of victims survive the lightning strike, up to 70% will suffer late organic or psychological effects.

The classical dermatological injury is an arborescent or feather-like lesion known as a Lichtenberg figure (Figure 27.2). Small burns at the site of metal objects held in the hands or pockets may also be evident.[9]

Therapy is directed toward management of the extracutaneous complications that include respiratory arrest, gastric dilatation, ileus, cerebral edema, rupture of the tympanic membrane, and fractures.

REFERENCES

1. Rajpura A. The epidemiology of burns and smoke inhalation in secondary care: a population-based study covering Lancashire and South Cumbria. Burns. 2002; 28:121–30.
2. Wallace AB. The exposure treatment of burns. Lancet. 1951; i:501–4.
3. Lund CC, Browder NC. The estimation of the areas of burns. Surg Gynaecol Obst. 1944; 79:352–8.
4. Hettiaratchy S, Papini R. Initial management of a major burn: I – overview. BMJ. 2004; 328:1555–7.
5. Papini R. Management of burn injuries of various depths. BMJ. 2004; 329:158–60.
6. Pham C, Greenwood J, Cleland H, et al. Bioengineered skin substitutes for the management of burns: a systematic review. Burns. 2007; 33:946–57.
7. Chi L, Ning YD, Jun QF, et al. Electrical injuries from graphite fishing rods. Burns. 1996; 22:638–40.
8. Campbell DC, Nano T, Pegg SP. Pattern of burn injury on hang-glider pilots. Burns 1996; 22:328–40.
9. Cherington M, McDonough G, Olson S, et al. Lichtenberg figures and lightning: case reports and review of the literature. Cutis. 2007; 80:141–3.

CHAPTER 28

Emergency Dermatoses of the Anorectal Regions

Yalçin Tüzün

Sadiye Keskin

ALTHOUGH THERE ARE some dermatological disorders that may affect the quality of life, the life-threatening dermatoses of the anorectal region are infrequently seen. When observed, bacterial infections would be the most serious, often being life threatening. For this reason, making the correct diagnosis and providing appropriate care is significant. Some of these disorders may be treated only with surgical treatment.

Emergency dermatoses in the anorectal region are listed in Table 28.1.

STAPHYLOCOCCAL CELLULITIS

The anorectal region can be susceptible to infection with *Staphylococcus aureus*. The high temperature, pressure, friction, and humidity of this area encourage colonization by staphylococci. Severe involvement with furunculosis and abscesses suggests an overlap with hidradenitis suppurativa. Cellulitis and abscess formation can complicate cysts, sinuses, and fistulas.[1]

Anorectal infections in patients with malignant disease are serious and potentially life threatening. Although some cases of anorectal cellulitis may respond to antimicrobials alone, necrotizing fasciitis and Fournier gangrene have a high risk. Swelling and fluctuation signifying abscess formation may develop. It is difficult to decide on the timing of surgery. Perianal infiltration, ulceration, or abscess occurs in 5% of hematological malignancies and may rarely be the presenting feature.[1]

STREPTOCOCCAL DERMATITIS/PERIANAL CELLULITIS

This syndrome is mostly seen in children between the ages of 1 and 8. Boys are affected more frequently than girls. Group A β hemolytic *streptococci* is the main cause (rarely *S. aureus*).[2] An association with acute guttate psoriasis has also been reported.[2]

The child presents with pruritus, painful defecation, anal soreness and redness, and satellite pustules of the buttocks.

Examination of the anus shows marked, sharply demarcated erythema and causes discomfort. Rarely, proctocolitis may be seen. Generally, systemic penicillin or topical mupirocin is used in the treatment of this disease. If the disease is clinically less acute, erythromycin may be selected, depending on resistance patterns.[1]

PERIANAL ABSCESS

Perianal and anorectal abscesses usually are seen with painful swelling and suppuration. They are commonly complicated by anal fistula. The usual cause of a perianal abscess is infection of the anal glands, but sometimes trauma or chronic illnesses (such as diabetes mellitus, Crohn disease, hidradenitis suppurativa, and rectal carcinoma) predispose to its development.[1]

ECTHYMA GANGRENOSUM

Ecthyma gangrenosum is a cutaneous manifestation of *Pseudomonas aeruginosa* in immunocompromised patients, such as those with leukemia, severe burns, pancytopenia or neutropenia, functional neutrophilic defect, terminal carcinoma, or some other severe chronic disease. Healthy infants may develop lesions in the perineal area after antibiotic therapy in conjunction with maceration of the diaper area. Ecthyma gangrenosum usually develops because of *P. aeruginosa* in the presence of bacteremia.

The clinical features are tender vesicles or pustules surrounded by narrow pink to violaceous halos. The lesions become hemorrhagic and violaceous and rupture to become round ulcers with necrotic black centers. The affected sites are usually the buttocks and extremities, but sometimes lesions can be seen in the anorectal region. The diagnosis is usually made by the presence of the classic vesicle. The contents of the vesicles will show gram-negative bacilli on Gram stain, and cultures will be positive for *P. aeruginosa*.

Treatment is the immediate institution of intravenous anti-*Pseudomonas* medications. Prognosis is poor if there is a delay in diagnosis and institution of appropriate therapy

TABLE 28.1: Urgent Dermatoses in the Anorectal Region

Staphylococcal cellulitis
Streptococcal dermatitis/perianal cellulitis
Perianal abscess
Ecthyma gangrenosum
Necrotizing infections

and if the neutropenia has not been resolved by the end of the course of antibiotics.[3]

NECROTIZING INFECTIONS (GANGRENOUS CELLULITIS, INFECTIOUS GANGRENE, CREPITANT SOFT-TISSUE WOUNDS)

These infections are characteristically rapidly developing, progressive, and accompanied by such constitutional symptoms as severe pain and tenderness, with changes in the skin that progress to bulla formation and frank necrosis. The process can be found in the superficial or deep fascia with secondary changes in the overlying soft tissues. Palpation of the lesions may reveal tenderness or gas in the area of involvement.[4]

There are a number of overlapping severe gangrenous and necrotizing diseases that may affect the anorectal and perineal region. They can be recognized and treated with appropriate therapy immediately as they are life-threatening diseases. Classification of necrotizing infections is shown in Table 28.2.

NECROTIZING FASCIITIS

Necrotizing fasciitis is a life-threatening infection that is characterized by necrosis of subcutaneous tissue and fascia. Necrotizing fasciitis can be divided into two groups: type 1 necrotizing fasciitis and type 2 necrotizing fasciitis.

Type 1 necrotizing fasciitis is more common in the anorectal region. This infection is generally caused by a

TABLE 28.2: Classification of Necrotizing Infections

1. Necrotizing fasciitis
   - Streptococcal gangrene (Type 2 necrotizing fasciitis)
   - Type 1 necrotizing fasciitis
   - Synergistic necrotizing cellulitis
   - Fournier gangrene
2. Clostridial soft-tissue infections
   - Anaerobic cellulitis
   - Anaerobic myonecrosis
   - Spontaneous, nontraumatic anaerobic myonecrosis
3. Meleney progressive bacterial synergistic gangrene
4. Gangrenous cellulitis in the immunosuppressed patient
5. Localized areas of skin necrosis complicating conventional cellulitis

Data adapted from (4).

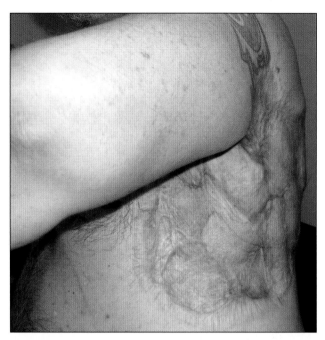

FIGURE 28.1: *Scar tissue after necrotizing fasciitis (Photo courtesy of Lawrence Charles Parish, MD, Philadelphia, PA).*

mix of facultative and anaerobic microbes, often found in the subcutaneous tissues following surgery, bowel perforation secondary to neoplasm or diverticulitis, trauma, or parenteral drug abuse. It often occurs in patients with diabetes mellitus or malnutrition.[4]

Type 1 necrotizing fasciitis most commonly occurs on an extremity, abdominal wall, and (rarely) perineum. Clinically, it is difficult to distinguish from streptococcal gangrene, but the initial pace of the illness may be slower than that of type 2 necrotizing fasciitis. The involved area may be painful at first and then evolve with objective findings, such as swelling, erythema, warmth, and tenderness. Within several days, the skin color becomes purple, bullae develop, and frank cutaneous gangrene is seen. At this stage the involved area is no longer tender due to destruction of superficial nerves in the subcutaneous tissues (Figure 28.1). Crepitation is often present, especially in patients with diabetes mellitus or if there are gas-forming anaerobes present.[4]

Type 2 necrotizing fasciitis or streptococcal gangrene is more common in the other regions of the body compared to the anorectal region. In this infection, group A β hemolytic *streptococci* alone are isolated in approximately 20% of patients. In perineal cases, there are almost always mixed infections. The major mechanisms of tissue destruction include deformation of erythrocytes and endothelial cell damage leading to thrombus formation, hemorrhage, and tissue necrosis. The combination of kinin activation, coagulation, and fibrinolysis leads to a disseminated intravascular coagulation–like picture. The many streptococcal enzymes such as hyaluronidase, streptolysins, and streptokinases also play a major role.[5]

The infection usually develops after minor trauma or surgery. Initially, a small region of cellulitis is present, but it expands rapidly, becoming dusky with bulla and a necrotic scar. Crepitation may be present, especially in mixed infections. The patient is ill with fever and extensive pain. There may be possible changes in mental status. The pain decreases as the disease progresses because the neurons are destroyed.[5]

In the histopathologic examination of necrotizing fasciitis, there is massive destruction of the soft tissue and fascia with thromboses and liquefaction. The muscle may be secondarily damaged.

The most important therapeutic approach is extensive surgical debridement. A complete removal of necrotic tissue is required; incision and drainage only or local debridement is not effective. For systemic therapy, penicillin G, 30 million units daily for at least 10–14 days, is combined with clindamycin 600 mg three times daily for 1–2 days because of anaerobe infections. Intravenous immunoglobulin is also recommended, as well as organ-specific supportive measures.[5]

Fournier Gangrene

Fournier gangrene is a localized variant of necrotizing fasciitis that is seen in the genitalia and perineum. Necrotizing gangrene of the genitalia and perineum is a fulminate, life-threatening infection. In 1883, Fournier described this condition in five patients. Since then, approximately 500 cases have been published. Infections may be idiopathic or secondary to local trauma or surgery and are usually polymicrobial. The organisms isolated include gram-negative bacilli, gram-positive cocci, and anaerobes.[6]

Fournier gangrene is 2 or 3 times more frequent in men than in women, and the average age of patients is 38–44 years. It is rare in children; cases after neonatal circumcision, however, have been observed. In men, infection typically affects the scrotum, occasionally invades the penis, and less frequently spreads to the perineum and abdomen. The muscles and testes are usually spared. In women, infection tends to involve both the vulva and the perineum.[6]

The true incidence of the infection is uncertain, although it seems to be higher in Asia and Africa. It is also more common in immunocompromised hosts, with diabetes mellitus, cancer, vascular disease, or neutropenia, as well as in human immunodeficiency virus–positive patients, alcoholics, and transplant recipients. In several series, 20%–40% of patients were diabetic and 35% were alcoholics.[6]

The onset of Fournier gangrene can be insidious, with a discrete area of edema, erythema, and necrosis on the scrotum, progressing to advancing skin necrosis rapidly over 1–2 days. Pain, swelling, and crepitation in the scrotum, perineum, or suprapubic region may be marked. Foul-smelling drainage occurs, indicating a contribution from anaerobes. Purplish discoloration of the scrotum and perineum, an

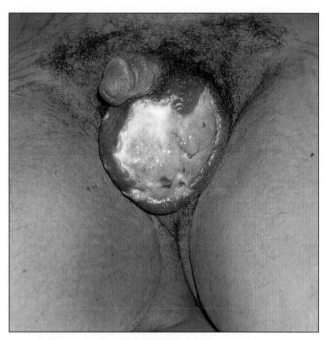

FIGURE 28.2: *Fournier gangrene (Photo courtesy of Lawrence Charles Parish, MD, Philadelphia, PA).*

initial "red flag," progresses to frank gangrene. The infection tends to be superficial, limited to skin and subcutaneous tissue and extending to the base of scrotum, but it may spread to the penis, perineum, and abdominal wall along fascial planes (Figure 28.2).[2,6]

Histologically, Fournier gangrene is characterized by obliterative endarteritis and thrombosis of the subcutaneous vessels, fascial necrosis, and leukocyte infiltration.

Although necrotizing gangrene of the genitalia and perineum is a clinical diagnosis, a biopsy showing necrosis, abscess formation, and vascular thrombosis is useful to confirm the disease and to obtain culture samples. Ultrasound imaging may reveal gas or testicular involvement and may help to identify *Clostridium* as the causal organism.[6]

Mortality rates of 25%–75% have been reported. Lower mortality rates of 0%–40% have been reported by others, possibly because of modern supportive measures.[6]

SYNERGISTIC NECROTIZING CELLULITIS (NECROTIZING CUTANEOUS MYOSITIS, SYNERGISTIC NONCLOSTRIDIAL ANAEROBIC MYONECROSIS)

This variant of necrotizing fasciitis is unique in that all soft-tissue structures, including muscle, can be involved in a painful, progressive, and polymicrobial infection that is highly lethal. This infection generally occurs in patients who are elderly, obese, or wasted, and have chronic illnesses, such as diabetes mellitus or various renal or cardiac diseases. The disease begins with a slow pain. Individuals are often afebrile or have only a low-grade fever, lacking systemic toxicity in the early stages. The initial skin

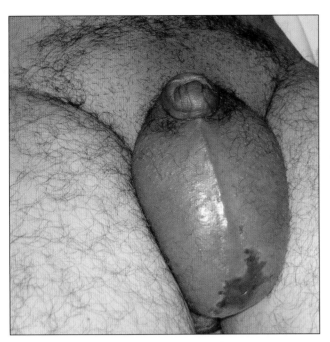

FIGURE 28.3: *Synergistic gangrene, following drainage of perianal abscess. (Photo courtesy of Hasan Kalafat, MD, Istanbul, Turkey.)*

lesion is a small area of necrosis or a reddish-brown blister with extreme local tenderness. Then a foul-smelling draining ulcer that rapidly expands is seen. Gram stain of the drainage reveals both gram-positive and gram-negative organisms and rare or absent neutrophils. Extensive gangrene of the superficial tissues and fat can be visualized by direct inspection through open areas or with skin incisions. Gas can be palpated in the tissues in approximately one quarter of patients. Organisms frequently isolated include anaerobes and facultative bacteria.[2,5,7]

The most common site of involvement is the perineum. The major predisposing factors are perirectal and ischiorectal abscesses. Treatment is similar to that for group A β hemolytic streptococcal necrotizing fasciitis, except that the antibiotic regimen must be adjusted to the culture results.[2,5,7]

PROGRESSIVE BACTERIAL SYNERGISTIC GANGRENE (MELENEY GANGRENE)

The name, synergistic gangrene, was coined by Meleney in the 1930s, based on studies done in vivo in rabbits. Microbi-ological studies confirm that this infection is usually associated with a microaerophilic *Streptococcus* or anaerobic *Streptococcus* at the advancing margin and *S. aureus* in the central, ulcerated area.[2]

This infection typically is seen in a drain site following an abdominal operation, in an incision in the chest wall following abdominal or thoracic infection, at the exit site of a fistulous tract, or in a chronic ulcer. Rarely, it may be seen in the perineum.[2]

The process usually begins with local redness, tenderness, and swelling that develops into a painful, superficial enlarging shaggy ulcer. Three zones of involvement become apparent: a central area of necrosis; a surrounding zone of violaceous, tender, edematous tissue with necrotic margins; and an outer zone of bright erythema and edema (Figure 28.3). Fever and systemic toxicity are minimal or absent. The process progressively enlarges if it is not treated with appropriate therapy as soon as possible. Treatment includes excision of the shaggy ulcer and necrotic margins and appropriate antimicrobials, guided by Gram stains and cultures.[2]

REFERENCES

1. Bunker CB, Neill SM. The genital, perianal and umbilical regions. In: Burns T, Breathnach S, Cox N, Griffiths C, editors. Rook's textbook of dermatology. Vol. 4, 7th ed. Oxford: Blackwell; 2004. pp. 68.1–68.104.
2. Odom RB, James WD, Berger TG, editors. Andrews' diseases of the skin clinical dermatology. Philadelphia: WB Saunders; 2000. pp. 307–57.
3. Matz H, Orion E, Wolf R. Bacterial infections: uncommon presentations. Clin Dermatol. 2005; 23:503–8.
4. Weinberg AN, Swartz MN, Tsao H, Johnson RS. Soft-tissue infections: erysipelas, cellulitis, gangrenous cellulitis, and myonecrosis. In: Freedberg IM, Eisen AZ, Wolff K, Austen KF, Goldsmith LA, Katz SI, editors. Fitzpatrick's dermatology in general medicine. 6th ed. New York: McGraw-Hill; 2003. pp. 1883–95.
5. Braun-Falco O, Plewig G, Wolff HH, Burgdorf WHC, editors. Dermatology. 2nd ed. Munich: Springer; 2000. pp. 128–244.
6. Cabrera H, Skoczdopole L, Marini M, et al. Necrotizing gangrene of the genitalia and perineum. Int J Dermatol. 2002; 41:847–51.
7. Bostancı S. Acil cerrahi tedavi gerektiren dermatozlar. Türk Klin J Surg Med Sci. 2006; 2:74–80.

CHAPTER 29

Emergency Management of Sexually Transmitted Diseases and Other Genitourethral Disorders

Michael Waugh

THIS CHAPTER is based on practical clinical experience of the author in the management of sexually transmitted diseases since 1969 in the United Kingdom (UK). In the UK, genitourinary medicine (sexually transmitted infections [STI] covers human immunodeficiency virus/acquired immune deficiency syndrome (HIV/AIDS) as well as does sexually transmitted diseases (STDs). It is a separate specialty and requires very considerable postgraduate study in all aspects of sexual health. Although emergencies in the acute internal or medical sense are rare, rapid and astute clinical management of many of the conditions encountered is necessary.

Patients are usually concerned when they think that they might have contracted an STD. Accurate diagnosis is needed so that necessary medication (whether it be antimicrobial, antifungal, or antiviral) may be given. Fast diagnosis is needed to abort infection, wherever possible, and to prevent immediate and long-term consequences to the patient. When an STI has been contracted, it is imperative that an easily understood explanation and education also be given to the patient with the reasons given why contact tracing (partner notification) must be pursued for sexual contacts. Follow-up is necessary not only to make sure that any immediate infection or infections are cured, but also to make sure that adequate care is taken to test for infections such as syphilis and HIV, which may well require testing not only on immediate presentation but also 1 month and 3 months after initial presentation. It is essential under any public health and legal system to maintain confidentiality of the patient and to explain, if necessary, to the patient what that means.

Many patients will nowadays use resources on the Internet to gain information. This method is frequent, and the good physician will work with that system and help the patient to enhance his or her knowledge rather than decrying Internet information. In the UK, the Department of Health has recognized the importance of early access to STD services and has set a goal that any patient should be offered an appointment within 48 hours of contracting the service, which must have well-publicized easy accessibility.[1]

NON-STD CONDITIONS

Conditions that are not STDs but that may present to venereologists and must never be missed include the following items.

Torsion of the Testicle

Torsion of the testis is not a common condition. The author has only seen one case presenting in almost 50 years in practice. It occurs with equal frequency in incompletely and fully descended testes. Taking into consideration that incomplete descent is present in less than 1% of men, it is obvious that torsion of an incompletely descended testis occurs relatively more frequently than that of a completely descended testis. The highest incidence is in men between 15 and 25 years old, and the second most common incidence is in infants.

The symptoms vary with the degree of torsion present. Most commonly the patient experiences sudden and agonizing pain in the groin and lower abdomen and vomits. In about one quarter of patients, the first symptom is a dull ache in the loin or hypogastrium. It is insufficiently appreciated that true testicular pain is situated in the lower abdomen at the level of the internal inguinal ring. It might be considered that the diagnosis is simple. It can be impossible to distinguish torsion of an imperfectly descended testicle from a strangulated inguinal hernia until the parts have been displayed by operation. Torsion of a completely descended testicle is a less difficult problem; sometimes, the actual twists in the cord can be felt thus establishing the diagnosis.

Torsion of the testicle may stimulate an acute epididymo-orchitis; after approximately 6 hours the skin of the scrotum becomes reddened and the temperature may be raised 37.2°C. Elevation of the scrotum usually relieves the pain in epididymitis but increases it in torsion.[2] Scrotal ultrasound is not a satisfactory way to make a diagnosis of torsion of the testicle, and if mumps and an acute infectious epididymo-orchitis are excluded surgical exploration should not be delayed by diagnostic imaging.[3]

Ectopic Pregnancy

Various degrees of pelvic inflammatory disease (PID), caused mainly by *Chlamydia trachomatis* and *Neisseria gonorrhoeae*, but also by *Mycoplasma hominis* and anaerobes, are frequently seen, but a condition in which there should be a high index of suspicion is ectopic pregnancy.[4]

By definition, ectopic pregnancy refers to any nonintrauterine pregnancy. Although ectopic pregnancies may be ovarian, cervical, or intraabdominal, the vast majority are tubal, having an incidence of 1:200–400 pregnancies. There may be a history of a previous ectopic pregnancy, previous surgery, pelvic infection, endometriosis, or in vitro fertilization, but approximately half occur with no predisposing cause.

Clinical Features. Clinical features range from no symptoms at all; to right, left, or bilateral lower abdominal pain; bleeding per vagina; intraabdominal hemorrhage (peritonism and shoulder tip pain); and collapse. Pelvic examination should be gentle to avoid tubal rupture. An ultrasound investigation is often useful. It should be noted that a gestational sac may be confused with a pseudosac (due to fluid in the thickened endometrium), which is seen in 20% of ectopic pregnancies and which lacks the echogenic ring of a gestational sac. A true sac is usually smooth with a double rim, is eccentrically placed, and may contain a yolk sac.

Management. Immediate referral for acute emergency gynecological assessment is essential. The management of shock and the setting up of two intravenous (IV) lines is urgent as is the setting up and patient cross-matching for 6 units of red cell concentrate.

PARAPHIMOSIS

Although this condition has none of the serious consequences of the previous two conditions, it is not infrequently seen turning up in young men attending STD clinics, especially in countries where men are uncircumcised. The tight prepuce has been retracted but cannot be returned, and it is constricting the glans, which is engorged and edematous. The patient is usually frightened. The diagnosis is apparent at a glance.

The surgical textbooks recommend injection of normal saline containing 150 turbidity units of hyalurodinase injected into each lateral aspect of the swollen ring of the prepuce. Usually, within 15 minutes the swelling is much reduced; this is, however, not always available. Soaking the swollen parts in ice water for the same amount of time and giving the patient 5 mg of diazepam while lying down usually allows the doctor to reduce the paraphimosis by bilateral gentle pressure of the thumbs on the glans while holding firmly but not painfully the prepuce proximal to the paraphimosis. The paraphimosis disappears. If that is impossible, or if the paraphimosis has been there too long or the patient will not relax, a urologist needs to be consulted for reduction under anesthetia and later circumcision.

SQUAMOUS CELL CARCINOMA OF THE PENIS

Although rare, this is a condition that must not be missed; it is a serious cancer with a high mortality. In STD clinics for men, one or two cases will turn up annually, usually in older men, often having noticed something wrong for some length of time but for one reason or another not having sought help from a doctor. Risk factors include being uncircumcised, smoking, and having contact with carcinogens such as oil, tar, and/or arsenic. There is a link with the human papillomavirus, and the condition may be found after phototherapy for psoriasis. I have seen it in three patients followed up for more than 20 years for lichen sclerosus et atrophicus (LSA). It accounts for approximately 0.5% male malignancies in western countries.

Symptoms often have been present for many years. Patients complain of itching, bleeding, irritation, and foreskin problems such as tethering and phimosis. Tumors may involve the glans penis in approximately 50% and prepuce in 20%, and in some patients both glans and prepuce are affected. There may be small nodules, nonhealing areas, and ulceration as well as phimosis and LSA. Palpable lymph nodes may be the first place for metastases. Referral to a urologist and specialist treatment center is needed. Diagnosis is by biopsy. Treatment is resection followed by radiotherapy and chemotherapy. Prognosis is poor.[5]

STDS

Although only a few complications of STDs could be considered to be emergencies, symptoms and signs suggestive of an STD should always be taken seriously. Accurate history taking and diagnosis or multiple diagnoses are necessary both for the purposes of effective therapy and appropriate partner notification (contact tracing), with follow-up to make sure the patient has been adequately cured. As the condition is infective, there is all the more reason why good diagnosis and treatment as a public health measure are imperatives. In many localities, there are also civil regulations that differ from country to country on treatment of STDs, aspects concerning confidentiality, their notification to public health authorities, and their situation within the legal framework of that country.

Here concise guidelines are given for management of gonorrhea, genital tract infection with *C. trachomatis*,

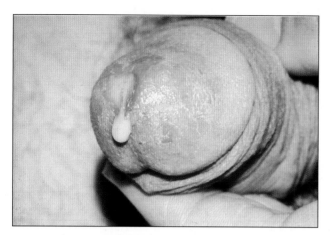

FIGURE 29.1: *Urethral gonorrhea.*

herpes genitalis, and syphilis, which may all have emergency elements in their presentations. These guidelines will generally follow those of the Clinical Effectiveness Group of British Association for Sexual Health.

Gonorrhea

Gonorrhea is an STD resulting from infection with *N. gonorrhoeae*, a gram-negative diplococcus. The primary sites of infection are the mucous membranes of the urethra (Figure 29.1), endocervix (Figure 29.2), rectum (Figure 29.3), pharynx (Figure 29.4), and conjunctiva. Transmission is by direct inoculation of infected secretions from one mucous membrane to another.[6]

In men, 80% have a mucopurulent urethral discharge and approximately 50% have dysuria if the urethra is infected. Most specialists will be only too aware of the man with acute gonorrhea entering the consulting room with a yellowish catarrhal urethral discharge. In a few, asymptomatic infection may occur. Pharyngeal infection is usually asymptomatic. Rectal infection in men who have sex with men (MSM) may be asymptomatic, but approximately 20% have anal discharge or perianal pain or discomfort.

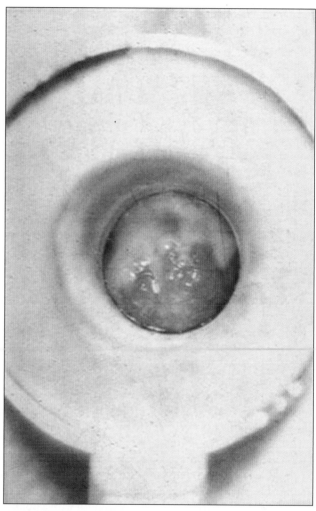

FIGURE 29.3: *Anorectal gonorrhea.*

In women, up to 50% with infection of the endocervix have no symptoms. Up to 50% may also have an increased vaginal discharge. If there is a degree of PID, lower abdominal pain may be found in up to 25%. Gonorrhea is also a rare cause of intermenstrual bleeding or menorrhagia. Twelve percent of women complain of dysuria but not frequency.

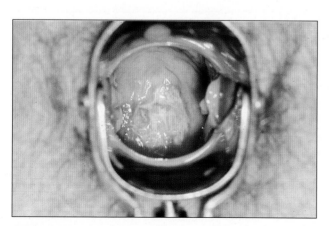

FIGURE 29.2: *Purulent cervicitis in gonorrhea.*

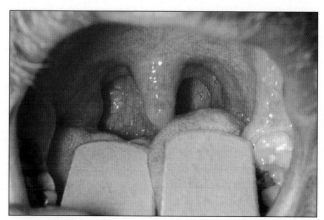

FIGURE 29.4: *Pharyngeal gonorrhea after fellatio.*

Rectal infection may occur after anal sexual intercourse or by spread from genital secretions. As with men, pharyngeal infection is usually asymptomatic.

It is important to realize that *N. gonorrhoeae* may coexist with *C. trachomatis*, *Trichomonas vaginalis*, and *Candida albicans*. If signs are present at all, up to 50% may have an endocervical discharge, but there may be few positive signs, the patient either presenting as a sexual partner of a man infected or presenting for a genital diagnostic check. Complications are transluminal spread of *N. gonorrhoeae* from the urethra to involve the epididymis and prostate in men (≤1%) and endometrium and pelvic organs (PID) in women, probably less than 10%. Hematogenous dissemination may also occur from infected mucous membranes (it is worth considering infection of the pharynx when this occurs), resulting in skin lesions, arthralgia, arthritis, and tenosynovitis. Disseminated gonococcal infection is uncommon, but in the 1960s outbreaks of gonococcal dermatitis arthritis syndrome were seen.[7]

Gonococcal Infection of the Eye. In adults, this infection is rare. It may occur from fomites but more likely as the result of sex play. The conjunctiva is swollen, red, edematous, and painful, and pus is pouring out. The possibility should always be considered that it was caught as a strain of penicillinase-producing *N. gonorrhoeae* and adequate cultures taken. It responds rapidly to appropriate antibiotics, and an ophthalmologic opinion should always be requested to exclude corneal ulceration.

In children, this infection is usually caught in places with poor hygiene, such as crowded tenements and refugee and nomad camps, but of course it may be after sexual interference with that child. Its appearance will be similar to that found in an adult.

Ophthalmia neonatorum in the UK is defined as a purulent discharge from the eyes of an infant within 21 days of birth. It is now much more common in babies infected with *C. trachomatis* than in those infected with *N. gonorrhoea*.

Diagnosis is made by identification of *N. gonorrhoeae* from an infected site. Microscopy with visualization of gram-negative diplococci is obviously the fastest way of making a presumptive diagnosis in men with symptomatic urethral gonorrhea, but in women microscopy from endocervical smears even with skilled technicians will pick up only approximately half the cases. Thus, cultures are also needed. Here again, specimens need to be adequately collected and selective culture medium containing antimicrobials are recommended to reduce contamination.[8] Culture tests help very much in diagnosis of gonorrhea from the pharynx, cervix, and anorectal canal as well as the urethra, and are the only way to monitor sensitivity and resistance patterns to antimicrobials in gonorrhea.

Nucleic acid amplification tests (NAATs) and nucleic acid hybridization tests are more sensitive than cultures and can be used for screening urine samples and self-taken vaginal swabs. Although probably adequate for pharyngeal and rectal specimens, long-term reliability still needs to be completely proven. Confirmation, especially in medical–legal cases, still requires adequate culture sampling. NAATs also do not show sensitivity patterns for antimicrobials. Screening for coincident STDs should always be performed in patients with gonorrhea.

Treatment. For 60 years since penicillin was first used, *N. gonorrhoeae* has shown capacity to develop reduced sensitivity and resistance to many antimicrobials. For instance, resistance to penicillin, tetracyclines, and ciprofloxacin is common.[9] Therapy should eliminate at least 95% of those presenting in the local community.[10]

Generally, the following treatments will work unless resistance has developed:

● Ceftriaxone 250 mg intramuscularly in or after (IM),
● Cefixime 400 mg orally with or after (PO),
● Spectinomycin 2 g IM.

Azithromycin is not recommended for the treatment of gonorrhea due to reports of developing resistance to it.[11]

***Co-Infection with* C. trachomatis.** Between 20% and 40% of men and women with gonorrhea will also be infected with *C. trachomatis*, so often combined therapy for both *N. gonorrhoea* and *C. trachomatis* is given at the same time. Thus, for the latter, azithromycin 1 g PO or doxycycline 100 mg twice daily for 7 days is recommended. When prescribing antibiotics, care should always be taken in pregnant women, patients with known antibiotic sensitivities or allergies, patients who are taking other medications, and (in the case of doxycycline) patients exposed to sunlight.

Sexual Partners. Partner notification is needed. It is a skill that requires diplomacy, and the patient will often be helped by a professional health adviser. Sexual partners should be treated for gonorrhea, preferably after evaluation as for STI.

Genital Tract Infection with *C. trachomatis*

This is the most common nonviral STD found in industrialized countries. It is thought that 5%–10% of sexually active women younger than 24 years and men in their late teens and early twenties may be currently infected.[12] Risk factors are being a young adult, having a new sexual partner in the last year, and lack of consistent use of condoms. There has been a pattern of serial monogamy. Although it usually causes a mild urethral discharge in men with variable dysuria (Figure 29.5), there may be few adequate symptoms in some men, and it is frequently asymptomatic in women. In women, when there are symptoms,

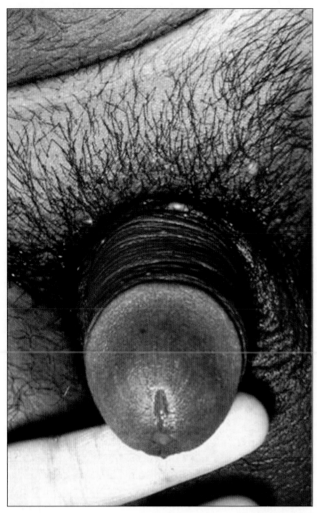

FIGURE 29.5: *Chlamydial urethritis with molluscum contagiosum.*

they are variable and may include postcoital or intermenstrual bleeding, lower abdominal pain, purulent vaginal discharge, mucopurulent cervicitis, and dysuria. Babies may be infected from mothers via the birth process (Figure 29.6). In men and women, after anal sexual intercourse there may

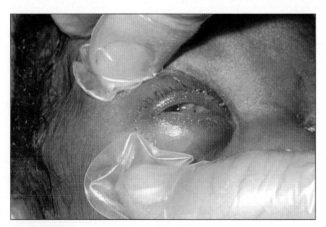

FIGURE 29.6: *Chlamydial ophthalmia in an infant.*

be a proctitis with anal discharge and anorectal discomfort. It is the complications that will cause the patient to seek help as an emergency.

Pelvic Inflammatory Disease (PID)

PID results when infections ascend from the cervix or vagina into the upper genital tract.[13] It includes endometritis, salpingitis, tubo-ovarian abscesses, and pelvic peritonitis. The main causes are *C. trachomatis* and *N. gonorrhoeae*, but *M. hominis* and anaerobes are also found. Even after laparoscopy, no bacterial cause may still be found.

Lower abdominal pain is the most common symptom, with increased vaginal discharge, irregular bleeding, deep dyspareunia, and dysuria also present in some women. The cervix may have a mucopurulent discharge with contact bleeding, indicative of a cervicitis. Adnexal and cervical motion tenderness on bimanual examination is the most common sign, but pyrexia and a palpable adnexal mass may also be present.

Diagnosis. Laparoscopy with microbiological specimens from the upper and lower genital tracts is considered the gold standard for diagnosis, but this is not always available. If laparoscopy is not available, the presence of lower abdominal pain, increased vaginal discharge, cervical motion, and adnexal tenderness on bimanual examination, together with confirmatory subsequent diagnosis from swabs taken from the lower genital tract, will give a diagnosis but only with a specificity of approximately 70%.

Treatment of PID. Prompt diagnosis and early treatment should reduce the risk of tubal damage and should be started before microbiology results are known. Regimens should cover all bacterial causes and may need to be given IV for the first few days.

A suitable regimen would be ceftriaxone 2 g IM plus doxycycline 100 mg twice daily or ofloxacin 400 mg twice daily plus metronidazole 400 mg twice daily for 14 days. Appropriate analgesia should be given. Partner notification is essential to prevent reinfection.

Other complications of genital *C. trachomatis* infection include Fitz–Hugh–Curtis syndrome (perihepatitis), transmission to the neonate (neonatal conjunctivitis, pneumonia), epididymo-orchitis, adult conjunctivitis, and sexually acquired reactive arthritis (SARA)/Reiter syndrome (more common in men). Of the complications mentioned, both epididymo-orchitis and SARA may present as emergencies and are discussed here.

Epididymo-Orchitis. An acute epididymitis may occur in older men (generally at least 35 years old) due to urinary tract infection usually caused by coliform organisms, although age does not preclude sexual activity and sexually transmitted causes of epididymitis should always be considered if there is an active sex life. In younger men under age 35, more frequently *C. trachomatis* and less frequently *N. gonorrhoeae* are the cause, although urinary tract infection, especially if there are underlying genital tract anomalies, should be considered. Rarer causes, but those still found in developing countries, are tuberculosis and leprosy. Mumps, especially where there are many youngsters living closely together, also should be considered. The differential diagnosis from torsion of the testicle has already been described. There does need to be a planned approach in centers where the symptomatic patient may well get to a venereal disease clinic but the asymptomatic patient gets to an urologist. Treatment includes excluding a urinary tract infection, giving necessary analgesics and scrotal support, and administering appropriate antibiotic therapy for either *N. gonorrhoeae* or *C. trachomatis* (in the latter case doxycycline 100 mg twice daily for 14 days). Partner notification for STD causes of epididymo-orchitis is a requisite.

If any group of young men presenting with epididymo-orchitis is analyzed, annually, there will be one or two who do not have an epididymo-orchitis but have, in fact, a malignant tumor of the testicle. The skilled clinician usually develops a sixth sense, and a high index of suspicion is needed for these cases when not presenting to an urologist. In my practice malignant tumors of the testicle are also more common in men with HIV infection. The usual signs of testicular cancer include a lump in the testicle, painless swelling, or altered consistency of the testis; any of these may be found on a medical examination. Ultrasound and nuclear magnetic resonance help in the diagnosis, and the patient needs to be seen rapidly by the appropriate team in a center that has specialist knowledge of testicular tumor management.

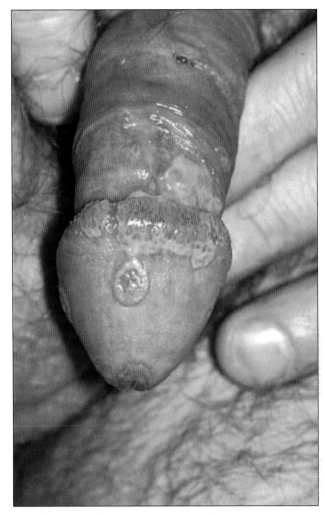

FIGURE 29.7: *Circinate balanitis.*

SARA/Reiter Syndrome. SARA/Reiter syndrome has been included as an emergency, as it may well have an insidious onset that can present to a variety of clinicians. It is often missed in its early stages; in practice, less would be seen if more often the early diagnosis of *C. trachomatis* (often asymptomatic in young men) was considered and appropriate therapy (best given as azithromycin 1 g PO) was instituted. Missing SARA may have disastrous effects in sportsmen with active sex lives when damages to the hip, knee, ankle, and small joints of the foot, as well as tenosynovitis, are short- and long-term side effects.

Circinate balanitis (Figure 29.7) may well occur a few weeks before other major symptoms and should act as a trigger for the dermatologist to screen for STDs (especially *C. trachomatis*) and to give appropriate antibiotic therapy with doxycycline or azithromycin. As any mucosa may well be affected, there is a need to look further than the genitals. Conjunctivitis occurs in approximately 30% of cases in the early stages as well as usually mild oral and buccal lesions in early SARA. In chronic SARA obviously the well-known classical signs of chronic arthritis, serious skin lesions, ker-atoderma blenorrhagica, onycholysis, and eye complications (such as an anterior uveitis) are all known but are not part of emergency presentation. The condition is far from common in women, but a vulvitis may occasionally present.

When considering the consequences and the differential diagnosis of *C. trachomatis* genital infection, it is necessary to consider the much more common and very frequently seen uncomplicated *C. trachomatis* genital infection.

Diagnosis and Treatment of* C. trachomatis *Genital Infection. Diagnostic tests are changing rapidly for *C. trachomatis*.[13] The tests for standard of care are NAATs. These are more sensitive and specific than enzyme immunoassays (EIAs). Suboptimal EIAs are no longer appropriate. No test, be it NAAT or EIA, is 100% sensitive or specific. The field of diagnosis changes so rapidly that ongoing specialist advice should be considered by those whose main specialty is not STDs.

It should be noted that, as yet, NAATs have not had U.S. Food and Drug Administration approval for specimens from rectal, pharyngeal, and conjunctival specimens

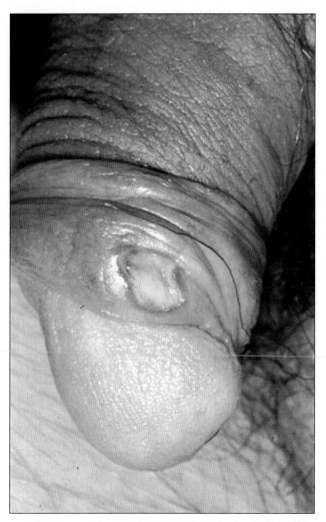

FIGURE 29.8: *Painful ulcer on penis, syphilis excluded, but herpes simplex virus type 2 isolated.*

in men or women; in the absence of culture tests, however, NAATs are usually taken from these sites. In Europe, in the last 5 years rectal lymphogranuloma venereum (LGV) has been seen not infrequently in MSM, and British guidelines recommend that when a rectal NAAT is found to be positive, it is sent for further testing for LGV typing to the appropriate laboratory. Rectal LGV was in recent years first seen in The Netherlands occurring in MSM who had passive anal sex without the use of a condom for protection against STIs. Since then, it has been found in MSM throughout Western Europe. The most common sign is a proctitis that may be not only purulent but bloody. There may be considerable alteration of bowel habits, perhaps being mistaken for irritable bowel syndrome, ulcerative colitis, or Crohn disease. There may be a fever, a general feeling of malaise, and inguinal regional lymphadenopathy. In contrast, there may be few symptoms. As would be expected, it may be found with other STIs in this region – namely, syphilis, rectal gonorrhea, anorectal herpetic infection, anal condyloma acuminata, HIV infection, and

hepatitis B and C – all of which should be investigated in this group of patients.

Treatment of Uncomplicated Genital C. Trachomatis Infection. Recommended treatment includes doxycycline 100 mg twice daily for 7 days, ofloxacin 200 mg twice a day for 7 days, or azithromycin 1 g PO, the latter being recommended by the World Health Organisation for pregnant women but not completely passed as being safe by all national health agencies, although it probably is.

In my own clinical practice, I have found azithromycin, although more expensive than doxycycline, much more acceptable for young adults. It needs to be taken only once, and, provided the partner is treated at the same time, a sex life will be started faster and safer without the risk of recurrent infection in one or the other (as may happen with doxycycline, where a week seems an incredibly long time for the eager young man to avoid sex).

Herpes Genitalis

As this condition is so often not only painful but comes as a most unpleasant shock to self-esteem in a world where young people are so media aware, it is the STD that most often gets the venereologist called outside his normal working day (Figures 29.8 and 29.9). Over the years it is often the parent of young persons who has realized that they are suffering from genital herpes who calls so often at weekends and public holidays.

Etiology. The two forms are herpes simplex virus type 1 (HSV-1), the usual cause of orolabial herpes and herpes simplex virus type 2 (HSV-2).

Natural History: What Do We Know about Herpes Genitalis? Infection may be primary or nonprimary. Disease episodes may be initial or recurrent and symptomatic or asymptomatic. Prior infection with HSV-1 modifies the clinical manifestations of first infection by HSV-2. After

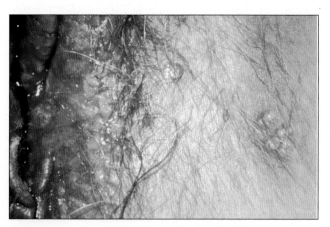

FIGURE 29.9: *Acute herpes genitalis in a woman.*

childhood, symptomatic primary infection with HSV-1 is equally likely to be acquired in the genital or oral areas.

Following primary infection, the virus becomes latent in local sensory ganglia, periodically reactivating to cause symptomatic lesions or asymptomatic (but infectious) viral shedding.

New diagnoses of genital herpes are equally likely to be caused by HSV-1 or HSV-2; the median recurrence rate, after a symptomatic first episode, however, is 0.34 recurrences per month for HSV-2 and 0.08 recurrences per month for HSV-1.[14] Recurrence rates decline over time in most individuals, although the pattern is variable.

The majority of individuals found to have asymptomatic HSV-2 infections subsequently develop symptomatic lesions. Asymptomatic perianal HSV shedding in HIV-negative HSV-2–seropositive MSM is common.[15] In HIV HSV-2–seropositive men, both symptomatic and asymptomatic shedding are increased, especially in men with low CD4 counts and in men who are also seropositive for HSV-1.[16]

As most modern information is available on the Internet, no wonder patients, their families, and friends get upset, when herpes genitalis is considered. So what are the clinical features, including ones that could be considered an emergency? In both sexes, there is painful genital ulceration often with local dysuria and urethral or vaginal discharge. There may be fever and myalgia. Unpleasant symptoms are more common in primary infection. Some patients are asymptomatic. Genital ulceration begins with an itchy vesicle that breaks down to form a shallow superficial painful ulcer, often in groups, on the genitals or cervix or in the anorectal canal (often very painful indeed). Complications include autonomic neuropathy resulting in retention of urine and aseptic meningitis.

Confirmation of Diagnosis. It is necessary but often difficult to isolate HSV from genital lesions. Successful diagnosis depends on using swabs taken directly from the base of the lesion, maintaining the cold chain (4°C), rapidly transporting specimens to the laboratory, and avoiding freeze–thaw cycles.

Serology. Most commercial tests for HSV antibodies are not type specific and are of no value in the management of genital herpes. Type-specific EIAs based on glycoprotein G (gG1, gG2) or western blot assays are becoming available. Type-specific immune responses can take 8–12 weeks to develop following primary infection. It is now becoming possible for serological evaluation of genital herpes, but that needs access to both HSV-1 and HSV-2 type-specific assays. Caution is needed in interpreting results because even highly sensitive and specific assays have poor predictive values in low-prevalence populations.

The clinical utility of these tests has not been fully assessed. Virus detection remains the method of choice, but the tests may be useful for the following conditions:

- Recurrent genital ulceration of unknown cause;
- Counselling patients with initial episodes of disease;
- Investigating asymptomatic partners of patients with genital herpes; and
- Evaluating genital herpes in pregnancy.

The Management of Genital Herpes and Its Complications

First Episode of Genital Herpes. The faster oral antiviral drugs are given preferably within hours of lesions forming. Acyclovir, valacyclovir, and famcyclovir all reduce the severity and duration of episodes. The availability of these drugs depends on local conditions. Manufacturers' recommendations regarding dosage should be followed. Antiviral therapy does not alter the natural history of the disease. Topical agents are less effective than oral ones. IV therapy is only indicated when the patient cannot swallow or tolerate oral medication because of vomiting. In addition, local bathing with normal saline solution and analgesia helps. Some clinicians recommend topical anesthetic agents, but then there is the danger of potential sensitization.

Regimens recommended for adults (all for 5 days) are acyclovir 200 mg five times a day; famciclovir 250 mg three times a day, or valacyclovir 500 mg twice daily.

Management of Complications. Hospitalization may be needed for urinary retention, meningism, and severe constitutional symptoms. If catheterization is needed, suprapubic catheterization is preferred because it prevents the risk of ascending infection and allows normal micturition to be restored without multiple removals and recatheterizations. Always, however, try sitting the patient in a warm bath and allowing him or her to try to pass urine in it before catheterization is attempted. It often works.

HIV-Positive Patients. In the early days of HIV, especially when dealing with gay men before the advent of highly active antiretroviral therapy (HAART), when often enormous painful and distressing perianal herpes was found, resistance of HSV to antivirals was found. With HAART, however, this condition is far less frequently seen.

Recurrent Genital Herpes. Although causing much personal distress to some patients, genital herpes cannot really be considered as an emergency. Most recurrences are self-limiting, but a good doctor–patient relationship can be supportive for the patient. Strategies for treatment include general support, treatment with antivirals episodically, and suppressive therapy. All of these management techniques need working out for each individual patient.

Management of Genital Herpes in Pregnancy.
Guidelines for genital herpes in pregnancy are categorized
into management of first episodes and recurrent episodes.
Accurate clinical classification is difficult. Viral isolation
and typing and the testing of paired sera (if a booking specimen is available) may be helpful. There are guidelines for
management depending on when genital herpes was first
acquired and in what trimester.[17] Basically, all guidelines
suggest continuous acyclovir in the last 4 weeks of pregnancy and an elective Caesarean section despite lack of evidence for its effectiveness. The risks of vaginal delivery for
the fetus are small and must be set against the risks to the
mother of Caesarean section.[18]

Syphilis

In this section, some of the pitfalls (mistakes) in making
a diagnosis and some of the side effects that may occur
in treatment are discussed. There are several good descriptions of syphilis in many dermatology and venereology textbooks that can be used for reference.

It was once said, "Always consider syphilis" (Sir William
Osler, 1909). That may well be almost as true now, but also
add on HIV infection. There are three main reasons why
syphilis is missed:

1) The patient does not know about it or fails to ask for
   medical advice;

2) the clinician (and this is far more serious) does not consider it in his differential diagnosis; and

3) public health authorities do not stress its importance.
   For the last 20 years the focus has been on HIV disease
   as the number one STI to consider.

Like much of medicine, a good history will consider
syphilis. Always take a sexual history in a quiet place out of
the earshot of others. Let the patient know that you will
keep confidences and be discreet. Do not show any sur-
prise at what you are told; all things human are within the
knowledge of a good clinician. Be candid and ask if the
patient is not forthcoming about his or her sexual practices. Start with simple questions, such as "Was a condom used?" If the patient is a man, find out if he had sex
with another man, a woman, or both sexes (if that has not
already been proffered). There has been a rise in homosexu-
ally (Figure 29.10) contracted early primary and secondary
syphilis in MSM in Europe, North America, and parts of
East Asia recently, often with HIV infection and pharyngeal and rectal gonorrhea. Early syphilis remains common
in Eastern Europe in heterosexuals and has been seen in
pockets all over Western Europe, often in groups related
to street drugs and/or prostitution (where sex workers are
brought in from Eastern Europe). Syphilis is no respecter
of social position, and perhaps the more money a person
has the easier it is to travel and meet others for sexual purposes. Always consider any genital sore to be syphilis until
proven otherwise (herpes genitalis is much more common),

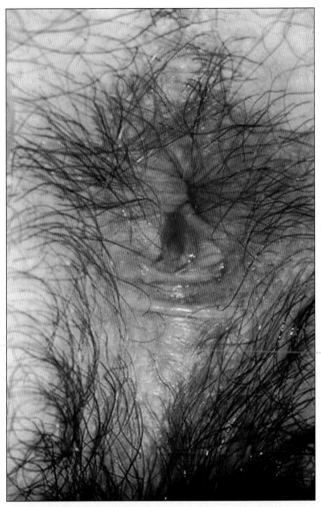

FIGURE 29.10:   Anal chancre.

and always consider syphilis in the differential diagnosis
of eruptions. Remember that most dermatology textbooks
in industrialized countries have used as photographs white
skins; presentation in brown, yellow, or black skins may
look different. The eruption may last for weeks but may be
fleeting and disappear before the patient has had a chance
to see a physician if the appointment is delayed. Remember
that the patient with secondary syphilis may feel unwell, be
running a fever, or even be jaundiced. Secondary syphilis
(Figure 29.11 and 29.12) may present with many different signs, some of them rare: meningism, uveitis, deafness,
arthralgia, periostitis, as well as skin signs easily missed such
as alopecia, snail track ulcers (buccal mucosal patches), and
condyloma lata around the mouth, axillae, inguinal regions,
and anus and toe webs. Generally, unless the patient is
severely immunocompromised standard serological tests
for syphilis will be reactive in secondary syphilis.

The Diagnosis of Primary Syphilis. The ulcer (chancre)
is said to be painless with rolled indurated edges but,
like many classical descriptions, this is not always so. If
the patient has applied antiseptic lotion or cream or has

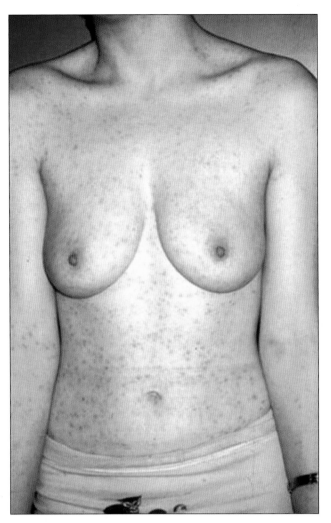

FIGURE 29.11: *Secondary syphilis.*

taken an antibiotic such as penicillin, tetracycline, or erythromycin prior to being seen, dark-field examination for *Treponema pallidum* is a waste of time as it will not be found. Dark-field examination for *T. pallidum* by a skilled observer when the chancre has not been modified is still an effective way of making a fast diagnosis, but it requires skill and much practice and is time consuming. Serological tests for syphilis need to be performed. If there is any doubt about syphilis, they need to be repeated at 1 month and 3 months. The initial test is likely to be an EIA; if reactive, the Venereal Disease Research Laboratory test or rapid plasma regain test, *T. pallidum* hemagglutination test, and fluorescent treponemal antibody absorption (FTA-ABS) test should be performed. It has to be remembered that, in the early stages of syphilis, there may be only *T. pallidum* seen on dark-field microscopy. One of the first blood tests to become reactive is FTA-ABS at about 2 weeks.

Remember that it may be difficult to tell if the patient has had either syphilis or a nonvenereal treponematosis (such as yaws or pinta) treated in the past, whether or not serological tests refer to the present or past infection. If in doubt, it is best to treat again.

Treatment. In parts of the world where there are good public health facilities staffed by specialists for the treatment of STDs, syphilis is best treated in such facilities; in other parts of the world, however, the dermatovenereologist will be responsible for treatment.

For early syphilis that is primary, secondary, or early latent, the following treatment is recommended: either benzathine benzylpenicillin 2.4 million units IM or procaine penicillin 0.6 million units IM daily for 10 days. If the patient is allergic to penicillin, doxycycline 100 mg twice daily for 14 days is recommended. The patient should be seen after a week to make sure that he or she is taking prescribed medication. *T. pallidum* is highly susceptible to penicillin – not requiring a high level, but rather a prolonged level of penicillin in tissues for it to be bactericidal, as penicillin only acts on dividing cells. Studies on doxycycline, tetracycline, erythromycin, azithromycin, and ceftriaxone all show efficacy in syphilis, but often the trials have been in the past and not conducted to modern criteria. There have also been reports of resistance to azithromycin, so it can not be recommended.

ANTIBIOTIC THERAPY AND SIDE EFFECTS

Acute Anaphylaxis after Treatment with Penicillin

This side effect is rare, and no patient should be given penicillin if there is any history of allergy to it. Desensitization takes time and is inappropriate in a busy clinic. Staff should be trained in resuscitation, and there should be the drugs and equipment present to give emergency treatment for acute anaphylaxis as well as the ability to summon immediate aid from resuscitation emergency services.

Jarisch–Herxheimer Reaction

This reaction occurs in more than half of patients when penicillin is given for early treatment of syphilis. Within

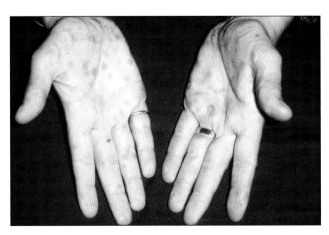

FIGURE 29.12: *Secondary syphilis, palms*

8 hours of an injection, the patient notices a febrile illness with malaise, headache, chills, and rigors. It clears quickly, but the patient should be told about it beforehand that it is not an allergic reaction. It is thought to be due to release of lymphokines including tumor necrosis factor and interleukins. In late syphilis, although rare, it may be potentially life threatening, so steroid cover is given for 3 days before treatment.

Procaine Reaction

This reaction will become rarer the more often benzathine benzylpenicillin is used instead of procaine penicillin. It is more common in men and is a sort of anaphylactoid reaction. The patient experiences auditory symptoms, a fear of impending death, seizures, and a violent behavioral reaction. It is thought to be due to inadvertent IV administration. It is much less common than it was 40 years ago when procaine penicillin was the treatment for gonorrhea. Most of the patients recovered without any therapy, although it usually needed all the clinic staff to hold the patients down in their struggles.

Stevens–Johnson Syndrome

Again, this has become infrequent in the treatment of STDs, because the use of sulfonamides (especially the long-acting ones) and cotrimoxazole has declined in the day-to-day treatment of conditions presenting in clinics. It is still seen, however, in the treatment of HIV disease after the use of non-nucleoside reverse transcriptase inhibitors such as nevirapine.

REFERENCES

1. British Association for Sexual Health and HIV: Department of Health. Genito-Urinary Medicine Clinics and the 48 hour Access Target. London: Department of Health, 2007. Gateway ref: 8930 [cited 2008 April 26]. Available from: http://www.bashh.org/whatsnew.asp
2. Bailey H. The testes and scrotum. In: Bailey H, Love McNeill, editors. A short practice of surgery. 12th ed. London: H.K. Lewis; 1962. pp. 1266–96.
3. Robertson DHH, McMillan A, Young H. Clinical practice in sexually transmitted diseases, 2nd ed. Edinburgh: Churchill Livingstone; 1989. pp. 244–53.
4. Drife J, Magowan BA. Clinical obstetrics and gynaecology. Edinburgh: W.B. Saunders Ltd.; 2004. pp. 171–3.
5. Shah M, De Silva A. The male genitalia: a clinician's guide to skin problems and sexually transmitted infections. Oxford: Radcliffe Publishing; 2008. pp. 60–2.
6. British Association for Sexual Health and HIV. National guideline on the diagnosis and treatment of gonorrhoea in adults 2005 [cited 2008 April 26]. Available from: http://www.bashh.org
7. Ackerman AB, Miller RC, Shapiro L. Gonococcemia and its cutaneous manifestations. Arch Dermatol. 1965; 91:227–32.
8. Jephcott AE. Microbiological diagnosis of gonorrhoea. Genitourin Med. 1997; 73:245–52.
9. Health Protection Agency (HPA). GRASP (The Gonococcal Resistance to Antimicrobials Surveillance Programme) – Annual Report 2004. London: Health Protection Agency, August 2005 [cited 2008 April 26]. Available from: http://www.hpa.org.uk/infections/topics az/hiv and ati/sti-gonorrhoea/publications/ GRASP 2004 Annual Report.pdf
10. FitzGerald M, Bedford C. National standards for the management of gonorrhoea. Int J STD AIDS. 1996; 7:298–300.
11. Tapsall JW, Schultz TR, Limnios EA, et al. Failure of azithromycin therapy in gonorrhoea and discorrelation with laboratory parameters. Sex Trans Dis. 1998; 25:505–8.
12. Fenton KA, Korovessis C, Johnson AM, et al. Sexual behaviour in Britain: reported sexually transmitted infections and prevalent genital Chlamydia trachomatis infection. Lancet. 2001; 358:1851–4.
13. Drife J, Magowan BA. Clinical obstetrics and gynaecology. Edinburgh: W.B. Saunders Ltd.; 2004. pp. 198–200.
14. British Association for Sexual Health and HIV. 2006 UK national guideline for the management of genital tract infection with chlamydia trachomatis [cited 2008 April 26]. Available from: http://www.bashh.org
15. Krone MR, Wald A, Tabet SR, et al. Herpes simplex virus type 2 shedding in human immunodeficiency virus-negative men who have sex with men; frequency, patterns and risk factors. Clin Infect Dis. 2000; 30:261–7.
16. Schaker T, Zeh J, Hu HL, et al. Frequency of symptomatic and asymptomatic herpes simplex virus type 2 reactivations among human immunodeficiency virus-infected men. J Infect Dis. 1998; 121:847–54.
17. British Association for Sexual Health and HIV. 2001 National guidelines for the management of genital herpes [cited 2008 April 26]. Available from: http://www.bashh.org
18. Mindel A, Taylor J, Tideman RL, et al. Neonatal herpes prevention: a minor public health problem in some communities. Sex Transm Infect. 2000; 76:287–91.

CHAPTER 30

Emergency Management of Environmental Skin Disorders: Heat, Cold, Ultraviolet Light Injuries

Larry E. Millikan

ENVIRONMENTAL SKIN disorders usually are associated with ambient changes (heat, humidity, intensity of ultraviolet [UV] solar rays) and new environments (ski slopes, beaches, jungles/rainforests, and areas with exotic animals unfamiliar to patients). Many of these new surroundings cause unique dermatologic reactions familiar to natives who understand the need for avoidance but unfamiliar to others who must seek dermatologic care.

PROPER AND EARLY MANAGEMENT

Proper and early management of skin disorders due to environmental factors might avert the ruin of a long anticipated trip or vacation. In some instances, the environmental exposure occurs at home before departure and then is manifested during travel to – or at – the destination. Such environmental exposures from contact allergens, toxins, and infections or infestations can be delayed. As a result, clinical manifestations are delayed and may not appear until several days after the return home. Likewise, the necessary therapy may be required in that wide window – the so-called incubation period. The challenge of many of the environmentally associated emergencies is to initiate therapy early, to achieve the best possible outcome, and, in some infectious complications, to be able to institute the now-delayed therapy to avoid great increases in morbidity and mortality.

HEAT EMERGENCIES

These emergencies are largely associated with ecotourism where the traveler is truly out in the environment – a marked departure from the usual life in "civilization" with its air-conditioned environment, dehumidification, and general protection from extremes.[1] These exposures, coupled with the "holiday" conditions of food and beverage excess (i.e., alcohol), impair the body's ability to maintain homeostasis, and, in extremes, regulation of body core temperature is lost. The resultant elevation of core temperature

can reach a potentially fatal level. Immediate care may be life saving. Simple measures – rehydration, cool water immersion, ice packs, and limiting of activities – are essential. Newer approaches (electrolyte replacement fluids and some drugs) reported in Olympic and world class sports may be the prevention as well as treatment in the future.[2] As these conditions are largely in primitive/remote areas, where access to professional assistance is limited if available at all, anticipation of heat stress is the primary step to avoid the serious sequelae (coagulopathy, etc.).[3] Obviously, these scenarios are not the domain of the dermatologist, but one should be aware of risk to encourage the patient to be alert to the symptoms and seek care, should they appear.

UV LIGHT

Here again, the key is environmental change. Essentials to anticipate include the enhanced UV exposure closer to the tropics and the effect of altitude on intensity of UV, especially with a pale, light-skinned traveler seeking respite from winter. The temptation of the sun during the long dark days is often too great, and careful planning and prevention are ignored or forgotten. Lower latitudes and higher altitudes are key to risk in the environment, as each enhances the intensity. The higher altitudes have thinner air filtering and less of the incoming sunlight, whereas the nearer the equator, the greater the direct effect of the rays.

An essential key is education in the use of sunscreens prior to departure and gradual increase of exposure to induce melanin formation. In addition, the late Harry Arnold who practiced for years in Hawaii was a proponent of planned/controlled tanning in his office prior to exposure to avoid the chance of burning (personal communication). Others (including myself) use this approach in certain selected cases (types 1 and 2 skin in particular).

Additionally, the present world of polypharmacy has greatly expanded the list of photosensitizing drugs, particularly for hypertensive and/or diabetic patients. The prototype in the past has been the group of furocoumarins and

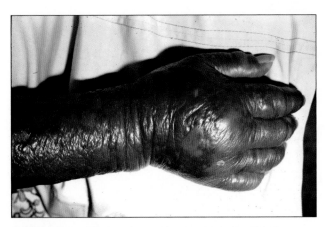

FIGURE 30.1: *Phototoxic reaction to a topical antibiotic.*

the sulfa-related drugs (Figure 30.1). Whereas the former group were used therapeutically, the latter are omnipresent in the treatment of infections, diabetes, and hypertension (diuretics) (Figure 30.2). The traveler should be aware of any drugs taken with such potential and use extra care. The personal physician and the pharmacist should be the best source for this information and obtain it before the patient travels. It should be noted that many busy general practitioners may not have the most recent information, whereas the pharmacist will have this information, usually on a computer program.[4]

Modern sunscreens are the real answer.[5] New guidelines for protection (sun protection factor [SPF]) are imminent and long overdue, as a consensus on UVA protection is essential for the informed and concerned consumer. The significance of UVA grows as data accumulate in its role in carcinogenesis, a far more insidious and significant "thief in the night" because of its much less obvious impact without the "sunburn" that inspires caution with UVB.[6] The significance of UVA relates to its greater penetration into the dermis (whereas UVB only penetrates superficially) and the immunosuppression it can cause. This problem is not emergent/acute but it is the cumulative exposure that is the

major cause/factor in the carcinogenesis. The acute problems are less associated with the risk for carcinogenesis; the immediate discomfort is the primary reason for the need for suncreens.

The early agents were effective protection but not aesthetically desirable and hence not well accepted. These agents included Red Vet Pet (red veterinary petrolatum), which had very good sunscreening properties and hence was standard in water survival kits when I was a flight surgeon in the U.S. Navy. Sudden loss of your ship put you on the open ocean in a life raft (if you were lucky) but often exposed to intense sunlight and sunburn. In this scenario, it could be life saving, and the greasy aspects of petrolatum were not a great concern – much different than applying it while on the sandy beach or by the pool. The total blockers such as titanium and zinc oxide have many, if the same, problems and hence are used primarily in medical conditions of very severe photosensitivity.

The first chemicals other than physical sunscreens such as *para*-aminobenzoic acid were primarily protective against UVB (and the sunburn sequelae) as that was the easiest to measure with SPF testing. Furthermore, it represented our best knowledge of the situation at the time. Of course, important prevention from UVB sunburn is the acute concern and would be key to avoid acute problems for the traveler. Much of the literature on sunscreens to date has dealt with UVB protection preventing sunburn, but it now is appreciated that the deeper penetration of the UVA rays into the dermis greatly enhances risk for carcinogenesis but poses a lesser risk for sunburn.

Newer agents such as avobenzone (Parsol 1789), one of the first with UVA screening, are now preferred because of broader spectrum A/B effect. They have greater acceptance but, in all instances, need to be used expectantly to prevent future acute episodes. This field is rapidly changing with the newer agents Helioplex®, Tinosorb M®, and Mexoryl XL®, which are just a few examples of this growing field. Even and repeat application is essential for protection, and the effectiveness is seen in Figure 30.3. The irregular tanning attests to protection potential.

Total disregard for usual "sun sense" can produce an emergency situation, especially when the results are near-second-degree burns, enhanced risk for infection, and significant morbidity. Acute treatment is instituted to prevent usual burn complications, fluid loss, infection, and systemic sequelae. Steroids may be of assistance in the first few hours, and nonsteroidal antiinflammatory drugs may be helpful in stopping the progression. These are primarily administered orally, but some newer preparations and concentrations of diclofenac gel are showing promise.[7]

CONTACT DERMATITIS

There are several groups of plants causing type 4 reactions that can be encountered, and most are widespread, if not

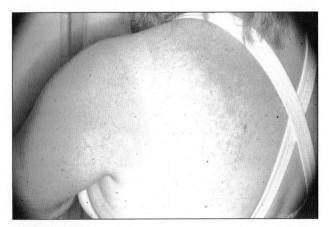

FIGURE 30.2: *Sulfonamide-associated photoreaction.*

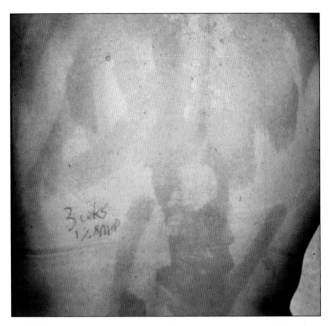

FIGURE 30.3: *Irregular pigmentation after uneven application of a sunscreen.*

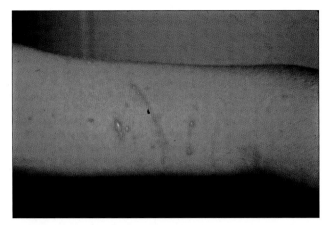

FIGURE 30.4: *Classical presentation of Rhus dermatitis.*

worldwide, in distribution. The *compositae* group of plants are the most widespread, but fortunately only few persons have allergic potential, and these are ones with extensive exposure, usually occupational, floriculture, and/or agriculture. The hallmark of the group is the daisy-like composite flower; the group also includes some popular herbal sources such as Echinacea. Even the common dandelion is in the same group. It is a vast group found everywhere, so they are difficult to avoid. The sesquiterpene lactones are the common antigens, and it has been recently documented with a higher incidence in children (4.2%) and adolescents (2.6%), primarily in those who are atopic.[8] This allergy further increases the risk, as atopic children are those with greatest morbidity in tropical dermatology from impetiginization and secondarily infected miliaria, seeming to double the risk for such children in the tropics.

The Rhus/Toxicodendron group has a much higher incidence of allergy but fortunately has a smaller range of distribution. Norman Goldstein wrote a classical article in *Cutis* documenting related plants that result in worldwide exposure – the very sensitive subject commences extensive travel, arrives in the tropics, and gets a perioral contact dermatitis from eating mango. Then on to the Orient, where dermatitis on the buttocks results from toilet seats finished with lacquer (the related Japanese lacquer tree as the source). In India, a dermatitis on the neck from laundry ink in the collar (the Indian marking nut tree). The different species have definite and limited range, but the oleoresin cross-reacts, and sensitivity then can even be widespread. Even cashews are related, but fortunately the usual processing inactivates the allergen.[9] Although frequently presenting as simple vesicles in a linear display (Figure 30.4), this

allergen also can result in the most dramatic vesicular and vesiculobullous reactions that can be widespread and are a frequent site for impetiginization. This secondary infection is the most frequent reason for emergency care as it progresses erysipelas and with certain nephritogenic streptococci symptomatic renal disease. As mentioned earlier in this chapter, exposure to contact dermatitis can be initiated even before departure or while on the trip. Either way, the morbidity can be such that it can nearly ruin the vacation/trip.

Alstroemeria is a newer problem largely due to the popularity of the plants in the flower and greenhouse industry. Although previously limited in range, the artificial nature of growth in the trade has greatly increased the exposure for persons in the business of floriculture. Previous sensitization and subsequent reexposure usually in the wild (primarily southern hemisphere) can give the same scenario as in the preceding paragraph in the seriously allergic individual.

Primula sensitivity seems to be largely limited to the United Kingdom, in gardeners, floriculturists, and so forth. The limited range of this group of plant species in cooler climes lessens the exposure to *primulin* and, furthermore, the cool environment usually results in clothing that limits the amount of bare skin exposure. Similar complications seen with other allergic contact dermatitis reactions are still possible. The usual clinical presentation with all of the previously mentioned allergens is so similar that often careful history taking and even patch testing may be necessary to discern the source of the contact dermatitis. Identification is essential to both educate the patient and prevent future exposure. Although some new barrier creams seem to have promise, there are none universally in use at present.

BEACH AND REEF: AQUATIC EXPOSURES

There are a few significant aquatic exposures that one can encounter; fortunately, most of the areas involved are well equipped to handle the problems as the shore, surf, and the coral reefs are primarily developed as resort facilities with

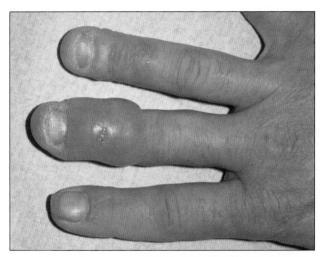

FIGURE 30.5: *Local reaction from toxins in spines of a scorpionfish.*

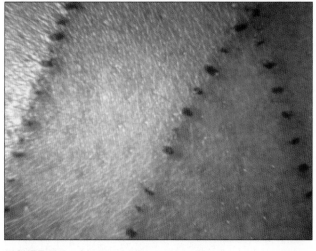

FIGURE 30.6: *Linear reaction to nematocysts.*

all the amenities, medical included. The reefs are associated with many fish having toxic spine, such as the scorpionfish (Figure 30.5).

The "aquatourists" also are usually well educated in risk, emergency care, and first aid – all part of the basic exposure to water safety, scuba diving, surfboarding safety, and, in some areas, the swimming education program. Perhaps, the primary impetus is the periodic headline on shark attacks and the previously mentioned death of Steve Irwin. He was an individual well versed in proper safety in such hostile environments. One can never be too prepared!

Although these large animals get the headlines, the smaller creatures – seeming innocents such as jellyfish – are the real cause of most problems.

Among coelenterates, two have the greatest impact. In the Western hemisphere, the Portuguese Man o' War (Physalia *physalis*) is a cause of reported deaths. The long tentacles of this creature can break off, and the unsuspecting swimmer suffers the consequences of the contact and subsequent reaction from the multiple nematocyst toxicity. This usually happens to swimmers with lack of knowledge of the problem; they get extensive stings and improper care (by fresh water exposure, massage, and other amateur first aid remedies), which results in continued "firing" of the nematocysts deposited in the characteristic linear arrays (Figure 30.6). The resort staff are usually available to assist. When managing these patients, it is also important to realize that broken tentacles can maintain toxicity for months, allowing for exposure over a broader window of time. Also, the nematocysts in the patient's dermis can fire off for variable periods of time after emergent care has been completed, a cause for morbidity in some patients.

In Southeast Asia, a much more serious threat is *Chironex fleckeri* (also occasionally reported in the Caribbean, but most of the publicity is from Australia). It is estimated that the fatality rate is between 15% and 20%.

The beaches in Australia (Queensland) have jugs of alcohol or vinegar strategically placed to provide emergency neutralization of the nematocysts – a potentially life-saving maneuver. Alternatively, experienced swimmers carry meat tenderizer as another approach to minimize morbidity. These creatures, colloquially sea nettles and sea wasps, are appropriately named.

The other headliner in this environment is the "deadly" cone shell. Here again, it has an estimated 15%–20% fatality rate that should be diminished by education. These attractive shells are sought by collectors in Australia, California, and Florida, often by occasional collectors unaware of the risk. With education on precautions (gloves, etc.), emergency symptoms from the neurotoxin can be avoided. Definitive treatment is still not standardized. The unusual nature of the venom is sparking interest to utilize it therapeutically and to approach better therapeutic avenues.[10]

Many other dermatoses have been described, from coral dermatitis to sea bathers eruption, which are acute, usually minor, and rarely prompt a visit to the emergency room. Alexander Fisher added a useful small atlas to the dermatologic literature,[11] which, when used along with the classic reference by Halstead,[12] one can easily master the dermatologic significance of these clinical challenges.

REFERENCES

1. Laws J. We're hot and unbothered. Occup Health Saf. 2008; 77:68–70.
2. von Duvillard SP, Arciero PJ, Tietjen-Smith T, Alford K. Sports drinks, exercise training, and competition. Curr Sports Med Rep. 2008; 7:202–8.
3. Levi M. Burning issues surrounding inflammation and coagulation in heatstroke. Crit Care Med. 2008; 36:2455–6.
4. Stein KR, Scheinfeld NS. Drug-induced photoallergic and phototoxic reactions. Expert Opin Drug Saf. 2007; 6:431–4.

5. Lautenschlager S, Wulf H, Pittelkow M. Photoprotection. Lancet. 2007; 370:528–37.

6. Antoniou C, Kosmadaki M, Stratigos A, Katsambas A. Sunscreens – what's important to know. J Eur Acad Dermatol Venereol. 2008; 22(9):1110–18.

7. New treatments for actinic keratoses. Med Lett Drugs Ther. 2002; 44:57.

8. Paulsen E, Otkjaer A, Andersen K. Sesquiterpene lactone dermatitis in the young: is atopy a risk factor? Contact Derm. 2008; 59:1–6.

9. Goldstein N, The ubiquitous urushiols, contact dermatitis from mango, poison ivy, and other "poison" plants. Hawaii Med J. 2004; 63:231–5.

10. Lewis RJ. Ion channel toxins and therapeutics: from cone snail venoms to ciguatera. Ther Drug Monit. 2000; 22:61–4.

11. Fisher AA. Atlas of aquatic dermatology. New York: Grune & Stratton; 1978.

12. Halstead BW. Poisonous and venomous marine animals of the world. Vol 1. Invertebrates. Washington, DC: US Government Printing Office; 1965.

CHAPTER 31

Endocrinologic Emergencies in Dermatology

Margaret T. Ryan

Vincent Savarese

Serge A. Jabbour

ENDOCRINE AND METABOLIC DISEASES, besides affecting other organs, can result in changes in cutaneous function and morphology and can lead to a complex symptomatology. Dermatologists may see some of these skin lesions first, either before the endocrinologist, or even after the internist or specialist has missed the right diagnosis. Because some skin lesions might reflect a life-threatening endocrine or metabolic disorder, identifying the underlying disorder is important, so that patients can receive corrective rather than symptomatic treatment.

In this section, we review a few endocrine and metabolic disorders in which patients may present to the dermatologist with various skin lesions and in which the diagnosis of the underlying condition must be made in a timely fashion before the patient ends up with complications that could be fatal.

HYPERPIGMENTATION AND ADDISON DISEASE

Addison disease, or primary adrenal insufficiency, can be caused by either infiltrative disorders that invade the adrenal cortex or by destructive disorders that attack the adrenal cells. In either etiology, the adrenal cortex is unable to produce and secrete adequate amounts of glucocorticoid and mineralocorticoid hormones. The most common etiology of Addison disease used to be tuberculous granulomatous disease, but with declining infection rates in the developed world, the most common cause of Addison disease today is autoimmune destruction of the adrenal glands. Other less common causes of Addison include other granulomatous fungal infections (histoplasmosis, coccidiomycosis), metastatic carcinoma infiltration of the adrenals, or bilateral adrenal hemorrhage.[1] Rarely, autoimmune Addison disease can be seen in association with certain inherited autoimmune polyglandular syndromes.

Clinical Features

The hallmark dermatologic feature of Addison disease is a darkening of the skin, particularly in sun-exposed areas. The hyperpigmentation of Addison disease is due to the melanocyte-stimulating activity of the high plasma levels of adrenocorticotropic hormone (ACTH).[2] This skin darkening may be homogeneous or blotchy and is observed in all racial groups, although it can be more difficult to see in darker-skinned individuals. Also seen is significant increased pigmentation in the palmar creases, the vermillion border of the lips, flexural areas, in recent scars, and in areas of friction such as pant waistlines. Mucous membranes such as the buccal, periodontal, and vaginal mucosa may show patchy areas of increased pigmentation. Women may have diminished axillary and pubic hair as their androgen production occurs primarily in the adrenal glands.[3,4] Patients with autoimmune Addison disease may also present with vitiligo or alopecia areata, from a similar autoimmune destruction of melanocytes and hair follicles, respectively.

Diagnosis

Diagnosis should be based on clinical presentation confirmed by laboratory testing. The presentation of a patient with chronic primary adrenal insufficiency is that of longstanding vague symptoms such as malaise, anorexia, joint aches, nausea, and fatigue, in addition the skin findings mentioned earlier. Patients may also report craving high-salt foods.[1] The acute presentation of adrenal insufficiency is that of orthostatic hypotension, confusion, circulatory collapse, and abdominal pain. This acute presentation is frequently precipitated by an acute infection.

Biochemical testing to confirm the diagnosis is done with a cosyntropin (synthetic ACTH) stimulation test. In this test, serum cortisol is measured immediately prior to and 60 minutes following injection of 250 μg of cosyntropin. A cortisol level at 60 minutes of 18–20 μg/dL or greater is considered a normal adrenal response. If the serum cortisol at 60 minutes is less than 18–20 μg/dL, the patient is diagnosed with adrenal insufficiency; however, this may be primary or secondary (pituitary/hypothalamic mediated).[5] Plasma ACTH should then be measured. In Addison disease (primary adrenal insufficiency), the ACTH will be elevated (>100 pg/mL) whereas in secondary adrenal insufficiency, the ACTH will be normal to low.[5] Other biochemical findings supporting a diagnosis of Addison disease include hyperkalemia, elevated renin activity, hyponatremia, hypoglycemia, and hyperchloremic metabolic acidosis. Measurement of a morning plasma cortisol is sometimes done instead of a cosyntropin stimulation test, as a morning serum cortisol greater than 18–20 μg/dL rules out the diagnosis of adrenal insufficiency and a value of less than 3 μg/dL makes it very likely. In many patients, serum cortisol falls within the intermediate range and further testing is required, making cosyntropin stimulation the preferred testing method for diagnosis.[5]

Treatment

Treatment of Addison disease includes replacing both glucocorticoids and mineralocorticoids. Typical dosing of glucocorticoids is prednisone 5–7.5 mg daily or hydrocortisone 15–20 mg in the morning and 5–10 mg in the evening. For mineralocorticoid replacement, fludrocortisone is given at a dose of 0.05–0.3 mg/day.[4] The fludrocortisone dose can be adjusted to normalize renin plasma activity, and the required dose is typically slightly lower in patients on hydrocortisone as opposed to prednisone, as hydrocortisone has some mineralocorticoid activity itself.[6] There is no easy way to assess the appropriateness of the glucocorticoid replacement dose as ACTH levels, although they do decline with appropriate treatment, generally do not normalize. Recurrent symptoms of adrenal insufficiency may suggest underreplacement whereas development of Cushingoid features may suggest overreplacement. Patients are typically advised to increase their dose of glucocorticoids during stressful events such as illnesses or surgery. The hyperpigmentation seen in untreated Addison disease should resolve with appropriate treatment.

Patients with Addison disease are also dehydroepiandrosterone (DHEA) deficient, and some studies show symptomatic improvement in women who are given DHEA replacement as well.[7] These findings, however, have not been consistently shown, and there is as of yet no consensus on whether DHEA replacement is appropriate.[1]

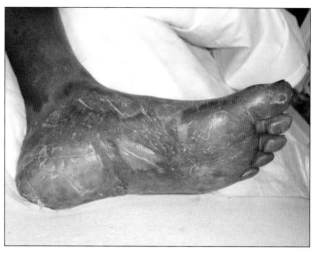

FIGURE 31.1: *Necrolytic migratory erythema on the foot, showing indurated areas with blistering, crusting, and scaling.*

NECROLYTIC MIGRATORY ERYTHEMA IN GLUCAGONOMA

Glucagonoma is a pancreatic tumor arising from the α cells of the pancreatic islets and causing increased secretion of the pancreatic hormone glucagon. The clinical syndrome classically associated with glucagonoma includes necrolytic migratory erythema (NME), cheilitis, diabetes mellitus, anemia, weight loss, venous thrombosis, and neuropsychiatric symptoms. Weight loss and NME are the most prevalent symptoms, occurring in approximately 65%–70% of patients by the time of diagnosis. The dermatitis may occasionally appear, prior to the onset of systemic symptoms, but most patients with rash usually have weight loss, diarrhea, sore mouth, weakness, mental status changes, or diabetes mellitus as well as hypoaminoacidemia and zinc deficiency on laboratory analysis.[8]

Clinical Features

NME is considered the hallmark feature of the glucagonoma syndrome[8,9] and is the clinical feature that leads to the diagnosis of glucagonoma syndrome in the majority of cases. NME is characterized by a painful and pruritic polymorphous rash. It begins as an erythematous macular and papular skin eruption that later develops into well-demarcated plaques with variable scaling and finally progresses to centrally forming vesicles and bullae that rupture leaving a crusted and eroded surface[8,9] (see Figure 31.1). NME has a relapsing remitting course. Individual lesions typically evolve over a period of time lasting 1–2 weeks, and patients will have multiple lesions in various stages of the cycle. These lesions are usually seen first in the groin, later progressing to the perineum, the buttocks, and the extremities.

NME is frequently complicated by secondary skin infections with *Candida albicans* or *Staphylococcus aureus* and, in fact, some patients are diagnosed incorrectly with chronic candidosis years before eventually being diagnosed with NME.[9]

Diagnosis

The differential diagnosis for NME is large and includes acrodermatitis enteropathica (AE), pemphigus foliaceus, psoriasis, and chronic mucocutaneous candidosis,[10,11] and should be differentiated on the basis of the larger clinical picture, histologic analysis, and laboratory findings. In patients in whom NME is suspected, one should check a glucagon level, and, if elevated, imaging should be done to look for a neuroendocrine tumor. Glucagon levels may be elevated in several conditions besides glucagonoma, including liver or kidney disease, prolonged starvation, or acute myocardial infarction, but a level greater than 1000 pg/mL is highly suggestive of glucagonoma.[9] Given the often long delay in diagnosis from initial presentation of NME, some authors argue that glucagon levels should be checked in all patients with diabetes mellitus and a chronic cutaneous eruption.[9]

Skin biopsy specimens should be taken from the inner edge of an advancing lesion. The characteristic finding is necrosis of the upper layers of the stratum spinosum with separation from the underlying epidermis, which is less affected.[8]

NME occasionally has been reported in patients without any evidence of glucagonoma. These patients, however, typically have hyperglucagonemia or amino acid deficiency of some other etiology and are often referred to as having pseudoglucagonoma syndrome.[12]

Treatment

The treatment of choice for NME is complete surgical removal of the α-cell tumor and is the only chance for a cure of the disease. After surgical resection, there is normalization of glucagon levels. The rash typically resolves rapidly, often within days, after removal of the tumor.[13] Unfortunately, the majority of glucagonomas are either too large for curative surgery or already metastatic at the time of diagnosis. Due to the slow growth of these tumors, even in metastatic disease, debulking surgery may achieve a prolonged resolution of symptoms although there is no evidence of prolonged survival.[14] If full surgical resection is not possible due to the size of tumor or distant metastases, chemotherapy is added to decrease tumor bulk and a long-acting somatostatin analog (a glucagon antagonist) such as octreotide is used to relieve symptoms of NME.[15,16] There have been case reports of successful surgical treatment of glucagonomas that are metastatic to

the liver with liver transplant in addition to resection of the primary tumor. The role of liver transplantation in patients with metastatic glucagonoma is, however, not yet clear.[17] Other treatments that have been tried with mixed results include intravenous amino acid and aggressive zinc supplementation.[18]

THYROID DYSFUNCTION

Thyroid disorders are common in the general population and can have varied dermatologic presentations based on the type and the severity of the thyroid dysfunction. Hyperthyroidism may be due to a transient thyroiditis, toxic nodules (either single or multiple), or, most commonly, Graves autoimmune thyroid disease. Hypothyroidism may be autoimmune Hashimoto, iodine-deficiency related, radiation induced, or postsurgical.

Clinical Features

Patients with hyperthyroidism have warm, moist, erythematous skin. Many patients develop onycholysis, and a significant percentage of them complain of scalp hair loss. Alopecia areata and loss of body hair may also be noted, but are less common.[4,19] In addition, patients with Graves disease may show evidence of Graves ophthalmopathy, pretibial myxedema, or acropachy. Pretibial myxedema can occur anywhere on the body but most commonly affects the anterior tibia and the dorsum of the feet. It is characterized by a nonpitting thickening and induration of the skin, and is present in 0.5%–4% of patients with Graves disease.[19] Acropachy is even less common, occurring in just 0.1%–1% of patients with Graves, and consists of a triad of digital clubbing, soft tissue swelling of hands and feet, and periosteal new bone formation.[19] Both pretibial myxedema and acropachy are seen almost exclusively in patients with Graves ophthalmopathy, and these two dermatologic manifestations are considered indicators of more severe autoimmune disease.[20] Vitiligo, a marker of autoimmune disease, is also frequently seen in Graves disease.[21]

Patients with hypothyroidism, by contrast, have pale cold skin that is typically dry, rough, scaly, and hyperkeratotic.[19] The skin may appear to have a yellowish discoloration, particularly in the palms, soles, and nasolabial folds, due to carotene deposition, and approximately 50% have a malar flush.[4,19] Myxedema, caused by mucopolysaccaride deposition in the dermis, is most pronounced in the periorbital regions, leading to nonpitting swelling around the eyes. Loss of sympathetic tone may lead to a drooping of the upper eyelid. Patients may lose hair on the outer third of their eyebrows, and scalp hair loss has been reported in about half of all hypothyroid patients. Hair becomes dry and brittle and nails are thin and grooved.[19]

Diagnosis

Serum TSH (thyroid-stimulating hormone) is the initial diagnostic test for either hyperthyroidism or hypothyroidism. In most cases of hyperthyroidism, the TSH will be suppressed, whereas in hypothyroidism the TSH will be elevated.[22] Thyroid peroxidase antibody may be checked in hypothyroid patients to evaluate for Hashimoto (autoimmune) thyroiditis. After a laboratory diagnosis of hyperthyroidism is made, patients should be sent for a 24-hour radioactive iodine uptake and scan to determine etiology, as an uptake and scan can differentiate between Graves, toxic nodules, and thyroiditis.

Treatment

Treatment of hypothyroidism is with levothyroxine weight-based dosing, typically 1.6 μg/kg/d, titrated to achieve a euthyroid state with TSH in the normal range.[4] Any symptomatic patient with hyperthyroidism may be given a beta blocker if there is no contraindication. Definitive treatment of hyperthyroidism varies depending on the etiology of the disorder. Thyroiditis typically resolves without treatment. In Graves disease or toxic nodules, radioactive iodine treatment is effective but frequently leads to hypothyroidism requiring levothyroxine therapy. In patients with Graves disease, antithyroid agents such as methimazole and propylthiouracil are other options; the remission rates after 18 months of medical treatment, however, are only 30%–40%, and these medications do come with the risk of allergic reactions or agranulocytosis.[23]

FLUSHING AND CARCINOID SYNDROME

Carcinoids are slow-growing tumors arising from the enterochromaffin or Kulchitsky cells and in most cases originate in the gastrointestinal (GI) tract or the lungs. Carcinoid tumors can secrete any number of bioactive substances, and their presentation is dependent on both the type of substances secreted as well as the location of the original tumor and any metastases. Carcinoid tumors typically produce large amounts of serotonin. In addition, they may also secrete histamine, corticotropin, dopamine, substance P, neurotensin, prostaglandins, kallikrein, and tachykinins.[24] Carcinoid syndrome is the term used to describe a constellation of symptoms caused by the secreted bioactive substances and is present in less than 10% of patients with carcinoid tumors. The bioactive products produced by carcinoid tumors are inactivated in the liver, so patients with GI carcinoids develop the carcinoid syndrome only if they have hepatic metastases leading to secretion of the substances into the hepatic veins, whereas patients with carcinoid of the lung can develop the carcinoid syndrome in the absence of metastatic disease.

Clinical Features

Episodic cutaneous flushing is the hallmark of the carcinoid syndrome and is seen in 85% of patients.[25] The flushing of carcinoid is typically confined to the face, neck, and upper trunk. Carcinoid tumors originating in the midgut (appendix, ileum, jejunum) produce what is known as the classical carcinoid flush, which is a rapid-onset cyanotic flush lasting approximately 30 seconds and associated with a mild burning sensation. Foregut carcinoids (stomach, lung, pancreas, biliary tract) produce a brighter pinkish-red flush that may be pruritic and can be more difficult to differentiate from physiological flushing. Flushing episodes may occur spontaneously or may be provoked by certain triggers, similar to the triggers of physiologic flushing (alcohol, cheese, coffee, exercise, or emotional stressors).[26,27] Carcinoid flushing often is associated with diarrhea and breathlessness or wheeze, and these associated symptoms are a method of differentiating the flushing of carcinoid from physiologic flushing.[28] Features of rosacea or vascular telangiectasias may develop after years of flushing. Severe flushing can be associated with a drop in blood pressure and tachycardia. A phenomenon known as carcinoid crisis can be precipitated by anesthesia or an interventional procedure and is characterized by a profound and prolonged hypotension with tachycardia.

Other clinical features of the carcinoid syndrome include niacin deficiency and hypoproteinemia from diversion of tryptophan for the synthesis of serotonin. Pellagra (glossitis, scaly skin, angular stomatitis, and confusion) as well as dependent edema may develop secondary to these deficiencies but are usually a later presentation of the carcinoid syndrome.[24,25,28] Scleroderma, without Raynaud phenomenon, also has been described in association with the carcinoid syndrome and is considered a poor prognostic indicator.[28]

Diagnosis

Symptoms of flushing, diarrhea, and bronchospasm, typically paroxysmal, may raise the suspicion for the carcinoid syndrome. Additional less specific symptoms may include GI discomfort, a palpable abdominal mass, GI bleeding, or heart failure. The symptoms of carcinoid are protean as they vary depending on the type of bioactive substances secreted and the location of the tumor. As such, patients are often initially misdiagnosed with other conditions, such as irritable bowel syndrome, asthma, or anxiety, and accurate diagnosis and treatment are delayed.

Although carcinoid may be suspected from the clinical presentation, the diagnosis must be confirmed with biochemical tests. The most specific test is a measurement of 24-hour urinary excretion of 5-hydroxyindoleacetic acid (5-HIAA), a degradation product of serotonin. The test for urinary 5-HIAA has a sensitivity of 75% and a specificity of 88%,[24] but there are some drawbacks. Certain serotonin-rich foods such as bananas, avocados, and tomatoes, can increase urinary 5-HIAA and lead to false-positive results. Serum chromogranin A (CgA) is another biochemical test commonly used for the diagnosis of carcinoid. CgA is a constitutive secretory product of most neuroendocrine tumors, and plasma CgA levels have a sensitivity of up to 99% in diagnosing carcinoid. Plasma CgA is thus a sensitive, but not specific, marker for carcinoid tumors as it may be elevated in several other neuroendocrine tumors as well as in cases of renal impairment, liver failure, and inflammatory bowel disease[24] or in patients on proton pump inhibitors.[29] A single recent study of the efficacy of plasma 5-HIAA in detecting carcinoid tumors demonstrated a sensitivity of 89% and a specificity of 97%,[30] but this test is not yet part of the standard armamentarium.

After carcinoid is confirmed by biochemical testing, localization of the primary tumor as well as any metastasis must be done; there are several different imaging modalities from which to choose. Octreotide scintigraphy, using In-111, is the initial modality of choice if it is available. Octreotide scintigraphy has an overall sensitivity of 80%–90% based on various studies.[31] In addition to the high sensitivity, octreotide scintigraphy allows imaging of the entire body in one session, thereby detecting primary tumors as well as metastasis (which may be missed with conventional imaging). Bone scintigraphy is used to detect bone metastases if they are suspected and ^{123}I-MIBG scintigraphy also can be used to localize carcinoid, although it appears to be less sensitive than octreotide scintigraphy, especially in detecting metastases.[31] Computed tomography and magnetic resonance imaging scans are frequently used for initial localization with a sensitivity for both of approximately 80%. Radiographic findings include mass lesions with calcification and stranding fibrosis. Other modalities frequently used for localization include positron emission tomography scan (sometimes in combination with octreotide scintigraphy), endoscopic ultrasound, and endoscopy.

Treatment

Surgery is the only curative treatment for carcinoid tumors. Unfortunately, curative surgery is possible only with nonmetastatic disease or in resectable nodal or hepatic metastases, and most patients have significant metastatic disease at the time of presentation. Even in patients who have metastic disease, surgery has a role for relief of mechanical obstructions and, in cases of carcinoid syndrome, debulking causes significant relief of symptoms. Similarly, reduction of hepatic metastases, via surgical resection or hepatic artery occlusion (ligation, embolization, or chemoembolization), has been shown to give symptomatic relief from the carcinoid syndrome, and some studies have shown survival benefits of up to 2 years.[32]

Medical treatment with somatostatin analogs (octreotide and lanreotide) has proven extremely efficacious for symptomatic relief, leading to resolution of flushing and diarrhea in 70%–80% of patients. In addition, urinary 5-HIAA levels were halved in 72% of patients.[33] Intravenous octreotide infusion has been used to successfully treat carcinoid crisis. The somatostatin analogs do not, however, appear to have any effect on tumor size or growth rate.[24,26] Other medical treatments commonly employed in metastatic carcinoid include interferon-α and chemotherapy agents. Lifestyle modifications to avoid the triggers of flushing episodes, such as alcohol, exercise, and spicy food, are also encouraged, and diet supplementation with nicotinamide may prevent the symptoms of niacin deficiency.

URTICARIA PIGMENTOSA AND MASTOCYTOSIS

Mastocytosis is a group of rare disorders affecting adults and children and is distinguished by a pathologic increase in mast cells.[25] This increase in mast cells may be seen in a variety of tissues including the skin, bone marrow, GI tract, spleen, liver, and lymph nodes. The symptoms of mastocytosis are heterogeneous[25] and tend to be related to the level of mast cell burden and the tissue type involved. Symptoms are typically related to mast cell mediator release. The mediators found within mast cells are legion, including histamine, prostaglandin D2, leukotrienes, interleukin-6, and many more. Patients with mastocytosis tend to experience symptoms in discrete attacks when mast cell mediators are released. Symptoms typically include pruritus, whealing, flushing, palpitations, and tachycardia. Bone marrow involvement, common in adult cases of mastocytosis, can lead to anemia and low bone density. If there is GI involvement, patients may experience diarrhea and abdominal pain. Strong stimuli of mast cell release can lead to anaphylactoid reactions with severe, prolonged hypotension. Mastocytosis can also present as idiopathic anaphylaxis in previously undiagnosed patients.

Clinical Features

The characteristic feature of mastocytosis is a rash known as urticaria pigmentosa (UP). UP is the presenting feature in the majority of patients with systemic mastocytosis but can also be present as a cutaneous mastocytosis, without any extracutaneous involvement. The classical lesion[34] is a hyperpigmented reddish-brown macule or papule (see Figure 31.2). Another feature seen in UP is the local whealing and development of edema around the lesions when rubbed or scratched. This is known as the Darier sign. In typical UP in adults, the lesions measure 3–4 mm individually and are symmetrically and randomly distributed, with the highest density of lesions seen on the trunk and thighs and with relative sparing of the palms, soles, and face. In extensive cutaneous disease, the lesions may become confluent. Children tend to present with larger lesions (5–15 mm), and their lesions are most prominent on the trunk.[34]

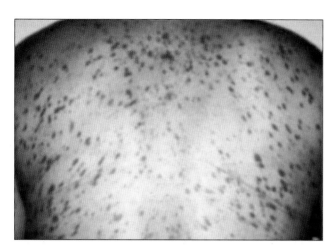

FIGURE 31.2: Urticaria pigmentosa on the back with hyperpigmented reddish-brown macules and papules.

TABLE 31.1: Diagnostic Criteria for Systemic Mastocytosis

Major criteria:
Multifocal infiltrates of mast cells in bone-marrow biopsy or in other extracutaneous organs

Minor criteria:
>25% of mast cells in bone-marrow biopsy or tissue specimens are spindle shaped or atypical

Detection of a codon 816 c-kit point mutation in blood, bone marrow, or lesional tissue

Mast cells in blood, bone marrow, or lesional tissue expressing CD25 or CD2

Baseline total tryptase level >20 ng/mL

Pruritus is typically associated with UP. Less common presentations of UP include telangiectatic, nonpigmented, nodular or plaque-like variations of the rash.[34] In rare cases, mastocytosis can present as a single large mastocytoma instead of the diffuse rash.

Diagnosis

The diagnosis of UP is based on clinical suspicion from the maculopapular lesions and a Darier sign, and is confirmed by histopathologic examination of a tissue specimen. Skin biopsy of a UP lesion typically shows aggregates of mast cells within the papillary dermis and extending into the reticular dermis,[35] particularly around blood vessels. Mast cells within skin biopsies show a characteristic spindle shape with metachromatic granules. Another characteristic of UP on skin biopsy is the absence of any inflammatory cells other than mast cells in the dermal infiltrate.[36] The most specific stain for mast cells in any tissue is immunohistochemical staining with tryptase.[37] The diagnosis of mastocytosis is occasionally made in patients lacking the typical rash, by bone marrow biopsy, typically done after unexplained anaphylaxis or flushing or for peripheral blood abnormalities.

When the diagnosis of UP is made, it is important to determine whether the patient has cutaneous mastocytosis alone or whether there is systemic involvement. A set of major and minor diagnostic criteria exist to diagnose systemic mastocytosis (see Table 31.1). A diagnosis of systemic mastocytosis requires the fulfilment of either one major criterion with one minor criterion or three minor criteria.[38,39] More extensive cutaneous disease tends to correlate with increased risk for systemic mastocytosis. Elevated levels of mast cell mediators such as tryptase and histamine also can be used to support the diagnosis of systemic mastocytosis. Serum tryptase levels greater than 20 ng/mL are suggestive of systemic mastocytosis, whereas patients with only cutaneous mastocytosis tend to have levels less than 14 ng/mL.[40] Histamine metabolites in a 24-hour urine collection also tend to be increased in systemic mastocytosis.[41] This test, however, is neither more sensitive nor more specific than the serum tryptase level.[42] Bone-marrow involvement is seen in the vast majority of patients with adult-onset mastocytosis. Thus, a bone-marrow biopsy is recommended in the evaluation of all patients with adult-onset disease, whereas in children with cutaneous disease bone-marrow biopsy is recommended only in the presence of other abnormal findings suggesting systemic involvement such as an abnormal complete blood count or an enlarged spleen or liver.

Treatment

Most patients, be they children or adults, have an indolent course and a good prognosis; however, there is no definitive treatment for mastocytosis. Treatment instead is directed toward the amelioration of symptoms related to the release of mast cell mediators and must be tailored to each patient's specific symptoms and organ involvement. All patients may be counseled in the avoidance of triggers such as exercise, rapid temperature changes, skin rubbing, or certain drugs including anesthesia medications. Histamine receptor blockers (H1 and H2) along with cromolyn are effective for pruritus and for episodes of flushing, diarrhea, or abdominal pain.[35] Topical glucocorticoids can be used for symptomatic skin lesions. Ultraviolet light irradiation (psoralen plus ultraviolet A) is used in the treatment of UP to decrease pruritus, whealing, and flare reactions.[43] Bone disease from marrow involvement can be treated similarly to osteoporosis of other etiologies, with calcium, vitamin D, and bisphosphonates. Patients with anaphylactic reactions are treated with epinephrine and should be given an epinephrine emergency pen to carry with them. For patients with more aggressive systemic disease, other treatments (such as chemotherapy, interferon-α, and splenectomy) have been tried with mixed results.

DIABETES MELLITUS

Diabetes mellitus is a group of disorders characterized by hyperglycemia due either to a deficiency of insulin secretion (type 1 diabetes), a resistance to insulin, or both (type 2 diabetes). Classic symptoms of diabetes include polyuria, polydipsia, and weight loss, but diabetes can be associated with several skin disorders both infectious and noninfectious in etiology.

Clinical Features

Common noninfectious skin findings in diabetics include acanthosis nigricans (AN), skin tags, vitiligo, necrobiosis lipoidica, and diabetic dermopathy. AN presents as hypertrophic, hyperpigmented velvety plaques seen in the body folds, most commonly in the axillae and the posterior neck. AN is generally asymptomatic and is more common in patients with type 2 diabetes, but it can be seen in other diseases that cause insulin resistance, such as acromegaly and Cushing disease. Skin tags, or acrochordons, are another skin manifestation of insulin resistance and 66%–75% of patients with skin tags have diabetes.[44] The skin tags are found most frequently on the eyelids, neck, and axilla. Vitiligo is an autoimmune disorder and, due to similar etiologies, is seen more frequently in type 1 (autoimmune) diabetes. Necrobiosis lipoidica (NL) is a rare but specific skin manifestation of diabetes. It occurs in only 0.3% of all diabetic patients, most of whom are insulin dependent at the time of presentation, and is more common in men.[4] NL consists of distinctive oval or irregularly shaped plaques with red or violaceous borders, central atrophy, and yellow pigmentation, typically occurring on the anterior shins. Up to 35% of these lesions result in ulceration.[4] Diabetic dermopathy, or shin spots, is seen in 40% of diabetic patients and is more common in men and in patients with evidence of other end-organ damage such as retinopathy, neuropathy, or nephropathy. The lesions of diabetic dermopathy begin as groups of red macules on the anterior shins that over time become shallow or depressed and hyperpigmented.

Skin infections are also common in diabetics, occurring in 20%–50% of all diabetic patients, more commonly in patients with type 2 diabetes and in patients with poor glycemic control, and can vary in severity from a simple superficial cellulitis to a necrotizing fasciitis.[44] Patients with poor diabetic control have both higher rates of colonization and higher rates of skin infection with *C. albicans, Staphylococcus* species, and *Streptococcus* species. Women with hyperglycemia and glycosuria frequently complain of recurrent vaginal yeast infections. Elderly diabetics can develop malignant external otitis, an invasive infection of the external auditory canal that typically occurs in immunocompromised patients, and *Pseudomonas aeruginosa* is the causative organism in more than 95% of cases.[45]

Diagnosis

The diagnosis of diabetes can be made one of three ways. The preferred method is the use of a fasting plasma glucose of 126 mg/dL (7.0 mmol/L) after a fast of at least 8 hours. Other acceptable criteria for diagnosing diabetes include symptoms of hyperglycemia (polyuria, polydipsia, weight loss) along with a random plasma glucose greater than or equal to 200 mg/dL (11.1 mmol/L) or an oral glucose tolerance test using a 75-g glucose load with a 2-hour plasma glucose level greater than or equal to 200 mg/dL.[46] The use of hemoglobin A1c for the diagnosis of diabetes is not currently recommended.

On histopathologic examination, acanthosis nigricans lesions appear hyperkeratotic with papillomatosis. The dark color of the lesions is due to the thickness of the superficial epithelium, but there is no change in melanocyte number or melanin content.[47] The lesions of diabetic dermopathy show basement membrane thickening, whereas NL is characterized by a degeneration of collagen with granulomatous inflammation of the subcutaneous tissues and blood vessels.[48,49] The yellow central area of the necrobiotic lesions is believed to be due to the thinning of the dermis, making subcutaneous fat more visible.[50]

Treatment

The treatment of diabetes focuses on normalization of blood glucose levels as well as aggressive management of known complications of diabetes, such as cardiovascular disease. Type 2 diabetes can be treated with oral medications (e.g., secretagogues, biguanides, and thiazolidinediones), with injectable drugs (e.g., exenatide, insulin, or pramlintide), or with a combination of both. Type 1 diabetes, however, must be treated with insulin; sometimes pramlintide is added. Improved glycemic control decreases the incidence of skin infections and delays progression to microvascular disease complications such as retinopathy and nephropathy.

Most of the noninfectious skin manifestations of diabetes are asymptomatic and do not require treatment. Acanthosis nigricans, diabetic dermopathy, and skin tags are generally asymptomatic and require no treatment. If desired, however, skin tags can be removed with laser or shave biopsy, and acanthosis may be ameliorated by weight loss. Necrobiosis lipoidica has no standardized treatment; however, most treatments use some form of glucocorticoid in topical, intralesional, or systemic form.[50]

PORPHYRIA CUTANEA TARDA

Porphyria cutanea tarda (PCT) is the most common of the porphyrias and is caused by a disruption of heme biosynthesis due to decreased activity of the enzyme uroporphyrinogen decarboxylase (UROD), the fifth enzyme in the heme biosynthetic pathway. PCT may be sporadic, inherited, or

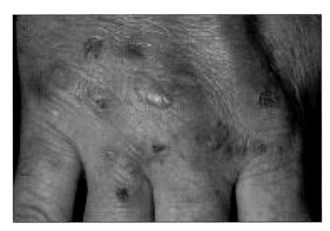

FIGURE 31.3: *Porphyria cutanea tarda with hand lesions presenting as vesicles, bullae, blisters, and sores.*

toxic in origin. Sporadic PCT makes up 80% of cases and is caused by an acquired deficiency of UROD activity in the liver, but not in any other tissues.[51] Twenty percent of cases are inherited as an autosomal dominant trait with low penetrance, and there are reports of PCT developing after exposure to certain chemicals such as fungicides, herbicides, and polyhalogenated hydrocarbons.[52–54] Most cases of PCT are associated with some sort of precipitant. Precipitants for PCT in susceptible individuals include alcohol, estrogens, viral infections (specifically, hepatitis C and human immunodeficiency virus [HIV]), and iron overload.[55] In addition, an association has been found between PCT and the hemochromatosis gene mutation C28Y.[56]

Clinical Features

PCT is characterized by photosensitive cutaneous lesions with increased skin fragility manifesting as vesicles, bullae, blisters, and sores (see Figure 31.3). The bullae rupture easily, crust over, and frequently become secondarily infected. Lesions are seen most commonly on the hands and forearms but can be found on any sun-exposed area and may heal with areas of hypopigmentation or hyperpigmentation or sclerodermatous changes.[57] Milia are frequently seen on the hands and fingers. Increased facial hair is common and is more noticeable in women.

Diagnosis

The characteristic finding of PCT on histopathologic examination is subepidermal bullae with minimal inflammation. The dermal papillae have an undulating base and are referred to as "festooned."[57] Liver biopsy findings include red autofluorescence under a Wood lamp as well as mild steatosis, siderosis, and focal lobular necrosis with pigment-laden macrophages. Birefringent needle-like cytoplasmic inclusions may be present in hepatocytes and are specific for PCT.[58] Serum iron levels are elevated in most patients with PCT. Urine studies will show a marked

increase in urinary uroporphyrins. An analysis of urinary porphyrins showing greater amounts of uroporphyrin versus coproporphyrin is consistent with PCT.[59]

Treatment

General measures in the management of PCT include avoidance of precipitating factors such as alcohol, estrogens, iron, and strong sunlight. If these measures are not sufficient, then phlebotomy is the treatment of choice for PCT. The goal of phlebotomy is to deplete body iron stores and produce a mild iron deficiency. Clinical improvement is typically seen starting 2–3 months after initiation of phlebotomy. If phlebotomy is contraindicated or unsuccessful, then chloroquine is an alternative treatment.[60]

CONGENITAL ICHTHYOSIS AND TYPE II GAUCHER DISEASE

Gaucher disease is the inherited autosomal recessive deficiency of lysosomal glucocerebrosidase. There is significant clinical heterogeneity within Gaucher disease related to the severity of the mutations affecting the glucocerebrosidase gene located at 1q21.[61] The disease is divided into three different types based on phenotypic presentation, including progression to neurologic manifestations. Type I is known as nonneuronopathic Gaucher disease. It is by far the most common type, and patients may remain asymptomatic or may present with cytopenia, hepatosplenomegaly, or bone involvement. Type II, acute neuronopathic Gaucher disease, is uniformly fatal with death typically occurring by early childhood; it is within this type that one can see presentations of congenital ichthyosis, or collodion baby syndrome. Type III, chronic neuronopathic Gaucher disease, presents with variable degrees of systemic involvement plus one or more neurologic manifestations.

Clinical Features

Type II Gaucher disease is the rarest and most severe form of the disease, and it is within this type that one can see presentations of congenital ichthyosis, or collodion baby syndrome. Congenital ichthyosis presents in neonates with red, dry, tight, hyperkeratotic, scaling skin throughout the body, often associated with joint abnormalities and contractures as well as other systemic signs of Gaucher such as hepatosplenomegaly and neurologic changes.[62] There have been case reports of patients presenting with congenital ichthyosis prior to neurologic deterioration that develop in subsequent months.[63]

Diagnosis

The skin changes in type II Gaucher disease are related to the loss of glucocerebrosidase leading to an increased ratio of glucosylceramide to ceramide in the lipid makeup of epidermal cells.[64] Ceramides are major components of the lipid bilayer in the normal epidermis, necessary for permeability barrier homeostasis. A paucity of ceramides leads to an inability to form a competent epidermal barrier, and, as a result, the lipid bilayer has a serrated, abnormal appearance.[64,65] Epidermal hyperplasia and hyperproliferation are also seen and have been hypothesized to be due to stimulation of cellular proliferation by the accumulated glucosylceramide.[66]

Histologic examination of skin from patients with congenital ichthyosis shows dense hyperkeratosis, epidermal hyperplasia, and inflammation. Ultrastructural examination reveals disruptions in the normal lamellar bilayer in the stratum corneum as well as a reversal of the normal ratio of sphingolipids in the stratum corneum, with much higher levels of glucosylceramide to ceramide in the type II Gaucher patients.[62,64] Significantly, these ultrastructural skin changes can be seen in all patients with type II Gaucher disease, whether or not they show skin changes clinically. In addition, these changes are seen only in type II Gaucher disease and are not present in type I or type III. These skin findings, thus, represent a method for early discrimination of type II from the other, milder types of Gaucher disease. Early differentiation of type II disease can aid in appropriate management and counseling, as neither enzyme activity nor genotypic analysis is able to determine the specific type of Gaucher disease.[64]

Treatment

There is, unfortunately, no treatment to halt or reverse the effects of type II Gaucher disease. Placental human glucocerebrosidase and recombinant glucocerebrosidase have been used as enzyme replacement therapy in type I and type III disease and have been effective at treating the visceral and hematologic manifestations, but these treatments have shown disappointing results in type II disease and do not appear to alter the course of neurologic deterioration.[62]

FABRY DISEASE

Fabry disease is a rare, X-linked lysosomal storage disease.[67] Patients with Fabry disease are deficient in the enzyme α-galactosidase A (α-gal A), which leads to the buildup of neutral glycosphingolipids in a range of tissues within the body. The clinical manifestations of Fabry disease are seen primarily in affected hemizygous men and to some extent in heterozygous women. The disease is slowly progressive; affected men have a shortened life expectancy of approximately 50 years, and heterozygous women have a life expectancy of 70 years with the main causes of death being renal failure, heart disease, or stroke.

Clinical Features

The characteristic dermatologic manifestation of Fabry disease is angiokeratoma. These lesions can occur at any time but typically first appear between 5 and 13 years of age.[67,68] The initial lesion is dark red, telangiectatic, and up to 4 mm across and does not blanch with pressure. Overlying hyperkeratosis may or may not be present. Lesions typically occur in symmetrical clusters and are seen most commonly in the areas between the umbilicus and the knees. In men, the first lesions are frequently seen on the scrotum. The number of lesions increases with age in the majority of patients, and the extent of cutaneous involvement correlates with the severity of the systemic manifestations of the disease.[69]

Other cutaneous findings in Fabry disease include telangiectasias, disorders of sweating, decreased body hair, and edema. Telangiectasias are characteristic of Fabry disease but are not specific as they can be seen in several other conditions. The most commonly reported sweating disorders are hypohidrosis or anhydrosis, associated with heat and exercise intolerance; hyperhidrosis has been reported as well.

In addition to cutaneous manifestations, several systemic effects are frequently seen, including multiple cardiac and cardiovascular manifestations such as hypertension, cardiomegaly and stroke, renal failure, neuropathic pain attacks, cataracts, and corneal dystrophy.

Diagnosis

In men, the diagnosis can be made based on the presence of cutaneous angiokeratomas in the setting of a positive family history, specifically of early deaths due to kidney or heart disease. Under light microscopy, angiokeratoma lesions are composed of a thin epidermis, below which the upper dermis is filled with dilated blood-filled vessels.[70] A hyperkeratotic stratum corneum may or may not be present. Further testing will reveal a deficiency of α−gal A in several tissues including serum, tears, and tissue specimens. Lipid inclusions with birefringent "Maltese crosses" as well as fat-laden epithelial cells may be seen in the urine.

In female heterozygotes, symptoms are seen only in a minority of affected patients and tend to be milder. The variability of presentations in female heterozygotes is believed to be due to variations in selective X-chromosome inactivation. Affected women may have α−gal A levels within the normal range, so genetic analysis is recommended.[67]

Treatment

Treatment of Fabry disease has been focused mainly on symptomatic relief up to this point; there is now, however, growing evidence of the effectiveness of enzyme replacement therapy. The mainstay of treatment for angiokeratomas has been the application of various types of laser systems. Recent trials of enzyme replacement therapy with two different preparations of bioengineered enzyme have shown beneficial effects on signs and symptoms such as pain, renal and cardiac complications, and overall quality of life.[71] In addition, enzyme replacement therapy has been shown to clear the deposits of neutral glycosphingolipids from the kidneys, hearts, and skin of patients with Fabry disease.[72]

ZINC DEFICIENCY

Zinc is an essential mineral for humans. It is present in more than 100 metalloenzymes, such as alkaline phosphatase and carbonic anhydrase, and appears to play an important role in protein and carbohydrate metabolism as well as cell proliferation, healing and tissue repair, and growth and development. Zinc is absorbed from the proximal small intestine and is excreted through intestinal and pancreatic secretions. It is also present in human breast milk.

Zinc deficiency can be either acquired or inherited. The inherited congenital form is known as acrodermatitis enteropathica (AE) and is a rare autosomal recessive partial defect in zinc absorption occurring in approximately 1 in 500,000 children.[73] In AE, patients present in infancy, within days if the infant is bottle fed and at the time of weaning if breast fed. Most acquired forms of zinc deficiency, however, do not present until later in development. Acquired zinc deficiency can be caused by inadequate dietary intake of zinc or from malabsorption of zinc, usually due to diseases such as celiac sprue, Crohn disease, cystic fibrosis, or short gut syndrome. Dietary zinc deficiency is common in certain parts of Southeast Asia and sub-Saharan Africa, but it is rare in the developed world. There are certain subpopulations, however, that are at increased risk; these include vegetarians, alcoholics, premature infants, and malnourished persons.[74]

Clinical Features

The dermatitis seen in zinc deficiency is similar in both the acquired and inherited forms and is also largely indistinguishable from the rash seen in glucagonoma, vitamin B3 (niacin) deficiency, and in other vitamin deficiencies. The dermatitis is characterized by eczematous, erythematous scaly plaques over the acral and periorificial areas. These plaques may become vesicular, bullous, or desquamative. The skin can become secondarily infected, typically with *C. albicans*. Other commonly seen features include angular cheilitis, stomatitis, and nail changes such as onychodystrophy, onycholysis, and paronychia.[75] If left untreated, these patients will go on to develop generalized alopecia as well as diarrhea.[76] Other possible findings are photophobia, irritability, loss of appetite, poor wound healing, growth retardation, and hypogonadism.

Diagnosis

Histopathologic examination of skin biopsy specimens is nonspecific and, again, indistinguishable from other vitamin deficiency dermatoses and glucagonoma. The most common findings are parakeratosis and necrolysis, the cytoplasmic pallor, vacuolization, and ballooning degeneration also seen in the NME of glucagonoma.[73] Diagnosis instead must be based on clinical suspicion and confirmed by laboratory testing. Plasma zinc level is the most commonly used test, although because only 0.1% of the body's total zinc stores is manifested in plasma zinc, it is an imperfect measure of total body zinc. A fasting morning plasma zinc level less than 50 μg/dL is suggestive of zinc deficiency. Other laboratory tests to support the diagnosis include a low level of serum alkaline phosphatase, a zinc-dependent metalloenzyme, and a low level of urinary zinc excretion.[77–79]

Treatment

Treatment of zinc deficiency is with zinc supplementation. It is important to distinguish acquired zinc deficiencies from AE because acquired deficiencies require only limited treatment durations, whereas inherited AE requires lifelong treatment. In AE, the recommended initial dosing starts at 3–10 mg/kg/d and maintenance dosing of 1–2 mg/kg/d, whereas the recommended dose for dietary deficiency is lower, at approximately 0.5–1 mg/kg/d.[73,80] Zinc can be administered in many preparations, but zinc sulfate appears to be the best tolerated.[75] Clinical improvement is typically seen within days to weeks of initiating zinc replacement therapy,[81] often long before a change in the plasma zinc levels can be seen. The most common side effect of zinc supplementation is GI irritation with resultant symptoms of nausea, vomiting, and gastric hemorrhage. Zinc has also been implicated in impaired copper absorption, so copper serum levels must be monitored as well in these patients.

VITAMIN DEFICIENCY

Vitamin A

Vitamin A is a fat-soluble vitamin found in meats, dairy products, and certain vegetables (e.g., carrots, spinach, kale, peas, cantaloupe). Because of the abundance of vitamin A in the food supply, deficiency of vitamin A is quite rare in Western countries, but is common in developing countries where malnutrition is prevalent. It also can be seen in patients with anorexia nervosa; in those with fat malabsorption syndromes, such as Crohn disease, celiac disease, pancreatic insufficiency, biliary disease, and cystic fibrosis; and in persons who have had GI surgery.[82–84]

Clinical Features. Deficiency of vitamin A typically presents with ocular findings, such as conjunctival xerosis, white patches on the sclera (known as Bitot spots), and night blindness, but it also can present with cognitive disturbances or growth failure.[82] Cutaneous manifestations of vitamin A deficiency may overlap with features of other nutritional deficiencies. The most common finding is phrynoderma, a form of follicular hyperkeratosis characterized by hyperkeratotic papules on the extensor surfaces of the limbs, shoulders, and buttocks. These papules tend to coalesce to form plaques, and, in severe phrynoderma, they can cover the entire body.[83] Phrynoderma was previously thought to result exclusively from vitamin A deficiency, but studies in recent years have associated the disease with deficiencies in B vitamins, vitamin E, essential fatty acids, and general malnutrition.[83–86]

Diagnosis and Treatment. Diagnosis of vitamin A deficiency is typically made by identification of typical ocular findings and confirmed by laboratory testing of serum vitamin A levels. Symptoms of deficiency typically resolve with vitamin A replacement. Phrynoderma traditionally has been treated with cod liver oil (which contains vitamin A),[83] and more recently treatment with safflower oil, vitamin B complex, and vitamin E have been associated with improvement in phrynoderma as well as visual symptoms.[86]

Riboflavin (Vitamin B₂)

Riboflavin deficiency is rare in developed countries, due to the abundance of this water-soluble vitamin in the food supply. Riboflavin is found in meats, fish, green leafy vegetables, dairy products, and fortified cereals. Riboflavin deficiency is typically seen in malnutrition states, and in Western countries it can be seen in liver disease and in infants treated with phototherapy for neonatal jaundice.[82,84]

Clinical Features. Typical cutaneous features of riboflavin deficiency involve the mucous membranes and frequently overlap with signs and symptoms of other vitamin deficiencies. Cutaneous manifestations of chronic deficiency include scaling of the lips, angular stomatitis, glossitis, monilial intertrigo, and scrotal dermatitis.[82,84,87]

Diagnosis and Treatment. Diagnosis can be made with plasma riboflavin concentration or erythrocyte glutathione reductase activity.[82,84] As other nutritional deficiencies may coexist, however, the diagnosis of riboflavin deficiency is commonly made based on clinical suspicion and confirmed by rapid improvement in symptoms and signs after repletion of riboflavin stores. Replacement of riboflavin is given as 1 mg/d in infants and 3 mg/d in children.[82]

Niacin (Vitamin B₃)

Similar to riboflavin, niacin is found in meats, dairy products, fortified cereals, and legumes, and is synthesized in the body from dietary tryptophan in the setting of vitamins B₁ and B₆.[83] In developed countries, niacin deficiency is typically seen in malabsorption syndromes, such as Crohn disease, anorexia nervosa, HIV, carcinoid syndrome, Hartnup syndrome, malnutrition secondary to alcoholism, and with use of medications such as isoniazid, 5-fluorouracil, and 6-mercaptopurine.[82,83]

Clinical Features. The clinical manifestation of niacin deficiency is pellagra. This is classically described in terms of the "three Ds": dermatitis, diarrhea, and dementia. The rash of pellagra is typically symmetric and in areas of sun exposure or friction. It tends to be erythematous and then hyperpigmented and scaly. A classic finding is Casal necklace – a scaling, hyperpigmented rash around the neck and chest. Bullous and depigmenting lesions also have been described,[83] as well as glossitis, stomatitis, and a facial rash with a butterfly distribution.[82]

Diagnosis and Treatment. Diagnosis of niacin deficiency is typically made after rapid improvement in clinical features with niacin supplementation, recommended at 50–100 mg/d.

Vitamin B₆ (Pyridoxine)

Vitamin B₆, or pyridoxine, is a water-soluble vitamin found in meats, bananass, and vegetables such as beans and potatoes. Deficiency in Western countries is typically seen in malnourished patients, chronic alcoholics, and patients taking isoniazid, penicillamine, or hydralazine.[82]

Clinical Features. Pyridoxine deficiency manifests as perioral and perianal skin changes similar to those seen in vitamin B₂ or zinc deficiency, and may resemble seborrheic dermatitis, stomatitis, or glossitis. GI symptoms and neurologic symptoms (such as weakness, confusion, or peripheral neuropathy) may be seen as well.[82,84] Blepharoconjunctivitis and atrophic tongue also have been described.[88]

Diagnosis and Treatment. Similar to that of other water-soluble vitamins, diagnosis can be made by serum levels, but may be made more commonly by prompt resolution of symptoms after treatment.

Vitamin C

Vitamin C, or ascorbic acid, is a water-soluble vitamin found in many citrus fruits, vegetables, and organ meats. It is obtained exclusively in the diet, as humans are unable to synthesize vitamin C. Like the deficiencies of other water-soluble vitamins, vitamin C deficiency is rare in developed countries, and is found in conditions of general malnutrition, such as in patients with alcoholism and/or drug addiction and in rare socially isolated elderly patients.

TABLE 31.2: Toxicity of Commonly Used Vitamins

Vitamin	Clinical features of vitamin toxicity	Minimum daily dose associated with adverse effect[93]
Vitamin A	Liver toxicity, cirrhosis, birth defects, benign intracranial hypertension[93,94]	Cirrhosis: 25,000 IU Birth defects: 10,000 IU
Niacin (B₃)	Flushing, nausea, vomiting, diarrhea, liver toxicity, fulminant hepatic failure (at least one case report)[93]	Flushing/gastrointestinal side effects: 10 mg Hepatotoxicity reported with 500 mg/d, but generally seen in doses >1000 mg/d
Vitamin B₆	Sensory neuropathy, photoallergic drug rash, acneiform rash, contact dermatitis[93,95–97]	300 mg
Vitamin C	Nausea, abdominal cramping, diarrhea; reports of increased incidence of oxalate kidney stones have not been substantiated[93,98,99]	1000 mg

Clinical Features. Deficiency of vitamin C causes the clinical entity of scurvy, with several classic cutaneous findings: follicular hyperkeratosis, perifollicular hemorrhages, and corkscrew-like, coiled hairs embedded in the hyperkeratotic follicular material. Also seen are petechiae and ecchymoses in dependent and friction-prone areas and swollen, inflamed gums (hemorrhagic hyperplastic gingivitis). Also seen in chronic vitamin C deficiency is a woody edema of the legs.[89–91]

Diagnosis and Treatment. Serum levels of ascorbic acid fall to almost zero rapidly after failing to meet sufficient dietary requirements, limiting the diagnostic value of serum testing. Diagnosis is typically made on clinical grounds, such as with a patient having signs of scurvy, or with improvement of symptoms with supplementation of vitamin C. In addition to its role in treatment of clinical deficiency, vitamin C, along with zinc and arginine, has been associated with improvement in the treatment of pressure ulcers.[92]

Vitamin K

Vitamin K is a fat-soluble vitamin found in green leafy vegetables and legumes. It is also synthesized by bacteria in the digestive tract. Deficiency is seen in malabsorptive states, such as Crohn disease, pancreatic insufficiency, and with medications such as antibiotics, anticonvulsants, isoniazid, rifampin, and cholestyramine.[89] It is also seen in patients with liver disease and in patients with poor diet.

Clinical Features. Deficiency of vitamin K is manifested by coagulopathy caused by deficiency of vitamin K–dependent clotting factors II, VII, IX, and X. As a result, patients with deficiency in vitamin K present with coagulopathy, with easy bruising, ecchymoses, or bleeding from the GI or genitourinary tract, or with excessive bleeding after injury, trauma, or surgery.

Diagnosis and Treatment. Diagnosis is made with the appropriate history and clinical findings, along with prolonged prothrombin time. The coagulopathy of vitamin K deficiency can be corrected with oral or subcutaneous supplementation. Cases with severe bleeding may require parenteral vitamin K supplementation and possibly transfusion of fresh frozen plasma.

VITAMIN TOXICITY

Potentially toxic levels of vitamins can be achieved easily in people who take very high potency vitamins. Water-soluble vitamins have an extraordinarily broad therapeutic ratio, with toxicity occurring only at doses thousands of times the daily value. Fat-soluble vitamins are generally more toxic than water-soluble vitamins. Table 31.2 summarizes some important points related to some vitamin toxicities.

REFERENCES

1. Nieman LK, Turner MLC. Addison's disease. Clin Dermatol. 2006; 24:276–80.
2. Dunlop D. Eighty-six cases of Addison's disease. BMJ. 1963; 5362:887–91.
3. Kim SS, Brody KH. Dehydroepiandrosterone replacement in Addison's disease. Eur J Obstet Gynecol Reprod Biol. 2001; 97:96–7.
4. Jabbour SA. Cutaneous manifestations of endocrine disorders: a guide for dermatologists. Am J Clin Dermatol. 2003; 4(5):315–31.
5. Grinspoon SK, Biller BM. Laboratory assessment of adrenal insufficiency. J Clin Endocrinol Metab. 1994; 79:923–31.
6. Oelkers W, L'age M. Control of mineralocorticoid substitution in Addison's disease by plasma renin measurement. Klin Wochenschr.1976; 54:607–12.
7. Libè R, Barbetta L, Dall'Asta C, et al. Effects of dehydroepiandrosterone (DHEA) supplementation on hormonal, metabolic and behavioral status in patients with hypoadrenalism. J Endocrinol Invest. 2004; 27:736–41.

8. Parker CM, Hanke CW, Madura JA, Liss EC. Glucagonoma syndrome: case report and literature review. J Dermatol Surg Oncol. 1984; 10:884–9.

9. Chastain MA. The glucagonoma syndrome: a review of its features and discussion of new perspectives. Am J Med Sci. 2001; 321:306–20.

10. Stone SP, Buescher LS. Life-threatening paraneoplastic cutaneous syndromes. Clin Dermatol. 2005; 23(3):301–6.

11. Tierny EP, Badger J. Etiology and pathogenesis of necrolytic migratory erythema: review of the literature. Med Gen Med. 2004; 6:4–13.

12. Marinkovich MP, Botella R, Datloff J, Sangueza OP. Necrolytic migratory erythema without glucagonoma in patients with liver disease. J Am Acad Dermatol. 1995; 32: 604–9.

13. Smith AP, Doolas A, Staren ED. Rapid resolution of necrolytic migratory erythema after glucagonoma resection. J Surg Oncol. 1996; 61:306–9.

14. Wynik D, Hammond PJ, Bloom SR. The glucagonoma syndrome. Clin Dermatol. 1993; 11:93–7.

15. Tomssetti P, Migliori M, Gullo, L. Slow-release lanreotide treatment in endocrine gastrointestinal tumors. Am J Gastroenterol. 1998; 93:1468–71.

16. Altimari AF, Bhoopalam N, O'Dorsio T, et al. Use of a somatostatin analog (SMS 201–995) in the glucagonoma syndrome. Surgery. 1986; 100:989–96.

17. Appetecchia M, Ferretti E, Carducci M, et al. Malignant glucagonoma. New options of treatment. J Exp Clin Cancer Res. 2006; 25:135–9.

18. Shepherd ME, Raimer SS, Tyring SK, et al. Treatment of necrolytic migratory erythema in glucagonoma syndrome. J Am Acad Dermatol. 1991; 25:925–8.

19. Ai J, Leonhardt JM, Heymann WR. Autoimmune thyroid diseases: etiology, pathogenesis, and dermatologic manifestations. J Am Acad Dermatol. 2003; 48:641–62.

20. Fatourechi V, Bartley GB, Eghbali-Fatourechi GZ, et al. Graves' dermopathy and acropachy are markers of severe Graves' ophthalmopathy. Thyroid. 2003; 13:1141–4.

21. Shong YK, Kim JA. Vitiligo in autoimmune thyroid disease. Thyroidology. 1991; 3:89–91.

22. Ross DS. Serum thyroid-stimulating hormone measurement for assessment of thyroid function and disease. Endocrinol Metab Clin North Am. 2001; 30:245–64.

23. Cooper DS. Antithyroid drugs. N Engl J Med. 2005; 352:905–17.

24. Lely AJ, Herder WW. Carcinoid syndrome: diagnosis and medical management. Arq Bras Endocrinol Metab. 2005; 49:850–60.

25. Jabbour SA, Davidovici BB, Wolf R. Rare syndromes. Clin Dermatol. 2006; 24:299–316.

26. Modlin IM, Kidd M, Latich I, et al. Current status of gastrointestinal carcinoids. Gastroenterology. 2005; 128:1717–51.

27. Kulke MH, Mayer RJ. Medical progress: carcinoid tumors. N Engl J Med. 1999; 340:858–68.

28. Bell HK, Poston GJ, Vora J, Wilson NJ. Cutaneous manifestations of the malignant carcinoid syndrome. Br J Dermatol. 2005; 152:71–5.

29. Sanduleanu S, De Bruïne A, Stridsberg M, et al. Serum chromogranin A as a screening test for gastric enterochromaffin-like cell hyperplasia during acid-suppressive therapy. Eur J Clin Invest. 2001; 31:802–11.

30. Carling RS, Degg TJ, Allen KR, et al. Evaluation of whole blood serotonin and plasma and urine 5-hydroxyindole acetic acid in diagnosis of carcinoid disease. Ann Clin Biochem. 2002; 39:577–82.

31. Modlin IM, Latich I, Zikusoka M, et al. Gastrointestinal carcinoids: the evolution of diagnostic strategies. J Clin Gastroenterol. 2006; 40:572–82.

32. Caplin ME, Buscombe JR, Hilson AJ, et al. Carcinoid tumor. Lancet. 1998; 352:799–805.

33. Kvols LK, Moertel CG, O'Connell MJ, et al. Treatment of the malignant carcinoid syndrome. Evaluation of a long-acting somatostatin analogue. N Engl J Med. 1986; 315:663–6.

34. Brockow K. Urticaria pigmentosa. Immunol Allergy Clin N Am. 2004; 24:287–316.

35. Escribano L, Akin C, Castells M, et al. Mastocytosis: current concepts in diagnosis and treatment. Ann Hematol. 2002; 81:677–90.

36. Soter NA. Mastocytosis and the skin. Hematol Oncol Clin North Am. 2000; 14:537–55.

37. Horny HP, Sillaber C, Menke D, et al. Diagnostic value of immunostaining for tryptase in patients with mastocytosis. Am J Surg Pathol. 1998; 22:1132–40.

38. Valent P, Horny HP, Escribano L, et al. Diagnostic criteria and classification of mastocytosis: a consensus proposal. Leuk Res. 2001; 25:603–25.

39. Valent P, Akin C, Escribano L, et al. Standards and standardization in mastocytosis: consensus statements on diagnostics, treatment recommendations and response criteria. Eur J Clin Invest. 2007; 37:435–53.

40. Schwartz LB, Sakai K, Bradford TR, et al. The alpha form of human tryptase is the predominant type present in blood at baseline in normal subjects and is elevated in those with systemic mastocytosis. J Clin Invest. 1995; 96:2702–10.

41. Keyzer JJ, de Monchy JG, van Doormaal JJ, van Voorst Vader PC. Improved diagnosis of mastocytosis by measurement of urinary histamine metabolites. N Engl J Med. 1983; 309:1603–5.

42. Schwartz LB. Clinical utility of tryptase levels in systemic mastocytosis and associated hematologic disorders. Leuk Res. 2001; 25:553–62.

43. Vella Briffa D, Eady RA, James MP, et al. Photochemotherapy (PUVA) in the treatment of urticaria pigmentosa. Br J Dermatol. 1983; 109:67–75.

44. Ahmed I, Goldstein, B. Diabetes mellitus. Clin Dermatol. 2006; 24:237–46.

45. Grandis JR, Branstetter BF, Yu VL. The changing face of malignant (necrotizing) external otitis: clinical, radiological, and anatomic correlations. Lancet Infect Dis. 2004; 4:34–9.

46. American Diabetes Association.. Clinical practice recommendations 2008. Diabetes Care. 2008; 31:s1–s110.

47. Hermanns-Le T, Scheen A, Pierard GE. Acanthosis nigricans associated with insulin resistance: pathophysiology and management. Am J Clin Dermatol. 2004; 5:199–203.

48. Fisher ER, Danowski TS. Histologic, histochemical, and electron microscopic features of the shin spots of diabetes mellitus. Am J Clin Pathol. 1968; 50:547–54.

49. Iwasaki T, Kahama T, Houjou S, et al. Diabetic scleroderma and scleroderma-like changes in a patient with maturity onset type diabetes of young people. Dermatology. 1994; 188:228–31.
50. Petzelbauer P, Wolff K, Tappeiner G. Necrobiosis lipoidica: treatment with systemic corticosteroids. Br J Dermatol. 1992; 126:542–5.
51. Elder GH. Porphyria cutanea tarda. Semin Liver Dis. 1998; 18:67–75.
52. Elder GH, Roberts AG, de Salamanca RE. Genetics and pathogenesis of human uroporphyrinogen decarboxylase defects. Clin Biochem. 1989; 22:163–8.
53. Cripps DJ, Peters HA, Gocman A, Dogramici I. Porphyria turcica due to hexachlorobenzene: a 20–30 year follow-up study on 204 patients. Br J Dermatol. 1984; 111:413–22.
54. Bleiberg J, Wallen M, Brodkin R, Applebaum IL. Industrially acquired porphyria. Arch Dermatol. 1964; 80:793–7.
55. Bleasel NR, Varigos GA. Porphyria cutanea tarda. Australas J Dermatol. 2000; 41:197–206.
56. Fodinger M, Sunder-Plassmann G. Inherited disorders of iron metabolism. Kidney Int Suppl. 1999; 69:S22–34.
57. Lambrecht RW, Thapar M, Bonkovsky HL. Genetic aspects of porphyria cutanea tarda. Semin Liver Dis. 2007; 27:99–108.
58. Cortes JM, Oliva H, Paradinas FJ, Hernandez-Guio C. The pathology of the liver in porphyria cutanea tarda. Histopathology. 1980; 4:471–85.
59. Badiu C, Cristofor D, Voicu D, Coculescu M. Diagnostic traps in porphyria: case report and literature review. Rev Med Chir Soc Med Nat Iasi. 2004; 108:584–91.
60. Kordac V, Jirsa M, Kotal P, et al. Agents affecting porphyrin formation and secretion: implications for porphyria cutanea treatment. Semin Hematol. 1989; 26:16–23.
61. Finn LS, Zhang M, Chen SH, Scott CR. Severe type II Gaucher disease with ichthyosis, arthrogryposis and neuronal apoptosis: molecular and pathological analyses. Am J Med Genet. 2000; 91:222–6.
62. Tayebi N, Stone DL, Sidransky E. Type 2 Gaucher disease: an expanding phenotype. Mol Genet Metab. 1999; 68:209–19.
63. Fujimoto A, Tayebi N, Sidransky E. Congenital ichthyosis preceding neurologic symptoms in two siblings with type 2 Gaucher disease. Am J Med Genet. 1995; 59:356–68.
64. Sidransky E, Fartasch M, Lee RE, et al. Epidermal abnormalities may distinguish type 2 from type 1 and type 3 of Gaucher disease. Pediatr Res. 1996; 39:134–41.
65. Elias PM, Williams ML, Holleran WM, et al. Pathogenesis of permeability barrier abnormalities in the ichthyoses: inherited disorders of lipid metabolism. J Lipid Res. 2008; 49:697–714.
66. Marsh NL, Elias PM, Holleran WM. Glucosylceramides stimulate murine epidermal hyperproliferation. J Clin Invest. 1995; 95:2903–9.
67. Mohrenschlager M, Braun-Falco M, Ring J, Abeck D. Fabry disease: recognition and management of cutaneous manifestations. Am J Clin Dermatol. 2003; 4:189–96.
68. Hurwitz S. Clinical pediatric dermatology. 2nd ed. Philadelphia: WB Saunders; 1993.
69. Orteu CH, Jansen T, Lidove O, et al. Fabry disease and the skin: data from FOS, the Fabry outcome survey. Br J Dermatol. 2007; 157:331–7.
70. Frost P, Tamala Y, Spaeth GL. Fabry's disease: glycolipid lipidosis. Histochemical and electron microscopic studies of two cases. Am J Med. 1966; 40:618–27.
71. Schiffman R, Kopp JB, Austin HA, et al. Enzyme replacement therapy in Fabry disease. JAMA. 2001; 285:2743–9.
72. Eng CM, Guffon N, Wilcox WR, et al. Safety and efficacy of recombinant human alpha-galactosidase A–replacement therapy in Fabry's disease. N Engl J Med. 2001; 345:9–16.
73. Maverakis E, Fung MA, Lynch PJ, et al. Acrodermatitis enteropathica and an overview of zinc metabolism. J Am Acad Dermatol. 2007; 56:116–24.
74. Prasad AS. Discovery of human zinc deficiency and studies in an experimental human model. Am J Clin Nutr. 1991; 53:403–12.
75. Perafan-Riveros C, Franca LF, Alves AC, Sanches JA. Acrodermatitis enteropathica: case report and review of the literature. Pediatr Dermatol. 2002; 19(5):426–31.
76. Dillaha CJ, Lorincz AL. Enteropathic acrodermatitis (Danbolt): successful treatment with diodoquin (diiodohydroxyquinoline). AMA Arch Dermatol Syphilol. 1953; 67:324–6.
77. Danks DM. Diagnosis of trace metal deficiency–with emphasis on copper and zinc. Am J Clin Nutr. 1981; 34:278–80.
78. Naber TH, Baadenhuysen H, Jansen JB, et al. Serum alkaline phosphatase activity during zinc deficiency and long-term inflammatory stress. Clin Chim Acta. 1996; 249:109–27.
79. Sandstrom B, Cederblad A, Lindblad BS, Lonnerdal B. Acrodermatitis enteropathica, zinc metabolism, copper status, and immune function. Arch Pediatr Adolesc Med. 1994; 148:980–5.
80. Mancini AJ, Tunnessen WW. Picture of the month. Acrodermatitis enteropathica-like rash in a breast-fed, full-term infant with zinc deficiency. Arch Pediatr Adolesc Med. 1998; 152:1239–40.
81. Neldner KH, Hambidge KM. Zinc therapy of acrodermatitis enteropathica. N Engl J Med. 1975; 292:879–82.
82. Prendiville JS, Manfredi LN. Skin signs of nutritional disorders. Semin Dermatol. 1992; 11:88–97.
83. Heath ML, Sidbury R. Cutaneous manifestations of nutritional deficiency. Curr Opin Pediatr. 2006; 18:417–22.
84. Barthelemy H, Chouvet B, Cambazard F. Skin and mucosal manifestations in vitamin deficiency. J Am Acad Dermatol. 1986; 15:1263–74.
85. Bleasel NR, Stapleton KM, Lee MS, Sullivan J. Vitamin A deficiency phrynoderma: due to malabsorption and inadequate diet. J Am Acad Dermatol. 1999; 41:322–4.
86. Maronn M, Allen DM, Esterly NB. Phrynoderma: a manifestation of vitamin A deficiency? . . . the rest of the story. Pediatric Dermatol. 2005; 22:60–3.
87. Roe DA. Riboflavin deficiency: mucocutaneous signs of acute and chronic deficiency. Semin Dermatol. 1991; 10:293–5.
88. Friedli A, Saurat J. Images in clinical medicine. Oculo-orogenital syndrome–a deficiency of vitamins B_2 and B_6. N Engl J Med. 2004; 350:1130.
89. Goskowicz M, Eichenfield LF. Cutaneous findings of nutritional deficiencies in children. Curr Opin Pediatr. 1993; 5:441–5.

90. Price NM. Vitamin C deficiency. Cutis. 1980; 26:375–7.

91. Catalano PM. Vitamin C. Arch Dermatol. 1971; 103: 537–9.

92. Frias Soriano L, Lage Vazquez MA, Maristany CP, Xandri Graupera JM, Wouters-Wesseling W, Wagenaar L. The effectiveness of oral nutritional supplementation in the healing of pressure ulcers. J Wound Care. 2004; 13:319–22.

93. Hathcock JN. Vitamins and minerals: efficacy and safety. Am J Clin Nutr. 1997; 66:427–37.

94. Lombaert A, Carton H. Benign intracranial hypertension due to A-hypervitaminosis in adults and adolescents. Eur Neurol. 1976; 14:340–50.

95. Tanaka M, Niizeki H, Shimizu S, Miyakawa S. Photoallergic drug eruption due to pyridoxine hydrochloride. J Dermatol. 1996; 23:708–9.

96. Sherertz EF. Acneiform eruption due to "megadose" vitamins B6 and B12. Cutis. 1991; 48:119–20.

97. Camarasa JG, Serra-Baldrich E, Lluch M. Contact allergy to vitamin B6. Contact Dermatitis. 1990; 23:115.

98. Curhan GC, Willett WC, Rimm EB, Stampfer MJ. A prospective study of the intake of vitamins C and B6 and the risk of kidney stones in men. J Urol. 1996; 155:1847–51.

99. Diplock AT. Safety of antioxidant vitamins and beta-carotene. Am J Clin Nutr. 1995; 62(6 Suppl):1510S–1516S.

CHAPTER 32

Emergency Management of Skin Torture and Self-Inflicted Dermatoses

Daniel H. Parish

Hirak B. Routh

Kazal R. Bhowmik

Kishore Kumar

TORTURE WRIT broadly is the intentional infliction of physical or psychological pain.[1] The term includes a wide variety of conduct ranging from that instigated by authorities to gain confessions or information to that caused by private actors in the course of domestic abuse or in the intimidation of neighbors or disliked ethnic or religious minorities. Most legal definitions of torture, however, restrict its definition by requiring an element of state action. Thus, for example, the United Nations Convention against Torture defines it as:

> **any act by which severe pain or suffering, whether physical or mental, is intentionally inflicted on a person for such purposes as obtaining from him or a third person information or a confession, punishing him for an act he or a third person has committed or is suspected of having committed, or intimidating or coercing him or a third person, or for any reason based on discrimination of any kind, when such pain or suffering is inflicted by or at the instigation of or with the consent or acquiescence of a public official or other person acting in an official capacity. It does not include pain or suffering arising only from, inherent in or incidental to lawful sanctions.[2]**

Similarly, the damage done by torture and the evidence of the same range widely. On the one hand, some persons torturing others seek to injure their victims in a way that is highly visible and consequently damaging to the victim's psyche (and serve as a threat to anyone who sees the victim). Cases in which perpetrators burn women chemically or thermally for failing to accept proposals or in defense of a family's "honor" will fall into this category. Such injuries can also lead to secondary complications such as skin infection and scar-related contractures. On the other hand, other forms of torture, although extremely painful

and devastating to the victim, are expressly designed to leave no visible mark on the skin whatsoever, in large part to allow the torturer to deny the torture. Without in any way diminishing the severity, horror, and tragedy of the latter, this chapter focuses on the former in the context of addressing such injuries in an emergency situation.

CLINICAL AND LABORATORY AIDS REQUIRED FOR DIAGNOSIS

In most cases that will fall under the rubric of torture, an especially detailed dermatologic history should be performed, as the exact location and description of wounds and scars can prove significant both for treatment and further legal proceedings. Any history of skin disease and lesions that predate the described torture should be noted. Lesions more consistent with torture will include those that are asymmetric, irregular linear lesions and those with well-demarcated borders.[3] All of this should be directed, in addition to providing treatment, to determining whether the physical findings on examination are consistent with a history of torture as presented.[4] A thorough examination of all skin areas should be conducted to the extent permitted, as a patient may have passed out during an episode of torture and not even know all affected portions of his or her body. It should be noted that torture, from the point of view of skin damage, will tend to be most extensive when the torturer did not expect that the patient would be leaving custody any time soon, if ever, and less so if a known court date or its equivalent had to be kept in the near future.[5] The exception, of course, lies in those cases where the visible damage is meant to frighten others or permanently scar the victim. Additionally, although one might suspect that a person in the position of potential asylum seeker or victim seeking redress might seek to overattribute every scar to torture, at least one physician who treats asylum candidates has noticed the exact opposite and that such victims tend to minimize rather than exaggerate.[5] Patients who have been brutalized and shamed may also be reluctant to permit full examinations, and although the wishes of the patient must ultimately be respected, the limitations of such an examination need to be noted.

The type of torture inflicted is also likely dependent upon the country or circumstances in which the torture took place. Although no fully accurate statistics of torture methods exist, one study found, for example, that electrical burns were extremely common in Bangladesh but not present in Iran, whereas foot beatings were the rule in Bangladesh and Syria but largely absent in Peru and Uganda.[6] A study of Sri Lankan victims showed that torturers beat nearly all victims with blunt weapons and burned 57% with cigarettes, whereas chemical and electrical burns, for example, were far less frequent.[7] The point is, however, that the examiner may detect patterns and injury based on the country or location in which the torture occurred.

Probably the most common form of injury in torture is that from blunt trauma, be it from stick, club, rod, or fist. Danielsen and Rasmussen[3] provide an excellent review of the consequences and manifestations of this form of torture. From the dermatologic perspective, such beatings may result in lacerations, abrasions, ecchymoses, and edema, although it may be rare for a torture victim to present with the immediate aftereffects of such trauma. Consequently, unless a wound reaches full thickness, there may well be little evidence of the trauma at the time the patient is brought to medical attention.[8] As is the case with suspected domestic abuse, it may be necessary to evaluate and document the trauma to the extent necessary to distinguish trauma from an accidental fall or other injury from more wanton and intentional violence (e.g., the custodial claim that the victim "simply fell" on his way out of the police car or "tripped" on his way into the interrogation room and hit his head on the table). Scars produced here will often appear nonspecific, although linearly patterned, hyperpigmented scars, such as from trauma from whippings or beatings with rods, may point strongly toward torture. Similarly, the tight binding of a victim around his or her arms or legs may produce characteristic linear scarring around the arms and ankles. In evaluating damage from possible blunt force with respect to scars, it must be kept in mind that a huge variety of causes can produce scarring throughout the body, from accidents at home and work and on playing fields to acne to earlier infections to stretch marks to vaccinations to prior surgery to ritual wounds, and although many of these scars are easily distinguished, it is not always the case; it is hard to tell if a kick to the legs came from torture or a soccer tackle.

The practice of bastinado (also known as falaka or falanga), the systematic beating of the feet, qualifies as a subset of blunt trauma and is another common torture with occasional dermatologic implications.[6] The practice is common among torturers, probably because it is easy to

carry out, is exquisitely painful, and generally produces little visible injury; nonetheless, above and beyond the pain of walking due to trauma to the soles, cases of atraumatic necrosis of the toes and necrotic ulcers on the feet also have been reported. The necrosis is, in part, a consequence of the damage to the subcutaneous tissue pads of the feet that can no longer cushion them while a patient is walking or standing.[4,9]

Moving along on the realm of blunt trauma, torturers will also often crush or remove nails, both because of the terrible pain such damage inflicts and because of the relatively minimal damage to the rest of the body. The consequence of such damage, after it heals, is a damaged nail bed that produces distorted nail growth, although such changes are not easy to distinguish from general nail trauma.[5] A differential of such damage may include, for example, psoriatic nail disease.

The various forms of burning – be they thermal, chemical, or electrical – are the most likely types of torture to produce skin damage and changes. Direct application of heat with a metal rod will tend to cause a brand, resulting in a full-thickness burn that demonstrates the shape of the object that caused the damage, with a scar forming in that shape.

Cigarette burns are likely the most common source of skin damage from burning. They follow the damage patterns of burns on any scale, ranging from superficial burns akin to moderate sun damage to full-thickness burns of the dermis and epidermis, albeit in circular patterns of 5–20 mm in diameter.[10] The damage caused will generally depend on the length of time the cigarette is applied to the skin, and may or may not be accompanied by a blister. The time needed to achieve the damage of a full-thickness burn is longer than the reflex time for withdrawal, indicating that such burns should be accompanied by a story of the affected body part being held in place while the burn was inflicted. Such injuries will generally heal in weeks to months, depending on the depth of injury, but are at risk for secondary infection. Cigarette burns inflicted in the course of torture are more likely to be on surfaces of the body visible to the victim, as no small portion of the pain and trauma from such burns comes from witnessing the event. Torturers also often burn victims this way in tight patterns as opposed to haphazard and irregular burns.[5,10] A differential diagnosis, depending on the case, may include impetigo, abscess formation, and pyoderma gangrenosum.

Chemical burns are an invidious form of torture, frequently associated with attempted disfigurement of a woman for refusal to marry or for some supposed disgrace visited on her family.[11] Such torture has been reported in India, Bangladesh (Figures 32.1–32.8), and Uganda, where sulfuric acid is the most common agent. In most cases, the face is involved, as the goal of the torture is, in no small part, to render the victim permanently disfigured, in order both to render her socially unacceptable and to let the victim

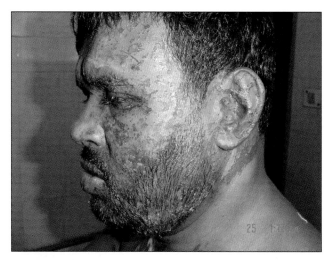

FIGURE 32.1: Domestic violence manifested by acid burns due to 50% sulfuric acid being thrown on the victim.

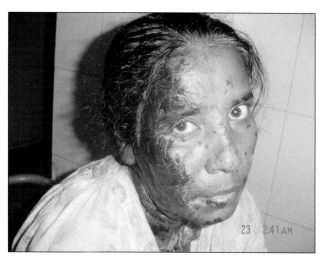

FIGURE 32.4: Domestic violence manifested by acid burns due to 50% sulfuric acid being thrown on the victim.

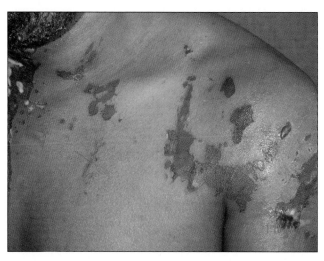

FIGURE 32.2: Domestic violence manifested by acid burns due to 50% sulfuric acid being thrown on the victim.

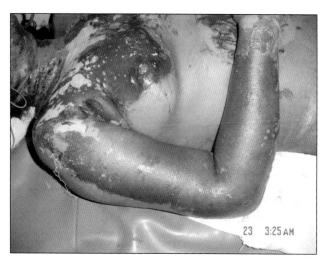

FIGURE 32.5: Domestic violence manifested by acid burns due to 50% sulfuric acid being thrown on the victim.

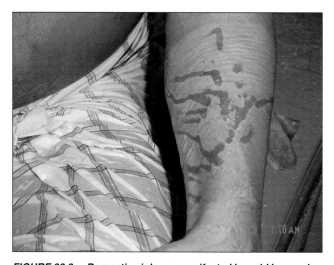

FIGURE 32.3: Domestic violence manifested by acid burns due to 50% sulfuric acid being thrown on the victim.

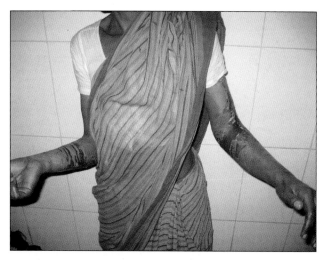

FIGURE 32.6: Domestic violence manifested by acid burns due to 50% sulfuric acid being thrown on the victim.

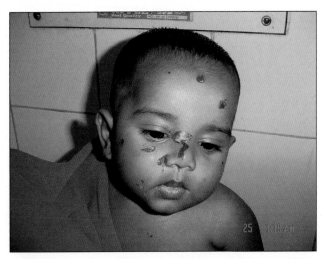

FIGURE 32.7: *Domestic violence manifested by acid burns due to 50% sulfuric acid being thrown on the victim.*

serve as a warning to others. When the burn is extensive, cosmetic surgery may have a role to play in ameliorating the damage, albeit not typically in the emergency context.

Electrical burns can occur when a torturer attaches electrodes to various parts of a person's body and runs current through the circuit, although such burns are usually incidental to the torture intended rather than its aim. These burn marks are usually small circular lesions that leave fine scars, although the wound will depend on the type of current and attachment used. Danielsen and Rasmussen[3] again provide an excellent overview of these differences. Broadening the foci of charge entry and emergence through the use of gels will render these marks even harder to find, if they exist at all.[4] A particular form of electrical torture common in Peru and other parts of South America ("picana," involving a wand that delivers a high-voltage but low-current shock) leaves clusters of tiny lesions covered with brown crusts and sometimes surrounded by a

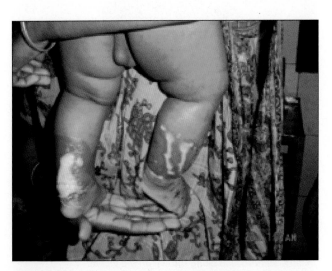

FIGURE 32.8: *Domestic violence manifested by acid burns due to 50% sulfuric acid being thrown on the victim.*

small erythematous ring. A differential diagnosis of such lesions may include contact dermatitis.[4] Biopsy and histological examination may have a role to play in the investigation of electrical torture. In the case of electrical burns, recently inflicted damage may show deposits of calcium salts on cellular structures that accords with the flow of an electric current, while perhaps also showing signs of burn damage due to the heat produced by the current.[3] One case series involving histologic examination of 11 patients seen after burns from defibrillation, however, showed no such evidence, implying that such evidence may be present less frequently.[12] Another study of 11 patients who suffered electrical fatalities (also not torture related) showed deposition of copper and iron on the skin in a significant number of histologic specimens from these patients, suggesting that staining for these metals might help to support a case of electrical torture.[13]

Torture can also potentially, as a result of stress induced, make a patient susceptible to flares of skin diseases from which he or she already suffers. Psoriasis and other diseases induced by various sorts of skin trauma may arise in response to torture via the Koebner phenomenon, while the psychological stress of the same may either provoke urticaria or the uncontrolled repetitive self-rubbing that can exacerbate or introduce disease.[3] Patients with other underlying diseases, such as diabetes mellitus and peripheral arterial disease, may also be more susceptible to ongoing effects from trauma to limbs and reduced healing. Patients who tend toward hypertrophic healing may develop keloids as a consequence of torture wounds. Finally, evidence of severe damage to the skin through torture may well indicate more internal damage that could result in rhabdomyolysis and consequently could warrant a check of renal function for signs of failure.[14]

THERAPY

Patients with extensive skin damage due to chemical or physical burns should be referred to a burn unit and ultimately for appropriate surgical intervention, if necessary. Care is otherwise commensurate with the damages and normal wound care. Depending on the age of the skin damage and how it was inflicted, it is also important to look for signs of infection and to treat the same if discovered.

In almost every situation in which a patient was the possible victim of torture, thorough documentation of the history and examination becomes extremely important, whether for asylum claims or conceivable future legal actions against a perpetrator. In some cases and countries, for example, it is essential for a physician to identify the victim through specific means for any possible legal redress to follow. One U.S. study has found that individuals who received medical evaluations from Physicians for Human Rights have obtained asylum at statistically significantly higher rates than have those without similar documentation.[15]

It is also important to ensure that social workers and psychiatrists or psychologists are involved in treatment when torture is suspected.[9] Similarly, a physician dealing with a patient who is suspected of suffering or claiming to be the victim of torture should be treated with great care. No matter how much the physician wishes to help, a person who has just been utterly mistreated by an authority figure and has suffered under questioning may be reflexively suspicious of answering the questions of a new authority figure. Women (and men) who may have been sexually brutalized may be ashamed to tell their whole story. Various forms of torture may also lead to impaired memory of the event. In any case, it may be necessary for additional visits for an adequate documentation of what has happened to the patient. Although these visits obviously should not take place in the emergency department setting, such a course of aftercare should be established to the extent possible.

COURSE AND PROGNOSIS

In cases of intentional mutilation, whether through chemical, electrical, thermal, or mechanical destruction of the skin, the patient's course and prognosis depend heavily on the extent of damage inflicted. Unless the patient was severely and significantly burned, most scars will follow a normal course of healing absent secondary infection or other complication. For the purposes of documenting torture, damage to the skin should be evaluated as near in time to the event as possible.

Of course, the goal of torture is ultimately not the infliction of the pain or disfigurement, per se, but the psychological repression of the victim. As such, much treatment will lie beyond the expert purview of the dermatologist and depend on ongoing social and psychological assistance. It is essential, therefore, that the patient does not simply shuttle through for evaluation of his or her skin condition.

The evaluation, depending on the situation, as noted previously, may be important for a patient's possible need or desire to seek asylum. All relevant symptoms should be documented, of course, and if there is no examination beyond the dermatologic that should be noted, lest evidence of the absence of such complaints be used against the patient. Even when treatment is being offered in situations where some limitations may be present in how far the patient may explain the torture (e.g., a prisoner brought in by his captors/torturers to seek medical treatment after a session of interrogation has gone too far) or the physician may express his or her opinions, documentation to the fullest extent, as well as an acknowledgment of any limitations, should be included.[16] Similarly, a full examination for the purposes of an asylum claim likely may well lie beyond the purview and time constraints of the physician delivering emergency care, and arrangements for a more extensive examination by someone more familiar with medical (and legal) aspects of such claims is likely in order.[17]

REFERENCES

1. Peel M. History of torture. In Payne-James J, Byard R, Corey T, Henderson C, editors. Encyclopedia of forensic and legal medicine. 1st ed. Amsterdam: Elsevier; 2005. pp. 520–4.
2. United Nations Convention against Torture and Other Cruel, Inhuman or Degrading Treatment or Punishment, Art. 1.
3. Danielsen L, Rasmussen OV. Dermatological findings after alleged torture. Torture. 2006; 16:108–27.
4. Pounder DJ. Torture: physical findings. In Payne-James J, Byard R, Corey T, Henderson C, editors. Encyclopedia of forensic and legal medicine. 1st ed. Amsterdam: Elsevier; 2005. pp. 297–302.
5. Forest DM. Examination for the late physical after effects of torture. J Clin Forensic Med. 1999; 6:4–13.
6. Moisander PA, Edston E, Torture and its sequel – a comparison between victims from six countries. Forensic Sci Int. 2003; 137:133–40.
7. Perera P. Physical methods of torture and their sequelae: a Sri Lankan perspective. J Forensic Leg Med. 2007; 14:146–50.
8. Forrest D. The physical after-effects of torture. Forensic Sci Int. 1995; 76:77–84.
9. Richey SL. Assessment and management of survivors of torture in the emergency department. J Emerg Nurs. 2007; 33:484–7.
10. Faller-Marquardt M, Pollak S, Schmidt U. Cigarette burns in forensic medicine. Forensic Sci Int. 2008; 176:200–8.
11. Routh HB, Parish LC, Sen SL, Bhowmik B. Skin torture. Clin Dermatol. 2005; 23:307–9.
12. Danielsen L, Gniadecka M, Thomsen HK, et al. Skin changes following defibrillation: the effect of high voltage direct current. Forensic Sci Int. 2003; 134:134–41.
13. Jacobsen H. Electrically induced deposition of metal on the human skin. Forensic Sci Int. 1997; 90:85–92.
14. Naqvi R, Ahmed E, Akhtar F, et al. Acute renal failure due to traumatic rhabdomyolysis. Ren Fail. 1996; 18:677–9.
15. Lustig SL, Kureshi S, Delucchi KL, et al. Asylum grant rates following medical evaluations of maltreatment among political asylum applicants in the United States. J Immigr Minor Health. 2008; 10:7–15.
16. Perera C. Review of initiatives adopted for effective documentation of torture in a developing country. J Clin Forensic Med. 2006; 13:288–92.
17. Forrest D, Knight B, Hinshelwood G, et al. A guide to writing medical reports on survivors of torture. Forensic Sci Int. 1995; 76:69–75.

CHAPTER 33

Skin Signs of Poisoning

Batya B. Davidovici

Ronni Wolf

CUTANEOUS POISONING syndromes produce a myriad of signs and symptoms. Poisoning may be acquired either accidentally or deliberately through inhalation, ingestion, or percutaneous contact of the toxic substances. It can affect all age groups, but children have an increased risk for adverse effects of these toxic agents.

Early diagnosis and therapeutic support may not always be achieved due to poor recognition of signs and symptoms. This realization emphasizes the importance of recognizing the signs of cutaneous poisoning syndromes and initiating adequate systemic therapy when indicated. The initial approach to poisoning entails a thorough clinical history, detailed physical examination, and institution of basic supportive measures. Primary and secondary prevention by way of public education and vigilant observation are essential.

One of the challenges in managing these patients is to identify the "needle in the haystack," the small percentage that may develop potentially serious clinical effects and require specific management without subjecting them to unnecessary procedures.

The focus of this review is on four major cutaneous poisoning syndromes, namely metallic poisoning (arsenic, mercury); excessive β-carotene (carotenoderma), which may present with diagnostic and therapeutic difficulties; carbon monoxide (CO) poisoning; and dioxin poisoning.

ARSENIC POISONING

Arsenic is a well-recognized poisonous metal due to its inexpensive cost, lack of odor, and tasteless quality. Arsenic can be contacted during the smelting of copper, gold, lead, and other metals. In smelting operations and in the manufacture of pesticides and herbicides, considerable contamination of the environment can be present, requiring extensive preventive measures. In the semiconductor industry, exposure to arsenic can occur during maintenance activities and especially during the handling of raw materials.

In children, the most common arsenic sources are medicinal and environmental.[1] Chronic arsenic toxicity due to drinking arsenic-contaminated water is a major environmental health hazard. Many aquifers in various parts of the world are contaminated with arsenic. Of these, the most noteworthy occurrences are in large areas of India, Bangladesh, Taiwan, and Northern China.[2] Although arsenic poisoning has been rarely reported in the pediatric population, a recent work analyzing the acute effects of arsenic poisoning showed that children as young as 1 year old may be affected.[3]

Arsenic can cause a persistent folliculitis, in addition to systemic poisoning. An increased incidence of skin cancer was also reported following ingestion of seafood and drinking water containing more than 0.6 mg of arsenic per liter.[4] There is additional evidence from human studies that chronic ingestion of inorganic arsenic causes skin, bladder, and lung cancer in adults.[5] Skin abnormalities, such as pigmentation changes and keratosis, have long been known to be hallmark signs of chronic arsenic exposure in adults. These lesions are the most common health effects found in populations exposed to arsenic-contaminated drinking water.

Clinical Manifestations

Arsenic poisoning may be classified as either acute or chronic. In a study on acute arsenic poisoning in Wakayama, Japan,[3] cutaneous manifestations from arsenic exposure in both children and adults appeared as soon as 3 months after exposure. Cutaneous findings, although rarely documented after acute arsenic poisoning, include facial edema and a mildly pruritic maculopapular eruption in the intertriginous areas, as well as acral hyperkeratosis with lamellar peeling. Transverse 1- to 2-mm-wide whitish fingernail bands, called Mees lines, become apparent after a 2-month incubation period and tend to be broader in children. Other cutaneous lesions such as urticaria, erythema multiforme lesions, a morbilliform eruption, periungual pigmentation, acral desquamation, and postinflammatory hyperpigmentation have also been reported.[6] With chronic low-level arsenic exposure, clinical signs and symptoms are subtle and difficult to detect initially but later can manifest as systemic signs and symptoms, including benign skin changes, skin cancer, or internal malignancy. Cutaneous signs from chronic arsenicism may present as facial and eyelid edema and blushing. Cutaneous melanosis with hyperpigmented patches has also been reported in the nipples, axillae, groin, and other pressure points.[7]. A 2003 study of an Argentinian population[1] showed that chronic arsenic exposure from contaminated well water ingestion presented with the principal skin manifestations of distinctive pigmentation and keratoses. The hyperpigmentation is marked by raindrop-shaped discolored spots, diffuse dark brown spots, or diffuse darkening of the skin on the limbs and trunk. Simple keratosis usually appears as bilateral thickening of the palms and soles, whereas in nodular keratosis, small protrusions appear in the hands, feet, or legs. Spotty depigmentation (leucomelanosis) also occurs in arsenicosis. In contrast to cancer, which takes decades to develop, these skin lesions are generally observed 5–10 years after exposure commences. The cutaneous malignancies reported were Bowen disease, basal cell carcinoma (BCC), and squamous cell carcinoma (SCC) with BCC being more common than SCC.[1]

Although limited epidemiological data exist, other reported clinical manifestations resulting from ingestion of arsenic-contaminated drinking water in adults include weakness, conjunctival congestion, hepatomegaly, portal hypertension, lung disease, polyneuropathy, solid edema of limbs, and anemia.[5]

Occurrence of chronic lung disease including pulmonary interstitial fibrosis was described in arsenic-exposed children in Chile. Influence on intellectual function is also reported from Thailand, Bangladesh, and India.

Diagnosis

Several diagnostic aids are available in detecting the presence of arsenic. Urine arsenic levels may be useful for acute poisoning due to rapid clearance of arsenic from the blood. Deposition of arsenic in hair and nails begins within 2 weeks of exposure and remains in the tissues for the next 1–2 years of life.[8] A few strands of hair, preferably from the pubic area, are necessary to reduce the likelihood of environmental contamination. Ancillary tests should also be done to rule out systemic involvement.

Management

Environmental control of arsenic exposure remains the major preventive measure against arsenic poisoning or morbidity. Seasonal variation, specifically dry periods, enhances toxicity. Chelation therapy with dimercaprol may enhance excretion of arsenic from the system. When carcinogenic effects of arsenic are evident, arsenic levels are minimal and chelation may prove to be inadequate treatment.[9] Oral retinoids have been used to reduce the risk of

internal malignancies as well as decrease the induction of multiple BCC formation.

MERCURY POISONING

Poisoning with mercury is now fortunately rare although it is still the second most common cause of heavy metal poisoning.[10] For more than 3000 years, mercury and its derivatives have been used in a variety of systemic medications, dermatologic creams, dental amalgams, and medications.[11,12] In addition, compounds of mercury have been widely used as fungicides, bactericides, and catalysts and in electrical parts, antifouling paints, and pulp and paper manufacturing. It is also found in a variety of household items, such as thermometers, light bulbs, batteries, and seafood products.[13] The reports highlighting the toxicity of mercury ranged from contaminated fish (Minamata disease–Japan, 1960)[14,15] to infected grains (Iraq, 1971).[16]

Clinical manifestations may vary, depending on the dose, type of mercury, method of administration, duration of exposure, and individual sensitivity.[17] Mercury toxicity can also cause a variety of cutaneous signs and manifestations. The effect of mercury on the skin depends on the mode of poisoning and extent of involvement. Mercury is also a moderate sensitizer and leads to contact sensitivity.

Elemental Mercury

Elemental mercury is commonly found in thermometers, mercury-laden latex paint, and dental amalgams. It is rapidly oxidized to mercuric ions and has a half-life of 60 days.[17] In pediatric patients, exposure to accidental breakage of thermometers is one of the common routes of mercury toxicity. Children are at a higher risk for elemental mercury poisoning because they attain much higher body concentrations of the element compared with adults for the same amount of exposure.[10] Clinical signs and symptoms are minimal after ingestion of elemental mercury because gastrointestinal absorption is negligible. Up to 80% of elemental mercury that is inhaled, however, is absorbed and diffuses rapidly across membranes, including the blood–brain barrier and placenta.[10] Acute toxicity results in three symptomatic stages.[18] Initially, a flu-like syndrome with fever, myalgia, and dryness of the mouth and throat occurs. After 2 weeks, the second stage ensues, mainly affecting the gastrointestinal and respiratory tracts. Symptoms include a metallic taste in the mouth, nausea, and vomiting. Fulminant interstitial pneumonitis, pulmonary edema, and even pulmonary failure may occur. Nephrotic syndrome has also been reported.[10] Chronic exposure to mercury produces a classic triad of intentional tremors, erethism (increased excitability), and gingivitis. Cutaneous manifestations include an erythematous papular eruption and bluish discoloration of the gingiva.

Organic Mercury

Organic mercury, in the form of methylmercury, is the most toxic form of mercury and is commonly found in processed wood, plastics and paper, insecticides, and vaccines containing thimerosal. It may also be found in seafoods that are exposed to mercury-contaminated water. Clinically, it causes irreversible damage to the central nervous system due to its lipid solubility allowing passage through the blood–brain barrier.[19] Demyelination, autonomic dysfunction, mental retardation, ataxia, and cerebral palsy have all been reported in methylmercury toxicity.[10]

Inorganic Mercury

Inorganic mercury is found in topical medications, such as antiseptic face creams and bleaching creams. Percutaneous absorption of lethal doses is possible. Women of childbearing age who use mercury-based skin whiteners may cause toxic effects on their unborn fetus.[20] Application of a mercury-containing cream to the face over many years can produce slate-gray pigmentation, especially on the eyelids, nasolabial folds, and neck folds (exogenous ochronosis),[21–23] and mercury granules lie free in the dermis or within macrophages.[24]

Inorganic mercury exposure sometimes causes a bluish linear pigmentation on the gums and tongue, which should be considered a marker for systemic poisoning.

Acrodynia

As early as the 1890s, a disease entity called "pink disease" was recognized in Australia, characterized by diffuse painful, occasionally itchy, redness of the hands, feet, and trunk.[11] Acrodynia or pink disease is a hypersensitivity condition of infancy and early childhood, which presents with both systemic and cutaneous symptoms due to chronic mercury exposure.[18] Acrodynia has been reported in some patients who were chronically exposed to calomel-containing teething and diaper powders, diaper rinses, termite-protected wood (mercury bichloride), batteries, cathartics, antihelminthics, ammoniated mercury ointments, wart treatment pills, antisyphilitic agents, and/or mercurial preservatives.[11] Acrodynia was also seen in a patient after inhalation of an accidental spillage of mercury onto the carpet where the child played frequently. In the more recent years, stricter industrial and commercial manufacturing measures have eliminated mercury in the production of many of these items, leading to a significant decline in the prevalence of acrodynia.

Clinical presentations may vary with children initially presenting with irritability, lethargy, and anorexia, as well as painful swelling of the hands and feet. Tips of the fingers and toes acquire a pink color and later become dusky, hence, the name "pink disease." Acrodynia is pathognomonically described as patients with "puffy, pink, painful, paresthetic, perspiring, and peeling hands."[18] Occasionally, excruciating pain of the digits leads to sleep deprivation, whereas persistent pruritus leads to lichenification and less often, trichotillomania. The skin is cool and moist due to hyperhidrosis. Patients also develop alopecia, photophobia, muscle weakness, excessive salivation with gum swelling, and diffuse hypotonia.

Mercury poisoning should be included in the differential diagnosis of atypical Kawasaki disease, although high fever pathognomonic for Kawasaki disease is the major differentiating factor.

The natural course of acrodynia is prolonged, although the prognosis is often good. A delayed presentation appears to be a good prognostic sign. Mortality approximates 10%.[11] Elevated urinary mercury level confirms the diagnosis. Treatment mainly involves removal of mercury from the patient's circulation and avoiding mercury exposure from the environment.

Mercury Poisoning from Fish Ingestion

Aside from neurotoxic effects associated with ingestion of mercury-containing food products, a recent report of a new cutaneous sign of mercury poisoning has been documented. Dantzig[25] described the appearance of nonpruritic or mildly pruritic, discreet, small (1–2 mm), flesh-colored or slightly erythematous papules and papulovesicles that correlated with blood mercury levels and responded well to lowering of the blood mercury levels. Children are 2–3 times more prone to mercury poisoning from seafood ingestion because of a higher food intake per kilogram of body weight.[19] Lesions are mostly found on the palms, soles, arms, and trunk. Lowering of blood mercury levels with a seafood-free diet in all patients and chelation therapy in seven patients resulted in clearing of the lesions.

Other Cutaneous Manifestations

In 2004, two distinct clinical patterns were reported in two pediatric patients in the form of acute generalized exanthematous pustulosis (AGEP) and symmetric flexural exanthema "baboon syndrome."[26]

AGEP is characterized by an acute eruption of widespread, nonfollicular pustules with underlying edematous erythema associated with fever (>38°C) and leukocytosis.[27] It is most frequently seen in association with drugs such as penicillins and macrolides. Although cases of mercury-related eruption have been reported, there is no definite conclusion regarding the existence of a cause–effect relationship. The baboon syndrome is a diffuse, symmetric, erythematous, maculopapular eruption of the flexural areas with a V-shaped pattern on the medial thighs and diffuse erythema of the buttocks. The syndrome occurs within a few days of exposure to mercury with no systemic symptoms.[28] Mercury exposure from topical disinfectants, ophthalmologic preparations, and antiparasitic powders was also reported to produce systemic reactions.[13,29] Patients recover with extensive exfoliation, particularly of the palmoplantar surfaces, after 2 weeks. Positive patch tests for delayed-type hypersensitivity were seen in 80% of cases, but serum mercury levels and cutaneous disease failed to show a correlation.[13,29]

Vaccine-Related Mercury Exposure

Neurodevelopmental disabilities, such as language delay, attention deficit hyperactivity disorder, and especially autism spectrum disorder[30,31] have been reported in vaccines containing thimerosal, a vaccine preservative. Thimerosal is 49.6% ethylmercury,[20] which may be found in diphtheria–tetanus–acellular pertussis, hepatitis B, and some *Hemophilus influenzae* type B vaccines.[32–34] It has emerged as a major source of mercury in children in their first 2 years of life.[17] Reports that idiopathic autism may be induced by early mercury exposure from vaccines that exceed the safety guidelines of thimerosal determined by the U.S. Food and Drug Administration (FDA) and the American Academy of Pediatrics[34] prompted studies validating this hypothesis. To date, there is no causal relationship between the timing of mercury administration via vaccines and the onset of autistic symptoms.[32] In July 1999, however, based on the rationale that cumulative doses of ethylmercury from multiple vaccinations may potentially exceed the recommended safety levels of mercury, the Environment Protection Agency responded by requesting manufacturers to remove thimerosal from vaccines. Although thimerosal has been recently removed from most children's vaccines, it is still present in flu vaccines given to pregnant women, elderly persons, and to children in developing countries.[31]

Diagnosis

An environmental history should be obtained when there is a high index of suspicion. Mercury intoxication can be identified with mercury-level assays from both blood and hair. Hair mercury analysis is a reliable and more acceptable means of detecting tissue mercury levels in children with chronic exposure because it reflects tissue accumulation of mercury for the past 2–3 months, whereas blood levels reflect a more recent exposure to mercury.[35] Histopathology is nonspecific. Urinary levels of vanillylmandelic and homovanillic acid are increased in acrodynia due to inhibition of catechol methyltransferase.

Management

Management mainly involves identifying and eliminating the source of mercury exposure. Removing the patient from the source of exposure alone may be sufficient to ameliorate or reverse the symptoms.[36] Chelation is recommended for symptomatic patients and those with toxic mercury levels in the blood or urine. Dimercaprol, which was previously the agent of choice, has now been found to exacerbate neurotoxicity and deemed unsuitable.[18] DMSA (2,3-dimercaptosuccinic acid), a water-soluble analog of dimercaprol, and/or D-penicillamine increase mercury excretion and are employed for aggressive elimination of serum mercury compounds. DMSA is, however, the only chelating agent approved by the FDA for use in the pediatric population.[36] There is a growing concern among some clinicians with regard to the use of chelation therapy in the treatment of mercury poisoning because of the lack of guidelines available to physicians and the paucity of controlled studies that show a clinical beneficial long-term outcome among patients.[36] The teratogenic effects of these agents also limit the use among pregnant women. Hemodialysis, peritoneal dialysis, and plasma exchange have been shown to have beneficial effects in previous reports.[37] Most patients improve after treatment, but long-term morbidity and death have been reported.[11] Treatment should be individualized, depending on severity and presentation.

CAROTENODERMA

Carotenoderma is a phenomenon, characterized by orange pigmentation of the skin, resulting from carotene deposition mainly in the stratum corneum. It is associated with a high blood β-carotene value and is regarded as a significant physical finding, but a harmless condition.

Von Noorden[38] described carotenemia in 1907. While investigating diabetes mellitus and its treatment, he noticed a carroty pigmentation in patients whose treatment involved special diets. A year later, Moro[39] noted the condition in infants. In 1919, Hess and Meyers[40] gave the term "carotenemia" to the condition consisting of increased carotene blood levels and yellow skin pigmentation.

During the last century, epidemics of carotenemia have occurred, usually as a result of carotene-rich diets. Food rationing during the Second World War forced the public to consume large quantities of carrots, which were nutritious and inexpensive. It was found to be transferred to infants by breast-feeding.[41] During the 1970s, carotenoderma was observed in many Japanese infants and in children who consumed high amounts of tangerines or tangerine juice.[42] Carotenemia is endemic in West Africa as a result of frequent use of red palm oil, which is rich in carotenoids.[43]

On histology, the stratum corneum has a high lipid content that has an affinity for carotene, so the carotene pigment is concentrated in the stratum corneum. On direct immunofluorescence it can autofluoresce in a pemphigus-like intercellular pattern, and thus be mistaken for pemphigus vulgaris.[44]

Carotenoids are found in a complex with proteins or in crystalline carotenoid complexes in vegetables and fruits.[45] β-carotene is not synthesized in the human body. Its source is food. It gives some fruits and vegetables their orange–yellow hue. In green vegetables, the yellow pigment is masked by chlorophyll. In a study done in a Brazilian population in 2005,[46] the authors showed that green vegetables, such as lettuce, contain a considerable amount of carotenoids.

About one third of ingested β-carotene is absorbed.[47] Absorbance is affected by the fiber content of food and by food processing. Mashing, cooking, and pureeing of fruits and vegetables cause rupture of cells and enhance the availability of β-carotene.[47] In the presence of bile acids it becomes incorporated into mixed micelles, from which it is absorbed by passive diffusion into the enterocytes in the small intestine mucosa. In the enterocyte, most of the β-carotene is converted into retinal by the enzyme 15,15′-dioxygenase.[48] Retinal reductase converts retinal to retinol[49] (vitamin A), which is then complexed with long-chain fatty acids to be transported to the liver as chylomicrons.[50] It is not clear how much intact β-carotene is absorbed. In the literature, estimates vary between 10% and 80%. The amount of intact β-carotene absorbed is affected by β-carotene intake and vitamin A stores. β-carotene that is directly absorbed, however, is transported to the liver via the portal circulation.[51,52] Although β-carotene is fat soluble, eating it with as little as 3–5 g of fat per meal can still increase its plasma levels.[53] Absorption is also enhanced by pancreatic lipase, bile acids, and probably by the thyroid hormone. Disturbance of fat absorption, infection, and intestinal disease may all impair β-carotene absorption.[54] High gastric pH levels interfere with absorption, probably by inhibiting passive diffusion into the enterocyte.[55] Certain constituents of food, such as sulfides and acids,[56] can destroy β-carotene. Pectin interrupts micelle formation and hence interferes with β-carotene absorption.[57] Lutein and canthaxanthin inhibit the conversion of β-carotene to retinal.[58]

β-carotene is stored in the liver and adipose tissues, and can also be found in high concentrations in the testes and in the adrenal glands. In healthy persons, there is a linear relationship between serum β-lipoprotein and serum β-carotene levels.[59]

Excretion of β-carotene occurs mainly through the colon and epidermis through sebaceous glands. A small amount is excreted through the urine.[60]

A number of mechanisms are presumed to be responsible for carotenemia. The most common is excessive dietary consumption of β-carotene. Carotenemia may be observed 4–7 weeks after initiation of a diet rich in carotenoids.[42] In these cases of carotenemia, serum levels of vitamin A may be normal or elevated, although never high enough to cause hypervitaminosis A. High blood levels of carotene are never high enough to cause hypervitaminosis A because conversion of carotene to vitamin A is slow.[47]

The linear relationship between β-lipoprotein and β-carotene may cause carotenemia in hyperlipidemia-associated disorders, such as diabetes mellitus, nephrotic syndrome, and hypothyroidism.[61,62] Carotenemia in anorexia nervosa is chiefly related to a diet that is rich in β-carotene sources. Some consider the cause to be an acquired defect in the metabolism or utilization of vitamin A. It may also be related to abnormalities of lipid metabolism, such as the decreased catabolism of β-lipoprotein[63] and hypothyroidism, which are observed in this disease.[64]

Liver disease may cause carotenemia due to impaired conversion of β-carotene into vitamin A. In these cases carotenoderma may be masked by jaundice.[54]

Kidney diseases, particularly nephrotic syndrome and chronic glomerulonephritis, may be associated with elevated serum levels of β-carotene. In nephrotic syndrome it is attributed to hyperlipidemia. An interesting finding is the absence of carotenoderma in patients who suffer from renal disease despite elevated serum β-carotene.[54]

Metabolic (idiopathic) carotenemia is thought to result from a relative or absolute deficiency of 15,15′-dioxygenase, which leads to accumulation of β-carotene and to low to normal vitamin A levels. This enzyme defect may be familial.[59] High β-carotene levels in Alzheimer disease are also suggested to arise from an abnormality in the conversion of β-carotene to vitamin A.[65]

Hypopituitarism and male castrates are conditions that have also been reported to be associated with carotenemia.[47] There is an anecdotal report of carotenemia and Simmonds disease.[54]

Clinical Manifestations

The yellow pigmentation of β-carotene appears when its concentrations in serum exceed 250 μg/dL. It is deposited mainly in the stratum corneum, in sweat, and in sebum, and hence pigmentation is noted in areas where sweating is marked, such as the nasolabial folds, palms, and soles. It can extend to the entire body. The sclerae are not affected, and this helps to distinguish carotenoderma from jaundice. Another typical sign of carotenoderma is its enhanced appearance under artificial light.[66]

Complications

There is a debate as to whether carotenemia is a harmless condition. Some authors report that long-standing carotenemia has been associated with weakness, weight loss, hepatomegaly, hypotension, neutropenia,[67] and amenorrhea.[68] Others report no abnormality with high serum β-carotene.[69] There is, however, an agreement that carotenemia is not associated with vitamin A toxicity.

Treatment

Treatment begins with reassurance that this is a benign condition. Dietary carotenemia is easily manageable within weeks to months on a low-β-carotene diet.[48] Carotenemia associated with hyper-β-lipoproteinemia is reversible by treatment of the underlying cause or with a lipid-lowering diet. There is not yet a satisfactory treatment for metabolic carotenemia.[50]

CO POISONING

CO poisoning causes organ damage as a result of cellular hypoxia. The toxic effects of tissue hypoxia were first described by Bernard in 1857[70]; then, in 1895, Haldane[71] described the underlying mechanism of CO toxicity. CO poisoning affects nearly all organs, including the central and peripheral nervous system, heart, kidney, skeletal, muscle, and skin. The clinical manifestations are diverse, and various complications and sequelae may develop following CO poisoning. Cardiac arrhythmias, such as ventricular fibrillations, however, constitute the major threats to life during acute exposure.[72–75]

Symptoms and signs become increasingly apparent as circulating levels of carboxyhemoglobin rise. Severe CO poisoning can also produce several types of lesions of the skin.[76–80] The lesions vary in degree from erythema and edema to marked vesicle and bulla formation. Vivid erythematous or edematous plaques appear, especially at pressure sites, within hours after CO poisoning.[81] Vesicles and bullae may develop, often in a geographical pattern.[82,83] The scalp lesion of edema and erythema may evolve into areas of alopecia.[77]

The lesions simulate those seen in burns, trauma, or barbiturate poisoning or after cerebral vascular accident or drug-induced coma. Histologically, the bullae show epidermal necrosis, intraepidermal vesiculation, and necrosis of the secreting portions of the sweat glands.[81] Pressure and hypoxia are probably the main factors in the pathogenesis.[79]

Spontaneous resolution occurs in persons who survive, in about 15 days.[81,84]

DIOXIN POISONING (CHLORACNE)

Chloracne is a rare, follicular, acneiform eruption that is a characteristic symptom of dioxin poisoning. Dioxins are polyhalogenated aromatic hydrocarbons that can be found in herbicides and wood preservatives.[85]

Dioxins are a group of chemicals, which include 75 different chlorinated molecules of dibenzo-p-dioxin and 135 chlorinated dibenzofurans. Some polychlorinated biphenyls are referred to as dioxin-like compounds. Of the chloracnegenic compounds, 2,3-tetrachlorodibenzo-para-dioxin (TCDD), or dioxin, is regarded to be the most harmful, associated with many harmful health effects, possessing potentially carcinogenic and teratogenic properties.[86] It is a normal by-product of numerous manufacturing processes and waste incineration.

Small amounts of TCDD (15–45 U/g body fat) are seen normally in humans because of its use in many common industries. It is tasteless but highly toxic.

More than 95% of human exposure to dioxin is through the diet. Air emissions of pollutants, including dioxin, settle on vegetation that is fed to livestock. Dioxin then accumulates in animal fatty tissue and is conveyed to humans through meat and dairy products. Fish and other aquatic organisms ingest dioxin that is washed into bodies of water from land, providing another potential pathway into the food chain. The average dietary intakes of dioxins have declined dramatically over the past 20 years in the United States and Western Europe due to better environmental regulations. As a result of this dramatic improvement in dioxin contamination, the average person born today in the Western world will receive his or her highest exposure to dioxins as a developing fetus and as a nursing infant. Much of that exposure comes from breast milk as the mother mobilizes fatty acids, where dioxin is sequestered, to form breast milk.

Acute dioxin poisoning is rare. Most of the experience with acute dioxin poisoning resulted from industrial accidents. In 1976, a large number of people in Seveso, Italy, were exposed to high levels of dioxins through contaminated cooking oil.

There is also the "Ranch Hand" study that examined the health of more than 1200 U.S. Air Force personnel who worked with Agent Orange. Dioxin was an ingredient in Agent Orange, a defoliant used during the Vietnam War. These servicemen have been followed for many years by the Department of Veterans Affairs and are still being monitored today. Many of them, particularly the ground technicians who loaded spray planes with Agent Orange, developed chloracne. Other episodes of dioxin poisoning occurred several years ago at places such as Love Canal, where hundreds of families needed to abandon their homes due to dioxin contamination, and Times Beach, Missouri, a town that was abandoned as a result of dioxin.

Dioxin, however, made worldwide headlines in September 2004, when Ukrainian President Viktor Yushchenko had been poisoned. His blood samples contained an abnormally high level of dioxin, 1000 times the accepted level. One year later, Yushchenko's face, with its strong jaw and movie-star features, remained badly pockmarked.

Clinical Findings

Dioxin taken in through the human diet dissolves in the fatty components of blood, eventually accumulating in fatty tissue. The human body eliminates dioxin slowly; at any given time, the dioxin concentration in the fatty tissue of a human body is a function of the competing rates of accumulation and elimination. Half a dose of dioxin gets eliminated every few years but never completely rids itself. Dioxin is eliminated also through sebaceous glands; as a result, the skin grows oily or pimply, resulting in chloracne. Chloracne is considered to be the hallmark of dioxin poisoning and represents a symptom of systemic poisoning by chemical chloracnegens and not just a cutaneous disorder.[87] It has been found to be 4 times more frequent in persons with plasma dioxin levels greater than 10 ppt.[88] Chloracne clinically presents a few months after ingestion, inhalation, or manipulation of the toxic agent. Cutaneous findings of chloracne include open and closed comedones and noninflammatory nodules and cysts, mostly on the malar crescent and in postauricular, axillary, and inguinal areas. With more severe dioxin exposure, cysts become inflammatory and may spread to the trunk and genitalia. The nose and limbs are usually spared. Scarring may be severe. It differs from acne vulgaris because of the paucity of pustules or nodules, atrophy of sebaceous glands, sparseness of *Propionibacterium* acnes,[87] frequent involvement of meibomian glands, and occurrence in any age group.[85]

A follow-up study on the Seveso, Italy, dioxin accident of 1976 done 20 years after the incident showed that dioxin toxicity was confined to acute dermatotoxic effects. Increased dioxin levels were still seen in 26.6% of the affected population – particularly in women, in persons who had ingested home-grown animals, and in individuals with older age, higher body mass index, and residence near the accident site. There was, however, an association between chloracne risk and light hair color as well as younger age (<8 years old) at the time of the accident.[88]

Dioxin also binds to cellular hormone receptors; thus, it has the potential to modify the functioning and genetic mechanism of the cell, causing a wide range of effects, from cancer to reduced immunity to nervous system disorders to miscarriages and birth deformity. Indeed, systemically chloracne may be associated with abnormal liver function, hyperhidrosis, conjunctivitis, transient peripheral neuropathy, encephalopathy, and porphyria cutanea tarda–like-features (pigmentation, hirsutism). In a study on the effects of dioxin in children involved in a major environmental accident near Seveso, Italy, in 1976, those exposed to the highest concentration of TCDD showed alterations in serum γ-glutamyltransferase and alanine aminotransferase activity compared with the control group. These changes were mild and disappeared with time.[89] In higher quantities, however, severe effects, such as spina bifida (split spine) and other birth defects, autism, endometriosis, reduced immunity, chronic fatigue syndrome, psychological disorders, and other nerve and blood disorders, have been reported.

Management

Management of chloracne may be challenging. It is important to identify and remove the source of exposure. Some lesions clear up spontaneously within 2 years while others may continue for decades. Persistent cases may be treated similarly to acne with topical retinoids, oral antimicrobials, or oral isotretinoin. A nondigestible, lipophilic dietary fat substitute called olestra has shown promise in reducing systemic dioxin levels by eightfold to tenfold and reducing the half-life from 7 to 1–2 years.[90] The most important means, however, is preventing contamination of the environment by strict legislation.

REFERENCES

1. Cabrera HN, Gomez ML. Skin cancer induced by arsenic in the water. J Cutan Med Surg. 2003; 7:106–11.
2. Mazumder DN. Effect of drinking arsenic contaminated water in children. Indian Pediatr. 2007; 44:925–7.
3. Uede K, Furukawa F. Skin manifestations in acute arsenic poisoning from the Wakayama curry-poisoning incident. Br J Dermatol. 2003; 149:757–62.
4. Blejer HP, Wagner W. Inorganic arsenic–ambient level approach to the control of occupational cancerigenic exposures. Ann NY Acad Sci. 1976; 271:179–86.
5. NRC (National Research Council). Arsenic in drinking water. Washington, DC: National Academy Press; 1999. pp. 83–149.
6. Schwartz RA. Arsenic and the skin. Int J Dermatol. 1997; 36:241–50.
7. Graeme KA, Pollack CV Jr. Heavy metal toxicity, Part I: arsenic and mercury. J Emerg Med. 1998; 16:45–56.
8. Madorsky D. Arsenic in dermatology. J Assoc Military Dermatol. 1977; 3:19–22.
9. Duker AA, Carranza EJ, Hale M. Arsenic geochemistry and health. Environ Int. 2005; 31:631–41.
10. Ozuah PO. Mercury poisoning. Curr Probl Pediatr. 2000; 30:91–9.
11. Dinehart SM, Dillard R, Raimer SS, et al. Cutaneous manifestations of acrodynia (pink disease). Arch Dermatol. 1988; 124:107–9.
12. Foulds DM, Copeland KC, Franks RC. Mercury poisoning and acrodynia. Am J Dis Child. 1987; 141:124–5.
13. Nakayama H, Niki F, Shono M, Hada S. Mercury exanthem. Contact Dermatitis. 1983; 9:411–17.
14. Grandjean P, White RF, Weihe P, Jorgensen PJ. Neurotoxic risk caused by stable and variable exposure to methylmercury from seafood. Ambul Pediatr. 2003; 3:18–23.
15. Harada M, Akagi H, Tsuda T, et al. Methylmercury level in umbilical cords from patients with congenital Minamata disease. Sci Total Environ. 1999; 234:59–62.
16. Amin-Zaki L, Elhassani S, Majeed MA, et al. Perinatal methylmercury poisoning in Iraq. Am J Dis Child. 1976; 130:1070–6.
17. Bernard S, Enayati A, Redwood L, et al. Autism: a novel form of mercury poisoning. Med Hypotheses. 2001; 56:462–71.
18. Boyd AS, Seger D, Vannucci S, et al.. Mercury exposure and cutaneous disease. J Am Acad Dermatol, 2000; 43:81–90.
19. Zahir F, Rizwi SJ, Haq SK, Khan RH. Low dose mercury toxicity and human health. Env Toxical Pharmacol 2005; 20:351–60.
20. Counter SA, Buchanan LH. Mercury exposure in children: a review. Toxicol Appl Pharmacol. 2004; 198:209–30.
21. Lamar LM, Bliss BO. Localized pigmentation of the skin due to topical mercury. Arch Dermatol. 1966; 93:450–3.

22. Prigent F, Cohen J, Civatte J. Pigmentation des paupieres probablement secondaire l'application prolongée d'une pomade ophtalmologique contenant du mercure. Ann Dermatol Vénéréol. 1986; 113:357–8.

23. Aberer W. Topical mercury should be banned - dangerous, outmoded but still popular. J Am Acad Dermatol. 1991; 24:150–1.

24. Burge KM, Winkelmann RK. Mercury pigmentation. An electron microscopic study. Arch Dermatol. 1970; 102:51–61.

25. Dantzig PI. A new cutaneous sign of mercury poisoning? J Am Acad Dermatol. 2003; 49:1109–11.

26. Lerch M, Bircher AJ. Systemically induced allergic exanthem from mercury. Contact Dermatitis. 2004; 50:349–53.

27. Roujeau JC, Bioulac-Sage P, Bourseau C, et al. Acute generalized exanthematous pustulosis. Analysis of 63 cases. Arch Dermatol. 1991; 127:1333–8.

28. Andersen KE, Hjorth N, Menne T. The baboon syndrome: systemically-induced allergic contact dermatitis. Contact Dermatitis. 1984; 10:97–100.

29. Barrazza V, Meunier P, Escande JP. Acute contact dermatitis and exanthematous pustulosis due to mercury. Contact Dermatitis. 1998; 38:361.

30. Geier DA, Geier MR. An assessment of the impact of thimerosal on childhood neurodevelopmental disorders. Pediatr Rehabil. 2003; 6:97–102.

31. James SJ, Slikker W 3rd, Melnyk S, et al. Thimerosal neurotoxicity is associated with glutathione depletion: protection with glutathione precursors. Neurotoxicology. 2005; 26:1–8.

32. Pichichero ME, Cernichiari E, Lopreiato J, Treanor J. Mercury concentrations and metabolism in infants receiving vaccines containing thiomersal: a descriptive study. Lancet. 2002; 360:1737–41.

33. Goldman LR, Shannon MW. American Academy of Pediatrics: Committee on Environmental Health Technical report. Mercury in the environment: implications for pediatricians. Pediatrics. 2001; 108:197–205.

34. Halsey NA. Limiting infant exposure to thimerosal in vaccines and other sources of mercury. JAMA. 1999; 282:1763–6.

35. Katz SA, Katz RB. Use of hair analysis for evaluating mercury intoxication of the human body: a review. J Appl Toxicol. 1992; 12:79–84.

36. Risher JF, Amler SN. Mercury exposure: evaluation and intervention the inappropriate use of chelating agents in the diagnosis and treatment of putative mercury poisoning. Neurotoxicology. 2005; 26:691–9.

37. Leumann EP, Brandenberger H. Hemodialysis in a patient with acute mercuric cyanide intoxication. Concentrations of mercury in blood, dialysate, urine, vomitus, and feces. Clin Toxicol. 1977; 11:301–8.

38. Von Noorden C. Die Zukerkrankheit und ihre Behandlung. 4th ed. 1907. p. 149.

39. Moro E. Karottensuppe bei Ernahringsstorungen Saulinge. Munch Med Wschr. 1908; 55:1637–40.

40. Hess AF, Meyers VC. Carotinemia: a new clinical picture. JAMA. 1919; 73:1743–5.

41. Almond S, Logan RFL. Carotenaemia. BMJ. 1942; 2:239–41.

42. Roe DA. Assessment of risk factors for carotenodermia and cutaneous signs of hypervitaminosis A in college-aged populations. Semin Dermatol. 1991; 10:303–8.

43. Person JR. Red palm and orange palms. Arch Dermatol. 1981; 117:757.

44. Palleschi GM, Knoepfel BR, Lotti T. Carotenoderma: a possible pit-fall in the immunopathologic diagnosis of pemphigus vulgaris. Int J Dermatol. 1992; 31:50–1.

45. Parker PS. Absorption, metabolism, and transport of carotenoids. FASEB J. 1996; 10:542–51.

46. Niizu P, Rodriguez-Abaya D. New data on the carotenoid composition of raw salad vegetables. J Food Comp Analysis. 2005; 18:739–49.

47. Lascari AD. Carotenemia. A review. Clin Pediatr. 1981; 20:25–9.

48. Stack KM, Churchwell MA, Skinner RB. Xanthoderma: case report and differential diagnosis. Cutis. 1988; 41:100–2.

49. Goodman DS, Huang HS. Biosynthesis of vitamin A with rat intestinal enzymes. Science. 1965; 149:879–80.

50. Vaughan Jones SA, Black MM. Metabolic carotenaemia. Br J Dermatol. 1994; 131:145.

51. Wouterson RA, Wolterbeed APM, Appel MJ, et al. Safety evaluation of synthetic beta carotene. Crit Rev Toxicol. 1999; 29:515–42.

52. Leung AK. Carotenemia. Adv Pediatr. 1987; 34:223–48.

53. van Het Hof KH, West CE, Weststrate JA Hautvast JG. Dietary factors that affect the bioavailability of carotenoids. J Nutr. 2000; 130:503–6.

54. Leung AK. Carotenemia. Adv Pediatr. 1987; 34:223–48.

55. Tang G, Serfaty-Lacrosniere C, Camilo ME, Russell RM. Gastric acidity influences the blood response to a beta-carotene dose in humans. Am J Clin Nutr. 1996; 64:622–6.

56. Dimitrov NV, Meyer C, Ullrey DE, et al. Bioavailability of beta-carotene in humans. Am J Clin Nutr. 1988; 48:298–304.

57. Paiva SA, Russel RM. Beta-carotene and other carotenoids as antioxidants. Am J Clin Nutr. 1999; 18:426–33.

58. Wouterson RA, Wolterbeed APM, Appel MJ, et al. Safety evaluation of synthetic beta carotene. Crit Rev Toxicol. 1999; 29:515–42.

59. Monk BE. Metabolic carotenaemia. Br J Dermatol. 1982; 106:485–7.

60. Greene CH, Blackford LM. Carotenemia. Med Clin North Am. 1926; 10:733–44.

61. Svensson A, Vahlquist A. Metabolic carotenemia and carotenoderma in a child. Acta Dermatol Venereol. 1995; 75:70–1.

62. Hoerer E, Dreyfuss F, Herzberg M. Carotenemic, skin colour and diabetes mellitus. Acta Diabetol Lat. 1975; 12:202–7.

63. Schwabe AD. Hypercarotenaemia in anorexia nervosa. JAMA. 1968; 205:533–4.

64. Gupta MA, Gupta AK, Haberman HF. Dermatologic signs in anorexia nervosa and bulimia nervosa. Arch Dermatol. 1987; 123:1386–90.

65. Singh S, Mulley GP, Losowsky MS. Carotenaemia in Alzheimer's disease. BMJ. 1988; 297:458–9.

66. Joseph WL. Carotenemia vs jaundice. JAMA. 1976; 236:2603.

67. Shoenfeld Y, Shaklai M, Ben-Baruch Net al. Neutropenia induced by carotenaemia. Lancet. 1982; 1:1245.

68. Kemmann E, Pasquale SA, Skaf R. Amenorrhea associated with carotenemia. JAMA. 1983; 249:926–9.

69. Mathews-Roth MM. Plasma concentrations of carotenoids after large doses of beta-carotene. Am J Clin Nutr. 1990; 52:500–1.

70. Bernard C. Lecons sur les effects des subtances toxiques et medicamenteuses. Bailliere, Paris, 1857.

71. Haldane J. The relation of the action of carbonic oxide to oxygen tension. J Physiol. 1895; 18:201–17.

72. Ehrich WE, Bellet S, Lewey FH. Cardiac changes from CO poisoning. Am J Med Sci. 1944; 208:1–23.

73. Corya BC, Black MJ, McHenry PL. Echocardiographic findings after acute carbon monoxide poisoning. Br Heart J. 1976; 38:712–17.

74. Shafer N, Smilay MG, MacMillan FP. Primary myocardial disease in man resulting from acute carbon monoxide poisoning. Am J Med. 1965; 38:316–20.

75. Penny DG, Stryker AE, Baylerian MS. Persistent cardiomegaly induced by carbon monoxide and associated tachycardia. J Appl Physiol. 1984; 56:1045–52.

76. Choi SA, Choi IS. Clinical manifestations and complications in carbon monoxide intoxication. J Korean Neurol Assoc. 1998; 16:500–5.

77. Long PI. Dermal changes associated with carbon monoxide intoxication. JAMA. 1968; 205:50–1.

78. Leavell UW, Farley CH, McIntyre JS. Cutaneous changes in a patient with carbon monoxide poisoning. Arch Dermatol. 1969; 99:429–33.

79. Nagy R, Greer KE, Harman LE Jr. Cutaneous manifestations of acute carbon monoxide poisoning. Cutis. 1979; 24:381–3.

80. Lee JB, Chang KH, Choi IS. Cutaneous manifestations of carbon monoxide poisoning. Korean J Dermatol. 1983; 21:279–83.

81. Achten G, Ledoux-Corbusier M, Thys JP. Intoxication a l'oxyde de carbone et lesions cutanées. Ann Dermatol Syphiligr. 1971; 98:421–8.

82. Long PI. Dermal changes associated with carbon monoxide poisoning. JAMA. 1968; 205:120.

83. Leavell UW, Farley CH, McIntyre JS. Cutaneous changes in a patient with carbon monoxide poisoning. Arch Dermatol. 1969; 99:429–33.

84. Mandy S, Ackerman AB. Characteristic traumatic skin lesions in drug-induced coma. JAMA. 1970; 213:253–6.

85. Sterling JB, Hanke CW. Dioxin toxicity and chloracne in the Ukraine. J Drugs Dermatol. 2005; 4:148–50.

86. Yamamoto O, Tokura Y. Photocontact dermatitis and chloracne: two major occupational and environmental skin diseases induced by different actions of halogenated chemicals. J Dermatol Sci. 2003; 32:85–94.

87. Pastor MA, Carrasco L, Izquierdo MJ, et al. Chloracne: histopathologic findings in one case. J Cutan Pathol. 2002; 29:193–9.

88. Baccarelli A, Pesatori AC, Consonni D, et al. Health status and plasma dioxin levels in chloracne cases 20 years after the Seveso, Italy accident. Br J Dermatol. 2005; 152:459–65.

89. Mocarelli P, Marocchi A, Brambilla P, et al. Clinical laboratory manifestations of exposure to dioxin in children. A six-year study of the effects of an environmental disaster near Seveso, Italy. JAMA. 1986; 256:2687–95.

90. Geusau A, Tschachler E, Meixner M, et al. Olestra increases fecal excretion of 2,3,7,8-tetrachlorodibenzo-p-dioxin. Lancet. 1999; 354:1266–7.

CHAPTER 34

Disaster Planning: Mass Casualty Management

Lion Poles

DISASTERS AND OTHER emergencies can strain and even damage – at least transiently – a health care system. The increased awareness of natural and manmade disasters has created a relatively new need for health care providers: preparedness and response for medical emergencies. To remain both robust and flexible, the medical systems must establish protocols, perform exercises, and learn from the experience of others. Facing threats since it was born 62 years ago, the Israeli medical system has conducted a comprehensive preparedness activity that has been tested in large-scale exercises and in large- and small-scale violent conflicts.

AN OVERVIEW OF THE ISRAELI MEDICAL SYSTEM

Israel has 24 public acute care hospitals in addition to its geriatric, psychiatric, and private hospitals. The hospital system serves both the civilian and the military population. Six are trauma centers (level 1) located in densely populated urban areas; 14 others are acute care medical centers without cardiosurgery or neurosurgery services (level 2), and the rest are relatively remote community hospitals (level 3) that can offer triage and limited surgical and surge capacity. All Israeli hospitals maintain continuous alert for mass casualty incidents (MCIs) in line with a unified national doctrine. Thus, we regard the hospitals as part of the first-responders system. In the extrahospital arena, there is a highly developed network of outpatient clinics, part of the four health maintenance organizations' (HMOs') network of primary care clinics.

As for other first-responders systems, Israel has a single national emergency medical service (EMS), a national police system, and a regionally based firefighting system. The national search-and-rescue unit and air evacuation systems are operated by the Israel Defense Forces (IDF). The leader of the medical system, which sets priorities in peacetime, during major disasters, and during wars, is the Supreme Health Authority (SHA); it is headed by the Director General of the Ministry of Health (MOH), the Surgeon General (member, IDF Medical corps) and the chief executive officer (CEO) of the largest HMO

(member). An advisory committee comprising the MOH senior executive officials, EMS, the Home Front Command (HFC) medical officer, and other organizations is consulted if necessary. The HFC medical department acts as an operational arm of the SHA. Main budgets of medical preparedness for MCIs originate from the MOH: Specific facilities such as decontamination sites, equipment (e.g., physical protection, respirators), pharmaceuticals, and new infrastructure are funded by the MOH.

EVOLUTION OF OPERABILITY OF THE HOSPITAL SYSTEM

The general hospitals have always been an integral part of Israel's national emergency response system. Most hospitals have participated in the management of injured soldiers and civilians during and between wars. Historically, lessons learned during wartime and through isolated conventional MCIs were gathered, but no comprehensive doctrine was established. In the 1980s, as lessons emerged from the war of 1973 and the perceived threat of chemical warfare (CW) increased, the heads of the medical system decided that a fundamental change was needed in the way hospitals prepare for crises.

Under the auspices of the SHA, a trilateral system was founded. The Emergency Division of the MOH was given overall responsibility and funding for infrastructure and procurement; and the IDF medical corps – acting on behalf of the MOH through a newly established Hospital Contingency Branch (HCB) and the Nuclear, Biological, and Chemical Medical Branch – led the development of doctrine and the implementation of new procedures. Representatives of the public general hospitals participated in planning and implementation through several steering committees. These committees were headed by hospital executives and were composed of subject-matter experts and representatives of the trilateral preparedness organization. Nominated specific committees included a contingency committee for conventional MCIs, a similar committee for CW hospital preparedness, and committees for human resources and for procurement. End products were presented and approved by the SHA, becoming official policies and backed up by the necessary budgets.

After Israel was attacked by Iraqi missiles during Operation Desert Storm in the Persian Gulf (1991), the HCB was designated as the leader for CW preparedness. Thereafter, new steering committees developed new directions, such as preparing for an accident at a nuclear reactor (1994) and preparing for a mass toxicological incident (1997, following the release of the nerve gas sarin by terrorists in Japan in 1994–1995). The principles of preparedness and the interrelationships of groups involved have remained since. Concomitantly, operational missions were transferred to the medical department of the HFC (established in 1994), which incorporated HCB in 1999. The emerging threat of biological warfare (BW) and a new crisis alert regarding Iraq in 1998 led to the development of an entirely new preparedness initiative – the "unusual biological incident." The evolving threats of BW, bioterrorism, and emerging infectious diseases necessitated different kinds of response and new partners, including the public health system, laboratory network, surveillance system, and ambulatory medical services. In the biological threat scenario, hospitals changed their role; rather than being the key factor, as in previous threats, they became just one component of a national interrelated response system that was developed within the MOH.

COMPONENTS OF PLANNING FOR EMERGENCY RESPONSE IN THE ACUTE CARE HOSPITAL

Israeli hospitals are regarded as part of the first-responder system because most of the medical management of victims and nearly all decontamination procedures are planned and actually have taken place within hospitals. In addition, the last decade's experience of the EMS has shown that, for most urban incidents, evacuation of all victims can last up to 90 minutes after the incident. Because natural and man-made MCIs can occur after hours, all hospital contingency plans base initial response on the emergency department, which is reinforced by any in-house staff available during those hours. Hospitals have developed redundant telecommunications and staff notification capabilities. The hospital standard operating procedure (SOP) plan is to provide effective triage, decontamination, and treatment in the first hour with these resources, until additional staff arrive and are incorporated into the crisis management activities. Specific means provided to hospitals by the MOH include decontamination infrastructure (e.g., communication, decontamination sites, and negative–positive pressure environments); power-driven level 3 respiratory protection sets with universal canisters (ABEK P3 type); mission-oriented protective posture 4 (MOPP4) protective garments or, alternatively, standard kits to protect against airborne biological agents; and specific sets of antidotes sufficient for the first 8–24 hours of treatment (to be supplemented from national stockpiles).

All prehospital and interhospital activities in times of large-scale emergencies are supervised and coordinated by the chief medical officer of the HFC (on behalf of the MOH) through a command and control center. Within the hospital, all emergency contingency activity is coordinated and supervised generally by a senior physician and nurse. Because emergency preparedness is principally a nonprofit activity funded by the hospital, in many places this physician is one of the hospital's deputy general managers. He or she heads an advisory committee – an emergency contingency committee – with representatives from nursing, logistics, security, and administration. Subcommittees are often established for specific scenarios (e.g., a bioevent committee comprising the infectious disease unit, the director of the microbiological laboratory, a security officer, and logistics and nursing executives). These subcommittees define and help to execute annual and ad hoc plans, updated according to MOH directives. As these officials are not primarily assigned to emergency preparedness, their activities usually reach a peak before planned or anticipated exercises or inspections of the regulatory bodies. Their most difficult task is maintaining continuous readiness among the staff, through intermittent individual or institutional training and small-scale drills.

In Israel, the public, the media, and the MOH expect hospitals to be able to handle any emergency, and hospital managers perform accordingly perhaps as a matter of self-esteem. Only recently has systematic analysis been done for the most likely wartime scenarios with which hospitals should prepare to cope. There is still no official specific analysis of hospitals' missions during terrorist events and natural disasters, and no procedures have been established for assessing hospitals' individual vulnerabilities to internal hazards. With respect to MCIs, all Israeli hospitals are expected to provide medical assessment, treatment, and continuing care for large numbers of patients and to identify and manage contaminated patients and patients who have been exposed to an unusual biological agent (this management includes protecting the hospital staff, patients, and others within the hospital). In general, such response and mitigation activities should not interfere with everyday emergency care.

According to lessons learned in Israel from mass casualty event MCIs, following a terrorist incident three waves of casualties arrive at emergency rooms: the most severely injured arrive by EMS ambulances or by private cars within 45 minutes in an urban location. Moderately or mildly injured victims arrive within 2 hours. The third wave consists of patients mildly injured and those experiencing acute stress reaction, all who arrive within 24 hours. Three systems of resources are involved in managing these patients: operational, medical, and informational. Hospitals need to assemble, evaluate, implement, and disseminate information quickly and accurately and deliver it to various internal and external customers, including local and state agencies.

To be efficient in response during a crisis, the hospital must be a part of a coordinated collaborative effort. Other members include other first responders, the media, local communities, the National Institute for Forensic Medicine, other hospitals, the MOH, and the HFC. Ideally, there should be one risk communication system for the public, for both informative and directive purposes. Practically, the media provide a medium for conveying information and sometimes directions to the public by senior officials in the hospital system or the MOH. As the hospitals' CEOs may be forced to address the media and share information with the public, providing updates on the situation, it is beneficial to train them in "risk communication" skills.

Target allocation and evacuation from the disaster or mass emergency area is done by the HFC's medical and the EMS control centers. They are also responsible for alerting hospitals of casualties that are on the way. This notification leads to activation of the hospitals' SOP.

Throughout the emergency, every hospital is planning to host a designated EMS liaison officer in its control center. His or her duty is to coordinate the activities of ambulances in the hospital both primarily from the scene and later for secondary allocation of victims. Another liaison is an officer from the HFC medical department who works with the hospital's incident command system to assist the hospital's needs – disseminate information within the hospital, the MOH, and the EMS networks; coordinate the air evacuation missions; and communicate about resources and support needed from other authorities and agencies.

The Israeli media plays a role in medical response in times of emergency, serving as a "first responder" for information. Hospital emergency plans incorporate designated areas for the media.

CURRENT POLICIES

Current policies – including policies for hospital emergency preparedness – are dictated by economic pressures and tight budgets, especially in the medical system. Moreover, there is a huge array of possible manmade and natural disasters. Consequently, there is a clear need for a cost-effective approach that can find a common denominator among many threats, so as to concentrate on generic solutions. Such denominators might include decontamination; surge capacity; multifaceted, multilevel triage; communication regarding risks and crises; and public relations. It is vital to consent on low- versus high-probability scenarios, so that preferences and resources can be allotted to

the latter (in toto) and critical steps in the response plan to the former. Hospital-specific hazards – both external and internal – should be analyzed, and emergency missions should be tailored accordingly and supported by appropriate resources.

Emergency scenarios can be classified as "rapid" or "slow" types. Rapid scenarios involve conventional events (e.g., mass trauma from explosives or airplane crashes), chemicals (including toxins), and quickly identifiable radiological exposure. These scenarios tend to be clearly bounded in time and place, with distinct victims or exposed individuals. Most of the rapid scenarios are easily perceived by human senses or simple monitoring equipment. Victims are managed mainly within the hospital system. The initial response phase is expected to be limited to 24 hours. Common problems in rapid scenarios include surge capacity, triage, decontamination, identification of hazards, treatment protocols, control and communication, public relations, intensive care, and personnel recruitment and management. The main principles of response planning for rapid scenarios are to apply the experience gained from the terror campaign of the last 15 years and to apply the conventional MCI model (modified as necessary for victims of contamination). It is pertinent that hospitals will maintain readiness for these type of emergencies, among others, by maintaining "just in case" annual training programs.

Slow scenarios include biological outbreaks and unidentified radiological exposure. These scenarios are not clearly bounded in space or time nor are the victims or exposed individuals distinct. Slow scenarios are not perceptible by human senses; thus relatively advanced or sophisticated diagnostic procedures are necessary. The response to a slow scenario is beyond the scope of the hospital system, and the response phase will last for several days or weeks. The main problems are similar to those in rapid scenarios: surge capacity, triage, contaminated victims, and so forth. Special consideration should be given, however, to detecting the event, to notification, to diagnostic procedures, and to relationships with external entities such as public health and ambulatory medical services. Specific criteria for a hospital's preparedness should be established. Local planning, staff training, and maintenance of emergency equipment are not funded by the MOH (preparedness activities tend to add expense but not to produce revenue); still, any new standards should be accompanied by appropriate resources or budget allocations. Finally, emergency contingency units should be founded and funded within the general hospital, ambulatory, and public health systems to ensure real commitment and productivity on the part of non-emergency medical organizations. For the slow scenarios, it is reasonable to maintain limited readiness – for the initial response only – and to prepare resources such as materials (manuals, presentations, etc.) for providing "just-in-time" training.

CONCLUSIONS

Some of these principles are already implemented or are expected to be implemented in the strategy of the MOH.

FURTHER READING

Hughes JM. The emerging threat of bioterrorism. *Emerg infect Dis*. 1999; 5:494–5.

Poles L. Contingency of the national hospitalization system for peacetime emergencies. *Harefuah*. 2001; 130:817–20. (Hebrew)

Shalala DE. Bioterrorism: how prepared are we? *Emerg Infect Dis*. 1999; 5:492–3.

Torok TJ, Tauxe RV, Wise RP, et al. A large cummunity outbreak of salmonellosis caused by intentional contamination of restaurant salad bars. *JAMA*. 1997; 278:389–95.

WuDunn S, Miller J, Broad WJ. How Japan germ terror alerted world. *New York Times*, 26 May 1998; Sect A: 1 (col 1), A: 10 (col 1–5).

CHAPTER 35

Catastrophes in Cosmetic Procedures

Marina Landau

Ronni Wolf

DERMATOLOGISTS HAVE performed surgery and cosmetic invasive procedures on the skin since the 19th century. They are responsible for developments in chemical peels, hair transplantation, dermabrasion, sclerotherapy, laser surgery, and liposuction. As with any medical treatment, those procedures carry inherent risk for possible complications.

"If you've been thinking of having your face or body rejuvenated, but have been scared off by the thought of major surgery, then maybe it's time to think again. A wealth of new techniques and technologies have transformed the field of cosmetic treatment. The common feature of all these new treatments is 'minimally invasive' – that is, less cutting, less open surgery, less risk and less downtime. Not only that – the cost is often far lower," says one (of many) Web sites (see http://www.shanghaiexpat.com/Article1103965.phtml accessed March 10, 2010). For individuals who choose a minimally invasive cosmetic procedure aimed at improving appearance, fighting the signs of aging, and restoring their youthful looks (as opposed to treating a "real" disease), any visual side effect is considered a "catastrophe." Therefore, we include in this chapter, aside from "true emergencies/catastrophes," what we call "aesthetic catastrophes."

SCARRING

A significant number of procedures in dermatology carry a risk of scarring. In some procedure scarring is inevitable, such as in surgical rhytidectomies and hair transplantations, whereas in others scarring is considered a complication, such as in chemical peels or laser surgery. The ultimate goal of a physician performing these interventions is to create a superior cosmetic outcome by avoiding or minimizing the scar.

Unfortunately, some cases result in hypertrophic scarring or keloids instead of a minimal scar. Those abnormally thickened scars are often painful or pruritic. The common locations for keloids and hypertrophic scars are on the upper trunk, neck, and upper extremities and over bony prominences of the face. Factors predisposing to the formation of such scars include race (skin of color and Asian), heredity, excessive wound tension, excessively deep dermal injury, wound infection, and foreign body reaction. The concomitant or recent use of oral vitamin A derivatives has been traditionally considered as a risk factor for bad scarring.[1,2] This opinion has been recently challenged.[3,4]

Despite the high prevalence of keloids in the general population, they remain one of the more challenging dermatologic conditions to manage. Because patients with a previous personal or family history of keloids are at increased risk for developing abnormal scars, they should avoid elective cosmetic procedures with a risk for scarring. If such a procedure is performed, wounds should be closed with minimal tension and the immediate use of silicone gel sheets should be started.

A wide range of therapies exists for keloids, with the most commonly used modalities being intralesional steroid injection, surgical excision, cryotherapy, laser therapy, radiation therapy, and the application of silicon gel sheets. Other treatments that have been used with variable success rates include imiquimod, 5-fluorouracil, bleomycin, retinoids, calcium channel blockers, mitomycin C, and interferon-α 2b. A recent meta-analysis of 39 studies, representing 27 different treatments, reported a 70% chance of clinical improvement with any type of treatment.[5]

INFECTIONS

Because dermatologic procedures disrupt skin integrity, they alter the body's protective barrier and predispose theoretically to cutaneous infections. Surprisingly, postoperative wound infections seldom complicate dermatologic procedures, ranging from 1% to 3%;[6] however, they have been rarely reported to complicate simple procedures such as excisions, biopsies, skin grafts, chemical peels, dermabrasion, laser resurfacing, liposuction, blepharoplasty, and filler injections.

Antimicrobials continue to be widely used in the setting of dermatologic surgery for the prevention of surgical wound infection, endocarditis, and late prosthetic joint infections. Debate regarding routine use of topical and systemic antibiotics is still ongoing. The literature suggests that, for most routine skin procedures, antibiotic use is probably not warranted. During prolonged Mohs procedures, delayed repairs, grafts, or any procedure that breaches a mucosal surface, decisions should be made on a case-by-case basis. Systemic prophylactic antibiotics for laser resurfacing and liposuction are also not routinely necessary.[7] For the prevention of surgical site infections, antimicrobials may be indicated for procedures on the lower extremities or groin, for wedge excisions of the lip and ear, skin flaps on the nose, skin grafts, and for patients with extensive inflammatory skin disease.[8]

Pooled data from four studies on the risk of bacteremia during dermatologic surgery including scalpel excision, electrodesiccation and curettage, Mohs surgery, hair transplantation, and flaps and grafts on clinically noninfected skin revealed a risk of bacteremia at 1.9%.[9–12] Despite a strong shift away from administration of prophylactic antibiotics in many dermatologic surgery settings, it is still needed for patients with high-risk cardiac conditions and for a defined group of patients with prosthetic joints at high risk for hematogenous total joint infection.[8]

BLEEDING

Although the overall incidence is low, bleeding complications in dermatologic surgery can occur and be the source of patient morbidity. It is particularly important because the use of blood thinners has increased dramatically in recent years among the general, and especially among the elderly, population. In addition, many patients are taking dietary supplements that may alter coagulation.[13] When these patients need to undergo cutaneous surgery, the surgeon might encounter a problem of increased bleeding tendency. Discontinuation of these medications may increase the risk of cerebral and cardiovascular complications; therefore, a question of safe continuation or discontinuation of anticoagulant and antiplatelet medications before surgery might be a major issue in dermatologic surgery.

Meta-analysis of controlled studies reporting bleeding and other complications among patients undergoing cutaneous surgery who were taking anticoagulant medications suggests that although low, the risk of bleeding among anticoagulated patients may be higher than baseline.[14] Until recently, discontinuation of anticoagulation and antiplatelet therapy before surgery was a rule.

In recent years, dermasurgeons have been more likely to continue medically necessary aspirin and warfarin, but to discontinue prophylactic aspirin, nonsteroidal antiinflammatory drugs (NSAIDs), and vitamin E.[15,16] There are no studies in the literature that examined the effects of combination anticoagulant therapy or the effect of herbal agents on postoperative risk of bleeding.

PROCEDURE-SPECIFIC COMPLICATIONS

Dermal Fillers

In 1899, Robert Gersuny, a Viennese surgeon, introduced mineral oil (Vaseline®) for correction of soft-tissue defects. The principle of the technique consisted in the injection of a product that becomes semiliquid by heating but solidifies when cooled. Later, Vaseline® was replaced with paraffin. Although serious complications were reported, it remained popular for the first 20 years of the 20th century. Unfortunately, even with initial good results, secondary or late severe complications appeared due to the dispersion of paraffin. There was formation of nodules, the paraffinomas that were very difficult to remove. The sequelae of paraffin injections were observed for several years.[17]

Since that time, soft-tissue augmentation using autologous or synthetic products has become the cornerstone of facial beautification and of antiaging treatment. The choice of commercially available dermal fillers is growing constantly.[18,19]

In the European Union, injectable fillers are certified as medical devices. Depending on the potential risk of each substance, a controlled clinical trial may be performed during the certification process; nevertheless, the process is completely different from that applied for U.S. Food and Drug Administration (FDA) approval. Not infrequently, the safety and efficacy of many CE-certified injectables are assessed only in the postmarketing process.

No matter what the origin of the fillers is, they are usually classified into resorbable and permanent groups. Resorbable materials, such as collagens and hyaluronic acids, are removed from the tissue by phagocytosis. Permanent fillers, such as silicone and ArteFill®, cannot be removed efficiently. Large microspheres of nonresorbable fillers are encapsulated with fibrous tissue and escape phagocytosis.

In 2004, a new classification of dermal fillers, taking into account the long-term safety and reversibility of the side effects, was proposed.[20] According to this classification, dermal fillers are nonpermanent and biodegradable (e.g., collagens and hyaluronic acids), semipermanent and biodegradable (e.g., polylactic acid), permanent and reversible (e.g., expanded poly tetrafluoroethylene), or permanent and nonreversible (e.g., liquid injectable silicone, polymethylmethacrylate).

Complications and adverse reactions can occur with all fillers and all filler procedures. The most common side effects include hematomas, ecchymoses, swelling, erythema, discoloration, visibility, or palpability of the filler. Hypersensitivity and tissue necrosis are rare and most distressing. Filler migration, granuloma formation, infection, and delayed inflammatory reactions do not usually occur with nonpermanent biodegradable fillers.

Hematoma and ecchymosis are due to extravasation of blood cells into the tissue due to needle injury of blood vessels. Alcohol consumption, blood thinners, NSAIDs, aspirin, vitamin E, omega 3, and probably other herbal agents facilitate the occurrence of hematoma. If these drugs are used prophylactically, proper discontinuation of their intake prior to the procedure, and refraining from alcohol consumption, may prevent some of the bleeding events. Firm pressure immediately after the injection and ice-pack application may minimize the bleeding, if it occurs. In general, collagen-based fillers (Zyderm, Evolence) are associated with less bleeding due to induction of platelet aggregation.

Transient swelling and redness occur immediately after a filler injection and usually last a few hours to a few days. These phenomena are probably secondary to the inflammation induced by the product itself, injection trauma, and tissue manipulation by massaging or molding. Some products are more prone to induce tissue swelling due to their hygroscopic properties (e.g., hyaluronic acid–based products). Certain facial areas, such as the lips, are specifically sensitive to injections and inevitably swell after the procedure. Prolonged icing of the area without direct contact between the ice cube and the skin can assist to diminish this phenomenon.

More prolonged swelling can signal overcorrection. Tear trough depression is especially sensitive to overcorrections. Permanent or periodic (usually in the mornings) swelling in this area may require dissolving the filler by enzyme hyaluronidase.[21]

Discoloration in the injection site is either induced by hemosiderin deposits following postprocedural hematoma or due to superficial implantation of the filler in a way that the original color of the product or its interaction with the tissue shows. A bluish tint in the areas where hyaluronic acid was implanted too superficially is known as the Tyndall effect.[22] This can be also successfully treated by hyaluronidase.

Visibility and palpability of the filler are also related to a bad injection technique.

Palpable nodularities after ArteFill® injection are observed as a result of uneven delivery of material due to clumping of the polymethylacrylate microspheres. This finding has nothing to do with granuloma formation.[23] Superficial implantation of Radiesse® may also create a visible whitish cord along the implantation route. To avoid this happening, an adequate practitioner's training is needed prior to the clinical work with the fillers. A physician has to adopt a proper technique of even delivery of the product to the mid-dermis or subdermally. In most cases, immediate postprocedural vigorous molding of the tissue will diminish filler palpability.

When a relationship between dermal filler injection methods and the incidence of the local adverse events was assessed, a higher rate of side effects was found with more tissue-traumatizing techniques, such as fanning, rapid injection rate, and higher volumes of the product.[24]

Necrosis of the overlying tissues after dermal filler implantation is elicited by vascular embolism, vascular injury, or compression. The overall estimate for necrosis with bovine collagen is 0.09% of treated individuals. Most of the cases were seen after injection of Zyplast® in the glabellar area.[25,26] The manifestations of intravascular injection are immediate blanching and pain. Completely identical symptoms and outcome are observed with hyaluronic acid.[27,28] When injecting into glabellar, periorbital, or nasal regions with any filler, caution is necessary to avoid intravascular injection. Aspiration when injected in these areas might be helpful. Different treatment modalities have been suggested to treat imminent necrosis, such as massaging, warm compresses, nitroglycerin paste, and systemic steroids, but their efficacy is not well established.[29] Local wound care, after necrosis settles in, is of paramount importance to reduce the extent of scar formation.

Hypersensitivity reactions and granuloma formation are the most distressing adverse effects occurring with soft-tissue augmentation. Every single filler material can cause this complication, but the risk rate differs among products. There are also patient-related factors that affect the incidence of the hypersensitivity. Allergic reactions to bovine collagen are well known (Figure 35.1). The collagen component of ArteFill® may evoke the same type of reactions in sensitive individuals. Since introduction of a double skin pretesting, the incidence of localized hypersensitivity at the test sites is 3%, and in treated patients, the numbers dropped to 1%–2%. These reactions resolve with time as the implant material is resorbed by the host. Circulating antibodies to bovine collagen can be demonstrated in the sera of a majority of patients (90%–100%) with local hypersensitivity. These antibodies are specific for bovine collagen and do not cross-react with human type I, II, or III collagen.[30]

The hypersensitivity reaction rate seems to be significantly lower with the recently developed cross-linked, porcine collagen implant, Evolence®. Because this implant has a low potential for hypersensitivity, intradermal skin testing before its use appears unnecessary.[31]

The rate of hypersensitivity reaction with most of the hyaluronic acid–based fillers is less than 1%. So far, approximately 40 cases of hypersensitivity to Restylane® were reported, and the global risk of sensitivity is estimated as 0.8%. Since 2000, the amount of protein in the raw product has decreased, and the incidence of hypersensitivity reactions has decreased to approximately 0.6%. Fifty percent of these reactions are immediate and resolved within less than 3 weeks. The risk of strong but transient, delayed reaction is approximately 0.3%.[32–35]

Whereas hypersensitivity reactions are self-limited with nonpermanent fillers, a completely different course is expected when such a reaction develops with permanent and nonreversible products (Figure 35.2). The liquid form of silicone, called dimethicone (dimethylpolysiloxane), has

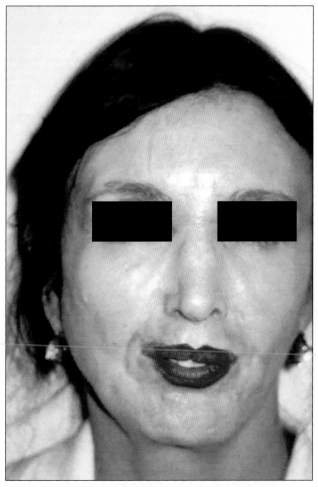

FIGURE 35.1: *Zyderm® -induced granulomatous reaction.*

been used extensively in some countries. Although considered biologically inert, this material has been reported as potentially inducing a granulomatous inflammatory response of variable severity. A remarkable paucity of reports about the development of complications after

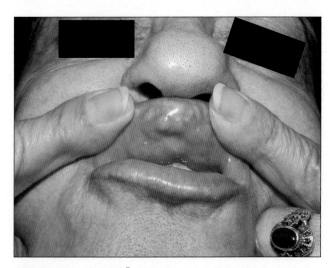

FIGURE 35.2: *ArteFill® -induced granuloma in the lip.*

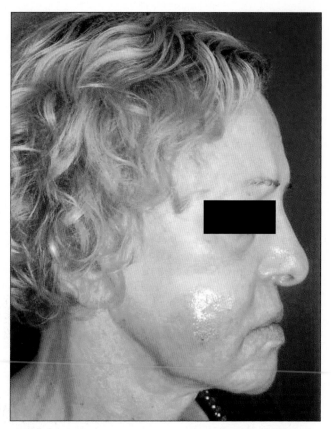

FIGURE 35.3: *Bio-Alkamid® -induced delayed inflammation.*

injections of liquid silicone is probably related to its illegal or semilegal use in most countries.[36] When using silicone in a microdroplet technique for lip enhancement, the incidence of granuloma formation is estimated to be approximately 2%.[37]

Nonreabsorbable gel polymers (Bio-Alkamid®, Aquamid®) are approved for use in Europe, but have not been released by the FDA. Those products may induce severe inflammatory/infectious granulomatous reactions at any point from the implantation time. In some cases, treatment of these adverse effects is extremely difficult (Figure 35.3).[38–41]

Botulinum Toxin A

Botulinum toxin A (BTXA) has become a widely used drug in cosmetic dermatology to treat hyperkinetic facial and neck lines and focal hyperhidrosis. The spectrum of possible adverse effects of BTXA is broad, but the effects are generally mild and transient. The major tools for preventing adverse effects from BTXA are knowledge and skill. Knowledge of the facial and extrafacial muscles allows physicians to select the optimal dose, time, and technique. The most common adverse effects of BTXA injections are pain, hematoma, flu-like syndrome, headaches, focal facial paralysis, and muscle weakness.[42,43] Severe side effects with

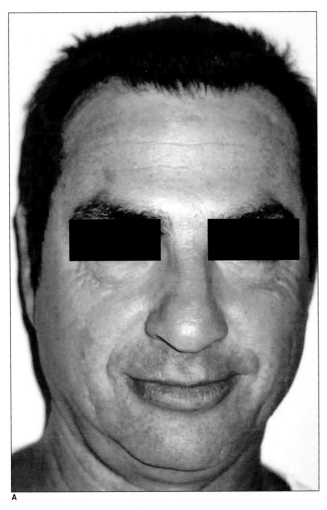
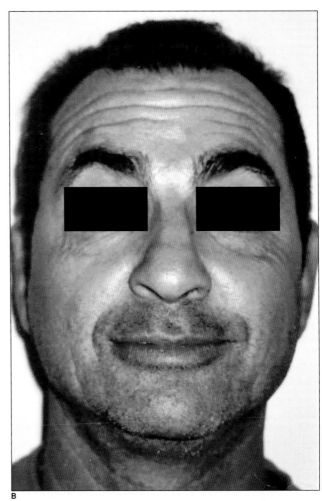

FIGURE 35.4: *Brow ptosis due to inadequate injection of botulinum toxin A to forehead before injection (panel A) and after injection (panel B).*

cosmetic use of BTXA are rare and related to extreme overdosing or illegal use of an unapproved toxin.[44–46]

The majority of BTXA-associated adverse reactions remain to be local and transient. In the glabellar area, the most important potential side effects used to be blepharoptosis and diplopia reaching approximately 5% in the early period of BTXA use. With better understanding of glabellar complex muscle function and a more precise dosing, this adverse effect had become extremely rare recently.[47] If it occurs, IOPIDINE® ophthalmic solution 0.5% is useful until the ptosis resolves.

While treating the forehead wrinkles, eyebrow ptosis and asymmetry are the major potential side effects.[48] A thorough analysis of the face animation is crucial to avoid injecting patients whose forehead wrinkles are related to the use of frontalis muscle to keep visual acuity (Figure 35.4). In most cases, co-injection of the forehead depressors (glabella complex) minimizes the risk of brow ptosis. Careful planning of injection doses and sites will decrease the risk of eyebrow position asymmetry. If it happens,

additional injection of the less deactivated muscle will correct it.

In the periorbital region, partial lip ptosis resulting from weakening of the zygomaticus major muscle is the most devastating complication, because it affects smile symmetry (Figure 35.5).[49]

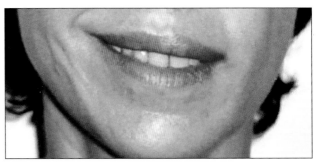

FIGURE 35.5: *Lip ptosis due to paresis of left zygomaticus muscle by periorbital botulinum toxin A injection.*

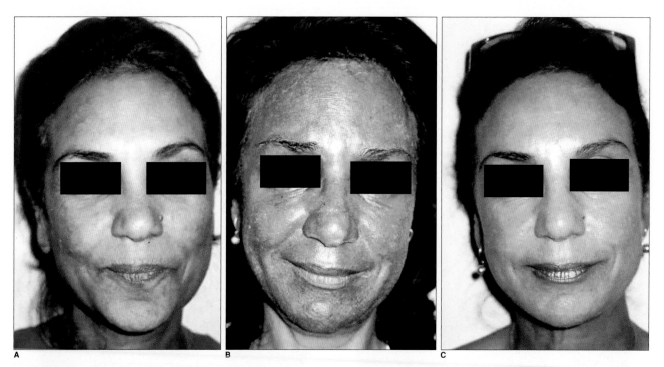

FIGURE 35.6: *Reactive hyperpigmentation after deep chemical peel in dark-skin patient before (panel A), 3 weeks after the peel (panel B), and 4 weeks after introduction of topical bleaching preparation (panel C).*

To avoid this happening, no toxin should be injected behind the zygomatic bone. BTXA can be used in the lower eyelid to improve wrinkles and widen the eye. In these cases, minute doses of the toxin are recommended because higher doses induce lower eyelid edema and incomplete sphincter function of the eyelids.[50] Although BTXA for lateral canthal rhytids usually does not suppress tear production, dry eye is a possible complication of this procedure. Treatment of dry eye and exposure keratitis is symptomatic and includes lubrication.[51] Another rare complication reported recently after BTXA injection in the lateral canthal area is proptosis associated with thyroid disease. Although proptosis represents progression of the patient's preexisting thyroid eye disease, cosmetic use of BTXA unmasks it.[52]

Procedures for the lower third of the face require a higher level of expertise because all the muscles there have specific functions. Different muscles in this zone interdigitate with others and, in some cases, act as antagonists. Thus, this region requires a rigorous evaluation by the physician, with precise diagnosis and technique of BTXA application.

Platysmal bands can be temporarily improved by BTXA with redundant skin being a limiting factor of this treatment success. Dysphagia and airway obstruction are the potential side effects related to the toxin dosing and diffusion.[53]

Hyperhidrosis refers to excessive and uncontrollable sweating beyond that required to return body temperature to normal. Although a broad spectrum of treatment modalities are available, including topical and systemic therapies, chemodenervation using botulinum toxin has emerged as a safe and effective treatment for both primary palmar and axillary hyperhidrosis in several clinical trials. This treatment is highly effective with a paucity of side effects. Fine motor impairment after palmar injection of BTXA has been rarely reported.[54]

Chemical Peels

Chemical peeling is a procedure used for cosmetic improvement of skin or for treatment of some skin disorders. A chemical exfoliating agent is applied to the skin to destroy portions of epidermis and/or dermis with subsequent regeneration and rejuvenation of the tissues. Chemical peels are divided into three categories, depending on the depth of the wound created by the peel. Superficial peels penetrate the epidermis only, medium depth peels damage the entire epidermis and papillary dermis, and deep peels create a wound to the level of midreticular dermis.

The list of potential complications of chemical peels includes pigmentary changes, infections, milia, acneiform eruption, scarring, and cardiotoxicity.

Reactive hyperpigmentation can occur after any depth of chemical peels (Figure 35.6). Usually lighter complected patients have a lower risk for hyperpigmentation, but genetic factors play an important role, and sometimes light patients with "dark genes" hyperpigment unexpectedly. Skin priming using a combination of hydroquinone and tretinoin cream (Kligman's formula) before the superficial and medium depth peels and early introduction of this

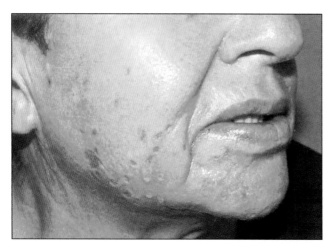

FIGURE 35.7: *Disseminated herpes simplex infection in patient after chemical peel.*

preparation after deep peels reduces the rate of this complication. Demarcation lines can be avoided if the boundaries of the peeling area are hidden under the mandibular line and feathered gradually to the normal skin. Hypopigmentation after phenol peels is proportional to the depth of the peel, amount of the solution used, number of drops of croton oil in the solution, inherent skin color, and postpeel sun-related behavior. Intradermal nevi can hyperpigment after deep peels.

Bacterial and fungal complications in chemical peels are rare. Patients with a positive history of herpes simplex infection are treated prophylactically with acyclovir or valacyclovir during medium and deep peels until full reepithelialization is achieved (Figure 35.7). Toxic shock syndrome has been reported after chemical peels.[55]

Milia or epidermal cysts appear in up to 20% of patients after chemical peels, usually 8–16 weeks after the procedure (Figure 35.8). Electrosurgery is simple and effective to treat this postpeel complication.

Acneiform eruption after chemical peels is not rare and usually appears immediately after reepithelialization. Its etiology is multifactorial and is either related to exacerbation of previously existing acne or is due to overgreasing of newly formed skin. Short-term systemic antibiotics together with discontinuation of any oily preparations will usually provide satisfactory results.

Scarring remains the most dreadful complication of chemical peels. The contributing factors are not well understood. The most common location of such scars is in the lower part of the face, probably due to more aggressive treatment in this area or to the greater tissue movement, because of eating and speaking, during the healing process. Delayed healing and persistent redness are important alarming signs for forthcoming scarring. Topical antibiotics and potent steroid preparations should be introduced as soon as this diagnosis is made.

The most important potential complication exclusive to phenol-based peels is cardiotoxicity. Phenol is directly toxic

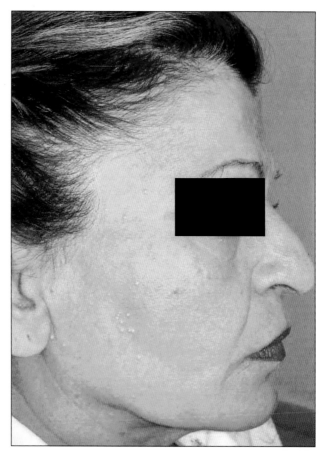

FIGURE 35.8: *Postpeel milia.*

to the myocardium. Studies in rats have shown a decrease in myocardial contraction and in electrical activity following systemic exposure to phenol.[56] Because fatal doses ranged widely in these studies, it seems that individual sensitivity of the myocardium to this chemical exists. In humans, sex, age, previous cardiac history, and blood phenol levels are not accurate predictors for cardiac arrhythmia susceptibility.[57] Cardiac arrhythmias in less than 30 minutes have been recorded in up to 23% of patients, when full face peel was performed.[58] Adequate patient management reduces this complication to less than 7%.[59] No hepatorenal or central nervous system toxicities have been reported in the literature with properly performed chemical peels.

CONCLUSIONS

Each one of the procedures in dermatology carries a risk of potential complications. They can be mild and reversible or severe and permanent. Most of them are avoidable and treatable.

REFERENCES

1. Zachariae H. Delayed wound healing and keloid formation following argon laser treatment or dermabrasion during isotretinoin treatment. Br J Dermatol. 1988; 118:703–6.

2. Katz BE, MacFarlane DF. Atypical facial scarring after isotretinoin therapy in a patient with previous dermabrasion. J Am Acad Dermatol. 1994; 30:852–3.

3. Tan SR, Tope WD. Effect of acitretin on wound healing in organ transplant recipients. Dermatol Surg. 2004; 30:667–73.

4. Khatri KA. Diode laser hair removal in patients undergoing isotretinoin therapy. Dermatol Surg. 2004; 30:1205–7.

5. Leventhal D, Furr M, Reiter D. Treatment of keloids and hypertrophic scars: a meta-analysis and review of the literature. Arch Facial Plast Surg. 2006; 8:362–8.

6. Hurst EA, Grekin RC, Yu SS, Neuhaus IM. Infectious complications and antibiotic use in dermatologic surgery. Semin Cutan Surg. 2007; 26:47–53.

7. Messingham MJ, Arpey CJ. Update on the use of antibiotics in cutaneous surgery. Dermatol Surg. 2005; 31:1068–78.

8. Wright TI, Baddour LM, Berbari EF, et al. Antibiotic prophylaxis in dermatologic surgery: advisory statement 2008. J Am Acad Dermatol. 2008; 59:464–73.

9. Zack L, Remlinger K, Thompson K, Massa MC. The incidence of bacteremia after skin surgery. J Infect Dis. 1989; 159:148–50.

10. Sabetta JB, Zitelli JA. The incidence of bacteremia during skin surgery. Arch Dermatol. 1987; 123:213–15.

11. Carmicahel AJ, Flanagan PG, Holt PJ, Duerden BI. The occurrence of bacteremia with skin surgery. Br J Dermatol. 1996; 134:120–2.

12. Halpern AC, Leyden JJ, Dzubow LM, McGinley KJ. The incidence of bacteremia in skin surgery of the head and neck. J Am Acad Dermatol. 1988; 19:112–16.

13. Dinehart SM, Henry L. Dietary supplements: altered coagulation and effects on bruising. Dermatol Surg. 2005; 31:819–26.

14. Lewis KG, Dufresne RG Jr. A meta-analysis of complications attributed to anticoagulation among patients following cutaneous surgery. Dermatol Surg. 2008; 34:160–4.

15. Kirkorian AY, Moore BL, Siskind J, Marmur ES. Perioperative management of anticoagulant therapy during cutaneous surgery: 2005 survey of Mohs surgeons. Dermatol Surg. 2007; 33:1189–97.

16. Alcalay J, Alkalay R. Controversies in perioperative management of blood thinners in dermatologic surgery: continue or discontinue? Dermatol Surg. 202004; 30:1091–4.

17. Glicenstein J. The first "fillers," vaseline and paraffin. From miracle to disaster. Ann Chir Plast Esthet. 2007; 52:157–61.

18. Haneke E. Skin rejuvenation without a scalpel. I. Fillers. J Cosmet Dermatol. 2006; 5:157–67.

19. Eppley BL, Dadvand B. Injectable soft-tissue fillers: clinical overview. Plast Reconstr Surg. 2006; 118:98e–106e.

20. De Boulle K. Management of complications after implantation of fillers. J Cosmet Dermatol. 2004; 3:2–15.

21. Andre P, Levy PM. Hyaluronidase offers an efficacious treatment for inaesthetic hyaluronic acid overcorrection. J Cosmet Dermatol. 2007; 6:159–62.

22. Douse-Dean T, Jacob CI. Fast and easy treatment for reduction of the Tyndall effect secondary to cosmetic use of hyaluronic acid. J Drugs Dermatol. 2008; 7:281–3.

23. Lemperle G, Hazan-Gauthier N, Lemperle M. PMAA microspheres (Artecoll) for skin and soft tissue augmentation. Part II: Clinical investigations. Plast Recostr Surg. 1995; 96:627–34.

24. Glogau RG, Kane MAC. Effect of injection techniques on the rate of local adverse events in patients implanted with nonanimal hyaluronic acid gel dermal fillers. Dermatol Surg. 2008; 34:S105.

25. Hanke CW, Higley HR, Jolivette DM, et al. Abscess formation and local necrosis following treatment with Zyderm and Zyplast collagen implant. J Am Acad Dermatol. 1991; 25:319–26.

26. American Academy of Dermatology Guidelines of care for soft tissue augmentation: collagen implants. J Am Acad Dermatol. 1996; 34:698–702.

27. Friedman PM, Mafong EA, Kauvar AN, Geronimus RG. Safety data on injectable nonanimal stabilized hyaluronic acid gel for soft tissue augmentation. Dermatol Surg. 2002; 28:491–4.

28. Inoue K, Sato K, Matsumoto D, et al. Arterial embolization and skin necrosis of the nasal ala following injection of dermal fillers. J Plast Reconstr Surg. 2008; 121:127e.

29. Glaich AS, Cohen JL, Goldberg LH. Injection necrosis of the glabella: protocol for prevention and treatment after use of dermal fillers. Dermatol Surg. 2006; 32:276–81.

30. Keefe J, Wauk L, Chu S, DeLustro F. Clinical use of injectable bovine collagen: a decade of experience. Clin Mater. 1992; 9:155–62.

31. Shoshani D, Markovitz E, Cohen Y, et al. Skin test hypersensitivity study of a cross-linked, porcine collagen implant for aesthetic surgery. Dermatol Surg. 2007; 33 Suppl 2: S152–8.

32. André P. Evaluation of the safety of a non-animal stabilized hyaluronic acid in European countries: a retrospective study from 1997 to 2001. J Eur Acad Dermatol Venereol. 2004; 18:422–5.

33. Bardazzi F, Ruffato A, Antonucci A, et al. Cutaneous granulomatous reaction to injectable hyaluronic acid gel: another case. J Dermatol Treat. 2007; 18:59–62.

34. Ghislanzoni M, Bianchi F, Barbareschi M, Alessi E. Cutaneous granulomatous reaction to injectable hyaluronic acid gel. Br J Dermatol. 2006; 154:755–8.

35. Patel VJ, Bruck MC, Katz BE. Hypersensitivity reaction to hyaluronic acid with negative skin testing. Plast Reconstr Surg. 2006; 117:92e–94e.

36. Ficarra G, Mosqueda-Taylor A, Carlos R. Silicone granuloma of the facial tissues: a report of seven cases. Oral Surg Oral Med Oral Pathol Oral Radiol Endod. 2002; 94:65–73.

37. Fulton JE Jr., Porumb S, Caruso JC, Shitabata PK. Lip augmentation with liquid silicone. Dermatol Surg. 2005; 31:1577–85.

38. Goldan O, Georgiou I, Grabov-Nardini G, et al. Early and late complications after a nonabsorbable hydrogel polymer injection: a series of 14 patients and novel management. Dermatol Surg. 2007; 33 Suppl 2:S199–206.

39. Jones DH, Carruthers A, Fitzgerald R, et al. Late-appearing abscesses after injections of nonabsorbable hydrogel polymer for HIV-associated facial lipoatrophy. Dermatol Surg. 2007; 33 Suppl 2:S193–8.

40. Niedzielska I, Pajak J, Drugacz J. Late complications after polyacrylamide hydrogel injection into facial soft tissues. Aesthetic Plast Surg. 2006; 30:377–8.

41. Kawamura JY, Domaneschi C, Migliari DA, Sousa SO. Foreign body reaction due to skin filler: a case report. Oral Surg Oral Med Oral Pathol Oral Radiol Endod. 2006; 101:469–71.

42. Cote TR, Mohan AK, Polder JA, et al. Botulinum toxin type A injections: adverse events reported to the US Food and Drug Administration in therapeutic and cosmetic cases. J Am Acad Dermatol. 2005; 53:407–15.

43. Alam M, Arndt KA, Dover JS. Severe, intractable headache after injection with botulinum a exotoxin: report of 5 cases. J Am Acad Dermatol. 2002; 46:62–5.

44. Souayah N, Karim H, Kamin SS, et al. Severe botulism after focal injection of botulinum toxin. Neurology. 2006; 67:1855–6.

45. Chertow DS, Tan ET, Maslanka SE, et al. Botulism in 4 adults following cosmetic injections with an unlicensed, highly concentrated botulinum preparation. JAMA. 2006; 296:2476–9.

46. Tugnoli V, Eleopra R, Quatrale R, et al. Botulism-like syndrome after botulinum toxin type A injections for focal hyperhidrosis. Br J Dermatol. 2002; 147:808–9.

47. Carruthers JD, Lowe NJ, Menter MA, et al. Double-blind, placebo-controlled study of the safety and efficacy of botulinum toxin type A for patients with glabellar lines. Plast Reconstr Surg. 2003; 112:1089–98.

48. Bulstrode NW, Grobbelaar AO. Long-term prospective follow-up of botulinum toxin treatment for facial rhytides. Aesthetic Plast Surg. 2002; 26:356–9.

49. Matarasso SL, Matarasso A. Treatment guidelines for botulinum toxin type A for the periocular region and a report on partial upper lip ptosis following injections to the lateral canthal rhytids. Plast Reconstr Surg. 2001; 108:208–14.

50. Flynn TC, Carruthers JA, Carruthers JA, Clark RE 2nd. Botulinum A toxin (BOTOX) in the lower eyelid: dose-finding study. Dermatol Surg. 2003; 29:943–50.

51. Matarasso SL. Decreased tear expression with an abnormal Schirmer's test following botulinum toxin type A for the treatment of lateral canthal rhytides. Dermatol Surg. 2002; 28:149–52.

52. Harrison AR, Erickson JP. Thyroid eye disease presenting after cosmetic botulinum toxin injections. Ophthal Plast Reconstr Surg. 2006; 22:397–8.

53. Kane MA. Nonsurgical treatment of platysmal bands with injection of botulinum toxin A. Plast Reconstr Surg. 1999; 103:656–63.

54. Pena MA, Alam M, Yoo SS. Complications with the use of botulinum toxin type A for cosmetic applications and hyperhidrosis. Semin Cutan Med Surg. 2007; 26:29–33.

55. Holm C, Muhlbauer W. Toxic shock syndrome in plastic surgery patients: case report and review of the literature. Aesthetic Plast Surg. 1998; 22:180–4.

56. Stagnone GJ, Orgel MB, Stagnone JJ. Cardiovascular effects of topical 50% trichloroacetic acid and Baker's phenol solution. J Dermatol Surg Oncol. 1987; 13:999–1002.

57. Litton C, Trinidad G. Complications of chemical face peeling as evaluated by a questionnaire. Plast Reconstr Surg. 1981; 67:738–44.

58. Truppman F, Ellenbery J. The major electrocardiographic changes during chemical face peeling. Plast Reconstr Surg. 1979; 63:44.

59. Landau M. Cardiac complications in deep chemical peels. Dermatol Surg. 2007; 33:190–3.

CHAPTER 36

Life-Threatening Dermatoses in Travelers

Larry E. Millikan

SEVERE SKIN reactions/conditions are of particular concern when the traveler is away from home and medical care is unfamiliar or of uncertain caliber. Perhaps the most significant of these conditions is Stevens–Johnson syndrome, which may occur after the use of antimalarials such as Fansidar® as prophylaxis while traveling in Africa. Travel remains a rapidly growing enterprise with more remote destinations appearing on the radar screen each year, making the previous review a basis for this update.[1]

More commonly, a serious dermatosis begins before the trip, progresses, and becomes significant while the traveler is away from usual medical care, not following his or her usual dietary and health habits, and often has a difficult time finding and/or communicating with medical personnel. Older patients (often the usual travelers with both time and means) have particular challenges – daunting lists of drugs and potential interactions, as well as the possibility of new drugs (and side effects) beginning around the time of the travel. The pediatric population is part of this new trend, and the smaller patients have higher risk in both toxic (venoms) and drug reactions.[1] The occasional traveler rarely keeps important medical documents with him or her, but they are necessary during an acute/life-threatening event, as the following example demonstrates.

there is minimal ascites. To obtain more information, the patient's wallet is examined, and of interest are the addresses of the two premier oyster houses in the New Orleans French Quarter. With this information and little else of medical history – plus signs of hypotension, fever, and sepsis – the dermatological consultants suggest the likelihood of infection from *Vibrio vulnificus* due to oysters. Intravenous ciprofloxacin is started approximately 3 hours after arrival at the hospital, when all of the preliminary data and consultations had been collated. Six hours later, after an up- and-down course during the night, the patient expires without ever regaining consciousness. On autopsy, *V. vulnificus* is confirmed with a septic vasculitis and advanced liver and kidney disease, as well as advanced coronary disease – all typical for the usual patient with life-threatening and usually fatal *Vibrio* sepsis.[2] More recently, Hurricane Katrina prompted other travel on the part of rebuilders of the Gulf Coast and at the same time resulted in a resurgence of the *Vibrio* problem.[3,4]

These types of events may have different outcomes if medical histories are made available when patients present to a major hospital in North America or Europe. Much more tenuous events can transpire in remote sites for ecotourism and in marginal medical facilities in so many developing countries.

CASE REPORT

A male tourist in his 50s is brought to the emergency room from the French Quarter in New Orleans, having been found confused, weak, tremulous, and unable to walk with a steady gait. He is placed in an emergency cubicle, where he is found to be hypertensive with a temperature of 38.5°C. As history taking commences, he becomes incoherent and lapses into a coma. Examination reveals moderate obesity, hypertension, and spreading waxy urticarial plaques (Figure 36.1) over most of his trunk.

He responds to pain and pressure with withdrawal, but otherwise he is unresponsive to verbal commands and questions. Preliminary laboratory studies reveal glycosuria, hyperglycemia, polymorphonuclear leukocytosis, and elevated erythrocyte sedimentation rate and C-reactive protein. The exam of the protuberant abdomen shows slight organomegaly of the liver and possibly the spleen, but

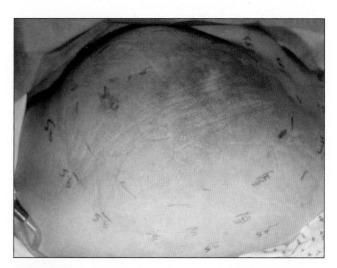

FIGURE 36.1: *Enlarging waxy plaques of* Vibrio vulnificus.

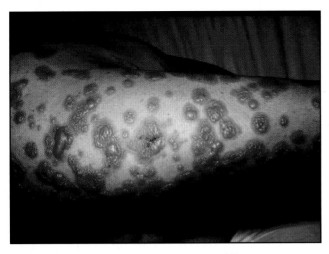

FIGURE 36.2: *Severe bullous erythema multiforme.*

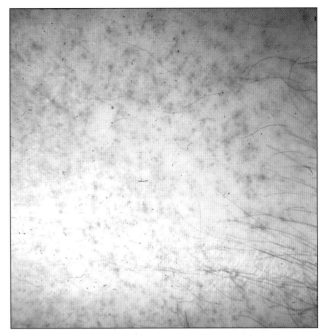

FIGURE 36.3: *Petechial lesions of drug vasculitis.*

Infectious Dermatoses

Infectious dermatoses are the first and most serious risk for the traveler, especially for one partaking of the exotic "out of the way" trips becoming in vogue as well as the popular ecotourism ventures, which as a routine are far from the fringes of civilization.

Food-Borne Infections

The case report underscores serious dermatologic conditions from food-borne infectious agents. Although it is more common to have the famous gastrointestinal (GI) sequelae – Montezuma's revenge, Tut's curse, and Delhi Belly are common descriptors – the primary challenge with these food-borne GI reactions is to restore fluid balance, which is difficult to do in some patients without hospitalization. Very young or infirm patients can be at mortal risk unless proper support is available. Of greater concern is the increase of contamination of the food chain in modern countries with various pathogenic agents, such as *Escherichia coli*, with widespread exposure in various fast food chains, where the usual assumption is safety and therefore caution is at a lower level. These same persons are ordinarily more careful while traveling, but as this evolves, concern that such adulteration of foodstuffs (as seen in animal foods in which potential toxic "expanders" were resulting in many pet deaths from renal failure) perhaps equals infection is a major concern.

It is reminiscent of the "porphyria Turcica"[5] from the ingestion of seed grains containing toxic antifungal powders – marked "not for ingestion" (in English), unintelligible to the rural people who desperately needed food and assumed that the grains were safe for cooking.[2] In the treatment phase, cutaneous sequelae may be an additional reason for the hospitalization – a result of reaction to the drugs prescribed (erythematous [EM] vide infra; Figure 36.2), sudden systemic collapse and sepsis complica-

tions such as vasculitis (Figure 36.3) and mechanobullous eruptions. These results are usually indicative of multiorgan involvement and potential organ failure and death. Cholera and typhoid fever are always risks to travelers, whether in the "first world" or "third world" because global sources of foods compromise the safety of the food chain, even in Europe and the Americas. An "ecotourist" may take all the right precautions in the country, only to become seriously ill on the way home!!!

ENVIRONMENTAL SOURCES

Traveling away from cities and civilization exposes one to many native infections and infestations that can be serious to those who are not natives and lack acquired immunity. Particularly susceptible are older patients, persons with immune deficiencies from pharmacotherapy (transplants, certain chemotherapy, etc.), and persons with infectious immunodeficiencies. The cutaneous presentations of these include petechiae (*Rickettsia*, *Meningococcus*, and some gram negatives – palpable purpura, ecthyma gangrenosum, and ulcers such as those seen in *Mycobacterium ulcerans* infections) (Table 36.1).[1]

This caveat is important: In an abnormal host, classical presentations seldom occur and diagnosis in atypical presentations requires a high index of suspicion and compulsive use of all diagnostic tests to provide confirmation of diagnosis. Many of these conditions require early aggressive treatment to ensure survival. Rickettsioses, as an example, respond best with early systemic therapy; late therapy is associated with a much lower survival rate.[3]

TABLE 36.1: Petechial/Purpuric Presentations

Rickettsia
Meningococcemia
Henoch–Schönlein purpura
Morbilliform
Rubella
Morbilla
Other viruses
Staphylococcal scalded skin syndrome
Many of the herpes viruses[1-9]
Drug eruptions

CASE REPORT

The patient is a 24-year-old former Peace Corps worker seen because of recurring problems in the amputee stump. He was working in Africa in the 60s during a time of increased greenery due to a wet phase in the weather. It was assumed that the initial event was trauma to the left leg from the sharp margins of the local grasses. The infection proceeded to an ulcer unresponsive to therapy: Thus began a scenario of repeated debridement, grafting, and recurrence – then ultimately amputation, below the knee, then above the knee, then at the hip. On examination, he appeared normal for his age except for his left lower quarter, where there were several EM and granulomatous arcuate lesions surrounding the scar from the last hip procedure. Biopsy of these granulomatous areas revealed heavy cellular infiltrate that was nearly magenta on the acid-fast stain, being loaded with organisms. Further surgery and trials of new antimicrobials were started.

Many of the atypical acid-fast organisms also are found on vegetation where they come in contact with animals. Many infections remain a challenge for chemotherapy. Although the effectiveness of clarithromycin has been documented, it usually needs some surgical assistance for the best results. This concerns life-threatening conditions; the prolonged course is debilitating to the patient – the only respite being the cryophilic nature of *M. ulcerans*, which does limit its spread to the body's core while the host remains in good health. Much later it has become apparent, concerning the extensive deforming spread of *Mycobacterium chelonae* and *Mycobacterium avium intracellulare*, that it begins to impinge on vital structures – thus a threat to life in addition to limb!

So the traveler can acquire infectious organisms that slowly destroy life as well as have much more acute episodes with infectious vasculitis, sepsis, and a stay in the intensive care unit (ICU)! Some of these organisms are from vegetation and others are from arthropods – *Plasmodia*, *Rickettsia*, and many others.[3]

Malaria remains a risk in much of the developing world, although the newer insecticidal curtains have been helpful in limiting the spread after the great increase without dichloro-diphenyl-trichloroethane (DDT) use. Cutaneous sequelae are less frequent. Usually, the patient in good health will usually survive and clear with appropriate treatment. Much more of a risk are the potential reactions to antimalarial prophylaxis. These have been documented – erythema multiforme, agranulocytosis with subsequent sepsis, and the dapsone syndrome. All of these outcomes have become serious if not treated early, intensively, and usually with hospitalization. The seriousness is compounded by the fact that the patient on malaria prophylaxis is usually far from medical care.

The most serious of infections are those of the filovirus group. They present with impressive cutaneous hemorrhagic findings, associated with a high mortality from, for example, the Marburg and Ebola viruses.[3] Fortunately, these infections are in remote areas and occur rarely in areas that are common tourist destinations. Hospitalization, isolation, and intensive care with precautions for the health care team (due to the high mortality and infectivity potential) are needed. Therapy is still on a case-by-case basis due to the lack of definitive antiviral therapy. Support therapy is the only usual approach, maintaining essential organ function until the patient recovers.

The usual bacterial and rickettsial infections also need to be considered for patients ill with petechial and/or morbilliform exanthems. The differential diagnoses need always to be reviewed to be sure that the diagnosis is not missed (Table 36.1). It is critical to establish the diagnosis and treat expectantly to be certain that the patient survives. Many of these infections respond only with early therapy. Early aggressive diagnosis and therapy are key!![8]

Allergic/Immunologic Reactions

Immediate/Immunoglobulin-Mediated Type I Anaphylactic/Immunoglobulin E. Anaphylaxis is the most significant of disorders affecting travelers and may result in death in a very short span of time. It may also be so sudden that more sophisticated medical facilities are not close enough to be able to offer their life-saving expertise. Patients who know of their risk are often prepared for emergencies with injectables, such as epinephrine carried with the person. This type of reaction (usually immunoglobulin E [IgE] mediated) can result from reexposure to antigens such as insect venom, drugs, or even contact antigens (usually environmental but can be due to personal care products including creams, sunscreens, and lotions). Initial presentation may be that of angioedema.[2,9,10]

When anaphylaxis occurs, the events are too rapid in sequence for dermatitis to appear, but the usual previous antigenic exposure is either urticarial or EM in nature. The patient's physician should alert the future traveler to reexposure risk and recommend prophylaxis such as antihistamines or epinephrine/antihistamine injection kits. Whereas the patient may be aware of the agent

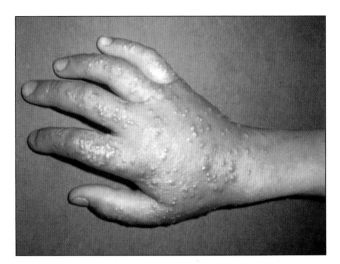

FIGURE 36.4: *Multiple pustules – Solenopsis/fire ant.*

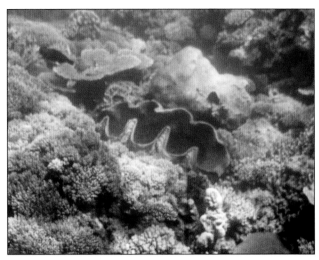

FIGURE 36.5: *Giant clam at the Great Barrier Reef.*

(arthropod, etc.) in the home environment, there may be related causes/agents encountered while traveling that are unfamiliar. It is important that the physician make an effort to educate the patient to these new threats (in other words, the different species of *Vespa, Apis, Latrodectus, Solenopsis*, etc. [Figure 36.4], the botflies, and other groups). This education can be life saving in the case of bee/hornet/wasp allergies. Avoidance is often far better than the prevention of anaphylaxis after exposure.[11,12]

Whereas airborne arthropods are the main cause for these venom reactions, there are others found at the seaside that vary from minor localized reactions to widespread skin involvement, predisposing to serious (and occasionally life-threatening) skin infections. Coelenterates are perhaps the most significant in this category and they can be ubiquitous and a serious health problem on the shores of Australia, where emergency care is available at the beach to neutralize the toxins and to avoid a trip to the hospital. Far more dramatic are the larger animals – sea snakes, giant clams (Figure 36.5), moray eels, barracuda, sharks, and various rays (such as the one that killed the zoologist Steve Irwin) – but it should be emphasized that these are extremely rare, and the morbidity is from trauma or venoms (not anaphylactic in nature). Most exposures at the beach – sea bathers eruption, swimmers itch, creeping eruption, and so forth – are sources of minimal morbidity unless large areas of skin are involved or an unusual allergic reaction occurs.

Type 2 or 3. Type 2 (vasculitis and the immuno-/mechanobullous dermatoses) and 3 (immune complex reactions) are rare in environmental exposure but hypothetically can occur after hypersensitivity to various venoms such as solenopsis[4] and subsequent exposure with possible intravascular dissemination of the venom with extensive immune complex formation and cascades of inflammatory mediators. These types can cause acute organ failure (liver,

kidney) and a picture not unlike infectious sepsis. These are rare and, in extreme cases, result in ICU stays.

Delayed/Cell Mediated. Delayed reactions can be just as serious as immediate reactions under the proper circumstances. Whereas atopic dermatitis is generally considered to be related to IgE, atopic patients seem to develop type 4 reactions to plants in increasing amounts as they age. The timing may be the significant factor. Many travelers have a vacation ruined by widespread rhus contact dermatitis (Figure 36.6); the patient, even under the best of care, cannot enjoy the destination city and its charms. Without proper care, and in certain climates, the heat and humidity can lead to secondary infection and the end result can approach the morbidity of a second-degree burn or worse. There are well-documented cases of nephrogenic streptococcus, resulting in acute renal complications, hospitalization, and rarely dialysis.

When the exposure takes place during the trip, the rapidity of the reaction often relates to the degree of sensitivity

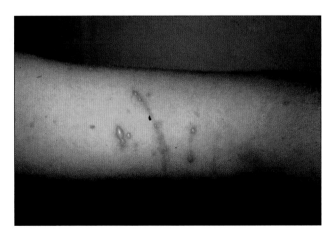

FIGURE 36.6: *Typical vesicular and linear lesions of rhus dermatitis.*

and the breadth of exposure. In many cases, the source is a related species unfamiliar to the traveler. The possibilities are immense. The main plant groups are Primula (mostly the in United Kingdom), Compositae (worldwide), Alstroemeria (largely acquired in the floral trades), Rhus (United States), Allium, and certain legumes that can be a source of allergy, largely manifested by food allergy, but occasionally cause type 1 and type 4 reactions. With a high degree of sensitivity, widespread vesiculobullous lesions increase the risk of infection and sepsis requiring hospitalization. The treatment varies with the infecting organism, but parenteral antibiotics are the main indication for hospitalization and are the most rapid means for quick recovery.

CONCLUSIONS

The current most significant trend in travel is "eco-tourism," which places the traveler directly in the environment and often in remote areas that make rapid response to severe and potentially life-threatening reactions a big challenge. Furthermore, travel is now more accessible to patients with significant morbidities such as diabetes, immunosuppression in transplant patients, and even advanced malignancies under chemotherapy. Minor environmental dermatoses and infections easily addressed at home can drastically evolve to threaten life when one is away from the usual medical support system. Evacuation and inherent delays in transfer can allow a minor and local condition to spread, impetiginize, and possibly secondarily involve internal organs mandating hospitalization. Dermatoses that respond to simple local measures normally become life threatening when care is delayed or complicated by measures in evacuation. The prepared traveler should have significant medical information available, especially when morbidities such as diabetes or other metabolic conditions predispose the traveler to greater risk and complicate usual recovery. Similarly, patients with a long list of

medications need to have documentation of it as well as an understanding of potential risks such as photosensitivity. Most major medical institutions now have travel medicine units that should be the first stop after the trip is finalized. This consultation educates the traveler as to risks and the necessary preparations, vaccinations, prophylactic drugs, as well as preparing him or her for environmental exposures.

REFERENCES

1. Millikan L. Life-threatening dermatoses in travelers. Clin Dermatol. 2005; 23:249–53.
2. Millikan L, Feldman M. Pediatric drug allergy. Clin Dermatol. 2002; 20:29–35.
3. Bross MH, Soch K, Morales R, Mitchell RB. Vibrio vulnificus infection: diagnosis and treatment. Am Fam Physician. 2007; 76:539–44.
4. Rhoads J. Post-Hurricane Katrina challenge: Vibrio vulnificus. J Am Acad Nurse Pract. 2006; 18:318–24.
5. Cripps DJ, Peters HA, Gocmen A, Dogramici I. Porphyria turcica due to hexachlorobenzene: a 20 to 30 year follow-up study on 204 patients. Br J Dermatol. 1984; 111:413–22.
6. Streit M, Bregenzer T, Heinzer I. Cutaneous infections due to atypical mycobacteria. Hautarzt. 2008; 59:59–71.
7. Wansbrough-Jones M, Phillips R. Buruli ulcer: emerging from obscurity. Lancet. 2006; 367:1849–58.
8. Walker DH. Rickettsiae and rickettsial infections: the current state of knowledge. Clin Infect Dis. 2007; 4:S39–44.
9. Carneiro SC, Cestari T, Allen SH, Ramos-e-Silva M. Viral exanthems in the tropics. Clin Dermatol. 2007; 25:212–20.
10. Dai YS. Allergens in atopic dermatitis. Clin Rev Allergy Immunol. 2007; 33:157–66.
11. Petitpierre S, Bart PA, Spertini F, Leimgruber A. The multiple aetiologies of angioedema. Rev Med Suisse. 2008; 4:1030–4, 1036–8.
12. Knight D, Bangs MJ. Cutaneous allergic vasculitis due to Solenopsis geminata (Hymenoptera: Formicidae) envenomation in Indonesia. Southeast Asian J Trop Med Public Health. 2007; 38:808–13.

Index

Note: The page numbers with "*f*" indicate the references to Figures, and the page numbers with "*t*" indicate the references to Tables.